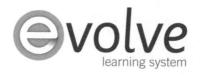

Pharmacology
Principles and Applications

THIRD EDITION

EUGENIA M. FULCHER
RN, BSN, EdD, CMA (AAMA)
Allied Health Instructor

ROBERT M. FULCHER
BS Chem, BSPh, RPh
Pharmacist
CVS Pharmacy
Waynesboro, Georgia

CATHY D. SOTO
PhD, MBA, CMA (AAMA)
Professor and Program Director
Medical Assisting Technology Program
El Paso Community College
El Paso, Texas

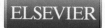

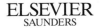

3251 Riverport Lane
St. Louis, Missouri 63043

Notices

Knowledge and best practice in this field are constantly changing. As new research and experience broaden our understanding, changes in research methods, professional practices, or medical treatment may become necessary.

Practitioners and researchers must always rely on their own experience and knowledge in evaluating and using any information, methods, compounds, or experiments described herein. In using such information or methods they should be mindful of their own safety and the safety of others, including parties for whom they have a professional responsibility.

With respect to any drug or pharmaceutical products identified, readers are advised to check the most current information provided (i) on procedures featured or (ii) by the manufacturer of each product to be administered, to verify the recommended dose or formula, the method and duration of administration, and contraindications. It is the responsibility of practitioners, relying on their own experience and knowledge of their patients, to make diagnoses, to determine dosages and the best treatment for each individual patient, and to take all appropriate safety precautions.

To the fullest extent of the law, neither the Publisher nor the authors, contributors, or editors, assume any liability for any injury and/or damage to persons or property as a matter of products liability, negligence or otherwise, or from any use or operation of any methods, products, instructions, or ideas contained in the material herein.

Library of Congress Cataloging-in-Publication Data

Fulcher, Eugenia M.
  Pharmacology : principles and applications / Eugenia M. Fulcher, Robert M. Fulcher, Cathy D. Soto.—3rd ed.
      p. ; cm.
  Includes index.
  ISBN 978-1-4377-2267-3 (pbk. : alk. paper)
  I. Fulcher, Robert M.   II. Soto, Cathy Dubeansky.   III. Title.
  [DNLM: 1. Drug Therapy—Problems and Exercises.   2. Pharmaceutical Preparations—Problems and Exercises. WB 18.2]
  LC classification   not assigned
  615'.1—dc23

                                                                                2011035202

Executive Editor: Susan Cole
Associate Developmental Editor: Laurie Vordtriede
Publishing Services Manager: Catherine Jackson
Senior Project Manager: Mary Pohlman
Senior Book Designer: Amy Buxton

Printed in the United States

Last digit is the print number: 9 8 7 6 5 4 3 2

We dedicate this third edition to our parents, Harold L. and Rosabel L. Mills and Robert M. and Lucy F. Fulcher, who gave us dreams and the desire for and the means to obtain professional educations, only wishing you were here to be proud. To our sons, Lee and Gene, and our grandchildren, Mac and Allie, we know you have dreams and we hope you will succeed in reaching them. We thank each of you for the love and support that you have provided during the preparation of this text. To our extended family, we appreciate all you have done to assist us. We also thank our students who have been supportive when we needed time to complete manuscript. To the many friends and instructors who have had suggestions, we have tried to include as many as possible so your dreams can be found within the text. To all allied health professionals who will use this text, may you achieve your professional dreams as both of us have, for almost fifty years—they can come true. You are the reason this text has been written—to provide the needed educational background for patient safety in health care.

Bobby and Genie Fulcher

I dedicate this third edition to the two men in my life for whom I will always be deeply grateful because of their unconditional love, encouragement, and continuous support in both my professional and personal lifelong journey. It was my father, Edward D. Dubeansky (1928-2009), a Korean War Veteran and paraplegic before I was born, who taught me to love God and family, to have dignity and respect toward everyone, to be self-disciplined, and to be a volunteer throughout life. My husband, Jose Soto III, has been by my side and my moral support for 35 years, who shared with me raising two beautiful daughters (Jenny and June), who drives me cross country for seminars, workshops, volunteer work, and of course to see our grandbabies (Victoria Anna, Fernando Miguel, and Murdock Lee), sons-in-law (Fernando and Ed), and all my siblings and their families. I will always treasure our times together!

Cathy D. Soto

Reviewers

Patricia G. DeBenedetto, CMA-CHI
Medical Assistant Program Instructor, CPR Instructor
Department of Medical Programs
Medical Career Institute
Ocean Township, New Jersey

Debra Downs, LPN, AAS, RMA (AMT)
Program Director, Instructor
Department of Medical Assisting
Okefenokee Technical College
Waycross, Georgia

Glenda Hatcher, BSN, RN, CMA (AAMA)
Medical Assisting Program Director
Department of Allied Health
Southwest Georgia Technical College
Thomasville, Georgia

MaryAnne Hochadel, PharmD, BCPS
Clinical Assistant Professor
Department of Pharmacy Practice
University of Florida
Gainesville, Florida;
Clinical Pharmacist
Department of Pharmacy Services
Bayfront Medical Center
St. Petersburg, Florida;
Editor Emeritus, Gold Standard
Tampa, Florida

Paul Juang, PharmD
Assistant Professor, Pharmacy Practice
St. Louis College of Pharmacy
St. Louis, Missouri

Julie P. Karpinski, PharmD, BCPS
Director, Drug Information
Assistant Professor, Pharmacy Practice
Concordia University Wisconsin
Mequon, Wisconsin;
Drug Information Pharmacist
Froedtert Hospital
Milwaukee, Wisconsin

Renee Koski, PharmD, CACP
Professor, Pharmacy Practice
Ferris State University College of Pharmacy
Marquette, Michigan

Donna Larson, EdD, MT (ASCP) DLM, MS, BA, BS
Dean, Allied Health
Allied Health Division
Mt. Hood Community College
Gresham, Oregon

Terri L. Levien, PharmD
Clinical Associate Professor
Department of Pharmacotherapy
Washington State University College of Pharmacy
Spokane, Washington

Ashley Moses, PhD
Assistant Professor of Mathematics
Mary Baldwin College
Staunton, Virginia

Joshua J. Neumiller, PharmD
Assistant Professor, Pharmacology
Washington State University
Spokane, Washington

Karen Snipe, CPhT, MEd
Department Head, Pharmacy Technician,
    Program Coordinator
Departments of Allied Health and Diagnostic &
    Imaging Services
Trident Technical College
Charleston, South Carolina

Rebecca Wright, EdD
Assistant Professor of Mathematics
Oakland City University
Oakland City, Indiana

Sandra Wright, MEd, PhD
Campus President
Department of Administration
Atlanta Medical Academy
Atlanta, Georgia;
CEO, Moaney Wright & Associates
Atlanta, Georgia

Preface

The goal of the third edition of *Pharmacology: Principles and Applications* is to help the student master not only the principles of pharmacology but also the critical thinking skills necessary to transfer this knowledge base to administer medications for patient safety. We have sought to achieve this in various ways, some of which are found in other pharmacology texts and others of which are unique to this text.

The purpose of this text has remained constant—to provide an introduction to pharmacology that gives allied health professionals an in-depth basic knowledge about medications that are used on a day-to-day basis in the ambulatory and some inpatient care settings. Dose amounts are shown as a single dose because administration in these settings would be in that form. The text includes information on medications used to stabilize a patient in outpatient emergency situations but not medications frequently used in inpatient emergency situations, such as intensive care units. Similarly, because medications that are used on a "stat," or immediate need basis, in specialized intensive care units, and in surgical areas are not typically used in ambulatory care settings, information about these drugs is not included or only limited information is provided.

As the world of medicine has evolved from a predominately inpatient setting for acute and chronic care to ambulatory care for many conditions previously seen on an inpatient basis, allied health professionals have integrated the skills needed to complete tasks ordered by the health care provider to provide safe, necessary patient care in the ambulatory setting. Because the tasks health professionals are legally permitted to perform vary from state to state, it is important for all health care personnel to understand state statutes in their particular employment setting while being aware of any changes as they occur. This text is designed to provide a solid background in pharmacology as well as the necessary skills to administer prescription and over-the-counter medications safely and with in the scope of practice. This is basic knowledge for a broad audience so the allied health professional should keep current with medications used in the place of employment and with the rules at the site of practice. Remember that local requirements may vary from those seen in this text, and local requirements should always set the basis for practice.

The organization of material by body system lends itself to the study of disease processes along with the study of medications used to therapeutically and prophylactically treat these diseases. This comprehensive study helps students achieve additional competency and critical thinking skills and helps prepare them for examinations that are required for licensure or certification. The depth of material is sufficient for critical thinking skills that can be readily transferred to patient care and patient teaching. If a review of materials such as anatomy and physiology are required for understanding, students should use an appropriate text for this information.

Because pharmacology is a specific science associated with many distinct health care fields, interaction among the professionals who work in these various health care settings is essential to ensure patient safety and compliance with therapeutic care. This professional intercommunication creates safeguards for the patient as well as checks and balances among professionals. It is essential for each professional—health care provider, pharmacist, and allied health professional—to keep his or her medication knowledge as current as possible. In addition, communication among health care workers is important because of the multitudes of medications released each year and the increase in indications for usage of established medications. Having all medications in this text is not realistic; however, the authors have tried to make the list of drugs for this text as current as possible; the constant release of new medications by the Food and Drug Administration and the new indications for older drugs makes this impossible. Always check current information for any changes that may seem to have occurred. The allied health professional must also be careful to ensure that correct medications are being charted in the medical record and are being relayed to the pharmacist as allowed by state laws.

ORGANIZATION OF THE TEXT

Pharmacology: Principles and Applications has been organized in a student-friendly manner intended to facilitate the study of pharmacology. Each chapter contains special elements that help make learning fun and easy.

Section I: General Aspects of Pharmacology

Section I, an introduction to pharmacology, gives a short history of the field and how it has changed our world. To ensure safety for both the student and patient, specific legislation and ethical issues related to pharmacology are stressed. The discussion also includes basic pharmacology terminology and provides an understanding of how drugs are used by the body and the skills needed to read and interpret medication orders and document medications appropriately.

Section II: Mathematics for Pharmacology and Dosage Calculations

Section II has a basic math review for the student who needs to practice rudimentary math skills and necessary content to calculate drug dosages so that medications are administered safely. The discussion covers the three systems of measurement used to prescribe medications and the conversions needed to change a medication order from one system to another. The calculation of dosages for adults and children and other special applications are also discussed.

Check Your Understanding math review boxes allow students to check the application and calculation concepts that they have learned as they work their way through each math module (answers to these sections are found in **Appendix A**).

Pretests gauge students' knowledge *before* each math chapter material is covered, allowing both instructors and students to identify areas of weakness. Further review of the material can be accomplished by retaking the pretest before completing the review section. This will indicate areas that need extra attention prior to completing the chapter-ending **Review Questions** that cover chapter concepts related to the ambulatory care setting.

Section III: Medication Administration

Section III presents the general principles of medication administration. The discussions about routes of medication administration are organized according to the CAAHEP/MAERB and ABHES curriculums, starting with enteral (routes that begin with introduction into the gastrointestinal tract), followed by percutaneous (routes

through the skin and mucous membranes), and ending with parenteral routes (by injection).

Procedures for drug dose calculation and administration are presented in storyboard format, displaying illustrations that present specific steps to assist the visual learner. The Procedure Boxes include **icons** that represent OSHA-mandated and methodology-related protocols that should be followed prior to administering medications. The following icons are presented:

 Handwashing required

 Gloves required

Sharps container required as indicated

3+7 Use the 3 "befores" and 7 "rights" of medication administration.

Section IV: Pharmacology for Multisystem Application and Section V: Medications Related to Body Systems

Sections IV and V are directly related to medications. Section IV presents medications that affect multiple body systems, such as analgesics, immunizations, antimicrobials, and antineoplastics. The rapidly growing use of herbs and nutritional supplements and their interactions with other medications are also addressed. Section V discusses medications specific to body systems. Tables are included in these sections that present both generic and trade names for drugs, usual adult dosage, typical routes of administration, and drug interactions.

Each chapter in these sections lists the **Common Signs and Symptoms of Diseases** found in the applicable body system. These can be compared to the **Common Side Effects of Medications** commonly prescribed for the diseases found in that system so that through critical thinking skills, the allied health professional will have the needed background for questioning a patient to provide the information needed for the evaluation by the health care provider. Using these tools, the allied health professional can learn to assist in distinguishing between disease progression and medication reactions by asking pertinent questions. This allows the allied health professional to teach patients which signs and symptoms must be reported to the health care provider and which they might expect as side effects—information that is critical for patient education. Medication safety is best reinforced when the patient becomes an active member of the medication administration process.

Easy Working Knowledge tables list medication classifications used with applicable body systems or systemic medications. This listing, which helps locate discussions of specific medication types, corresponds to the quick reference of drug classifications found inside the text's cover. The student can learn to group medications by systemic disease processes to help with accurate documentation of medicines. When the student knows the medications used for specific body systems and specific disease process, the potential for drug errors is reduced.

Icons representing the body systems are located next to associated medication names. These icons, listed below, help students begin to identify drugs as they relate to particular body systems.

 Medications used for sensory system disorders

Medications used for infectious diseases

Medications used for immune system disorders

 Medications used for endocrine system disorders

Medications used for musculoskeletal disorders

Medications used for gastrointestinal system disorders

Medications used for respiratory tract disorders

 Medications used for circulatory disorders

Medications used for blood disorders

Medications used for urinary system disorders

 Medications used for reproductive system conditions

 Medications used for mental disorders

Medications used for neurological conditions

Medications used for pain management

Medications used as antineoplastics

Medications used as nutritional supplements

Medication used for substance abuse

WORKBOOK

The *Workbook* includes multiple review questions and practice problems to not only promote continued learning, but to also offer thought-provoking, critical thinking questions on how a variety of realistic situations would be handled safely by the allied health professional.

INSTRUCTOR'S RESOURCE MANUAL WITH TEACH

The *Instructor's Resource Manual with TEACH*, accessed through the Evolve web site, contains answer keys to the text and workbook, a test bank and answer key, as well as detailed lesson plans and lecture outlines. The lesson plans are linked to each chapter and are divided into 50-minute units in a three-column format. The lecture outlines in PowerPoint provide talking points, thought-provoking questions, and unique ideas for lectures. The electronic resource includes all the instructor's resource manual assets plus the test bank in ExamView, and PowerPoint slides to help the instructor save valuable preparation time and create a learning environment that fully engages the student.

PURPOSE OF THE TEXTBOOK

Our goal has been to provide a student-friendly pharmacology text that helps the allied health professional administer medications accurately and safely and to teach patients to administer ambulatory medications safely at home. The book's early introduction of drugs to their corresponding body systems is designed to help the student begin to recognize the drugs that are most often used with a specific body system. The introductory section on body system and systemic-related medications is designed to assist the allied health professional accurately record information about medications administered for diseases of that system and to obtain information from the patient that will assist the health care provider in deciding on the appropriate medications for the specific patient. This multidisciplinary process must be directed to each individual patient, with the health care provider, pharmacist, and allied health professional providing a system of checks and balances for patient safety.

As authors, we hope that the third edition of *Pharmacology: Principles and Applications* provides students with an enjoyable and basic in-depth way to learn how to administer medications safely, document medications in the medical record, and relay needed information to other health care professionals and patients who are a part of the medication therapy process.

Acknowledgments

Having worked in the medical field for almost 100 years combined, we have seen the importance of having a strong background in pharmacology to ensure patient safety and education. As health professionals—an ambulatory care nurse and a pharmacist—we understand that safe patient care is only as strong as the individuals involved in medication administration. This book is intended to provide the foundation for that knowledge.

We give special thanks to some special people at Elsevier. To Jamie Augustine and Laurie Vordtriede, our Developmental Editors, who have been our friends, mind-readers, and consultants, we give a big thanks for a job well done. To Susan Cole, Executive Editor, we acknowledge the time you have taken to ensure the text is as it should be. We do appreciate your understanding of time needed to complete two text revisions at the same time. To Andrew Allen, Vice President and Publisher, your continuous support of our endeavors is so appreciated. You have been a guide that has produced a light to increase our writing abilities for many years. To Sue Hontscharik, Administrative Assistant—you are friend in need and a friend indeed. Your encouraging words on so many occasions helped us complete this text. To Mary Pohlman in production, you have been wonderful to work with; you have spent hours being sure the text is the best it could be and we do appreciate you. We thank all of the Elsevier staff for being there for us when we needed assistance. You are the greatest!

To our reviewers, we say a big thank you for providing guidance throughout the publication of this text. To those who reviewed previous editions and gave suggestions for the new edition—know that we have tried to incorporate your ideas. To those who reviewed the chapters during the production of this edition, thank you for providing many ideas and guidance for this text you are special people to take time to give us the needed assistance. To the instructors who have used the text and have provided guidance we hope that we

have helped you with teaching the information to your students.

We also must thank some special individuals who have provided background materials and direction, as well as moral support when needed. To our personal physicians who provided much guidance in the choice of medications to be presented, thanks. To Don Balasa at the American Association for Medical Assistants, we owe our gratitude for providing information about the medical practice acts of the states. To Judy Jondahl at Medical Assisting Education Review Board, thanks for being a friend who gave us moral support during this busy time. To all who have provided encouragement and guidance, a heartfelt thanks. Special kudos to our sons, Lee and Gene, for their patience and support throughout the entire project. To our grandchildren (and they are really grand), Mac and Allie, you have been the light that made the long days seem shorter. Thanks for being such great children during the times that we were busy writing and you were visiting with us. Through the love, understanding, and patience of all who have helped with this book, our dream continues to be a reality—a reality that we will assist allied health students now and in the future.

Genie and Bobby Fulcher

I wish to acknowledge Man Tai Lam, MD, El Paso, Texas, in Private Practice for Internal Medicine and Infectious Diseases, and Medical Director for El Paso Community College's Medical Assisting Program. For the past 12 years, Dr. Lam has participated in every Advisory Board meeting. Thank you, Dr. Lam for your continued words of encouragement and professional support.

I would also like to acknowledge my co-authors, Genie and Bobby, as well as the staff at Elsevier for all their hard work that went into this edition.

Cathy D. Soto

Critical Thinking Scenario
These scenarios stimulate class discussion by introducing the real world aspect of pharmacology to students.

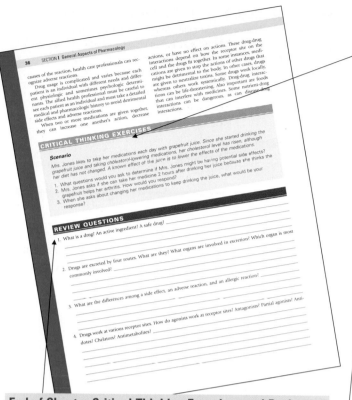

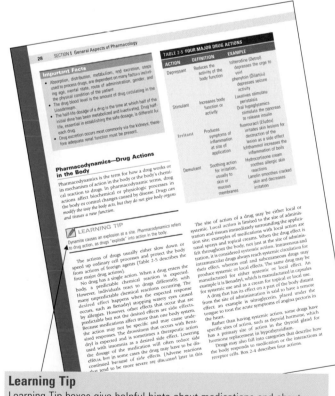

End of Chapter Critical Thinking Exercises and Review Questions
End of chapter Critical Thinking Exercises and Review Questions offer challenging, thought-provoking questions on how a variety of realistic situations would be handled by the allied health professional.

Did You Know? box
Did You Know? Boxes provide enrichment facts about relevant topics of interest, such as new medical trends, history, diagnostics, treatments, and diseases.

Clinical Tip box
Clinical Tip boxes provide information about the clinical administration of medications.

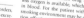

Learning Tip
Learning Tip boxes give helpful hints about medications and about studying pharmacology.

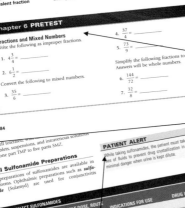

Important Facts box

Important Facts boxes contain bulleted summations of previously learned material that provide an at-a-glance resource for students to consult in reviewing important topics.

Patient Education for Compliance box

Patient Education for Compliance boxes contain information pertinent to instructing patients on medication administration and about possible side effects or adverse reactions.

Extensive Math Review

All math chapters begin with a pretest that highlights material covered within the chapter. If a student masters the pretest with a 90% or better, the student should then move on to the review questions. If a student can score 90% or better on both, he or she is ready to move on to the next chapter. Students are encouraged to go back to the pretest when studying the chapter to check for mastery of the chapter's contents.

Patient Alert box

Patient Alert boxes highlight important information that the allied health professional should communicate to the patient when he or she is receiving treatment.

Medication Alert box

Medication Alert boxes contain facts about specific drugs, the goals of their administration, and any potential adverse reactions.

Contents

SECTION V
MEDICATIONS RELATED TO BODY SYSTEMS

APPENDIXES

General Aspects of Pharmacology

CHAPTER 1

Introduction to Pharmacology and Its Legal and Ethical Aspects

OBJECTIVES

After studying this chapter, you should be capable of the following:

- Describing the role of the allied health professional in pharmacotherapy and the role of each participant in medication delivery.
- Explaining the need of the allied health professional's knowledge base as a safeguard in medication administration.
- Understanding folk medicine and its effects on medicine today.
- Differentiating among major governmental agencies and the role and regulations of each in medication development and delivery.
- Identifying the legal aspects of the Comprehensive Drug Abuse Prevention and Control Act of 1970 and describing the five schedules for controlled substances found therein.

- Describing the registration and documentation process for compliance with the Drug Enforcement Administration with regard to administering, dispensing, and prescribing controlled drugs.
- Describing the role of the Food and Drug Administration in medication safety.
- Differentiating among drug dependence, drug abuse, drug misuse, and habituation.
- Listing and describing signs of drug abuse and ethics involved in addressing these problems with patients and medical professionals.
- Identifying ethical procedures regarding prescriptions, including who may prescribe medications, and the use of protocol to ensure that these measures are followed.

Judy, a new allied health professional, has little background in pharmacology. Sara, a young mother of a 2 year old, calls and states that her child has a cold with fever. She asks Judy to call in a prescription to the local pharmacy for the child. Judy does not think that it is necessary to ask any further questions about the child's condition because "a cold is a cold." Judy does pull the medical record and sees that the child is allergic to penicillin but was given Augmentin previously. So, without consulting the physician, Judy orders the same antibiotic. The next day Sara calls to say the child has a rash covering the entire body and cannot breathe properly. Judy tells Sara to continue the medicine because it sounds like the child has measles and will be fine. Later that day Judy learns that the child is in intensive care at the local hospital with an adverse reaction.

What are some of the implications for Judy?
What has she done that could be grounds for litigation?
Should she have called in the prescription without consulting the physician? Explain your answer.
What is the physician's responsibility?
What is the pharmacist's responsibility?

KEY TERMS

Administer	Drug abuse	Food and Drug	Physical dependence
Adverse reaction	Drug addiction	Administration	Physiology
Anatomy	Drug dependence	(FDA)	Placebo
Bioequivalence	Drug efficacy	Generic drug	Prescribe
Brand-name drug	Drug Enforcement	Homeostasis	Prescription
Bureau of Narcotics	Administration	Legend drug	Psychologic drug
and Dangerous	(DEA)	Medication	dependence or
Drugs (BNDD)	Drug purity	Narcotic	habituation
Clinical pharmacology	Drug quality	National Formulary	Respondeat superior
Controlled substance	Drug sample	(NF)	Side effect
Dangerous drug	Drug standardization	Over-the-counter (OTC)	Standardization
Dispense	Drug standards	drug	*United States*
Dosage	Drug strength or drug	Pathology	*Pharmacopoeia*
Dose	potency	Pharmacology	*(USP)*

An important responsibility of allied health professionals is understanding drugs, their interactions, and routes of administration. All health care professionals should know answers to questions about **medications** such as the following: What is the correct **dose** to be given? Is the **dosage** within normal limits? What are signs of drug overdose? What are the interactions with the drug? What **side effects** or **adverse reactions** can occur when drugs are given singly or in combination with other drugs? How do routes of administration affect the drug's effectiveness? With knowledge of medications, health care professionals can prepare the patient for a realistic expectation and safe outcome.

Did You Know?

The word *pharmacology* comes from the Greek *pharmakon*, which has three related meanings: claim, poison, and remedy.

Pharmacology changed immensely in the last half of the twentieth century. Many medications used today were not available as recently as 10 years ago. New medicines and new uses of older medicines are constantly being researched and approved by the **Food and Drug Administration (FDA)** for use. Developments in pharmacology require constant and diligent study for safe medication administration.

PHARMACOLOGY AND HEALTH SCIENCES

Drawing on many health care disciplines, **pharmacology** is the study of drugs, their uses, and their interaction with living systems. **Anatomy** and **physiology** provide essential information about body parts and normal physical body function. **Pathology** describes changes from normal structure and function as well as the function of medications when the person is out of **homeostasis**. *Psychology* provides an understanding of how a person's mental state and lifestyle influence medication compliance. Allied health professionals must integrate established knowledge in the basic health sciences with information from the rapidly advancing field of pharmacology.

Important Facts

- Pharmacology is the study of drugs and their uses.
- Pharmacology draws information from many scientific disciplines.

Why Study Pharmacology?

Before administering medications safely, health professionals must know forms of drugs available and what patient factors could affect actions of the drugs. The knowledge includes the expected action and correct dosage of drugs, methods and routes of administration, symptoms of abnormal reactions, and appropriate patient education for safe delivery of the medication.

The allied health professional functions as a link in the health care chain to ensure that the physician is aware of all medications, both prescription and **over-the-counter (OTC)**, that the patient is taking (Figure 1-1). A complete history of medication use must be documented with each patient encounter to assist the physician in safely and effectively prescribing medications. Because the names of some medications are spelled similarly or sound alike, the professional must ensure

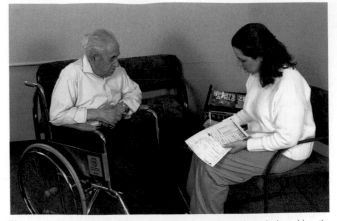

Figure 1-1 The allied health professional plays a major role by taking the patient's complete medication and health history.

accuracy in documentation. Use of alcohol, recreational drugs, and alternative medications such as herbals and vitamins should also be recorded. These actions alone assist in preventing legal and ethical problems for the physician.

Did You Know?

Sound-alike–look-alike drugs are labeled with high alert warnings for verification at the time of dispensing medication.

In many cases allied health professionals will reinforce patient teaching about a drug's purposes, its method and route of administration, and regimen for medication efficacy, especially with initial drug prescriptions, for patient safety.

With the growing number of OTC drugs, the availability of information concerning their actions and their interactions with **prescription** medications (or **legend drugs**) will prevent reactions detrimental to the patient. People today frequently use OTC drugs previously available only by prescription, to treat themselves for common ailments or illnesses such as allergies, colds, arthritis, and gastric conditions, without consulting a physician. These OTC items are mandated to be noted in the patient's medical record as medications being taken.

Role of Professionals in Medication Administration

According to guidelines of the **Drug Enforcement Administration (DEA)**, each person in the medication pathway has a specific duty. A physician **prescribes** a drug to be filled by the pharmacy in an outpatient setting or an order in an inpatient setting. The pharmacist **dispenses** or distributes the drug in a correctly labeled container with specific instructions for the patient on

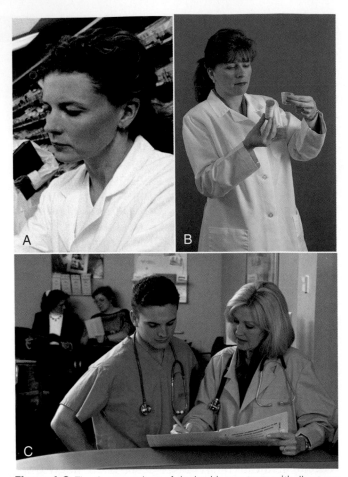

Figure 1-2 The three members of the health care team with direct use of pharmacology for patient safety. **A,** Pharmacist; **B,** allied health professional; **C,** physician.

how and when to take the medication (Figure 1-2). To **administer** a drug means to give the medication by the route prescribed. Drug administration may be done by the patient personally or by a health care professional in a medical facility (see Figure 1-2, *B*). The patient is the most important figure in the drug administration triangle. Patient safety for all members involved in drug therapy focuses on the patient (Figure 1-3).

The physician, who is a central figure in drug administration because he or she determines the specific drug therapy required for a specific patient in a specific situation, may also dispense sample medications or administer some drugs, such as antipyretics for fever or analgesics for pain, in his or her medical facility.

Sixty percent of visits to a physician result in a prescription; therefore pharmacists are involved not only in providing the correct drug product, but also in helping to ensure its proper use. The pharmacist ensures that the course of therapy prescribed is safe, effective, and correct in every detail. If a question concerning the therapy is evident, the pharmacist will contact the physician for verification.

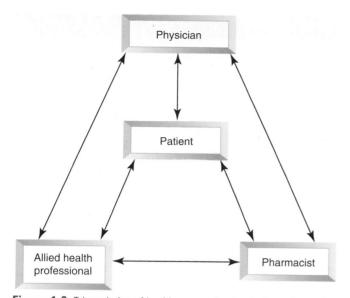

Figure 1-3 Triangulation of health care professionals for patient safety with medication use.

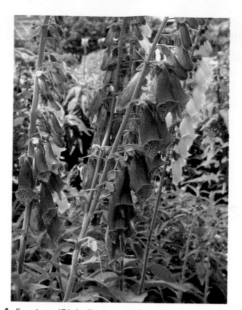

Figure 1-4 Foxglove *(Digitalis purpurea)*, used for cardiac disorders, is an example of plant materials that have been used as medications for many centuries.

The allied health professional begins patient education in proper drug use while also functioning as a liaison between the physician and pharmacist. The allied health professional usually is the person who receives phone calls from patients with questions about their prescriptions or is the first person in the team to hear that the medication has caused problems or has not had the expected results. Most patients discuss medications that have not had the desired effect with other health care professionals such as a pharmacist or office staff member rather than the physician. Therefore, important roles for allied health professionals are to provide knowledgeable answers and to include other health care professionals such as physicians and pharmacists in safe patient care. The pathway of medication delivery requires that the entire team know medications and their uses and misuses, as well as the patient who will be using the drugs. Just as the physician and staff must know the medical needs of patients, so the pharmacist must keep updated records of all medications being taken by a patient to ensure drug safety.

Important Facts

- A complete medication profile, including both prescription and over-the-counter drugs, must be documented for all patients.
- Allied health professionals must continue to learn about new medications as they are released and keep current on new uses for older drugs.
- Basically, physicians *prescribe*, pharmacists *dispense*, and allied health professionals (depending on state law) may *administer* medications and be a liaison to other health care

Important Facts—cont'd

professionals. Therefore the physician, pharmacist, and allied health professional must cooperate in a system of checks and balances to ensure patient safety.
- Allied health professionals must have a working knowledge of all medications used at the site of employment, including new drugs and new applications of established drugs.

HISTORY OF PHARMACOLOGY

Ancient civilizations recorded use of drugs more than 2000 years ago. Through trial and error, humans discovered which plants might be used for food and which had medicinal value. Folk remedies largely did, and still do, use herbs and other plants. In previous generations, serious illnesses were considered to be of supernatural origin as a result of spells cast on the victim by an enemy, a demon, or an offended god. Ancient medicine men using frog bile, pig teeth, spider webs, and sour milk were actually witch doctors, wise men, "root doctors," *curanderos,* shamans, or sorcerers who treated the whole body. Herbal treatments for illnesses became a part of every cultural heritage, with many cultural communities choosing healers and with culture members seeing these men as having "cures" because of their special knowledge of plants. Over the years, folk uses of plants and other natural remedies became the basis for certain modern medicines used in pharmacology today. For example, the digitalis plant, also called *foxglove (Digitalis purpurea),* is the basis of the commonly used cardiac medication digoxin (Figure 1-4).

BOX 1-1 TIME LINE OF MEDICATIONS

Pre–sixteenth century	Egyptians collected plants for treatment of specific diseases and used molded bread for treatment of infection. India's version of *Materia Medica* was written as a drug formulary of plants used for treating diseases.
Sixteenth century	Chinese devised a 52-volume formulary of concoctions prepared to restore and maintain body harmony. Reserpine *(Rauwolfia)* was prescribed for high blood pressure, and ginseng as a diuretic.
Seventeenth century	Greek physicians, and especially Hippocrates, used opium for pain, herbal remedies such as belladonna (atropine) for nausea and vomiting, and Jesuit's bark (quinine) for malaria. Greeks used natural cures for dieting. Romans began use of prescriptions for obtaining patient medications.
Eighteenth century	Edward Jenner developed first vaccine for immunity against cowpox (smallpox).
Nineteenth century	Morphine (1806), strychnine (1817), quinine (1820), and nicotine (1828) were created.
1865	During American Civil War, carbonic acid was used for surgical asepsis.
1897	During Spanish-American War, typhoid vaccines were administered to troops.
Twentieth century	
Early 1900s	Prontosil (1908, forerunner of sulfa drugs), Salvarsan (1910, synthetic arsenic for syphilis), and phenobarbital (1912, for epilepsy) were created.
1916	Insulin was isolated.
1914-1918 (World War I)	Tetanus antitoxin was developed and used for military personnel.
1920s	Diphtheria vaccine (1922) was created.
1930s	Sulfa (antiinfective), phenytoin (Dilantin, for epilepsy), and yellow fever vaccine were created.
1940s (World War II)	Penicillin (antiinfective), Benadryl (1945, antihistamine), cortisone (1948, immunosuppressant), antibiotics, chemotherapeutic agents, and influenza vaccine were introduced.
1950s (Korean War)	Medications to treat mental illness were introduced. Salk vaccine (1954, polio vaccine) and oral contraceptives were introduced.
1960s	Sabin oral polio vaccine was introduced. Vaccines for rubella, measles (rubeola), and mumps were created. Beta blockers were developed to treat hypertension. Clotting factors were developed for hemophilia.
1970s	Cimetidine for treatment of peptic ulcers and ibuprofen for treatment of inflammation were introduced.
1980s	DNA-produced insulin (1980) was the first DNA-produced medication. Chickenpox vaccine, medications for cardiac arrhythmia and benign prostatic hypertrophy, and angiotensin-converting enzyme (ACE) inhibitors were developed.
1990s	Acquired immunodeficiency syndrome (AIDS) medications and chemotherapy developed at a rapid pace to treat these devastating illnesses. Newer forms of medications were developed to treat peptic ulcers, impotence, and diabetes, especially newer forms of insulin with fewer reactions.
Twenty-first century	New drug administration techniques are being developed, such as insulin delivered via nasal spray, continuous oral contraception, and inhaled antibiotics. A vaccine for AIDS, microchips for drug administration, and gene therapy are on the horizon, and antivirals and antibiotics for drug-resistant microbe are increasing in numbers.

Many medications have been introduced during times of war or as technology has advanced. See Box 1-1 for an annotated history of pharmacology.

In the twenty-first century, transdermal patches and small dots are increasingly being used for medication administration for smoking cessation, hormone replacement therapy, contraception, and even treatment of attention-deficit/hyperactivity disorder (ADHD) because of convenience. Insulin pumps for type 1 diabetes mellitus and nasal sprays for treating acute or chronic illnesses are commonly used. Inhalation medications using aerosol particles are used to treat bronchial diseases.

Important Facts

- By trial and error, early civilizations found plant sources that could be used to treat disease processes. This was a precursor to folk medicine.
- In the sixteenth century, the Chinese created the first pharmacopoeia, which listed drugs of animal, vegetable, and mineral origin that were used to maintain body harmony.
- At the end of the nineteenth century and beginning of the twentieth century, many laws were enacted in the field of pharmacy to protect the public.
- Medications for previously fatal chronic illnesses were introduced during the first half of the twentieth century. Many of

Society and the Need for Drug Regulation

Throughout history, some members of societies have chosen to misuse or even abuse medicinal substances from herbs to chemicals. As societies became more progressive, governing bodies saw the need to establish regulations to control use of these substances by enacting laws and regulations.

Government has also taken steps to ensure that the consumer has high-quality drugs providing the expected therapeutic properties. Before the twentieth century, drug legislation would have been almost impossible—detailed information about drugs was not available because there was no means to analyze drugs as they were developed. A **drug's potency or strength,** or concentration of active ingredients, varied with the conditions under which the drug was prepared. The drug consistency might vary from one bottle of medication to the next; thus patients' reactions to medication also varied, affecting even patient safety. Since the beginning of the twentieth century, however, research methods mandated by legislation have resulted in consistent manufacture of medications and thus safety in their preparation and effectiveness. Legislation now also requires that all new medications undergo stringent testing before release to ensure **drug standardization** of these therapeutic agents and therefore consistency with use. Over the past quarter century the public has become more knowledgeable about medications as the number of OTC medications has increased, making patient education about drug interactions and adverse reactions an important patient issue.

Pharmaceutical companies spend vast amounts of money on drug development and advertising. Therefore legislation is necessary to protect consumers and companies and to enforce quality control of the medication. Advertisements for medication stress their positive effects to increase sales. However, by law, adverse reactions, drug interactions, and other negative effects are required to be given equal coverage so people are given sufficient information to make informed choices about the value of the therapeutic agent. Because of today's information highways such as the Internet, the U.S. government continues to investigate ways to ensure that information gathered from computer sources is accurate and complete.

Controls for ensuring safety and promoting informed choices have been a direct result of legislation at federal, state, and local levels. State and local regulations, such as classification of certain controlled drugs, are usually more stringent and precise than federal regulations. Restrictions found in policy and procedure manuals of individual offices or medical facilities may be even more stringent than government regulations. Allied health professionals *must* have a working knowledge of regulations at all levels to comply with all restrictions.

DRUG STANDARDS AND PATIENT SAFETY

Drug standards assure consumers that they are receiving safe medications. Legislation requires that *all* drugs with the same name and dosage be of uniform strength, quality, and purity so each prescription filled for a given medication is the same in all pharmacies. Drug manufacturers must meet standards set in the *United States Pharmacopeia–National Formulary* (USP-NF) for quality, efficacy, strength or potency, and purity of a drug. **Drug purity** specifies the type and concentration of a chemical substance present in a drug. Most products are combinations of active ingredients with the fillers, buffers, and solvents necessary to give form to tablets and capsules, to make the product more palatable, or to change the absorption rate of the medication. Purity standards also ensure that excessive contaminants are not found in the medication. **Drug potency** or strength is the concentration of active ingredients in the preparation measured by chemical analysis. **Drug quality** ensures that consumers receive medications that achieve the standards required by the federally approved USP-NF. **Drug efficacy** refers to the ability of a drug to produce the desired chemical change in the body. Clinical trials are used to compare the response of volunteer individuals to the drug with other volunteers' response to a **placebo.**

Did You Know?

Because of the strict regulation of safety standards for new drugs in the market, drugs are often available in other countries before they are found in the United States.

Even OTC drugs are studied to make sure they are safe for administration without professional guidance if the manufacturer's directions are followed and that labels bear sufficient warnings and instructions. By 1983 OTC medications were either found safe or were removed from sale except by prescription. One of the problems in medicine today is that vitamin and herbal supplement standards are not enforced by the FDA; rather, these supplements are supervised as food products according to the less strenuous restrictions of the Department of Agriculture. These supplements may not have the same purity and quality with each manufacturer or batch; therefore consumers must be careful to choose reputable companies and to carefully read labels to lower risks of taking poor-quality supplements.

In the illicit drug market, the consumer does not enjoy the protection of these standards, resulting in inherent dangers similar to those found in the time of the medicine man. The use of illegal drugs has resulted in overdoses and death among those willing to take the risks involved.

Important Facts

- Drug standards ensure that consumers will receive safe medications that are the drugs that were expected.
- Drug purity specifies that the correct active ingredient is present and manufactured without excessive contaminents.
- Drug potency or strength is the concentration of active ingredient.
- Drug quality ensures that the consumer receives drugs that meet the standards published in the *United States Pharmacopeia–National Formulary.*
- Drug efficacy is the ability of the drug to produce the desired chemical change in the body.
- Over-the-counter medications must meet the same standards as legend drugs.

International, Federal, and State Statutes for the Regulation of Medications

The international control of medications comes under the authority of the World Health Organization of the United Nations. This group provides technical assistance in the drug field and promotes research on drug abuse. Because no world judicial groups enforce laws concerning drugs, drug control varies from country to country. Some nations have more stringent laws than statutes of the United States. Harsh punishments including long prison sentences and even death are imposed for possession of illegal drugs or drug trafficking in some countries. Other countries have lenient laws and enforcement concerning drug possession, even to the point of allowing use of some drugs that are illegal in the United States.

Before the twentieth century, many drugs containing opium and the new miracle drug morphine did not require a prescription, and pharmacists and physicians were not required to hold a license. Labeling of ingredients on medication bottles was not a requirement. Use of many nonstandardized **dangerous drugs** resulted in injury or death from their use, addiction, or inconsistency in manufacture.

Did You Know?

Before 1906, patent medicines were sold by medicine men in traveling shows, by mail order, in stores, by trained physicians, and even by individuals who just called themselves "doctors." Medications with names like *Dr. Smith's Miraculous Cough Medicine* or *New Age Miracle Soothing Syrup* were popular. For example, John S. Pemberton, a pharmacist in Atlanta, first made *French Wine Coca—Ideal Nerve and Tonic Stimulant* in 1885. In 1886 Pemberton used coca leaves and caffeine from the African kola nut as ingredients in a product called *Coca-Cola.* Advertised as a "therapeutic agent" and "sovereign remedy," the "quicker picker-upper" became known by the nicknames "Dope" and "Coke."

Federal Legislation Related to Drugs

- *Pure Food and Drug Act* of 1906
  - Earliest regulation included many loopholes and lack of enforcement abilities.
  - Drugs found in interstate commerce could not be labeled as curative if the claims were false and misleading, but advertisement by word of mouth or printed materials was not covered.
  - The USP and the NF were created as the compendia containing the official standards for strength and purity during manufacturing, including a label showing the eleven specific dangerous chemicals present that may cause drug addiction.
- *Shirley Amendment* of 1912
  - Prevented fraudulent therapeutic claims by drug manufacturers.
- *Harrison Narcotic Act* or *Federal Narcotic Drug Act* of 1914
  - Established the word *narcotic* and required the use of a stamp on the containers of these drugs.
  - For patient safety, regulated the importation, manufacture, sale, and use of opium, codeine, and their derivatives and compounds.
- *Food, Drug, and Cosmetic Act* of 1938
  - Provided safety testing on all drugs.
  - The FDA was formed to enforce the laws, seize goods that were improperly manufactured or packaged, and undertake criminal prosecution of the responsible persons or firms.

- Required pharmaceutical firms to report all adverse effects associated with their drugs at regular intervals.
- Required that all new drugs be tested for toxicity before approval.

Did You Know?

In the late 1930s sulfanilamide, an antibacterial agent in a raspberry-flavored base, was a lethal elixir because the base was not known to be toxic. With no need for approval of safe chemicals used in manufacture, the company did not use an alcohol base that was indicated for an elixir, but made the drug using an industrial-strength toxic liquid solvent, diethylene glycol—a major ingredient in antifreeze. More than 100 children died after ingesting less than an ounce of the medicine, and in excess of 350 more children were poisoned.

- *Durham-Humphrey Amendment* (1951) replaced laws of 1938
  - Indicated regulations for prescription orders or dispensing by designating prescription and OTC medications, with labeling of prescription medications being met by placing an "Rx" on the label of the manufacturer's bottle.
  - Required that all prescriptions be labeled "Caution: Federal law prohibits dispensing without a prescription."
  - Designated the OTC drugs that were considered sufficiently safe not to require a prescription.
  - Required warning labels on drug packaging.
- *Kefauver-Harris Amendment* (1962)
  - Was passed because drug companies were making large profits and engaging in misleading and even false drug promotions.
  - Required proven effectiveness of a drug before marketing, with old and new drugs requiring proof testing.

Did You Know?

The manufacturer of thalidomide, a hypnotic that was taken by pregnant women early in pregnancy, claimed it was a miracle drug for the nausea of pregnancy and a sleeping aid without realizing the associated dangers of severe deformities in fetuses, leading to a wave of "thalidomide babies." These infants were born with severe deformities, especially of limbs. Some pregnant women in the Northeast were prescribed the drug, but the tragedy was more a "might-have-been" catastrophe than a widespread, actual one because a U.S. Food and Drug Administration employee was suspicious of the drug and wanted more information before approving it for use in the United States. Sadly, the chemist who developed the drug later committed suicide.

- *Comprehensive Drug Abuse Prevention and Control Act of 1970* (also called *Controlled Substances Act* of 1970)
  - Repealed the 50 laws passed between 1914 and 1970 concerning drug control.
  - Regulated manufacture, distribution, and dispensing of drugs with the potential for abuse.
- Indicated drugs that had potential for abuse, and placed these medications in five schedules sorted by potential for abuse or addiction to prevent indiscriminate use of these drugs by limiting their use.
  - Required security of **controlled substances** by anyone who dispenses, receives, sells, or destroys controlled substances using special DEA forms to show current inventory.
  - Regulated use of controlled substances to only legitimate handlers to help reduce the widespread illicit use of these drugs.
  - Provided for prevention of **drug abuse** and **drug dependence** and for treatment and rehabilitation of abusers and drug-dependent persons.
- Two important agencies had a role in the enforcement of this act:
  - The **Bureau of Narcotics and Dangerous Drugs** (BNDD), in existence from 1968 to 1973, with the following responsibilities:
    - To register all persons who manufacture, dispense, prescribe, or administer any controlled substances.
    - To provide for necessary revision of schedules and classes of controlled drugs.
  - The **Drug Enforcement Administration (DEA)** was established in 1973 to continue regulation and enforcement of manufacturing and dispensing of dangerous and potentially abused drugs. (See section on DEA that follows.)
- *Poison Prevention Packaging Act* of 1970
  - Created standards to ensure that both prescription and OTC medications were in child-resistant packages.
- *Drug Listing Act* of 1972
  - Established National Drug Code for use by the FDA to identify a drug's manufacturer, including the drug formulation and the size of the packaging, by using a unique and permanent code for drugs.
- *Drug Regulation and Reform Act* of 1978
  - Allowed for briefer investigation of new drugs and to allow for faster access by the consumer.
- *Orphan Drug Act* of 1983
  - Established in response to the removal of drugs because of potential dangers or the lack of research.
  - Established funding for research for use of these drugs in the treatment of rare chronic illnesses through grant monies and tax incentives to find

new drugs and new uses for older drugs for conditions with so few patients that the manufacturer would be unlikely to recoup expenses once the drug could be marketed.

Did You Know?

Thalidomide, which caused severe birth defects in the 1960s, has been found today to be effective for leprosy, multiple myeloma, acquired immunodeficiency syndrome, and other rare conditions because of the enactment of the Orphan Drug Act.

- *Drug Price Competition and Patent Term Restoration Act* (1984)
  - Eased requirements for marketing generic drugs by allowing generic drug companies to prove bioequivalence without having to duplicate trials.
  - Extended length of time of patents to compensate for the time lost in premarketing trials.
- *Omnibus Budget Reconciliation Act* of 1990 (OBRA 1990)
  - Mandated that OTC drugs be considered an important part of the medical record and that they be documented.
- *Anabolic Steroids Control Act* of 1990
  - Placed anabolic steroids under umbrella of the Controlled Substances Act of 1970.
- *Prescription Drug Amendments* of 1992
  - Allowed rapid approval of medications by the FDA, especially for life-threatening diseases and debilitating conditions.
- *Food and Drug Administration Modernization Act* (1997)
  - Allowed rapid approval of medications by the FDA, especially for life-threatening diseases and debilitating conditions.

Other laws may come from regulatory agencies such as the Federal Trade Commission, which regulates business practices in the medical field, and the Consumer Products Safety Commission, which has a routine that must be followed, such as for drug packaging to prevent poisoning in children.

Did You Know?

During the widespread outbreak of H1N1 influenza in 2009, the FDA allowed emergency use of the experimental drug peramivir for hospitalized patients who had not responded to the FDA-approved antivirals.

Over the years, federal legislation has established standards for medicines that provide patient safety. Citizens of the United States can feel assured that their medications have been tested and found effective with minimal adverse reactions and that all prescriptions for the same medication will contain the same therapeutic ingredients.

Did You Know?

The use of the Internet for medications has brought ethical and safety dilemmas of its own. New consumer safety regulations are being put into place to ensure safety for patients who fill medication prescriptions by using the Internet or providers in other countries. The government is even looking into ways to ensure that such Internet sites provide patient safety and that the medications are those specified and protected by regulations pertaining to the manufacture and distribution of the drugs.

At the state level, almost all states have laws governed by the state boards of pharmacy concerning the substitution of **generic drugs** for **brand-name drugs.** Some states and some insurance companies permit generic substitution by the pharmacist, although the person prescribing the medication, usually a physician, retains the right to require the dispensing of a brand-name drug by writing "brand necessary" on the prescription. If the state has mandatory substitution, the pharmacist is required to use less expensive generic drugs for dispensing. If a generic name is used on the prescription, the pharmacist may use his or her discretion to select the drug with a bioequivalence to the brand-name medication. A generic medication must go through testing to ensure that the inert ingredients provide bioequivalence and that the active ingredients have not changed from those in the trademarked drug.

THE FOOD AND DRUG ADMINISTRATION AND THE INTRODUCTION OF NEW DRUGS

As an agency of the U.S. Department of Health and Human Services, the FDA is responsible for reviewing the testing of all drugs before they are released to the public (Table 1-1). The development process is lengthy, taking 6 to 12 years, and is expensive. At the end, only about one drug emerges for each 5000 to 10,000 different compounds tested. (See Box 1-2 for the drug testing process.) At any time during the process or even after approval, the FDA may ask for additional information from the manufacturer, for revisions in the trials, or for the medication to be returned to the company for further research or testing. Therefore manufacturers that develop a drug are given a 20-year patent on the medication to cover the time and expense of trials necessary to show that the

TABLE 1-1 AGENCIES RESPONSIBLE FOR DRUG SURVEILLANCE

AGENCY AND SUPERVISING DEPARTMENT OF U.S. GOVERNMENT	CONCERN	RESPONSIBILITY
Food and Drug Administration (FDA) under Department of Health and Human Services	General safety standards in the production of drugs, foods, and cosmetics	Approves and removes products on the market Regulates labeling and advertising of prescription drugs; cooperates with Federal Trade Commission on regulation of nonprescription drugs Regulates drug manufacturing practices Engages in postmarketing surveillance to detect unanticipated adverse and therapeutic effects of drugs
Drug Enforcement Administration (DEA) under Department of Justice	Controlled substances only	Enforces laws against unlawful drug activities Assigns identification numbers (DEA numbers) for those entities that prescribe, dispense, and manufacture scheduled drugs Monitors scheduled drugs for need to change possible abuse level

BOX 1-2 STEPS IN THE DEVELOPMENT OF NEW DRUGS

Development of a New Compound by a Pharmaceutical Company
↓
Preclinical Testing in Animals
Drugs are tested for toxicity, use of drug in the body, and possible useful effects.
Animal testing: range of 1 to 3 years, usually 18 months
↓
Food and Drug Administration (FDA) safety review of testing results
↓
Investigational New Drug Status if Approved
(Go back to earliest research if not approved.)
↓
Clinical Trials in Humans
Range of 2 to 7 years, usually 5 years
Testing for safety, effectiveness, dosage range, and therapeutic use
Phase 1 trials—test of an experimental drug or treatment in a small group of people (20-80) for evaluation of safety, safe dosage range, and identify side effects
Phase 2 trials—experimental study of drug or treatment to larger group of people (100-300) to further evaluate effectiveness and safety

Phase 3 trials—experimental study of drug or treatment to larger group of people (1000-3000) to confirm effectiveness, monitor side effects, compare to commonly used treatments and collect information that will drug or treatment to be used safely
Phase 4 trials—post-marketing studies delineate additional information including the drug's risks, benefits, and optimal use
↓
New Drug Application (NDA) Sent to FDA
FDA review: Range of 2 months to 7 years, usually 24 months
↓
FDA Approval of NDA
(If not approved, return to manufacturer for further initial testing or further research.)
↓
Postmarketing Surveillance
Drug is released for use, permitting observation in large numbers of patients.
Surveys, sampling, and inspections by FDA and physicians using the medication are performed.
Adverse reactions are reported to FDA for analysis and reevaluation.

drug has the intended therapeutic purpose in humans. The process of FDA approval uses up to half of the patent time, leaving the company with about 10 years of marketability under patent, or trade name. At the end of that time, another company may manufacture the drug under another **brand name** or use the generic name that has been assigned by the USP.

Did You Know?

Many brand names may be available for the same generic drug. For example, ibuprofen is sold under the brand names Motrin, Nuprin, and Advil, and naproxen is sold as Naprosyn at prescription strength and as Aleve at over-the-counter strength.

The FDA also reviews proposals for new indications for already approved drugs, with the clinical testing process being performed as for a new drug. A new indication for an already patented drug extends the time of the patent on the medication. Conversely, if a drug appears to be associated with too many adverse reactions, the FDA or manufacturer has the right to withdraw the drug from the market after approval has been granted.

Did You Know?

Drugs that are deemed unsafe may be removed from the market, as occurred with the voluntary withdrawal of the cyclooxygenase-2 (COX-2) inhibitors Vioxx and Bextra, after they were found to increase the risk of multiple adverse reactions such as heart attack and stroke.

Many prescription medications are becoming OTC drugs at strengths decreased below the legend strength. An OTC drug is a medication, and as such, the consumer must use it as the FDA has approved it for OTC use. Educating the patient to follow directions is an important element in the safe use of OTC drugs. See Table 1-1 for the role of the FDA in drug regulations.

Important Facts

- The DEA, an agency of the U.S. Department of Justice, is responsible for monitoring controlled substances. The Food and Drug Administration (FDA), an agency of the U.S. Department of Health and Human Services, is responsible for regulating the manufacture and safety of drugs.
- The development of a new drug is a lengthy process, taking up to 12 years, and only one of up to 10,000 compounds tested may reach the stage of a new drug.
- A company introducing a new drug has approximately 10 years of exclusive use of the drug.
- Preclinical and clinical testing must be done on a new medication to ensure its safety. Any adverse reactions to medications, especially newly marketed drugs, should be reported to the FDA.

The Drug Enforcement Administration and Controlled Substances

Controlled substances became regulated by the DEA through the Controlled Substances Act, Title II of the Comprehensive Drug Abuse Prevention and Control Act of 1970 (see Table 1-1). The drugs are classified according to their established abuse potential, which applies not only to pain relievers but also to drugs with the

potential to be addictive or habit forming, such as steroids, depressants, and stimulants. Criteria for placement on the list include the following:

- Evidence that the substance is being used in sufficient amounts to pose a medical threat to individuals or a hazard to the community
- Significant diversion of the substance from legitimate use to illegal drug trafficking
- Tendency of consumers to take the substance on their own initiative rather than on medical advice
- A new drug with an action related to the action of a drug already on the controlled substances list until a decision is made concerning its abuse potential

The controlled substances are grouped into five categories, or schedules, each with its own prescription and dispensing restrictions (Table 1-2). Medications with highest potential for abuse and with no accepted medical use are placed on Schedule I. Those with least abuse potential are placed on Schedule V. A drug may be moved from one schedule to another or may be removed from the list on reevaluation of abuse potential by the DEA. Any revision of the list is sent to practitioners to keep the health professional's knowledge current.

Because the DEA strictly enforces regulations pertaining to scheduled medications, precise and complete records are required for Schedule II medications. These records must indicate the flow of the medicines from time of arrival at the facility until they are administered.

Important Facts

- Controlled substances are placed in one of five groups, or schedules, each with restrictions on prescribing and dispensing, based on the danger of abuse or misuse.
- DEA controlled substances may be moved between schedules on the controlled substances list. A current inventory of all Schedule II medications should be kept; if Schedule III medications are dispensed by the facility, an inventory of those is also necessary.
- Controlled substances can be abused and misused with or without prescription use.

The Drug Enforcement Administration and Controlled Substances in the Medical Office

Controlled substances are labeled so that they can be easily identified. A large C shows that the drug is a controlled drug, with the Roman numeral of the schedule (I through V) appearing within the C. For example, a

TABLE 1-2 DRUG CLASSIFICATIONS ACCORDING TO THE CONTROLLED SUBSTANCES ACT OF 1970

DRUG SCHEDULE	CHARACTERISTICS	PRESCRIPTION REGULATIONS	EXAMPLES
Schedule I	High potential for abuse, severe physical or psychologic dependence For research use only	No accepted use in United States Marijuana may be used in cancer and glaucoma for research and may be obtained for patients in research situations	Narcotics—heroin Hallucinogens—peyote mescaline, PCP, hashish, amphetamine variants, LSD Cannabis—marijuana, THC Designer drugs—ecstasy, crack, crystal meth
Schedule II	High potential for abuse, severe physical or psychologic dependence Accepted medicinal use with specific restrictions	Dispensed by prescription only Oral emergency orders for Schedule II drugs may be given, but physician must supply written prescription within 72 hr Refills require a new written prescription from physician	Narcotics—opium, codeine. morphine, methadone, hydromorphone (Dilaudid), meperidine (Demerol), oxycodone (Oxycotin), fentanyl (Duragesic), pentobarbital (Nembutal) Stimulants—amphetamines, amphetamine salts (Adderall), methylphenidate (Ritalin) Depressants-pentobarbital (Nembutal)
Schedule III	Moderate potential for abuse, high psychologic dependence, low physical dependence Accepted medicinal uses	Dispensed by prescription only May be refilled five times in 6 mo with prescription authorization by physician Prescription may be phoned to pharmacy	Narcotics—paregoric (opium derivative), certain codeine combinations (with acetaminophen) Depressants—pentobarbital (Nembutal) (rectal route) Stimulants—benzophetamine (Didrex)
Schedule IV	Lower potential for abuse than Schedule III drugs Limited psychologic and physical dependence Accepted medicinal uses	Dispensed by prescription only May be refilled five times in 6 mo with physician authorization Prescription may be phoned to pharmacy	Narcotics—pentazocine (Talwin) Depressants—chloral hydrate (Noctec), phenobarbital, diazepam (Valium), chlordiazepoxide (Librium), alprazolam (Xanax), clorazepate (Tranxene), benzodiazepines (lorazepam [Ativan], flurazepam [Dalmane]), midazolam (Versed), meprobamate (Equanil), temazepam (Restoril), Stimulants—phentermine (Adipex-P)
Schedule V	Low potential for abuse Abuse may lead to limited physical or psychologic dependence Accepted medicinal uses	OTC narcotic drugs may be sold by registered pharmacist depending on state laws Buyer must be 18 years of age, show identification, and sign for medications	Preparations containing limited quantities of narcotics, generally cough and antidiarrheal preparations—cough syrups with codeine, diphenoxylate hydrochloride with atropine sulfate (Lomotil) and attapulgite (Parepectolin)

From the Drug Enforcement Administration (DEA), U.S. Department of Justice, Washington DC. Local DEA offices can provide current lists of medications on these schedules.

LSD, Lysergic acid diethylamide; *OTC,* over the counter; *PCP,* phencyclidine hydrochloride; *THC,* tetrahydrocannabinol.

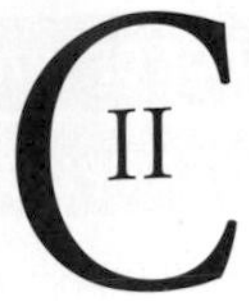

C II

Figure 1-5 Symbol that indicates a drug is a controlled substance in Class II (Schedule II).

Schedule II medication would be shown as appears in Figure 1-5.

Physicians or other health professionals (such as dentists) who administer, dispense, or prescribe controlled substances must have a current state license, must register with the DEA and be assigned a DEA number, and in some states must have a state controlled-substance license. Exceptions to this ruling are physicians who are interns, residents, in the armed services, from a foreign country, or on the staff of a Veterans Administration facility, who dispense and prescribe using a special code under the registration of the hospital or institution. At the appropriate time for renewal (every 3 years), the DEA will automatically send a renewal form 45 days before the renewal date. If this form is not received, it is the responsibility of the physician to notify the DEA.

Ordering and Securing Controlled Substances

Schedule II substances for use in the medical office or in the physician's medical bag must be ordered from suppliers using the Federal Triplicate Order (DEA Form 222). When scheduled medications are ordered, one copy of the form goes to the DEA, the second copy goes to the supplier, and the third copy is retained by the physician. On receipt of the drugs, the physician attaches the documentation showing receipt of the medication to the retained copy. This documentation could be a packing slip with cash receipt showing payment for the medication or invoice and a copy of the check showing payment. Good record keeping not only is invaluable to the physician, but also assists the physician in following state and federal regulations related to controlled substances.

Schedule II drug records must be kept separate from other medical records and must be readily available for at least 5 years for inspection by the DEA or government agencies interested in drug administration. Records of other scheduled drugs may either be kept separately or be easily retrievable from professional records.

To purchase controlled substances on Schedules III through V, the physician does not use Form 222 but may purchase these medications through local pharmacies. However, the records of the suppliers' invoices with date of receipt and quantity of drug received and a logbook of the administration of the medication must be kept for 2 years.

Schedule II controlled substances must be kept separate from other drugs and be placed in a securely locked area. Some states require a double lock on opioid products. The stock of controlled substances should be kept to a minimum. For the office needing large amounts of controlled substances, higher security measures such as an alarm system, should be in place. The physician or his or her designee should keep the key. The statutes of each state provide guidelines on the handling of controlled substances.

If theft of inventory occurs, it is significant and the local DEA office must be notified. If theft has occurred, it is *required* that the local police department be notified first, as well as the state bureau of narcotic enforcement. If damage to or contamination of significant amounts of controlled substances occurs, the local DEA office should be contacted for appropriate disposal instructions.

Record Keeping and Inventory Control

As controlled substances are received, the medication should be recorded on a special inventory form (Figure 1-6). The receipt should be signed by two employees and should show the exact amount of stock medication received. To take an inventory count, the allied health professional counts the amount of the medication on hand and compares this with the amount ordered and the amount either administered or dispensed to patients. The total of the medications on hand plus the dispensed medications should equal the inventory received.

An inventory with invoices or copies of invoices from the drug suppliers is required by the DEA every 2 years. This inventory must contain the following information:

- The name and quantity of each controlled substance
- The name, address, and DEA registration number of the physician
- The date and time of the inventory process
- The signature of the person(s) taking the inventory; preferably two persons should take the inventory

If a medication for controlled substances is administered in the facility and none is dispensed, then the medical record of the patient must show medication administration and must be easily available for DEA review. If controlled substances are administered and dispensed, records must be maintained separate from medical charts and must be readily available for inspection. States vary as to the exact requirements of record keeping, and allied health professionals should be aware of the state regulations where they practice.

Registrant Name: Lawrence Merry, M.D.	DEA Reg #: AD0000000
Address: 4th Street and Jones Ave.	Inventory of Schedule: II ✓ III,IV,V ___
City/St. Zip: Holly, GA 00111	Inventory Date: 11/01/01
	Inventory Time: Opening of business ✓ Close of business ___

Drug/Preparation	# Containers	Contents*	CS Contents**
morphine sulfate	bottle	100 tabs	15 mg
Demerol HC1 ampule	10	1.0 mL	25 mg
Percocet	1 bottle	50 tabs	5/325 mg

The above stock controlled substances was inventoried by the person(s) signed below, who attest that the above inventory is maintained at the location appearing at the top of this inventory and has been maintained at the location appearing at the top of this inventory for at least two years.

June Smith, CMA
Inventoried by

Jane Joy, CMA
Inventoried by

* Number of grams, tables, ounces, or other units per container.
** Controlled substance content of each unit.

Drug Name	Patient	Dose	Date	Hour	MD	MA

Reviewed by
_____, CMA

Reviewed by
_____, MD

Figure 1-6 Typical form for inventory of controlled substances.

Disposing of Scheduled and Nonscheduled Drugs

To dispose of controlled drugs, such as expired drugs, call the nearest DEA office for instructions. If the drug must be mailed, the allied health professional should be sure that registered mail is used to ensure safe shipment. Once drugs have been destroyed, the DEA will issue a receipt that the physician must place with controlled substance records.

Outdated, noncontrolled medications do not come under these stringent regulations. Depending on the state law, they may be flushed down the toilet, washed down a sink, or placed in the trash. If placed in the trash, the physician should maintain security to ensure these medications do not fall into the hands of the public. Incineration may be necessary for medications such as topicals or injectables that are difficult to destroy.

Important Facts

- Stock labels for controlled substances are marked with *C*, with the schedule number (in Roman numerals) within the letter.
- DEA has specific forms that must be used when applying for a DEA number. Forms obtained from the DEA must be used to order Schedule II medications. Medications on Schedules III through V do not require the special form.
- The physician has the specific responsibility of renewing his or her DEA registration every 3 years.

Continued

Preventing Drug Dependence and Drug Abuse

Substance abuse is a national and international problem that affects all of us. Health care workers have a responsibility to patients and society to assess the chances for abuse or misuse of medications. A patient's frequent request for a given drug and "doctor-hopping" may be signs of potential abuse or misuse. A pharmacist may make the medical office aware of the patient's use of multiple medical facilities for prescriptions and will provide the information to prevent further abuse. The medical office professional should be sure the physician is aware of any information provided by other health care professionals. Other signs that may indicate substance abuse include pinpoint pupils, lethargy, or a change in or unusual behavior.

Drug dependence may be both **physical dependence** and **psychological drug dependence,** or **habituation.** The physical dependence begins with use of a medication over a prolonged period of time and is a normal adaptation to continued drug use. The medication may involve a drug used to relieve pain or to control physical or emotional problems, or it may be one used for such conditions as blood pressure or respiratory disease. Psychologic drug dependence is a craving of a drug for pleasure or to relieve discomfort and a psychologic crutch used to relieve anxiety. However, **drug addiction** is compulsive use of a drug despite physical harm and is therefore a dysfunctional behavior.

Drug abuse depends in part on why a drug is taken and what is culturally defined as acceptable drug use. What is considered abuse in one culture may not be considered abuse in another. Drug abuse is use of a drug in a way that is not consistent with medical or social reasoning or administration of drugs in quantities over an excessive time that is inconsistent with accepted medical practice. (See Chapter 31 for a discussion of drug abuse and misuse.)

Some actions by patients may indicate possible abuse, as with the patient who asks for a particular medication and is not satisfied without that specific drug. Drug abusers, or those with drug-seeking behaviors, usually know which drugs they want and will continue to ask for a specific drug rather than accept the medical care offered by the physician. Many times a drug-seeking person will state that he or she has lost a previously obtained prescription or lost the medication after the prescription was filled and therefore needs a new prescription. The health care professional should follow office protocol exactly by checking medical records for signs of possible misuse of medications, such as repeated prescriptions for pain medications, sedatives, or behavior-altering medications. Documenting all prescriptions precisely is of utmost importance for all patients so that the physician can detect early signs of possible misuse.

Finally, prescription pads should be safeguarded at all times. Prescription pads should never be used as note pads or for orders other than those for prescription medications. Signature lines may have the imprint of the health care professional's signature, and drug abusers may copy the imprint made by signing multiple times and forge a prescription. A prescription pad should never be left in an examining room unattended. The patient who abuses medications may be able to obtain drugs more easily by stealing prescription blanks. Although all prescriptions should be documented in the medical record, another safeguard is to copy all prescriptions leaving the medical office and place copies in the medical records. The patient seeing this procedure would certainly be less likely to forge a prescription because the pharmacist could easily confirm that the prescription had been written. Medical office personnel are an important link in preventing drug abuse and misuse by participating in the checks-and-balances system between the physician and pharmacist. This system often is the first line of defense as early warning signs are observed and proper action is taken.

ROLE OF ALLIED HEALTH PROFESSIONALS IN MEDICATION ADMINISTRATION

The medical practice act of each state in compliance with federal regulations provides the guidelines for prescribing, administering, storing, and dispensing of medications by allied health professionals. Because some allied health professionals perform tasks under the legal premise of **respondeat superior,** the physician also needs a working understanding of state and federal laws governing legal job performances in his or her state of practice. Any legal interpretation of the law must come from the agency in each state that enforces the medical practice act. As agents or representatives of the physician, allied health professionals work under the laws of the state in which they practice their profession and have a legal and ethical responsibility to know what is allowed under that state's medical practice act. When federal and state laws concerning medications differ, which law prevails? The stricter laws, whether they are federal or state, prevail. The office policy and protocol concerning who may handle prescriptions and administer medicines in the medical office must be in compliance with state and national laws.

Some states allow allied health professionals to write prescriptions for a physician's signature or allow a physician's agent, such as a nurse practitioner, to sign. In other states this practice is illegal. Some states allow medication administration by allied health workers; other states do not. Because many medications have similar names, health care professionals should be sure that their knowledge of medications is adequate to perform telephone transmittal of prescriptions with accuracy. (See the Evolve site for sound-alike and look-alike names.) For commonly prescribed medications, health care professionals should know indications, normal dosage, side effects, adverse reactions, and what patient education is necessary before handling telephone orders. New medications should be researched before health care professionals administers or relays orders for these.

Important Facts

- The allied health worker must understand laws as they pertain to the medical practice in the state where he or she is employed.
- Federal and state laws concerning medications and prescriptions must be followed.

Ethics of the Health Professional in Medication Management

Ethically, the person administering a medication must also have a working knowledge of the medication—its dosage, strength, physical appearance, side effects, and adverse reactions. If there is any doubt about the physician or health care professional's order, the person administering the medication should ask for clarification. With a written or phoned prescription, this accountability becomes a responsibility of the pharmacist. The ultimate goal in medication administration is safety of the patient and reduction of possible mistakes.

All health professionals must use confidentiality in all areas of medications and their administration. Some drugs indicate certain conditions such as a human immunodeficiency virus (HIV) infection, and the health professional must carefully protect prescription information from anyone who does not have a need or does not have the patient's permission to see them. If prescriptions are sent by facsimile equipment or electronically sent to pharmacies, a protocol must be in place to safeguard confidentiality. The procedure will vary among medical offices, but it must be in place to protect the provider against the possibility of legal actions and invasion of privacy.

Drug Samples and Ethics

Drug samples are a manufacturer's way of promoting sales by providing free supplies of medications to health care professionals; drug samples should not be sold. Sample drugs requiring a prescription are marked "sample" and bear the federal legend ℞. These medications must be inventoried before being left with the physician. Manufacturers may also supply drug coupons for a discounted price of prescribed drugs. These coupons may not be sold or traded for use on a drug other than the one identified on the coupon.

Samples are distributed to health care professionals (prescribers) only when the physician provides a written request for any sample and identifies the desired quantity of the drug, manufacturer's name, and prescriber's name. Medical personnel in the physician's office may not sign for samples; the physician must sign the required form to receive samples. (Box 1-3 outlines the protocol for receiving drug samples and the DEA surveillance of controlled substances.)

BOX 1-3 DRUG SAMPLES AND DRUG ENFORCEMENT ADMINISTRATION (DEA) SURVEILLANCE

Responsibilities of Manufacturer
- Supply samples.
- Provide documentation to DEA for scheduled medications.

Responsibilities of Sales Representative
- Inventory drugs on receipt and yearly.
- Show place for safe storage.
- Maintain records of distribution.
- Report theft or loss.
- Verify current valid DEA registration of health care professionals receiving samples.

Responsibilities of Medical Office
- Provide prescription or representative's form signed by the health care professional.
- Safeguard against theft and misuse by storing in secure area not accessible to patients.
- Document that samples are supplied to patients.
- Dispose of unused or outdated samples properly.
- Retain samples at office once signed for; do not return to manufacturer's representative.
- Obtain authorization from health care professional to use prescription samples.
- Do not repackage samples.
- Do not charge for samples.

Samples should be immediately stored in an area that is not accessible to patients and should be organized by indication of use or disease process and expiration date. Samples approaching their expiration date should be placed toward the front of the storage area so they are used first. Office personnel should assist the physician in being sure that only those medications that will be used are left by the sales representative. Destruction of medications that are not used or distributed by expiration date may be accomplished by flushing the medication down the toilet, pouring liquid medications into sink drains (followed by flushing with water), or incinerating. Drug destruction requires time and effort and should be avoided if at all possible. Distributed drugs may *not* be returned to sales representatives.

Finally, drug samples must be provided to the patient in the manufacturer's package.

Medical personnel should always ask permission from the physician, and office protocol should be followed before distribution to patients or for personal use.

Ethics of Medications with Medical Personnel

Because of the easy availability of medicines in the medical office, health care workers are at risk for drug abuse and misuse. Many medications, especially sample medications, are found in the outpatient setting, which can lead to the indiscriminate use of drugs. Career pressures such as stress and lower back pain place professionals at greater risk of drug abuse and misuse. Many people begin the road to drug abuse by having medications prescribed for legitimate health problems, only to find they have become chemically-dependent health care workers.

The impaired health care professional is a danger not only to himself or herself but to the patient. The patient is in danger because of erratic behavior that causes errors in judgment and accidents. The impaired health care worker is also a problem for co-workers because they cannot depend on the person to perform assigned duties. How the problem is handled is an ethical matter (and in some states a legal issue) that must be faced with each situation. When the problem is confronted head-on, patient safety is protected and the impaired worker has the opportunity to receive needed care.

Important Facts

- Allied health professionals must have a working knowledge of all medications used in the office of employment. Health professionals with questions about a drug should investigate the drug prior to any administration.
- Have a working knowledge of drug samples. Be sure to follow office protocol when distributing these samples.

Important Facts—cont'd

- Know the signs of drug abuse, and work within a legal framework to be sure you do not provide a way for drug abuse with the medical office staff or with patients.
- Work with pharmaceutical sales representatives to gain knowledge of new medications, new uses for medicines, and information on drug samples left at the office.
- Drug samples should be suitable for the physician's practice and should be organized by their use for disease processes or drug categories. All similar drugs should be grouped together; those with the nearest expiration date placed in front.
- Health care professionals are at risk of drug abuse or misuse because of the ready availability of medicinal agents, such as drug samples, and the tensions of the profession.
- Drug abuse or misuse by health care professionals is a physical issue but more importantly an ethical problem because of the impact on patient care.

SUMMARY

As partners with pharmacists and physicians, allied health professionals are a major link in the medication delivery pathway in today's health care environment. The administrative assistant must know medications in order to refer medication questions appropriately to other members of the health care team. Knowledge of drugs, their actions, their interactions, their side effects, and their adverse reactions is necessary for appropriate patient care. Depending on the laws of individual states, allied health professionals may administer medications, whereas physicians prescribe and pharmacists dispense. The ideal working relationship among all of these professionals provides a system of checks and balances for patient safety. All medications, whether prescription or OTC, should be documented in the medical record to prevent overdosing or adverse reactions from multiple medications from multiple providers. Through education about the importance of providing information to all physicians and taking medications as ordered, the patient becomes an active participant in pharmacologic therapy, and this role will only increase in the future.

Today's health market has come a long way from the early twentieth century, when medicine men hawked their wares from wagons. Those wares were not subject to quality assurance oversight for ingredients or the manufacture of the drug. One bottle of medication might do wonders, but the next might be ineffective or deadly. Today with federal and state legislation, people can be assured that the medication prescribed and dispensed will be of the same strength and purity every time they fill the prescription or receive the medicine in the physician's office. Through multiple statutes, the FDA continues to follow previously recognized drugs and studies proposals of new uses of medications by manufacturers while watching closely as new medications are developed. The process is long, time-consuming, and expensive, but the public can feel reassured that drugs are safe. If for any reason safety is questioned, drugs are recalled or taken off the market until their quality and safety can be established.

Controlled substances have the potential to be abused, and through stringent laws these drugs are watched closely by drug enforcement agencies. Written prescriptions are required for drugs with the greatest potential for abuse, and it is unlawful for a person to possess a controlled substance without a valid prescription. The 1970 Controlled Substances Act was designed to provide increased research into prevention of drug abuse and drug dependence. It also required special labels for drugs with potential for abuse, dependence, or both to ensure they would be administered or dispensed by legal drug handlers and not used illicitly. To avoid illegal use of these controlled substances, the public should be aware of potentially abusive or dependent drugs and signs of abuse or dependency.

Health care workers must know federal and state laws because ignorance of the law is not a defense in court if mishandling or poor administration of drugs occurs. The allied health professional must know the laws in the state of employment, because medical practice acts vary from state to state. Allied health personnel often work under the doctrine of *respondeat superior,* with the physician assigning a protocol that is appropriate to a given situation.

Ethics in the medical office requires ensuring confidentiality for the patient, safeguarding prescription pads, and handling drug samples properly. By working with other health care professionals such as physicians and pharmacists, the allied health professional can be effective for patient safety. Because drugs are readily available in the medical field, the allied health professional should be extremely careful about drug misuse and drug abuse and be observant for early signs and symptoms of misuse.

CRITICAL THINKING EXERCISES

Scenario

Mary Ann, an administrative allied health professional, is manning the phone at Dr. Merry's office. Janelee calls to say that she has been to the pharmacy to get her medication and has read on the patient information sheet that the drug prescribed should not be taken with aspirin, which she takes daily.

1. What should Mary Ann do first?
2. Should she make a decision, or should she ask Dr. Merry?
3. The pharmacist had called earlier and asked to speak to Dr. Merry, but Mary Ann took a message and did not give the message to Dr. Merry. Why is it important that the information be given to the physician as soon as possible?
4. What should be provided to the physician at the time the message is relayed?

REVIEW QUESTIONS

1. Define:

Pharmacology _____

_____

Drug _____

_____

Medication _____

_____

OTC _____

_____

Dispense _____

_____

Prescribe _____

Administer _____

Prescription drugs _____

Legend drugs _____

Drug abuse _____

Drug dependence _____

Drug standards _____

Drug Enforcement Administration (DEA) _____

Food and Drug Administration (FDA) _____

2. The three health professionals in the medication pathway are _____, _____, and
   _____. Describe the role of each in the system of checks and balances for safe medication use. _____
   _____
   _____

3. Name and define the five schedules found in the Controlled Substances Act. Place common medications that fall
   under this legislation in the correct schedule. _____
   _____
   _____
   _____
   _____
   _____
   _____
   _____
   _____

4. Drug abuse, drug dependence, and habituation are real problems in the medical office. Describe signs that patients
   are abusers or are dependent on certain drugs. What measures can the medical office take to assist the patient yet
   ensure that the office does not aid in further abuse or dependency? _____
   _____
   _____
   _____

5. Why are ethics in handling and dispensing of medication samples so important to health care workers? _____
   _____
   _____

CHAPTER 2

Basics of Pharmacology

OBJECTIVES

After studying this chapter, you should be capable of doing the following:

- Providing definitions of the keywords using the glossary or a medical dictionary.
- Stating health care workers' responsibility with regard to adverse reactions, side effects, and toxic reactions.
- Defining *drug*.

- Describing the five fundamental categories of pharmacology and how these factors influence medications.
- Describing indications for medicines.
- Explaining drug interactions with other drugs, nutrients, and diseases.

Joyce works in a physician's office that has several patients who do not think that going to a physician is necessary until an illness becomes life-threatening. These patients often see folk healers and use herbal supplements and over-the-counter (OTC) preparations rather than prescription medications. Joyce does not think it is necessary to document herbal supplements and OTC medications in the medical record.

What harm may Joyce cause these patients?
Thinking that the patient is taking medications as ordered, the physician cannot understand why the maintenance dose is not working and increases the dosage. What are the dangers of cumulation (accumulation), synergism, and antagonism?

KEY TERMS

Absorption	Chelator	Drug blood level	Local action
Active ingredient	Clinical pharmacology	Drug half-life	Metabolism
Addiction	Contraindication	Drug interaction	Mucosal
Adverse reaction	Cumulation	Enteral	Pharmacodynamics
Agonist	(accumulation)	Excretion	Pharmacognosy
Alkaloid	Curative (healing)	First-pass effect	Pharmacokinetics
Allergic reaction	medication	Free or unbound drug	Pharmacotherapeutics
Analgesic	Demulcent	Habituation	Potentiation
Anaphylaxis	Dependence	Hypersensitivity	Prophylactic
Antagonism	Depressant	reaction	Receptor site
Antagonist	Desired therapeutic	Ideal drug	Recombinant DNA
Antidote	effect or desired	Idiosyncratic drug	technology
Antiinflammatory	effect	reaction	Safe drug
Antimetabolite	Destructive agent	Indication	Side effect
Antipyretic	Distribution	Inert ingredient	Solubility
Biotransformation	Drug	Irritant	Summation

KEY TERMS—cont'd

Supportive
  medication
Synergism

Synthetic or
  manufactured drug
Systemic action

Therapeutics
Tolerance
Toxic

Toxicology
Usage

With the possible exception of computers, in no area of life during the twentieth and twenty-first centuries has technology transformed everyday living more than with pharmacology. Drugs are not new; they have been used since prehistoric times through all eras of civilization. With the introduction of many new drugs and new uses for older drugs, the allied health professional is responsible for being current on the action of drugs within the body; routes of administration; forms of drugs for administration; desired side effects; and **toxic** effects and adverse reactions of drugs on patients of all ages. The allied health professional's understanding of pharmacology can be critical to the patient–health professional relationship, as well as to the employer–employee relationship.

A drug assists in maintaining or restoring homeostasis after a decline in body functions caused by illness. Drugs can become dangerous if they are used to create unnecessary dependence or irreversible harm, but when used intelligently they provide a lifesaving benefit.

When patients and prescribers use medications appropriately, medications can restore health, prolong life, and increase quality of life for patients.

WHAT IS A DRUG?

The word *drug* comes from the Dutch word *droge,* meaning dry. The term is appropriate because for centuries most drugs used for treatment came from dried plants. Today a drug is considered to be any substance that causes chemical changes within the body. Virtually all chemicals, including such substances as tea and coffee, may be classified as drugs. In this book, a **drug** is any chemical used for a therapeutic application such as treating an illness or relieving a symptom or for diagnostic testing. Drugs are chemical substances that can help or harm individuals, altering the biochemical function in the body.

Researchers today build on the accumulated knowledge of the past to produce major new advances. Through the years, increasing knowledge about disease processes has led to the need for refined medications and to rapid changes in the field of pharmacology. **Pharmacology** will continue to change rapidly in the future as medical research makes innovative studies. However, the four basic terms used in pharmacology—*drug, pharmacology, clinical pharmacology,* and *therapeutics*—will remain the same (Box 2-1).

Most drugs contain various components—active and inactive (or inert) ingredients. An active ingredient is the pure, undiluted form of chemical that produces an effect but is rarely given alone. Usually it is combined with one or more **inert ingredients** (or vehicles) that assist in the drug's action and may also contain ingredients such as preservatives, colorings, and flavorings.

An **ideal drug,** a theoretical construct, is one that has only qualities of effectiveness and safety and produces no **side effects** or **adverse reactions.** Although no ideal drug exists, some characteristics, such as the following, help a drug draw near to ideal:

- Predictability—Drug will produce the same effect each time the same dose is given.
- Ease of administration—Drug is simple to administer, convenient to use, and requires only one dose a day, to help the patient follow the directions for the medication.
- Inexpensive—Low cost will help lighten the financial burden of taking medications over prolonged

BOX 2-1 FOUR BASIC TERMS IN PHARMACOLOGY

1. **Drug**—Any chemical that can affect living processes. Under this broad definition, all chemicals are considered drugs when given in amounts large enough to alter or affect life.
2. **Pharmacology**—Study of drugs and their interactions with living systems. The definition includes the study of physical and chemical properties of drugs, as well as their effects on the body. It also includes the history of drugs, their sources and uses, and how they are used by the body. This is a broad field, and this book will consider only those areas of pharmacology relevant to an ambulatory medical setting.
3. **Clinical pharmacology**—Study of drug absorption and metabolism in humans, including those who are healthy as well as those who are not in homeostasis.
4. **Therapeutics**—Use of drugs to diagnose disease *(diagnostic agents)*, prevent disease or a condition such as pregnancy *(prophylactic agents)*, or treat disease *(therapeutic drugs)*. This definition, simply stated, is the medical use of drugs, even though some may cause adverse reactions. (Adverse reactions are those effects that are undesirable or unintended.) The term *therapeutics* also encompasses the basic reasons for giving a particular drug to a particular patient, in a particular dosage, by a particular route, and on a particular schedule. Knowledge of pharmacology helps show what strategies will promote beneficial drug effect while minimizing undesired effects.

periods. Because of ongoing expense, even moderately priced drugs can be financially devastating.

- Identification—a name that is easy to pronounce and remember.

No drug is completely safe, because all drugs have side effects, but selectivity in prescribing reduces the chance of side effects and possible injury. A **safe drug** produces only the response for which it is given, causing no harmful effects when taken over a long period of time. The drug response may be difficult to predict from person to person and may change if the patient takes other medications. The health care team should work together to ensure that medications are producing the **desired effect,** or intended results, to minimize the chance of a drug-induced injury.

Important Facts

- Medications aid in keeping the body in homeostasis and are of lifesaving benefit when used correctly and with discrimination. If used incorrectly, drugs can cause irreparable harm.
- No ideal drug exists. All drugs cause some side effects or adverse reactions. The allied health professional must be aware of these effects and acquire an adequate medication knowledge base for patient safety.
- Safe drugs are those that can be taken in adequate doses over long periods of time with no harmful effects.

FIVE BASIC CATEGORIES OF PHARMACOLOGY

Medicines are foreign matter to the body and are capable of causing unexpected results, as well as **desired therapeutic effects.** Medications change body chemistry or function to diminish disease processes causing the symptoms rather than eliminating the cause of the symptoms. Terms used in pharmacology are **pharmacognosy,** or origins of drugs; **pharmacokinetics,** or how drugs are processed; **pharmacodynamics,** or actions of drugs; **pharmacotherapeutics,** or effects of drugs; and **toxicology,** or the study of toxic or poisonous effects of drugs.

Important Facts

The fundamental divisions in pharmacology are as follows:
- Pharmacognosy—Origin of drugs
- Pharmacokinetics—How the body processes drugs (what the body does to the drug)
- Pharmacodynamics—Drug actions on the body (what the drug does to the body)
- Pharmacotherapeutics—Effect of drugs in treatment of disease
- Toxicology—Poisonous effects of drugs on the body

Pharmacognosy—Origins of Drugs

Drugs come from basically five sources: plants, animals (including humans), minerals or mineral products, synthetic or chemical substances, and modern engineering. No longer is the drug industry bound to natural substances in either crude or natural states. Today, chemicals and even human tissues, such as in stem cell therapy, can be manipulated to increase drug sources.

The early *crude drugs* came from all dried plant parts and had unknown purity and varying strength. Often, undesired materials entered the plants and produced toxic effects. Later, active ingredients were separated from the plant, resulting in more reliable substance administration. (Table 2-1 shows examples of plant sources.)

Minerals from the earth and soil are used as they occur in nature or combined with other ingredients for drugs. An example is coal tar, an acid that yields salicylic acid, which was first used to manufacture aspirin (see Table 2-1).

Drugs can be derived from animal sources including vaccines, oils, and fats used in treatment of endocrine system diseases and for immunizations. Human extracts such as enzymes and hormones, may be used for treating diseases or potential conditions—for example, RhoGAM for possible erythroblastosis fetalis (see Table 2-1).

Chemists are producing drugs from living organisms (organic substances) or nonliving materials (inorganic substances) in ever-increasing numbers. Chemically developed drugs are free of the impurities found in natural substances and are called **synthetic or manufactured drugs.** Some drugs are both organic and inorganic (e.g., propylthiouracil, an antithyroid hormone) (see Table 2-1).

Did You Know?

Infection was the leading cause of death before the isolation and production of penicillin in a laboratory in 1942.

Recombinant DNA technology, the fastest growing area in the pharmaceutical world, uses artificially manipulated DNA segments from different organic sources by transferring a cell from a different species to a host cell to change the way the cell reproduces. In effect, the cell becomes a small-scale protein factory that creates genetic instructions leading the organism to produce chemical substances for use as drugs. These medications are specifically targeted outside cells, although the source of the disease proteins is inside cells where the disease begins (Figure 2-1). DNA research is now focusing on finding ways to deliver enzymes and proteins inside the cell for repair of diseased cells. The newer forms of insulin have been produced by this technique, as have skin grafts for

TABLE 2-1 DRUG SOURCES

SOURCE	DRUG
PLANTS	
Purple foxglove (digitalis)	digoxin
Rose hips	vitamin C
Cinchona bark	quinidine
Opium poppy	morphine, codeine, paregoric
Periwinkle (vinca)	vinCRIStine
Snakeroot	reserpine
Grapefruit	methylcellulose
Belladonna	atropine, scopolamine
Willow bark	aspirin
Castor bean	castor oil
MINERALS	
Gold	Solganal, auranofin
Zinc	zinc oxide
Calcium	Os-Cal, Cal-Bid, Citracal, Rolaids, Tums
Magnesium	milk of magnesia, Mylanta, Maalox
Aluminum	Amphojel, Gelusil
ANIMALS	
Codfish	cod liver oil
Urine of mares	conjugated estrogen
Stomachs of hogs	pepsin
Animal thyroid glands	thyroid hormone
Placenta	hair products
SYNTHETICS AND SEMISYNTHETICS	
Inorganic	sulfonamides, oral contraceptives, barbiturates meperidine (Demerol)
Organic	penicillin, cephalosporins
RECOMBINANT DNA TECHNOLOGY	
Drugs such as insulin	Humulin
Erythropoietin	Epogen

Step 1

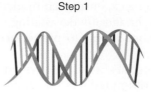

GENE IS SPLICED
Genes for a disease-fighting protein are inserted into the cells of a living organism.

Step 2

CELLS EXTRACTED
The cells containing the new protein are then removed from the organism.

Step 3

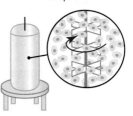

COPIES MADE
The cells multiply slowly at first, then in increasingly larger quantities to supply amounts needed for manufacturing of medications.

Step 4

HARVESTED
The desired proteins are extracted from the rest of the cell, purified, and made into biologic medicines.

Figure 2-1 Making of DNA technologic medications and substances. (Redrawn from Marsiglio D: New miracle drugs, AARP The Magazine, Nov-Dec 2009.)

as hepatitis C have been introduced. Many others will be brought to market in the future through methods such as cloning of salivary gland cells to produce insulin to treat diabetes (see Table 2-1).

Did You Know?

The reason that DNA-technology–produced biologic drugs and grafts are not used more often is that these medicines are so expensive—sometimes over $100,000 per year—and patients cannot afford the price. It is predicted that by 2014, many of the top 100 drugs will be biologics.

Important Facts

The origin of drugs that began with use of natural plant and animal substances has now moved into the laboratory, where scientists manufacture drugs synthetically from chemical compounds.

burns and other wounds that are produced from the foreskin of the penis (Apligraf).

Another biotechnologic method of drug production is use of cells from animals with antigens to produce hybrid cells that produce antibodies to attack tumors and permit diagnosis of many conditions, from anemia to syphilis. These drugs are also used as antirejection medications after organ transplantation. Through biotechnology, drugs to promote blood clotting in hemophiliacs and interferons to combat viral infections such

Pharmacokinetics—How the Body Processes Drugs

The word *pharmacokinetics* comes from the Greek words *pharmako*, meaning drugs, and *kinesis*, meaning motion; hence, *pharmacokinetics* refers to the movement of drugs

BOX 2-2 FACTORS THAT AFFECT DRUG ACTIVITY

Drug administration—Patient compliance or medication errors

Disintegration or dissolution of drug—Availability of drug for absorption

Pharmacokinetics—How body processes drugs

Pharmacodynamics—Drug-receptor cell interactions

Intensity of response—Individual differences in response to drugs related to physiologic (e.g., age, gender), psychologic, genetic, and dietary factors; disease states; and interactions with other drugs

BOX 2-3 FOUR BASIC PROCESSES OF PHARMACOKINETICS

Absorption

- Active ingredients are absorbed and transported to sites of action.
- Amount of absorption depends on drug's ability to cross cell membranes.

Distribution

- Drug molecules are transported to various body areas via circulating body fluids.
- Permeability of capillaries to the drug determines rate of distribution.

Metabolism (Biotransformation)

- Drug is chemically altered by the action of enzymes in the blood, liver, lungs, kidneys, and intestines to convert drug molecules into water-soluble compounds or metabolites for the body's use or elimination.

Excretion

- Unused drug molecules are removed from their sites of action, usually through the urinary tract, respiratory tract, gastrointestinal tract, or skin.

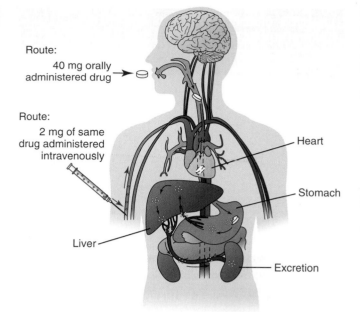

Figure 2-2 Pharmacokinesis is the movement of drugs through the body via absorption, distribution, metabolism, and excretion. (From Klieger DM: *Saunders essentials of medical assisting*, ed 2, St Louis, 2010, Elsevier.)

TABLE 2-2 RATE OF DRUG ABSORPTION BY ROUTE OF ADMINISTRATION

ROUTE	RATE OF ABSORPTION* FROM FASTEST TO SLOWEST
Enteral	Rectal → Nasogastric → Oral
Parenteral	Intravenous → Intramuscular → Subcutaneous → Intradermal
Percutaneous or mucosal	Inhalation (lungs) → Sublingual (tongue) → Transdermal (through skin) → Topical (on skin)

*Rate of absorption is specific to each route of administration.

through the body. The four processes involved in pharmacokinetics are absorption, movement of a drug from its site of administration into the blood; distribution, movement of a drug from the blood into the tissues and cells; metabolism (or biotransformation), physical and chemical alteration of the drug in the body; and excretion (or elimination), removal of waste products of drug metabolism from the body (Figure 2-2; Boxes 2-2 and 2-3).

 LEARNING TIP

Kinesis means motion or movement (recall "kinetic exercises"). Pharmacokinetics is the way drugs move through the body.

Absorption

The rate of absorption of a medication is directly related to the route of administration and the drug's solubility or its ability to dissolve (Tables 2-2 and 2-3). Absorption is dependent on the form of the drug and the amount of blood flow in the area; some medications dissolve rapidly, whereas others dissolve slowly. Primary sites of absorption are the mucosa of the mouth, lungs, stomach, small intestines, and rectum and blood vessels in the muscles and subcutaneous tissues. Examples include nitroglycerin, placed under the tongue next to blood vessels; albuterol (Ventolin HFA), taken into the lungs by inhalation; and dextrose in water, administered intravenously directly into the bloodstream (see Box 2-3).

TABLE 2-3 ORAL PREPARATIONS AND THEIR ABSORPTION RATES

PREPARATION	RATE
Syrups, elixirs, liquids	Fastest
Suspensions	
Powders	
Capsules	
Tablets	
Coated tablets	
Enteric-coated tablets	
Timed-release capsules	Slowest

Table 2-4 shows routes of administration versus time for absorption of medications.

Other factors that may cause variation in the absorption rate include the following:

Incorrect administration—Poor technique in giving a medication may destroy the drug before it reaches the bloodstream or its site of action. Specific directions for administration must be given and followed to enhance absorption.

pH—Drugs of an acidic pH such as aspirin are easily absorbed in the acidic surroundings of the stomach, whereas alkaline medications such as Maalox are more readily absorbed in the alkaline environment of the small intestine.

TABLE 2-4 DRUG ADMINISTRATION ROUTE AND RATE OF ABSORPTION OR ACTION

ROUTE	TIME INVOLVED	WHEN USED	EXAMPLES
ENTERAL ROUTES			
Oral	30-60 min	As often as possible	Most medications
		Safest and most convenient	Tablets, capsules
Sublingual	Several sec to several min	Rapid effect	Nitroglycerin for angina
Buccal	Several min	Rapid effect	Fentanyl for pain
Rectal	15-30 min, depending on contents of rectum	When oral medications cannot be used (e.g., with nausea/vomiting) and parenteral route is not indicated	Suppositories for nausea/ vomiting or for constipation
		For local effect	Preparation H for hemorrhoids
PARENTERAL ROUTES			
Subcutaneous (SC)	Several min; 20-30 min	Medications inactivated by gastrointestinal tract or when fast absorption is not indicated	Insulin, vaccines
Intramuscular (IM)	Several min, shorter than SC route; 15-25 min	Medications with poor absorption or when more rapid effects are desired— higher blood levels are obtained faster	Narcotics for pain, antibiotics, hormones
Intravenous (IV)	Approximately 1 min; administered directly into bloodstream	When immediate effects are necessary; when absorption in muscles is not adequate or is damaging to tissues	Cancer medications, cytotoxics
Intraarterial	Approximately 1 min	Local effects within an internal organ	Select cancer medications
PERCUTANEOUS OR MUCOSAL ROUTES			
Transdermal	30-60 min	Convenient to provide continuous absorption and systemic effects over hours	Nitroglycerin, estrogen, and fentanyl
Intrathecal	Several min	Local effects in spinal cord	Spinal anesthesia, epidurals
Inhalation	Approximately 1 min	Local effects on respiratory tract	Medications for asthma, chronic obstructive pulmonary disease; oxygen
Topical	Approximately 1 hr	Local effects on skin, ears, eyes	Creams, ointments, drops
Vaginal	15-30 min	Local effects	Creams, foams, suppositories
Urethral	15-30 min	Local effects	Gels, jellies

Min; Minute(s), *Sec;* second(s).

Food in stomach—Food in the stomach slows the absorption rate and decreases irritation, whereas an empty stomach increases the rate of absorption and irritation in most medications. Some drugs require food in the intestinal tract for absorption to take place.

Fat or lipid solubility—Drugs that are highly soluble in fats or lipids, such as alcohol and alcohol-containing substances, are readily absorbed in the gastrointestinal tract, whereas those with low lipid solubility are better absorbed when given by other routes.

Length of contact—Absorption of topical drugs is influenced by the length of contact time with the skin, size of contact area, skin thickness, and hydration of tissues at the site of application.

Inhalation factors—Depth of respirations, surface area of mucous membranes, hydration of the patient, blood supply to the lungs, and drug concentration influence the rapidity of absorption. Inhalation is actually one of the most rapid forms for medication absorption.

Drug concentration—High concentrations of drugs tend to be absorbed more rapidly; thus initial or first doses may be larger than maintenance or daily doses (see Box 2-3).

Distribution

Drug blood level is the amount of drug circulating in the bloodstream ready to travel through body fluids to its site of action or distribution. Areas with an extensive blood supply receive a drug rapidly, whereas areas with less blood supply have a delay in distribution. *Although a drug is delivered to the organ or tissues through blood vessels and capillaries, the effect of the drug is in the tissues, not in the blood vessels.* The rate at which a drug enters different areas of the body depends on the permeability of the capillaries to the drug's molecules and to the chemical makeup of the drug, amount given, size of the person, and amount of protein in blood.

Two factors that influence drug distribution are fat solubility and protein binding. A sustained pharmacologic effect is the result of the body providing storage reservoirs in the fatty tissues for fat-soluble drug accumulation. Because little blood flows through fat tissue, the storage site for the drug is established and a relatively stable reserve of the drug is maintained. Lipid-soluble drugs, such as hormones given by injection in an oil base, tend to have a longer-lasting effect.

Plasma protein binding is attaching of drugs to proteins in the blood, decreasing the amount of **free or unbound drug** circulating in the body and thus limiting the amount of drug at the site of action. As the body uses the free drug, the protein-bound drug breaks down for use. Because of this process, sulfa drugs remain in the body with antiinfective action for longer periods of time than other antibiotics.

Some drugs cannot pass through certain types of cell membranes. With the blood-brain barrier, the brain is protected by the barrier's restriction of entry of water-soluble electrolytes, but lipid-soluble drugs are allowed distribution into the brain and cerebrospinal fluid because the brain is composed of many lipids. The placental barrier, another membrane, is less selective in the distribution of medications, allowing water- and lipid-soluble drugs to cross. Many medications given to a mother may also reach the fetus, producing either a therapeutic effect (such as cardiac drugs that may be necessary for the fetus) or harmful effects (such as anesthetics, alcohol, and narcotics). Other drugs may be distributed to selected specific sites—for example, sending human chorionic gonadotropin (hCG) to the ovaries to treat infertility (see Box 2-3).

Metabolism or Biotransformation

Metabolism, or biotransformation, is a series of chemical reactions that alter and convert drugs into water-soluble compounds for excretion. Most drugs are detoxified, or turned into a relatively harmless substance, to allow the body to rid itself of the drug. Without metabolism, the drug would continue to have an effect on the body and could eventually cause harm to the person by accumulation to toxic levels.

Although other organs can contribute to metabolism of drugs, the liver is the primary site for drug metabolism. The amount of the drug that may be metabolized during an initial pass through the liver varies from a small amount to a substantial portion of the drug, leaving only a limited amount of the medication to reach the site of action. This is called the **first-pass effect.** Drugs that are administered parenterally or sublingually do not undergo a first-pass effect; therefore lower doses may be required than for drugs given by enteral routes (see Figure 2-2).

The rate of metabolism is an important issue in drug dosage. The **drug half-life** is the time the body takes to metabolize half of the available drug. Older adults or persons with impaired liver or renal function may have inefficient or insufficient metabolism of the drug and may be at risk for drug toxicity because the drug's half-life is prolonged (see Box 2-2).

Excretion or Elimination

The rate of excretion or elimination depends on the chemical composition of the drug, rate of metabolism, and route of administration (see Tables 2-2, 2-3, and 2-4). The functionality of excreting organs such as the kidneys also determines how quickly and completely excretion occurs.

Important Facts

- Absorption, distribution, metabolism, and excretion, steps used to process drugs, are dependent on many factors including age, mental state, route of administration, gender, and the physical condition of the patient.
- The drug blood level is the amount of drug circulating in the bloodstream.
- The half-life dosage of a drug is the time at which half of the initial dose has been metabolized and inactivated. Drug half-life, essential in establishing the safe dosage, is different for each drug.
- Drug excretion occurs most commonly via the kidneys; therefore adequate renal function must be present.

Pharmacodynamics—Drug Actions in the Body

Pharmacodynamics is the term for how a drug works or its mechanism of action in the body or the body's chemical reaction to drugs. In pharmacodynamic terms, drug actions affect biochemical or physiologic processes in the body or control changes caused by disease. *Drugs can modify the way the body acts, but they do not give body organs and tissues a new function.*

✎ **LEARNING TIP**

Dynamite causes an explosion at a site. *Pharmacodynamics* refers to drug action, as drugs "explode" into action in the body.

The actions of drugs usually either slow down or speed up ordinary cell processes and protect the body from actions of foreign agents (Table 2-5 describes the four major drug actions).

No drug has a single action. When a drug enters the body, a predictable chemical reaction is expected. However, individuals react to drugs differently, with many unpredictable chemical reactions occurring. The desired effect happens when the expected response occurs, such as Benadryl stopping watery eyes caused by allergies. However, other effects that occur that are predictable but not the desired effects are side effects. Because medications affect more than one body system, the action may not be specific and may cause undesired responses. The drowsiness that occurs with Benadryl is expected and is sometimes a therapeutic action used with insomnia as a desired side effect. Lowering the dosage of the medication will often reduce side effects, but in some cases the drug may have to be discontinued because of side effects. (Adverse reactions that tend to be more severe are discussed later in this chapter.)

TABLE 2-5 FOUR MAJOR DRUG ACTIONS

ACTION	DEFINITION	EXAMPLE
Depressant	Reduces the activity of the body function	tolterodine (Detrol) depresses the urge to void phenytoin (Dilantin) depresses seizure activity
Stimulant	Increases body function or activity	Laxatives stimulate peristalsis Oral hypoglycemics stimulate the pancreas to release insulin
Irritant	Produces symptoms of inflammation at site of application	fluorouracil (Efudex) irritates skin lesions for destruction of the lesion as a side effect Ichthammol increases the inflammation of boils
Demulcent	Soothing action for irritation, usually to skin or mucous membranes	Hydrocortisone cream soothes allergic skin reactions Lanolin smoothes cracked skin and decreases irritation

The site of action of a drug may be either local or systemic. **Local action** is limited to the site of administration and tissues immediately surrounding the application site; examples of medications with local action are nasal sprays and topical creams. When the drug effect is felt throughout the body, not just at the site of administration, it is considered **systemic action.** Intravenous and intramuscular drugs always reach systemic circulation for their effect, whereas oral and subcutaneous drugs may produce systemic or local effects. The same drug may be manufactured for either systemic or local effect. An example it is Benadryl, which is manufactured in capsules for systemic use and as a cream for topical or local use.

A drug that has its effect on a part of the body distant from the site of administration is said to have a remote effect; an example is nitroglycerin, placed under the tongue to treat the acute symptoms of angina pectoris in the heart.

Rather than having systemic action, some drugs have specific sites of action, such as thyroid hormone, which has a primary site of action in the thyroid gland for hormone replacement in hypothyroidism.

Drugs may also fall into categories that describe how the body responds to medication or the interactions at receptor cells. Box 2-4 describes four actions.

BOX 2-4 FOUR MAJOR CATEGORIES OF DRUG ACTIONS

- *Depressant*—A lessening or suppression of some body function or activity (e.g., omeprazole [Prilosec] to suppress gastric acid secretions)
- *Stimulant*—An increase in or stimulation of some body function or activity (e.g., bisacodyl [Dulcolax] to increase peristalsis in the colon for excretion of waste)
- *Irritant*—The production of inflammation, generally by drugs applied to mucous membranes or the skin (e.g., fluorouracil [Efudex], used topically to irritate keratosis for destruction of proliferating cells)
- *Demulcent*—Relief of irritation or the production of a soothing effect (e.g., calamine lotion to relieve itching and irritation of chickenpox)

Important Facts

- Drugs do not have a single action, although each drug has an expected action or desired effect. Because drugs may not be specific to a single body system, side effects may occur when another system is influenced.
- Drug action is also related to the site of action. A drug that is not absorbed into the bloodstream but works at the site of application is said to act *locally*. *Systemic action* refers to a total-body effect of a drug that is absorbed into the bloodstream. *Remote action* refers to the effect of a drug on the body at a site distant from the site of administration.
- Four major drug actions are stimulant, depressant, irritant, and demulcent.

Pharmacotherapeutics—Indications for or Effects of Medication Use

Different from drug *action* of *how* and *where* a drug acts in various body systems, the *effect* of a drug is the sum of the biologic, physical, and psychologic changes that occur in the body, or the result of the drug's action. Effects that are not part of the desired therapeutic response do occur with drugs given systemically because more than one type of body tissue, not just the target receptor site, can be affected.

LEARNING TIP

If we have therapy of any kind, we expect it to affect or change our body in some way. *Pharmacotherapeutics* refers to how a drug changes what is occurring in the body or the therapeutic effect of the medication to treat symptoms or diseases such as a headache or cough.

Drug therapy is one part of the physician's total treatment plan for the medical condition, but it does not stand on its own. Illnesses manifest with signs and symptoms, which may then become **indications,** or reasons, for treatment with certain medications, or pharmacotherapy for the specific condition. **Usage** is prescribing and applying or administering a medication for a given purpose. Many drugs produce therapeutic effects in several ways while still having the same indications and usage. For example, aspirin is used as an **analgesic** and **antipyretic,** but it is also used to slow blood clotting and as an **antiinflammatory** agent. Diuretics may be used both to relieve edema and to lower blood pressure, in this way affecting both the urinary and circulatory systems. A final example is ibuprofen, which was first introduced for the relief of arthritic pain and is also used as an antipyretic and analgesic.

As the field of pharmacology has evolved, a new classification of indications for medication use has come into being. The broad terms *therapeutic, diagnostic, destructive, pharmacodynamic,* and *prophylactic* represent the spectrum of drug indications (see Table 2-6 for an explanation of these terms).

When a drug enters the body, a predictable chemical reaction is expected. This intended response and expected therapeutic result is called the desired effect.

Because a medication may influence more than one body system at a time, it may produce unpredictable reactions, called side effects, which are usually mild but sometimes annoying responses to the medication. In some therapeutic cases, medications are used for the side effects—for example, minoxidil (Rogaine), with its side effect of hair growth, or drowsiness caused by antihistamines. The incidence of side effects may decrease when the medication is taken over an extended period of time. Lowering the dosage of the drug may reduce some side effects. In some instances, the drug must be discontinued or stopped because of the annoying response.

Important Facts

- The effect of a drug in the treatment of disease is referred to as *pharmacotherapeutics* or *pharmacotherapy* and is a combination of the biologic, physical, and psychologic changes induced as a result of the drug's action.
- Drugs do not have a single action, although each drug has an expected action or desired effect. Because drugs may not be specific to a single body system, side effects may occur when another system is influenced.
- Side effects may be annoying responses to a medication or may be an indication for the medication's use.

TABLE 2-6 MEDICATION INDICATIONS

INDICATION	EXPLANATION OF TERM	USAGE
Therapeutic	Maintain homeostasis, relieve symptoms, fight illness, and reverse disease processes	Promotion of normal growth and functioning Replacement of hormones Antiinfectives for infections Alleviation of pain Treatment of mental illness
Diagnostic	Aid in diagnosing diseases, aid in examination of the patient, and permit discovery of the nature or extent of disease conditions	Barium for x-ray studies Dyes for diagnostic radiologic studies Acetic acid for use during colposcopy to detect abnormal cervical tissue
Destructive	Destroy cells and tissues	Radioisotopes to treat hyperactive glands Bactericidals and antiseptics to destroy bacteria Chemotherapeutics for destruction of malignant cells
Pharmacodynamic	Alter normal body function	Anesthetics for either sleep or numbness Contraceptives to alter hormone balance Aspirin for blood "thinning" Digitalis to increase heart muscle contractions
Prophylactic	Prevent occurrence of illnesses or diseases	Antihistamines for allergies Vaccines, toxids, immunizations

Toxicology—Poisonous Effects of Drugs on the Body

All drugs or chemicals have a toxic level; when taken in excess, they act as poisons. A single dose of a medication can mean the difference between a therapeutic or toxic effect. The goal of pharmacology is to select a medication in a dose that is therapeutic and to avoid medications and doses that produce toxic effects. The difference between a therapeutic dose and a toxic dose is considered the margin of safety. Just a small increase in drug levels can cause toxicity, whereas slightly lowering the blood levels of other drugs may cause therapy failure. When the toxicity level has been exceeded, another drug used as an **antidote** may be given to stop the toxic effect.

Adverse reactions usually imply problems or symptoms more severe than side effects. Adverse reactions are unintended, undesirable, and often unpredictable effects that cause unintentional pain or discomfort or unwanted symptoms. When Benadryl causes unexpected hyperactivity, the reaction is adverse, versus the side effect of drowsiness. Because the Food and Drug Administration (FDA) requires substantial testing of drugs before allowing them to be marketed, common adverse reactions may be predictable. The allied health professional has a responsibility to monitor a patient for adverse reactions. The physician takes the necessary action for reporting adverse reactions to appropriate authorities as designated by law.

> **CLINICAL TIP**
>
> All adverse reactions should be documented (usually in red) in the patient's record and should be noted in an obvious place to prevent the patient from receiving the same drugs again, either in the office or as a prescription.

Allergic reactions are a type of **hypersensitivity reaction** that may occur after only one dose of a drug has been taken; these reactions occur either because the drug was taken many years before or because the person is allergic to a similar antigenic substance. The antigen-antibody reaction appears with single- or multiple-dose administration of the drug and may be mild to severe to life-threatening. Signs and symptoms of allergic reactions are itching; rashes; hives; difficulty breathing; wheezing; and swelling of eyes, lips, or tongue. Some reactions occur almost immediately, whereas others may be delayed for hours or days. Those that occur rapidly are usually more serious. The patient should be educated to report all mild adverse reactions before another dose of the same medication is administered.

> **CLINICAL TIP**
>
> The allied health professional must use extreme caution when giving any medication for the first time to a person with known allergies to medications, foods, or other substances. People with allergies are more susceptible to drug allergies.

Anaphylaxis, or anaphylactic shock, is a severe, potentially fatal adverse reaction occurring a short time after drug administration to a person who is sensitive or allergic to the medication. Initial symptoms are rapid swelling of the mouth and throat with difficulty breathing. Angioedema, a medical emergency requiring immediate medical attention, is the accumulation of fluid in the subcutaneous tissues of the eyelids, lips, mouth, throat, hands, and feet. The symptoms of anaphylaxis are hives, reddened skin, bronchospasm, initially elevated blood pressure followed by a drop in blood pressure, cyanosis, dyspnea, vascular collapse, loss of consciousness, cardiac arrhythmias, and cardiac arrest. Anaphylaxis has been noted most often after administration of antibiotics, especially penicillin and its derivatives, and dyes used in diagnostic studies, especially those containing iodine, but it could potentially occur with any medication at any time. Insect stings and some foods such as shellfish, peanuts, and eggs may also produce anaphylaxis.

Patient Education for Compliance

All patients who have had severe allergic reactions to medications should wear a medical alert bracelet or tag to identify the allergenic substance. All allergies should be listed on a card and placed in the wallet of a hypersensitive person. Some people allergic to insect stings or bites may even be prescribed a small kit of emergency medications containing Benadryl and epinephrine to carry with them when they might be exposed to the significant allergen. An example is the stinging insect kit for persons allergic to bee stings whose work or activities outdoors might put them in contact with bees or other stinging insects.

Important Facts

- Toxic effects can occur with all drugs. A small dosage change of a medication may separate a therapeutic effect from a toxic effect.
- Adverse reactions can be an indication of hypersensitivity to a drug in response to changes in the immune system. These reactions have unpredictable effects including allergic reactions and anaphylaxis.
- Anaphylaxis is the most serious and dangerous of the adverse reactions.

IDENTIFYING UNDESIRABLE EFFECTS OF DRUGS

About 50% of adverse reactions occur in patients older than 60 years of age. Deciding whether the patient is experiencing adverse reactions or some other symptom

BOX 2-5 QUESTIONS FOR DETERMINING ADVERSE REACTIONS

- Did the patient follow the directions accurately?
- When did the symptoms first occur? How long after the first use of the drug?
- Has the patient started anything else new or changed something (such as adding herbals or vitamins)? Has a new household product, such as a new detergent, been used?
- If the drug was discontinued, did the signs and symptoms disappear?
- If the drug was restarted, did the same effects return?
- Could the illness cause the symptoms? Are the signs and symptoms consistent with the diagnosis?
- Could other drugs or products that are being used concurrently cause the reaction?
- Is there a possibility of a drug-drug or drug-food interaction?

BOX 2-6 REDUCING DRUG-DRUG INTERACTIONS

- Consult physician or pharmacist before taking new drugs, including over-the-counter drugs and dietary supplements. Discuss any disorders present and any prescriptions being taken.
- Keep a list of all drugs being taken and disorders being treated and discuss with physician on a periodic basis. Make sure all physicians know all drugs being taken.
- Select a pharmacy that provides comprehensive services, including checking for possible interactions, and that maintains a drug profile on each person. Have all prescriptions filled at this site.
- Learn purpose, actions, and possible side effects of all drugs prescribed.
- Learn how to take medications as instructed, what time of day they are to be taken, and whether they can be taken during the same time period as other drugs.
- Report to the physician and/or pharmacist any new symptoms that may be related to drug use.

of an illness may be difficult. The questions found in Box 2-5 will assist in helping the professional make this decision. If the drug regimen has caused no problems in the past, then perhaps a new medication recently added could be the cause.

Remember that **idiosyncratic drug reactions**—unwanted reactions that occur with the first dose of a drug or when a subsequent dose is given—are unpredictable and may be from genetic predispositions. For drug safety, risks of the drugs and probable benefits to the patient should be evaluated, and a balance sought during drug therapy. See Box 2-6 for means to decrease undesirable drug effects.

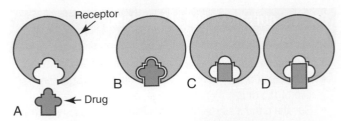

Figure 2-3 A, Drugs act by forming a chemical bond with specific receptor sites, similar to a key and lock. **B,** The better the "fit," the better the response. Those with complete attachment and response are called *agonists.* **C,** Drugs that attach but do not elicit a response are called *antagonists.* **D,** Drugs that attach, elicit a small response, and also block other responses are called *partial agonists.* (From Clayton BD, Stock YN, Cooper S: *Basic pharmacology for nurses,* ed 15, St Louis, 2010, Mosby.)

DRUGS AND THEIR RECEPTOR SITES

For drugs to be effective, the medication must attach appropriately to a **receptor site.** If the drug only moves about the body in the blood, the desired effect cannot take place. For a drug to be therapeutic, chemicals found in that drug must selectively attach to the specific cell receptor site—*selective action.* The receptor site on the cell wall and the drug chemical fit together like pieces of a jigsaw puzzle (Figure 2-3). The better the fit of the drug and receptor site, the better the expected response to medication. If the pieces do not fit together, the stimulation of receptor sites may not occur and the drug may block another medication from being effective. Thus drugs at receptor sites may either mimic or block action of a medication. A drug's selectivity of a specific receptor site, however, does not guarantee its safe medicinal use.

When the medication stimulates the receptor site, the drug works with the body to mimic its function, or is called an **agonist.** When drugs are attached strongly and do not produce a chemical reaction but do prevent agonists from binding at the receptor site, the medication is called an **antagonist.** Antagonists that prevent other drugs from binding to receptor sites counteract the expected effects of other drugs.

A weak bond that prevents other chemicals or drugs from binding to receptor sites on the cell wall is called a *partial agonist.* Some drugs act by changing cell wall permeability, whereas others act as enzyme inhibitors. Examples are antidotes, used to neutralize toxic substances; **chelators,** used to treat metal poisonings; and **antimetabolites,** used with cancer to disrupt essential cell metabolic process, either by inhibiting enzymes or by interrupting DNA replication and function.

MECHANISMS OF DRUG INTERACTIONS

Drugs interact in various ways with other drugs and nutrients. When multiple drugs are given together, some interactions are desirable but others are undesirable. Some medications are prescribed together to achieve a desired response. Other drugs may counteract or augment each other's effect if given together; may be wholly incompatible together; and may interfere with the absorption, metabolism, or excretion of medications. Interactions must be addressed, or they may result in permanent bodily damage or even death.

Drug interactions, or the combined effect of drugs administered together, may take the form of **synergism, potentiation,** or **antagonism.** In addition to drug-drug interactions, there may also be nutrient-drug and disease-drug interactions. For example, tetracyclines interact with milk, and alcohol interacts with many drugs, especially hypnotics, sedatives, and antianxiety medications. It is important to note that vitamins, minerals, and herbal supplements can interact with prescribed medications, such as cabbage with **warfarin sodium** (Coumadin).

Drug-Drug Interactions

When two or more medications are prescribed together, (1) the drugs have no effect on each other's action, (2) the drugs increase the effect, or (3) the drugs decrease the effect of each. Most drugs do not interact with other drugs or food, but when such interactions do occur, some may be life-threatening. Because patients are taking more than one medication for more than one disorder, the potential for duplications and interactions increases.

Some terms for drug effects in drug-drug interactions are synergism and antagonism, which may be desirable or undesirable. Potentiation and **tolerance** refer to how the expected effect occurs in the long term. See Figure 2-4 and Table 2-7 for definitions and explanations of drug-drug interactions.

CLINICAL TIP

Drug-drug interactions can change the outcome of drug therapy significantly. The chance of undesirable interactions can be lowered by reducing the number of medications taken. If a patient taking multiple drugs has unusual symptoms, the possibility of a drug interaction should be considered. The allied health professional should take a thorough history and assist by documenting all possible medications and in finding ways to decrease the number of medications being taken.

Addition of ingredients

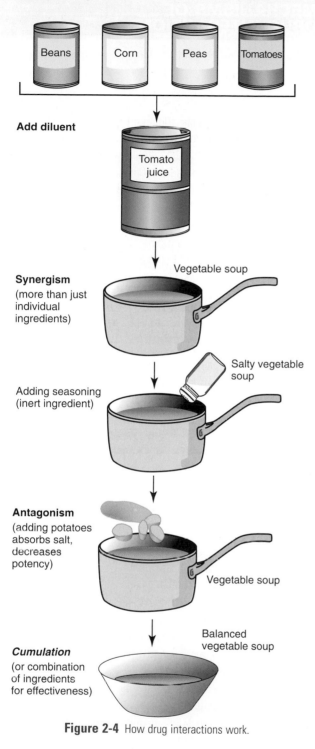

Figure 2-4 How drug interactions work.

BOX 2-7 COMMON NUTRIENT DRUG INTERACTIONS

Food/Drug	Effects
Milk and calcium products/tetracycline	Tetracycline becomes insoluble, and antibacterial properties are ineffective with binding to calcium
High-fiber diets with wheat bran and oats	Reduce the absorption of many drugs
Grapefruit, grapefruit juice/"statin" drugs for hypercholesterolemia and sildenafil (Viagra)	Reduces effectiveness and raises blood levels of many medications such as statins; with other medications, stop the action of the drug; juice seems to affect drug metabolism even if medication and juice are taken at different times; the greater the amount of juice consumed, the greater the inhibition of medications
Wine, yogurt, cheese/monoamine oxidase inhibitors (MAOIs that act as antidepressants)	Cause potential toxic effects when used together
Caffeine or caffeine-containing foods/central nervous system stimulants	Toxic stimulation of nervous system
Salt substitutes/potassium-sparing diuretics	Dangerously high potassium levels
Citrus juices (orange juice)/aluminum-based antacids	Excessive absorption of aluminum
Broccoli, Brussels sprouts, cabbage/warfarin sodium (Coumadin)	Inactivate the medication because they contain vitamin K
All foods/bisphosphonates	Decreased absorption and drug effectiveness with any food; drug ususally taken with water 30-60 minutes before eating or drinking any other food substance

Nutrient-Drug Interactions

Nutrient-drug interactions are poorly understood. They can induce toxic effects and/or cause failure of therapy. The absorption of drugs can be significantly changed by food in the stomach. Some medications must be taken on an empty stomach for more rapid absorption, whereas other medications are taken on a full stomach to maximize the absorption rate. See Box 2-7 for common nutrient-drug interactions.

TABLE 2-7 EFFECTS OF DRUGS IN THE BODY

EFFECT	REACTION IN BODY	EXAMPLES
Agonism (desired effect)	Drug stimulates the desired response at the receptor site	epinephrine for allergic reactions
Synergism	One drug brings about a stronger effect of another drug when taken together	
Desirable synergism		meperidine (Demerol) for pain and promethazine (Phenergan) for nausea—combination prolongs the effects of each
Undesirable synergism		warfarin sodium (Coumadin) and aspirin—combination increases bleeding tendencies
Potentiation	Drug increases the effect of another drug in the body	
Desirable potentiation		meperidine (Demerol) and pentazocine (Talwin) to prolong analgesic effects
Undesirable potentiation		cimetidine (Tagamet) and theophylline; Tagamet increases the effects of theophylline
Antagonism	Drugs weaken or stop the effects of one another when given together	
Desirable antagonism		vitamin K decreases effects of warfarin
Undesirable antagonism		aspirin and ibuprofen when given together decrease action of both; tetracyclines and antacids cause decrease in absorption of tetracyclines
Summation or addition	Combining two drugs and achieving expected medicinal effects of each by adding drugs together	Antihistamine plus antibiotic for sinus infection
Cumulation	Drug has stronger effect than expected because previous dose has not been metabolized or excreted from the body	Hyperactivity caused by excessive caffeine ingestion
Pseudoaddiction	Abnormal behavior developing as direct result of inadequate pain management	Drug-seeking behavior; Patients asking for pain management can be mistaken for having an addiction
Tolerance	Drug has less effect than expected; body gets used to drug (may be acquired or congenital)	Need for increased dosage of opioids for relief of pain
Idiosyncrasy	Drug produces different effect than expected	Allergic reaction
Dependence, addiction, **habituation**	Body dependent on drug to function	Need for more and more pain medication to obtain the same result
Psychologic dependence	Emotional attachment to or craving for drug	Using sleep preparations without having insomnia
Physical dependence	Physiologic dependence with possibility of withdrawal symptoms	Using pain medications over a long period of time, especially scheduled drugs
Allergy	Hypersensitivity to drug; body develops antigen-antibody reaction	Most common is the allergic reaction to penicillin, including rash, difficulty breathing, and possible anaphylaxis
Interference	One drug promotes the rapid excretion of another, reducing the activity of the first	Taking a laxative with an antacid

Disease-Drug Interactions

Sometimes drugs used for one disease are harmful with regard to another disorder or disease present. Diabetes, high or low blood pressure, an ulcer, glaucoma, an enlarged prostate, poor bladder control, and insomnia are particularly important because these conditions are more likely to cause disease-drug interactions. For example, some beta blockers taken for heart disease or hypertension can worsen asthma and make it difficult for the person with diabetes to tell when his or her blood sugar is too low. Some cold preparations can worsen glaucoma. These interactions are more common with older adults, who tend to have more diseases and an increased use of drugs. Awareness of all diseases by the physician before prescribing medications is most important for drug safety.

SUMMARY

A drug is a chemical compound used to prevent, cure, or treat disease or to diagnose abnormal conditions. No drug is ideal because chemicals interact differently in each person because of the distinct body functionality of each person. A drug with the fewest side effects and adverse reactions and the greatest efficacy is considered the medication of choice.

Drugs may occur in natural substances such as plants, minerals, or animals or may be made in chemical laboratories with synthesis of new drugs, including the manipulation of genes with recombinant DNA techniques. The study of the origins of medicines is *pharmacognosy*, one of the five fundamental pharmacologic categories. The way drugs are processed by the body—through absorption, distribution, metabolism, and excretion—is their *pharmacokinetics*. Age, weight, gender, route of administration, and disease processes will affect how a particular drug acts. *Pharmacodynamics* refers to how and where drugs act in the body to produce a therapeutic or diagnostic action. The sites of action—local, systemic, selective, remote, and specific—are where drugs act on target cells or tissues. *Pharmacotherapeutics* refers to the physiologic changes brought about by a drug. Drugs are selected to cure or prevent a disease, palliate symptoms, or reveal a diagnosis. Drugs may also produce toxic effects including adverse, allergic, idiosyncratic, and anaphylactic reactions. Potential side effects and adverse reactions are reported in drug inserts for health care professionals' awareness.

No matter how careful the physician or how compliant the patient, undesirable reactions may occur. Deciding whether an adverse reaction or an undesirable effect is occurring may be difficult, but by eliminating possible causes of the reaction, health care professionals can recognize adverse reactions.

Drug usage is complicated and varies because each patient is an individual with different needs and different physiologic and sometimes psychologic determinants. The allied health professional must be careful to see each patient as an individual and must take a detailed medical and pharmacologic history to avoid detrimental side effects and adverse reactions.

When two or more medications are given together, they can increase one another's action, decrease actions, or have no effect on actions. These drug-drug interactions depend on how the receptor site on the cell and the drugs fit together. In some instances, medications are given to stop the actions of other drugs that might be detrimental to the body. In other cases, drugs are given to neutralize toxins. Some drugs work locally, whereas others work systemically. Drug-drug interactions can be life-threatening. Also important are foods that can interfere with medicines. Some nutrient-drug interactions can be dangerous, as can disease-drug interactions.

CRITICAL THINKING EXERCISES

Scenario

Mrs. Jones likes to take her medications each day with grapefruit juice. Since she started drinking the grapefruit juice and taking cholesterol-lowering medications, her cholesterol level has risen, although her diet has not changed. A known effect of the juice is to lower the effects of the medications.

1. What questions would you ask to determine if Mrs. Jones might be having potential side effects?
2. Mrs. Jones asks if she can take her medicine 2 hours after drinking her juice because she thinks the grapefruit helps her arthritis. How would you respond?
3. When she asks about changing her medications to keep drinking the juice, what would be your response?

REVIEW QUESTIONS

1. What is a drug? An active ingredient? A safe drug? _____

_____

_____

_____

2. Drugs are excreted by four routes. What are they? What organs are involved in excretion? Which organ is most commonly involved? _____

_____

_____

_____

3. What are the differences among a side effect, an adverse reaction, and an allergic reaction? _____

_____

_____

_____

4. Drugs work at various receptor sites. How do agonists work at receptor sites? Antagonists? Partial agonists? Antidotes? Chelators? Antimetabolites? _____

_____

_____

_____

_____

5. Drug-drug interactions occur when medications are taken together. Some interactions are wanted; others are undesirable and even life-threatening. Give two reasons for giving medications together, and cite two types of dangerous drug interactions. _____

_____

_____

_____

_____

_____

6. What role do OTC drugs play in drug-drug interactions? _____

_____

_____

_____

7. Define *synergism, antagonism, potentiation, idiosyncratic drug reaction, cumulative effect,* and *drug tolerance.* _____

_____

_____

_____

_____

_____

_____

8. Describe what happens in drug-food interactions. Give examples of drug-food interactions. _____

_____

_____

_____

9. What is meant by *drug-disease interaction?* Why is this found more often in older adults? _____

_____

_____

_____

_____

10. Why is DNA technology so important in today's medical practice? _____

_____

_____

_____

CHAPTER 3

Drug Information and Drug Forms

OBJECTIVES

After studying this chapter, you should be capable of doing the following:

- Determining different means of classifying medications.
- Discussing what is meant by *off-label medications.*
- Contrasting drug nomenclature.
- Using main sources of drug information.
- Identifying and describing drug forms.

Susan works in a local physician's office that specializes in gerontology. Mrs. Elder has come to see the physician about a small, painful wound on her leg that will not heal. Dr. Merry asks Susan to apply a dressing to Mrs. Elder's leg using an ointment. Unable to find an ointment in the medicine cabinet, Susan uses a cream. When Mrs. Elder tries to change the dressing, it has stuck to her leg.

Is it permissible for Susan to swap an ointment and a cream? Why or why not?

Mrs. Elder has difficulty swallowing pain medication because her mouth is dry. Would you suggest that she take medications in a capsule or a tablet form? Why?

What difference would an ointment have made in this scenario?

KEY TERMS

Aerosol
Aerosol foam
Ampule
Buccal tablet
Buffered tablet
Caplet
Capsule
Chewable tablet
Colloid suspension/ solution
Cream
Delayed-release capsule
Dispersion
Douche
Drug Facts and Comparisons
Drug nomenclature

Effervescent powder
Elixir
Emulsion
Enteric-coated tablet
Gel/Gelcap
Granule
Gum
Implant
Insulin pen
Legend drug
Liniment
Lotion
Lozenge
Magma
Medicated enemas
Metered dose inhaler
Nebulizer

Off-label use
Ointment
Package insert
Paste
Pellet
Physicians' Desk Reference (PDR)
Plaster
Powder
Premeasured cartridge
Reconstitution
Shelf life
Solution
Spirits
Spray
Sublingual tablet
Suppository

Suspension
Sustained-release (controlled-release) tablet
Sustained-release capsule
Syrup
Tablet
Tampon
Tincture
Topical
Transdermal
Transdermal patch/ disk
Troche
Vial
Viscous

Drugs can be named and classified in several ways. Sources of information concerning medications, their names, and their classifications are available to provide safe dosages for each patient. In this text drugs are classified according to the body system where the therapeutic effect is expected. Icons for body systems will be used throughout the remainder of the book to assist in identifying medications with receptor sites in the body's organ system. Other drugs such as antibiotics and analgesics with systemic effect will be placed in chapters without relationship to a specific body system.

Medication forms vary according to route of administration and speed at which the body needs to absorb the drug for therapeutic effects. In this text medication forms are considered as enteral to include all routes involving the gastrointestinal (GI) tract; parenteral to include all medications injected into the bloodstream (intravenously [IV]), into the muscle (intramuscularly [IM]), or under the skin (subcutaneously [SC] or intradermally [ID]); or percutaneous for drugs that are absorbed through the skin. Refer to Tables 2-2 through 2-4 for the rates of absorption by route.

DRUG CLASSIFICATIONS

Classifying drugs is complex and difficult because a drug may be indicated for use in treating conditions in several body systems. One classification is based on a drug's therapeutic action on body organs; examples are diuretics used to relieve edema and analgesics used to relieve pain. Drugs may also be classified according to their general use, in which case the classification is similar to their therapeutic action, involving such terms as *diuresis* and *analgesia*. Families of drugs may also be used for classification, such as penicillins used as antibiotics or thiazides for diuresis. It should be remembered that some medications have more than one use and may have therapeutic effects on more than one body system such as diuretics, which are used for diuresis and to lower blood pressure, and aspirin, used for analgesia, to reduce inflammation and as an antithrombotic (to prevent blood clots) with coronary disease. Classifications by therapeutic effect and by drug family are usually found in drug reference materials.

Important Facts

- Drugs are classified by their medicinal uses and their therapeutic actions, as well as by therapeutic family. A single drug may have more than one classification, may affect more than one body system, and may be used in several ways in treatment of illnesses and conditions.
- Most drug classifications are based on medical terminology for the symptoms or disease processes for which the drugs are used.

"OFF-LABEL" USES FOR MEDICATIONS

Drugs are used for Food and Drug Administration (FDA)–approved conditions found on the package insert. However, some medications have off-label uses, which means a medication can be indicated and prescribed therapeutically for a condition that has not been studied by the manufacturer for FDA approval. The off-label use of drugs is becoming more widespread as physicians use medications and report their unexpected effects after initial FDA approval, resulting in a new therapeutic indication and use. Some drugs used in the past now have FDA approval for off-label indications because of financial gain from required further testing. Examples are Rogaine, originally developed as a blood pressure medication and now used to prevent or slow balding. However, some of the older medications are truly used as off-label therapy because of the money necessary for extra studies for FDA approval and success of nonapproved use in the past. An example is **cyproheptadine** (Periactin), an antihistamine, used for weight gain, usually in geriatric patients.

DRUG NOMENCLATURE

Drugs are named in a variety of ways, including names that include the family of drugs. For example, "cillin" in *amoxicillin* indicates that the drug is a penicillin derivative. With the FDA assigning names to any drug approved in the United States, all drugs manufactured with the same *generic* or *official* name must have the same chemical name and structure. Listings of official drug names or drug nomenclature can be found in drug reference books such as the *United States Pharmacopoeia–National Formulary* (USP–NF).

✐ CLINICAL TIP

Health professionals must check the exact spelling of all medications to be administered or prescribed. Some drug names look and sound alike or are spelled similarly, leading to mistakes in documentation when correct drug nomenclature is not used. See the Evolve website for a full list of Do Not Confuse drugs.

Each drug has several ways of being named:

- The *chemical name* of a drug identifies the exact chemical compound of a medication and its molecular structure.
- The *generic* or *nonproprietary name*, also called the *common name*, is the one given a drug when a manufacturer first proposes it to the FDA for approval. The generic name is never capitalized, is easier to remember than the chemical name, and is not the property of the manufacturer. Generic drugs are often used when prescribing in preference to proprietary drugs because they tend to cost less, have the lowest potential for errors, and identify the drug no matter what manufacturer.
- Several interchangeable terms for *trademarked* drugs exist. *Trade name, brand name,* and *proprietary name* all refer to a drug name owned by a specific manufacturer and can be used only by the original manufacturer. The symbol ® follows a trade name, indicating that the name is a registered trademark and is restricted to use by the owner of the name, usually the manufacturer that owns the patent. Trade names are designed to be easily remembered (e.g., Viagra, Claritin). The first letter of a trade name is capitalized, and the name may suggest some special feature of the drug, such as Skelaxin, a skeletal muscle relaxant. Confusion is possible when trade names are used because names for entirely different compounds may be pronounced or spelled similarly.

Examples of drug nomenclature follow:

Chemical name—2-(4-isobutylphenyl) propionic acid

Trade name—Motrin

Generic name—*ibuprofen*

Over-the-counter (OTC) drug name—ibuprofen, Advil, Nuprin, Motrin IB (the last three are also proprietary names)

Chemical name—*N*-cyano-*N*′-methyl-*N*″-[2-[[(5-methyl-1*H*-imidazol-4-yl)methyl]thio]ethyl] guanidine

Trade name—Tagamet

Generic name—*cimetidine*

OTC drug name—Tagamet HB (also a proprietary name)

Legend drug is the name for drugs sold only by prescription, such as *meperidine* (Demerol) and *diazepam* (Valium). So named, these drugs must bear the federally mandated warning or legend—"Caution: Federal law prohibits dispensing without a prescription"—thus the name *legend drug.*

OTC drugs do not require a prescription. They are found on the shelves of pharmacies, grocery stores, and the like and are sold in doses that are considered safe if manufacturer's directions are followed. Usually the doses are lower than found with prescription strengths of the same drug.

Patient Education for Compliance

1. Health care professionals should teach patients to read all ingredients and drug interactions listed on packaging before taking OTC drugs.
2. Generic and trade named drugs contain the same formulation even if the drug is manufactured by different companies (e.g., Amoxil by Beecham is the same *amoxicillin* as Trimox by Apothecon).

CLINICAL TIP

OTC drugs being used are medications and must always be listed in the clinical record, as these drugs can interact with prescription medications.

Important Facts

- *Drug nomenclature* refers to all the names by which a drug can be identified—all drugs have a chemical name, an official or a generic name, and a trade name, and may have an OTC name.
- The trade name belongs to the company that developed the drug. The company also owns the right to be the sole manufacturer of the new drug for 20 years after the patent has been filed.

SOURCES OF DRUG INFORMATION

The USP–NF, the official drug list recognized by the U.S. government, is revised annually with supplements twice a year to keep it updated. Its primary purpose is to provide official standards adopted by the FDA regarding identity, quality, strength, and purity of medications and quality control of medications and nutritional supplements produced in the United States.

Before a new drug is marketed, the manufacturer must develop an FDA-approved package insert (Figure 3-1). The insert provides a comprehensive and concise description of the drug (Table 3-1) and must accompany each package of the product for dispensing, whether in bottles for pharmacy use or on samples at the physicians' offices.

The *Physicians' Desk Reference (PDR)* is published yearly by Medical Economics Publishing and is financed by the pharmaceutical industry. The publication includes information about drugs in an easily accessible form, making it a frequently used reference in a physician's office. The company also provides several supplements per year with revised information and information on new products. Another PDR for OTC drugs is also available. All drugs are cross-referenced by manufacturer, trade and generic names, and drug classification.

The PDR consists of seven sections, each separated by color for easy access:

- Section I (white), Manufacturer Index: This section includes an alphabetic listing of each manufacturer with the manufacturer's address, an emergency phone number, and a partial list of available products.
- Section II (pink), Brand and Generic Name Index: This section is a comprehensive alphabetic listing of medications by generic and trade names for drugs found in the Product Information Section (Section V, white).
- Section III (blue), Product Category Index: This section subdivides medications by therapeutic class (e.g., antibiotics, antiarthritics, analgesics).
- Section IV (gray), Product Identification Guide: Each manufacturer supplies full-color photographs of actual-size tablets, capsules, and other drug forms. This section is invaluable for identifying brand (trade) name products.
- Section V (white), Product Information Section: This section contains information found on package inserts. The section is alphabetized by manufacturer and then by product.
- Section VI (white), Diagnostic Product Information: This section includes an alphabetic listing of many of the diagnostic test medications and products used in hospitals and physicians' offices.
- Section VII (white), Miscellaneous: This section assembles miscellaneous information including the following:
  - Key to controlled substances categories
  - Key to FDA use-in-pregnancy ratings
  - List of Poison Control Centers
  - FDA telephone directory
  - Drug information centers
  - Look-alike, sound-alike drug names
  - Adverse event report forms

Pharmacists use *Drug Facts and Comparisons,* a loose-leaf binder source for comparison and evaluation of medications, which is updated monthly. The manufacturer, form of packaging, and comparison tables of medications are included, along with a section on orphan drugs, diagnostic aids, and drugs in developmental stages.

Other references include books and electronic drug information sources such as Micromedex and Lexi-Comp's *Drug Information Handbook.* Manufacturers also include information on their websites concerning the drugs they manufacture. Reliable medication websites such as RxList, MedlinePlus, and WebMD rapidly provide information for the Internet user.

Pharmacists are another professional source of information. They keep current on medications and have access to the package inserts found on each medication bottle. With each prescription, pharmacists give patients drug information sheets about their prescriptions (Figure 3-2).

Allied health professionals should make drug cards for medications used at their employment setting. It is vital that anyone giving medications be knowledgeable about any drugs being administered. Trade and generic names, as well as usual dosage, should be included, along with side effects and adverse reactions. These drug cards should be readily available for answering questions before administration of medications. New drug cards should be prepared as new medications are introduced for clinical use.

Drug handbooks and textbooks with information on medications are available at different levels of detail. Because information in books may not be completely current, journal articles and news releases, as well as the Internet should be read to update the information. Some material that passes for information on Internet sites is not accurate; therefore health professionals should be selective in sites they review. Good sites are those associated with medical, nursing, and pharmacy schools, as well as the FDA, National Institutes of Health, American Heart Association, and similar associations, making specialized and accurate information from manufacturers and government agencies only a click away.

Knowing all there is to know about drugs on the market is impossible, but the health care professional must know how and where to obtain the necessary information to ensure patient safety and compliance with medications.

Important Facts

Drug references including drug package inserts, the *United States Pharmacopoeia–National Formulary* (USP–NF), the *Physicians' Desk Reference* (PDR), drug handbooks, and drug cards are important to ensure proper administration of medications and safety in drug usage. The allied health professional should be knowledgeable about all medications to be administered.

DRUG FORMS AND DRUG DELIVERY SYSTEMS

Drugs come in many dosage forms that differ in their rate of action, site of action, and amount of medication delivered at the site of action. Dosage forms may be solid, semisolid, liquid, or gas. The route of delivery influences efficiency and action of the drug. The drug may be given orally (enterally), or through the GI tract; parenterally, or through routes outside the enteral route (although this route is usually considered to be by

Rx only

WARNINGS:

1. **ESTROGENS HAVE BEEN REPORTED TO INCREASE THE RISK OF ENDOMETRIAL CARCINOMA IN POSTMENOPAUSAL WOMEN.**

Close clinical surveillance of all women taking estrogens is important. Adequate diagnostic measures, including endometrial sampling when indicated, should be undertaken to rule out malignancy in all cases of undiagnosed persistent or recurring abnormal vaginal bleeding. There is no evidence that "natural" estrogens are more or less hazardous than "synthetic" estrogens at equi-estrogenic doses.

2. **ESTROGENS SHOULD NOT BE USE DURING PREGNANCY.**

There is no indication for estrogen therapy during pregnancy or during the immediate postpartum period. Estrogens are ineffective for the prevention or treatment of threatened or habitual abortion. Estrogens are not indicated for the prevention of postpartum breast engorgement.

Estrogen therapy during pregnancy is associated with an increased risk of congenital defects in the reproductive organs of the fetus, and possibly other birth defects. Studies of women who received diethylstilbestrol (DES) during pregnancy have shown that female offspring have an increased risk of vaginal adenosis, squamous cell dysplasia of the uterine cervix, and clear cell vaginal cancer later in life; male offspring have an increased risk of urogenital abnormalities and possibly testicular cancer later in life. The 1985 DES Task Force concluded that use of DES during pregnancy is associated with a subsequent increased risk of breast cancer in the mothers, although a causal relationship remains unproven and the observed level of excess risk is similar to that for a number of other breast cancer risk factors.

DESCRIPTION:

Estropipate, (formerly piperazine estrone sulfate), is a natural estrogenic substance prepared from purified crystalline estrone, solubilized as the sulfate and stabilized with piperazine. It is appreciably soluble in water and has almost no odor or taste - properties which are ideally suited for oral administration. The amount of piperazine in Estropipate Tablets is not sufficient to exert a pharmacological action. Its addition ensures solubility, stability, and uniform potency of the estrone sulfate. Chemically estropipate is represented by estra-1,3,5(10)-trien-17-one, 3-(sulfooxy)-, compound with piperazine (1:1). The structural formula may be represented as follows:

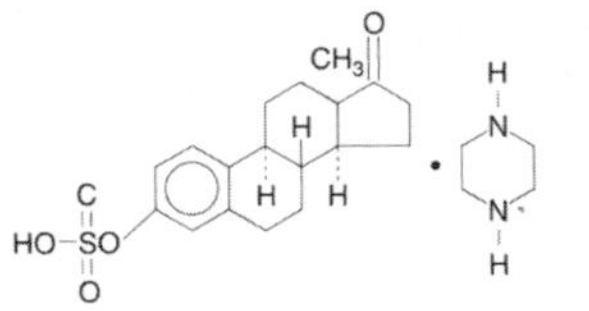

$C_{18}H_{22}O_5S.C_4H_{10}N_2$ **Molecular Weight: 436.58**

Estropipate Tablets are available for oral administration containing 0.75 mg, 1.5 mg or 3 mg estropipate (calculated as sodium estrone sulfate 0.625 mg, 1.25 mg and 2.5 mg, respectively).

Inactive Ingredients: Colloidal silicon dioxide, crospovidone, lactose monohydrate, magnesium stearate, and pregelatinized starch. The 0.75 mg also contains D&C yellow no. 10 aluminum lake and FD&C yellow no. 6 aluminum lake. The 1.5 mg also contains FD&C yellow no. 6 aluminum lake. The 3 mg also contains FD&C blue no. 2 aluminum lake.

CLINICAL PHARMACOLOGY:

Estrogen drug products act by regulating the transcription of a limited number of genes. Estrogens diffuse through cell membranes, distribute themselves throughout the cell, and bind to and activate the nuclear estrogen receptor, a DNA-binding protein which is found in estrogen-responsive tissues. The activated estrogen receptor binds to specific DNA sequences, or hormone-response elements, which enhance the transcription of adjacent genes and in turn lead to the observed effects. Estrogen receptors have been identified in tissues of the reproductive tract, breast, pituitary, hypothalamus, liver, and bone of women.

Estrogens are important in the development and maintenance of the female reproductive system and secondary sex characteristics. By a direct action, they cause growth and development of the uterus, Fallopian tubes, and vagina. With other hormones, such as pituitary hormones and progesterone, they cause enlargement of the breasts through promotion of ductal growth, stromal development, and the accretion of fat. Estrogens are intricately involved with other hormones, especially progesterone, in the processes of the ovulatory menstrual cycle and pregnancy, and affect the release of pituitary gonadotropins. They also contribute to the shaping of the skeleton, maintenance of tone and elasticity of urogenital structures, changes in the epiphyses of the long bones that allow for the pubertal growth spurt and its termination, and pigmentation of the nipples and genitals.

Estrogens occur naturally in several forms. The primary source of estrogen in normally cycling adult women is the ovarian follicle, which secretes 70 to 500 micrograms of estradiol daily, depending on the phase of the menstrual cycle. This is converted primarily to estrone, which circulates in roughly equal proportion to estradiol, and to small amounts of estriol. After menopause, most endogenous estrogen is produced by conversion of androstenedione, secreted by the adrenal cortex, to estrone by peripheral tissues. Thus, estrone—especially in its sulfate ester form—is the most abundant circulating estrogen in postmenopausal women. Although circulating estrogens exist in a dynamic equilibrium of metabolic interconversions, estradiol is the principal intracellular human estrogen and is substantially more potent than estrone or estriol at the receptor.

Estrogens used in therapy are well absorbed through the skin, mucous membranes, and gastrointestinal tract. When applied for a local action, absorption is usually sufficient to cause systemic effects. When conjugated with aryl and alkyl groups for parenteral administration, the rate of absorption of oily preparations is slowed with a prolonged duration of action, such that a single intramuscular injection of estradiol valerate or estradiol cypionate is absorbed over several weeks.

Administered estrogens and their esters are handled within the body essentially the same as the endogenous hormones. Metabolic conversion of estrogens occurs primarily in the liver (first pass effect), but also at local target tissue sites. Complex metabolic processes result in a dynamic equilibrium of circulating conjugated and unconjugated estrogenic forms which are continually interconverted, especially between estrone and estradiol and between esterified and non-esterified forms. Although naturally-occurring estrogens circulate in the blood largely bound to sex hormone-binding globulin and albumin, only unbound estrogens enter target tissue cells. A significant proportion of the circulating estrogen exists as sulfate conjugates, especially estrone sulfate, which serves as a circulating reservoir for the formation of more active estrogenic species. A certain proportion of the estrogen is excreted into the bile and then reabsorbed from the intestine. During this enterohepatic recirculation, estrogens are desulfated and resulfated and undergo degradation through conversion to less active estrogens (estriol and other estrogens), oxidation to nonestrogenic substances (catecholestrogens, which interact with catecholamine metabolism, especially in the central nervous system), and conjugation with glucuronic acids (which are then rapidly excreted in the urine).

When given orally, naturally-occurring estrogens and their esters are extensively metabolized (first pass effect) and circulate primarily as estrone sulfate, with smaller amounts of other conjugated and unconjugated estrogenic species. This results in limited oral potency. By contrast, synthetic estrogens, such as ethinyl estradiol and the nonsteroidal estrogens, are degraded very slowly in the liver and other tissues, which results in their high intrinsic potency. Estrogen drug products administered by non-oral routes are not subject to first-pass metabolism, but also undergo significant hepatic uptake, metabolism, and enterohepatic recycling.

INDICATIONS AND USAGE:

Estropipate tablets are indicated in the:

1. Treatment of moderate to severe vasomotor symptoms associated with menopause. There is no adequate evidence that estrogens are effective for nervous symptoms or depression which might occur during menopause and they should not be used to treat these conditions.
2. Treatment of vulval and vaginal atrophy.
3. Treatment of hypoestrogenism due to hypogonadism, castration or primary ovarian failure.
4. Prevention of osteoporosis.

Since estrogen administration is associated with risk, selection of patients should ideally be based on prospective identification of risk factors for developing osteoporosis. Unfortunately, there is no certain way to identify those women who will develop osteoporotic fractures. Most prospective studies of efficacy for this indication have been carried out in white menopausal women, without stratification by other risk factors, and tend to show a universally salutary effect on bone. Thus, patient selection must be individualized based on the balance of risks and benefits. A more favorable risk/benefit ratio exists in a hysterectomized woman because she has no risk of endometrial cancer (see Boxed **WARNINGS**).

Estrogen replacement therapy reduces bone resorption and retards or halts postmenopausal bone loss. Case-control studies have shown an approximately 60 percent reduction in hip and wrist fractures in women whose estrogen replacement was begun within a few years of menopause. Studies also suggest that estrogen reduces the rate of vertebral fractures. Even when started as late as 6 years after menopause, estrogen prevents further loss of bone mass for as long as the treatment is continued. The results of a double-blind, placebo-controlled two-year study have shown that treatment with one tablet of estropipate 0.75 mg daily for 25 days (of a 31-day cycle per month) prevents vertebral bone mass loss in postmenopausal women. When estrogen therapy is discontinued, bone mass declines at a rate comparable to the immediate postmenopausal period. There is no evidence that estrogen replacement therapy restores bone mass to premenopausal levels.

At skeletal maturity there are sex and race differences in both the total amount of bone present and its density, in favor of men and blacks. Thus, women are at higher risk than men because they start with less bone mass and, for several years following natural or induced menopause, the rate of bone mass decline is accelerated. White and Asian women are at higher risk than black women.

Early menopause is one of the strongest predictors for the development of osteoporosis. In addition, other factors affecting the skeleton which are associated with osteoporosis include genetic factors (small build, family history), endocrine factors (nulliparity, thyrotoxicosis, hyperparathyroidism, Cushing's syndrome, hyperprolactinemia, Type I diabetes), lifestyle (cigarette smoking, alcohol abuse, sedentary exercise habits) and nutrition (below average body weight, dietary calcium intake).

The mainstays of prevention and management of osteoporosis are estrogen, an adequate lifetime calcium intake, and exercise. Postmenopausal women absorb dietary calcium less efficiently than premenopausal women and require an average of 1500 mg/day of elemental calcium to remain in neutral calcium balance. By comparison, premenopausal women require about 1000 mg/day and the average calcium intake in the USA is 400-600 mg/day. Therefore, when not contraindicated, calcium supplementation may be helpful.

Weight-bearing exercise and nutrition may be important adjuncts to the prevention and management of osteoporosis. Immobilization and prolonged bed rest produce rapid bone loss, while weight-bearing exercise has been shown both to reduce bone loss and to increase bone mass. The optimal type and amount of physical activity that would prevent osteoporosis have not been established, however in two studies an hour of walking and running exercises twice or three times weekly significantly increased lumbar spine bone mass.

CONTRAINDICATIONS:

Estrogens should not be used in individuals with any of the following conditions:

1. Known or suspected pregnancy (see Boxed **WARNINGS**). Estrogens may cause fetal harm when administered to a pregnant woman.
2. Undiagnosed abnormal genital bleeding.
3. Known or suspected cancer of the breast except in appropriately selected patients being treated for metastatic disease.
4. Known or suspected estrogen-dependent neoplasia.
5. Active thrombophlebitis or thromboembolic disorders.

WARNINGS:

Induction of Malignant Neoplasms:

Endometrial Cancer: The reported endometrial cancer risk among unopposed estrogen users is about 2 to 12 fold greater than in non-users, and appears dependent on duration of treatment and on estrogen dose. Most studies show no significant increased risk associated with use of estrogens for less than one year. The greatest risk appears associated with prolonged use—with increased risks of 15 to 24-fold for five to ten years or more. In three studies, persistence of risk was demonstrated for 8 to over 15 years after cessation of estrogen treatment. In one study a significant decrease in the incidence of endometrial cancer occurred six months after estrogen withdrawal. Concurrent progestin therapy may offset this risk but the overall health impact in postmenopausal women is not known (see **PRECAUTIONS**).

Breast Cancer: While the majority of studies have not shown an increased risk of breast cancer in women who have ever used estrogen replacement therapy, some have reported a moderately increased risk (relative risks of 1.3 - 2.0) in those taking higher doses or those taking lower doses for prolonged periods of time, especially in excess of 10 years. Other studies have not shown this relationship.

Congenital Lesions with Malignant Potential: Estrogen therapy during pregnancy is associated with an increased risk of fetal congenital reproductive tract disorders, and possibly other birth defects. Studies of women who received DES during pregnancy have shown that female offspring have an increased risk of vaginal adenosis, squamous cell dysplasia of the uterine cervix, and clear cell vaginal cancer later in life; male offspring have an increased risk of urogenital abnormalities and possibly testicular cancer later in life. Although some of these changes are benign, others are precursors of malignancy.

Gallbladder Disease:

Two studies have reported a 2- to 4-fold increase in the risk of gallbladder disease requiring surgery in women receiving postmenopausal estrogens.

Cardiovascular Disease:

Large doses of estrogen (5 mg conjugated estrogens per day), comparable to those used to treat cancer of the prostate and breast, have been shown in a large prospective clinical trial in men to increase the risks of nonfatal myocardial infarction, pulmonary embolism, and thrombophlebitis. These risks cannot necessarily be extrapolated from men to women. However, to avoid the theoretical cardiovascular risk to women caused by high estrogen doses, the dose for estrogen replacement therapy should not exceed the lowest effective dose.

Elevated blood pressure:

Occasional blood pressure increases during estrogen replacement therapy have been attributed to idiosyncratic reactions to estrogens. More often, blood pressure has remained the same or has dropped. One study showed that postmenopausal estrogen users have higher blood pressure than nonusers. Two other studies showed slightly lower blood pressure among estrogen users compared to nonusers. Postmenopausal estrogen use does not increase the risk of stroke. Nonetheless, blood pressure should be monitored at regular intervals with estrogen use.

Hypercalcemia:

Administration of estrogens may lead to severe hypercalcemia in patients with breast cancer and bone metastases. If this occurs, the drug should be stopped and appropriate measures taken to reduce the serum calcium level.

PRECAUTIONS:

General:

Addition of a Progestin: Studies of the addition of a progestin for ten or more days of a cycle of estrogen administration have reported a lowered incidence of endometrial hyperplasia than would be induced by estrogen treatment alone. Morphological and biochemical studies of endometria suggest that 10 to 14 days of progestin are needed to provide maximal maturation of the endometrium and to reduce the likelihood of hyperplastic changes.

There are, however, possible risks which may be associated with the use of progestins in estrogen replacement regimens. These include: (1) adverse effects on lipoprotein metabolism (lowering HDL and raising LDL) which could diminish the purported cardioprotective effect of estrogen therapy (see **PRECAUTIONS** below); (2) impairment of glucose tolerance; and (3) possible enhancement of mitotic activity in breast epithelial tissue, although few epidemiological data are available to address this point (see **PRECAUTIONS** below).

The choice of progestin, its dose, and its regimen may be important in minimizing these adverse effects, but these issues remain to be clarified.

Cardiovascular Risk: A causal relationship between estrogen replacement therapy and reduction of cardiovascular disease in postmenopausal women has not been proven. Furthermore, the effect of added progestins on this putative benefit is not yet known.

In recent years many published studies have suggested that there may be a cause-effect relationship between postmenopausal oral estrogen replacement therapy without added progestins and a decrease in cardiovascular disease in women. Although most of the observational studies which assessed this statistical association have reported a 20% to 50% reduction in coronary heart disease risk and associated mortality in estrogen takers, the following should be considered when interpreting these reports:

(1) Because only one of these studies was randomized and it was too small to yield statistically significant results, all relevant studies were subject to selection bias. Thus, the apparently reduced risk of coronary artery disease cannot be attributed with certainty to estrogen replacement therapy. It may instead have been caused by life-style and medical characteristics of the women studied with the result that healthier women were selected for estrogen therapy. In general, treated women were of higher socioeconomic and educational status, more slender, more physically active, more likely to have undergone surgical menopause, and less likely to have diabetes than the untreated women. Although some studies attempted to control for these selection factors, it is common for properly designed randomized trials to fail to confirm benefits suggested by less rigorous study designs. Thus, ongoing and future large-scale randomized trials may fail to confirm this apparent benefit.

(2) Current medical practice often includes the use of concomitant progestin therapy in women with intact uteri (see **PRECAUTIONS** and **WARNINGS**). While the effects of added progestins on the risk of ischemic heart disease are not known, all available progestins reverse at least some of the favorable effects of estrogens on HDL and LDL levels.

(3) While the effects of added progestins on the risk of breast cancer are also unknown, available epidemiological evidence suggests that progestins do not reduce, and may enhance, the moderately increased breast cancer incidence that has been reported with prolonged estrogen replacement therapy (see **WARNINGS** above).

Because relatively long-term use of estrogens by a woman with a uterus has been shown to induce endometrial cancer, physicians often recommend that women who are deemed candidates for hormone replacement should take progestins as well as estrogens. When considering prescribing concomitant estrogens and progestins for hormone replacement therapy, physicians and patients are advised to carefully weigh the potential benefits and risks of the added progestin. Large-scale randomized, placebo-controlled, prospective clinical trials are required to clarify these issues.

Physical Examination: A complete medical and family history should be taken prior to the initiation of any estrogen therapy. The pretreatment and periodic physical examinations should include special reference to blood pressure, breasts, abdomen, and pelvic organs, and should include a Papanicolaou smear. As a general rule, estrogen should not be prescribed for longer than one year without reexamining the patient.

Hypercoagulability: Some studies have shown that women taking estrogen replacement therapy have hypercoagulability, primarily related to decreased antithrombin activity. This effect appears dose- and duration-dependent and is less pronounced than that associated with oral contraceptive use. Also, postmenopausal women tend to have increased coagulation parameters at baseline compared to premenopausal women. There is some suggestion that low dose postmenopausal mestranol may increase the risk of thromboembolism, although the majority of studies (of primarily conjugated estrogens users) report no such increase. There is insufficient information on hypercoagulability in women who have had previous thromboembolic disease.

Familial Hyperlipoproteinemia: Estrogen therapy may be associated with massive elevations of plasma triglycerides leading to pancreatitis and other complications in patients with familial defects of lipoprotein metabolism.

Fluid Retention: Because estrogens may cause some degree of fluid retention, conditions which might be exacerbated by this factor, such as asthma, epilepsy, migraine, and cardiac or renal dysfunction, require careful observation.

Uterine Bleeding and Mastodynia: Certain patients may develop undesirable manifestations of estrogenic stimulation, such as abnormal uterine bleeding and mastodynia.

Impaired Liver Function: Estrogens may be poorly metabolized in patients with impaired liver function and should be administered with caution.

Information for the Patient:

See text of Patient Package Leaflet below.

Laboratory Tests:

Estrogen administration should generally be guided by clinical response at the smallest dose, rather than laboratory monitoring, for relief of symptoms for those indications in which symptoms are observable. For prevention and treatment of osteoporosis, however, see **DOSAGE AND ADMINISTRATION** section.

Drug/Laboratory Test Interactions:

Accelerated prothrombin time, partial thromboplastin time, and platelet aggregation time; increased platelet count; increased factors II, VII antigen, VIII antigen, VIII coagulant activity, IX, X, XII, VII-X complex, II-VII-X complex, and beta-thromboglobulin; decreased levels of anti-factor Xa and antithrombin III, decreased antithrombin III activity; increased levels of fibrinogen and fibrinogen activity; increased plasminogen antigen and activity.

Increased thyroid-binding globulin (TBG) leading to increased circulating total thyroid hormone, as measured by protein-bound iodine (PBI), T4 levels (by column or by radioimmunoassay) or T3 levels by radioimmunoassay. T3 resin uptake is decreased, reflecting the elevated TBG. Free T4 and free T3 concentrations are unaltered.

Other binding proteins may be elevated in serum, i.e., corticosteroid binding globulin (CBG), sex hormone-binding globulin (SHBG), leading to increased circulating corticosteroids and sex steroids respectively. Free or biologically active hormone concentrations are unchanged. Other plasma proteins may be increased (angiotensinogen/renin substrate, alpha-1-antitrypsin, ceruloplasmin).

Increased plasma HDL and HDL-2 subfraction concentrations, reduced LDL cholesterol concentration, increased triglycerides levels.

Impaired glucose tolerance.

Reduced response to metyrapone test.

Reduced serum folate concentration.

Carcinogenesis, Mutagenesis, Impairment of Fertility:

Long term continuous administration of natural and synthetic estrogens in certain animal species increases the frequency of carcinomas of the breast, uterus, cervix, vagina, testis, and liver. See **CONTRAINDICATIONS** and **WARNINGS**.

Pregnancy:

Teratogenic Effects: Pregnancy Category X: Estrogens should not be used during pregnancy. See **CONTRAINDICATIONS** and Boxed **WARNINGS**.

Nursing Mothers:

As a general principle, the administration of any drug to nursing mothers should be done only when clearly necessary since many drugs are excreted in human milk. In addition, estrogen administration to nursing mothers has been shown to decrease the quantity and quality of the milk.

ADVERSE REACTIONS:

The following additional adverse reactions have been reported with estrogen therapy: (see **WARNINGS** regarding induction of neoplasia, adverse effects on the fetus, increased incidence of gallbladder disease, cardiovascular disease, elevated blood pressure, and hypercalcemia.)

Genitourinary System:

Changes in vaginal bleeding pattern and abnormal withdrawal bleeding or flow; breakthrough bleeding, spotting.

Increase in size of uterine leiomyomata.

Vaginal candidiasis.

Change in amount of cervical secretion.

Breasts:

Tenderness, enlargement.

Gastrointestinal:

Nausea, vomiting.

Abdominal cramps, bloating.

Cholestatic jaundice.

Figure 3-1 Typical drug insert showing a warning box. See Table 3-1 as a guide for interpreting the insert. (Reprinted with permission of Barr Laboratories, Pomona, New York.)

TABLE 3-1 READING A PACKAGE INSERT

ITEM	MEANING
Drug form	Tablet, syrup, elixir, etc.
Drug trade name followed by ® (capitalized first letter)	Manufacturer's registered name for drug
Drug generic name (lowercase first letter and in parentheses)	USP–NF official name
Chemical description and structural formula	Indicates chemical compound of drug
Clinical pharmacology	Purpose of the drug and expected effects on the body
Indications and usage	Therapeutic actions of the drug; conditions or disease processes for drug use
Contraindications	Conditions in which drug should not be used
Warnings	General risks when taking drug; include drug interactions, potential toxic effects, and possible diseases or conditions that might be potentiated Black box indicates possible life-threatening interactions or effects
Precautions	Reasons to adjust dosage or to discontinue use of drug, and pregnancy category
Adverse reactions	Compilation of possible reactions to the drug
Drug abuse and dependence	Information present only for drugs with potential for abuse or dependence DEA scheduled drug; if no "C," not scheduled
Overdosage	Effects and treatment of overdosage
Dosage and administration	Usual dosage and route of administration
How supplied	Dosage of drug; description of its forms and how they are supplied, with NDC number for each supply source; how to store; also shows marking on drug for identification
Drug company	Name, address, and logo of the drug manufacturer
Date of package insert	Information on when insert was written or last revised

DEA, Drug Enforcement Administration; *NDC,* National Drug Classification; *USP–NF, United States Pharmacopoeia–National Formulary.*

Rx/pharmacy
505 South Bell St
Holly, GA
00111-0000

#44 Ph:001-555-4444
www.Rx.com

05-23-20XX
Prscbr: Lawrence, Merry
Refills: 12

PATIENT PRESCRIPTION INFORMATION
IF YOU HAVE ANY QUESTIONS ABOUT YOUR
MEDICATION, PLEASE CONTACT YOUR PHARMACIST:
Foster, Richard

ZETIA 10 MG TABLET M/S
MERCK/SCHERING
TAKE 1 TABLET BY MOUTH EVERY DAY

This is a WHITE, OBLONG-shaped, TABLET imprinted with 414 on the front.
EZETIMIBE - ORAL (eh-ZET-ih-mibe)

COMMON BRAND NAME(S): Zetia

USES: This medication is used either alone or with other drugs (e.g., HMG-CoA reductase inhibitors or "statins"), along with a low cholesterol/low fat diet, to help lower cholesterol in the blood. Reducing cholesterol helps prevent strokes and heart attacks. Ezetimibe works by reducing the amount of cholesterol your body absorbs from your diet.

HOW TO USE: Read the Patient Information Leaflet provided by your pharmacist before you start taking this medication and each time you get a refill. If you have any questions regarding the information, consult your doctor or pharmacist. Take this medication by mouth usually once daily with or without food. If you are also taking a bile acid sequestrant (e.g., cholestyramine, colestipol), take ezetimibe at least 2 hours before or at least 4 hours after the bile acid sequestrant. It may take up to 2 weeks before the full benefit of this drug takes effect. Use this medication regularly in order to get the most benefit from it. Remember to use it at the same time each day. It is important to continue taking this medication even if you feel well. Most people with high cholesterol do not feel sick.

SIDE EFFECTS: Dizziness, headache, diarrhea, back pain may occur. If any of these effects persist or worsen, notify your doctor or pharmacist promptly. Remember that your doctor has prescribed this medication because the benefit to you is greater than the risk of side effects. Many people using this medication do not have serious side effects. Tell your doctor immediately if any of these serious side effects occur: chest pain, fatigue, stomach pain. This drug can very rarely cause muscle damage. Tell your doctor immediately if you experience the following: muscle pain/tenderness/weakness (especially with fever or unusual tiredness). A serious allergic reaction to this drug is unlikely, but seek immediate medical attention if it occurs. Symptoms of a serious allergic reaction include: rash, itching, swelling, dizziness, trouble breathing. If you notice other effects not listed above, contact your doctor or pharmacist.

PRECAUTIONS: Before taking ezetimibe, tell your doctor or pharmacist if you are allergic to it; or if you have any other allergies. This medication should not be used along with a statin agent if you have certain medical conditions. Before using this medicine, consult your doctor or pharmacist if you have: active liver disease. Before using this medication, tell your doctor or pharmacist your medical history, especially of: liver disease (moderate to severe). This medication should be used only when clearly needed during pregnancy. Discuss the risks and benefits with your doctor. It is not known whether this drug passes into breast milk. Consult your doctor before breast-feeding.

DRUG INTERACTIONS: Your doctor or pharmacist may already be aware of any possible drug interactions and may be monitoring you for them. Do not start, stop, or change the dosage of any medicine before checking with them first. Before using this medication, tell your doctor or pharmacist of all prescription and nonprescription products you may use, especially of: "blood thinners" (e.g., warfarin), cyclosporine, fibrates (e.g., fenofibrate, gemfibrozil).

OVERDOSE: If overdose is suspected, contact your local poison control center or emergency room immediately. US residents can call the US national poison hotline at 1-800-222-1222. Canadian residents should call their local poison control center directly.

NOTES: Do not share this medication with others. Laboratory and/or medical tests (e.g., cholesterol levels) should be performed periodically to monitor your progress. When ezetimibe is given with a statin agent, liver function tests should be performed to monitor for side effects. Consult your doctor for more details. For best results, this medication should be used along with exercise and a low cholesterol/low fat diet. Consult your doctor.

MISSED DOSE: If you miss a dose, use it as soon as you remember. If it is near the time of the next dose, skip the missed dose and resume your usual dosing schedule. Do not double the dose to catch up.

STORAGE: Store at room temperature at 77 degrees F (25 degrees C) away from light and moisture. Brief storage from 59-86 degrees F (15-30 degrees C) is permitted. Do not store in the bathroom. Keep all medicines away from children and pets. Properly discard this product when it is expired or no longer needed. Consult your pharmacist or local waste disposal company for more details about how to safely discard your product.

Information last revised April 2007
Copyright(c) 2007 First DataBank, Inc.

Figure 3-2 Drug information sheet.

injection); or percutaneously, by medications applied to the skin or mucous membranes (including instillations into body orifices).

Oral Medications

The oral route, in which medication is taken by mouth and swallowed, is the simplest way to administer medications. It is usually more convenient, economical, and safer than other routes. A drug taken by mouth is subject to actions of the GI tract and may be affected by variations in peristalsis, gastric secretions, and other GI functions. Vomiting and diarrhea may alter medication availability for absorption and may even be reason to avoid the oral administration. The disadvantage of the oral route is that drugs administered orally are absorbed slowly and at an unpredictable rate because of patient-to-patient differences in gastric function. Some drugs, such as insulin, are destroyed by digestive fluids and must be administered by other routes.

Oral drug forms include solids, liquids, powders, and other miscellaneous forms. The terms *tablet* and *capsule* have replaced the term *pill*, a term that should not be used today.

Solid Oral Preparations

Tablets are dried powder forms of medication that have been compressed into a small disk or solid mass available in many shapes, colors, and sizes (Table 3-2). In addition to active ingredients, tablets contain inactive ingredients such as binders (adhesives to hold the substances together), disintegrators (substances that encourage dissolving in the body), lubricants (to give the tablet a sheen for ease in swallowing and to assist with the manufacturing process), and fillers (inert ingredients that make the tablet a convenient size). Some oral medications can be mixed with food for a more acceptable taste, some must be taken with food, whereas others must be taken on an empty stomach (Box 3-1).

Capsules are two-pieced cylindric gelatin containers that fit together. This form is a convenient way for giving medications with an unpleasant odor or taste. Capsules usually contain powder, granules, or a combination of the two and may have one or more active ingredients. In most cases capsules also contain an inert filler substance and do not need flavorings because the medication is enclosed.

✐ CLINICAL TIP

Except for sustained-release capsules, capsules may be pulled apart and the entire contents added as powder to foods for patients who have difficulty swallowing, if permissible. Never mix medications in whole servings of food because the person may not eat all of the food.

BOX 3-1 Important Facts about Solid Oral Preparations

1. Drugs that may dissolve in mouth and discolor teeth should not be given orally.
2. Oral medications should not be given to someone who is unconscious, vomiting, or unable to swallow.
3. Enteric-coated tablets should be swallowed whole, not crushed or chewed, because the desired place of absorption is in the intestines.
4. Sustained-release tablets should not be crushed because crushing changes the absorption rate and may result in an overdose.
5. Patients should not swallow or chew buccal or sublingual tablets, nor should these tablets be taken with water because water would dissolve tablet too rapidly and prevent desired absorption rate.
6. Oral dissolving tablets should be allowed to dissolve in the mouth and should not be swallowed whole. Mouth must have sufficient moisture to allow tablet to disintegrate.
7. Timed-release products should never be opened; they should be swallowed whole to maintain manufacturer's expected rate of absorption and prevent an overdose; opening capsule will alter absorption rate and could result in an overdose of the medication.

Troches or lozenges are hard medications in a candy or fruit base designed to dissolve in the mouth for local effect. Examples of lozenges are cough drops used for relief of a sore throat.

Liquid Oral Preparations

Liquid oral preparations consist of one or more active ingredients placed in a liquid medium. Most oral liquids are divided into two major categories—solutions and dispersions—although some are oils or combinations with other forms, such as gelcaps, a cross between capsule and liquid medications. Solutions are medications in which the active ingredient has been dissolved in a liquid vehicle. In dispersions, the medication is not dissolved in a liquid but instead is distributed as particles throughout the liquid. The most common type of dispersion is a suspension (Table 3-3 and Box 3-2).

Miscellaneous Oral Medications

Miscellaneous oral products include powders and granules containing finely ground drug particles. Granules are larger and of irregular shape, making them better suited than powders for use in solutions because powders tend to float on the surface of a liquid. Laxative granules, such as Metamucil, are used to relieve constipation. Effervescent powders are coarsely ground agents with an effervescent salt that releases carbon dioxide for a bubbling action when mixed with liquid. Examples are analgesics, such as BC Powder and Alka-Seltzer.

TABLE 3-2 SOLID ORAL PREPARATIONS

FORM	DESCRIPTION	EXAMPLE
TABLETS		
Unscored tablet	Tablets intended to be swallowed whole	aspirin
Scored tablet	Tablets that allow for partial doses by breaking tablet on scoring line(s)	furosemide (Lasix)
Enteric-coated tablet	Tablets with special coating so drug dissolves in intestines rather than stomach	enteric-coated aspirin (Ecotrin)
Coated tablet	Tablet coated with sugar for taste enhancement or with film-coating for ease of swallowing	erythromycin 300 mg (EES-300)
Chewable tablets	Medications in a flavored or sugar base designed to be chewed	antacids (Tums), chewable vitamins
Sublingual tablets	Tablets designed to dissolve under the tongue for short-term release of medication	nitroglycerin
Buccal tablets	Tablets placed between cheek and gum to dissolve and be absorbed through buccal membrane for short-term release of medication	fentanyl (Fentora) for pain
Buffered tablets	Tablets with antacids added to active ingredients to prevent irritation of stomach and gastrointestinal tract	aspirin (Bufferin)
Sustained-release (controlled-release) tablets	Tablets manufactured with a matrix that releases medication over a period of time; may allow ingredients to be found in layers or a wax matrix to be released at different times; allows incompatible active ingredients to be given in one medication for release in stages	loratadine-pseutdoephedrine (Claritin-D 12 Hour)
Caplets	Tablets shaped as capsule for ease of swallowing	acetaminophen (Tylenol)
Oral dissolving tablets	Tablets designed to dissolve in mouth	desloratadine (Clarinex) soluble tablets
CAPSULES		
Capsule	Gelatinous containers that hold powdered medications	amoxicillin (Amoxil)
Sustained-release capsules	Medications within a capsule delivered over a specified period of time	venlafaxine (Effexor XR)
Delayed-release capsules	Capsules prepared to release drugs at a particular site; some of these medications contain beads designed for release at different times or at a particular site to meet metabolism of the body; these capsules provide a steady flow of medications over a period of time	theophylline (Theo-24)
GUMS		
Gums	Gums are usually polysaccharides that produce thick substances and are sticky when wet and hard when dry, attracting and holding water for formation of gelatin-like agents	nicotine (Nicorette)

TABLE 3-3 LIQUID ORAL MEDICATIONS

FORM AND BASE	DESCRIPTION	EXAMPLE
GELCAP		
Liquid gelcap	Cross between capsule and liquid (liquid within a gelatin shell) that should not be chewed; may be squeezed into mouth with physician's permission	docusate sodium (Colace)
SOLUTIONS		
Syrups, aqueous (water-based)	Solutions sweetened with sugar or sugar substitute to disguise medicinal taste; may also contain flavorings, color, and aromatic agents	guaifenesin (Robitussin)
Elixirs (alcohol and water)	Sweetened, flavored medications containing alcohol and water to improve solubility; if solution is mainly water, sweetener is natural sugar; if solution is mainly alcohol, sweetener is artificial	diphenhydramine (Benadryl)
Extracts and fluid extracts (water or alcohol, or both)	Highly concentrated preparations that move desired materials into a solution and then evaporate to leave a syrup, mass, solid, ointment-like substance, or dry powder; fluid extracts are from plant sources used in syrups; extracts are used in compounding medications	vanilla extract, peppermint extract
Tinctures (alcohol or hydroalcohols)	Potent medications or pure chemicals or extracts from plants	camphorated tincture of opium (Paregoric)
Spirits (alcohol or hydroalcohols)	Solution containing volatile aromatic ingredients that may be diluted with water before administration; aromatic spirits containing oils and other substances are easily released into the air to provide a pleasant smell and are therefore used in vaporizers and humidifiers	spirits of ammonia, peppermint spirit
OIL		
Oil	Thick, sometimes greasy liquid, that may have an odor or bad taste	mineral oil
DISPERSION		
Suspension	Undissolved particles of medication mixed with, but not dissolved in, a solvent; most are suspensions requiring reconstitution using purified or distilled water	amoxicillin suspension (Amoxil Oral Suspension)
Emulsion	Water-in-oil mixture in which one liquid is dispersed in another; liquids do not mix readily	Fat emulsion used in total parenteral nutrition; whole milk with cream, oil in vinegar
Gel	A semisolid jelly-like product containing large amount of water; thick viscous liquid that easily penetrates without a residue	Orajel
Magma	Viscous suspensions of medications containing ultrafine particles blended in liquid	milk of magnesia, aluminum hydroxide (Aludrox)

BOX 3-2 Important Facts about Oral Liquid Medications

1. The patient's mouth needs to be moist for the patient to be able to swallow a gelcap; the gelcap will adhere to the dry mucous membranes of the mouth.
2. If syrups are added to juice or milk, the person must drink the entire amount to receive the total dose. Be careful in using milk, because the medication may change flavor of milk and a child might refuse to drink milk. Milk may also change a property of the drug.
3. Because of the high sugar content of elixirs, care should be taken when used with people having diabetes. Because of the alcohol content, persons who are alcohol dependent should not take these medications, especially patients taking disulfiram (Antabuse).
4. Elixirs may have to be diluted for children. The medication should be diluted one dose at a time to prevent active ingredients from precipitating out if water is added to the entire bottle.
5. Camphorated opium texture should always be diluted before administration.
6. A suspension should always be shaken before administration. If a suspension is not shaken, the active ingredient will settle to the bottom of container and will not be administered correctly.
7. After a suspension has been reconstituted, it has a short shelf life (usually 7 to 14 days) at room temperature. Some must be under refrigeration for a 14-day shelf life, such as amoxicillin. The drug label will specify instructions.
8. Because a residue is expected on the spoon, medicine cup, or other means used to administer a suspension, the container for administration should be cleaned between doses to ensure proper dose with each administration.
9. Oral emulsions may be diluted with water immediately before administration. Shaking well ensures mixing of medications just before dispensing.
10. Oral liquid iron preparations for children are given by dropper or straw to prevent staining of teeth.

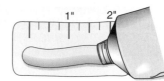

Figure 3-3 Paper for measuring transdermal nitroglycerin ointment.

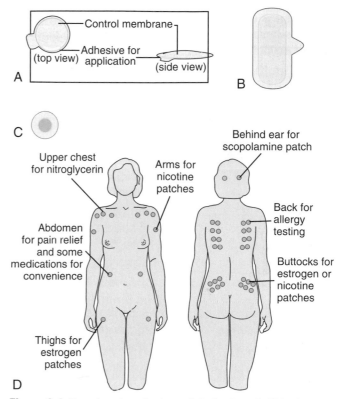

Figure 3-4 Transdermal applications of medications. **A,** Side view of a transdermal patch. **B,** Transdermal patch. **C,** Transdermal spot. **D,** Sites for transdermal medical applications and the medications typical for each site.

Did You Know?

Transdermal patches were used by astronauts on the space shuttle to prevent nausea. Patches have found a growing market as treatment for conditions such as angina, smoking cessation, chronic pain, and estrogen replacement therapy and for allergy testing.

Percutaneous Medications

Percutaneous or topical medications (Table 3-4 and Box 3-3) are those applied to the skin and mucous membranes for local effect. Many are OTC drugs that are not absorbed systemically, but some preparations are absorbed into the bloodstream from the topical application. Topical refers to application of medications directly to any body surface. Transdermal refers to absorption of a drug through the skin using a form of topical application, such as a patch or spot impregnated with a medication (Figures 3-3 to 3-4).

CLINICAL TIP

- Eardrops should be warmed to body temperature to prevent vertigo (dizziness). Holding the medication bottle in the hand for a few minutes will do this.
- When otic preparations are applied, the head should be tilted away from the affected side to prevent drainage of the medication from the ear.
- Shake ear medication in a suspension for 10 seconds to place the active ingredient back into suspension.

TABLE 3-4 PERCUTANEOUS MEDICATIONS

FORM	DESCRIPTION	EXAMPLE
Liniments	Drugs containing oil, soap, water, or alcohol applied to skin to produce heat for relief of muscular aches and pains	BenGay
Colloid suspension/ solution	Gluelike suspension or solution containing particles dispersed in solvents such as water, volatile ether, or alcohol and leaving residue on skin	Suspension—Aveeno oatmeal bath; Solution—Compound W and flexible collodion
Tinctures	Alcohol-based liquids that evaporate to disinfect skin	Tincture of iodine
Lotions	Free-flowing liquids or suspended ingredients in water	Hand lotions, calamine lotion for itching
Creams	Semisolid preparations in water base that are absorbed into tissues for slow, sustained drug release	Bactroban cream (antiinfective) and corticosteroid cream; Solarcaine
Ointments (see Figure 3-3)	Semisolid greasy preparations in oil base that are not easily absorbed into skin; prevent adherence of bandages to the skin	Triple antibiotic ointment; eye preparations
Pastes	Semisolid preparations that are stiffer than ointments because they contain more solid materials; apply more thickly	Toothpaste
Gels	Semisolid preparation with high proportion of water with a drug plus a thickening agent; used to reduce friction and provide lubrication	Antiseptic, antifungal, and contraceptive gels and lubricants; topical anesthetics
Plasters	Solid or semisolid medicated or unmedicated preparations that adhere by means of a backing	Salicylic acid spots for removal of corns or warts
Aerosol foams	Water-in-oil emulsion that disperses as spray and slows vaporization in air	Vaginal preparations, hair products
Transdermal patches and disks (see Figure 3-4)	Drug-containing reservoirs of medication applied to skin for absorption of medication through skin	Nicotine patches, fentanyl patches; estrogen patches for menopause and contraception
Suppositories (see Figure 3-6)	Medication placed in a base of cocoa butter, hydrogenated vegetable oil, or glycerinated gelatin to form solid dose for insertion into a body orifice; some have local action, others have systemic action	Glycerin suppositories, vaginal suppositories
Sprays	Emit a fine dispersion of liquids, solids, or gaseous materials Nasal—solutions designed for both local and systemic effects in alcohol or water pump-type dispenser Translingual—used under the tongue Topical—applied to skin	Decongestants, fluticasone (Flonase); nitroglycerin; sunscreens; hormones to treat postmenopausal symptoms
Aerosols	Liquid in a pressurized can that releases fine mist or coarse liquid spray	Primatene mist aerosol
Metered dose inhalers	Fine mist of medications that are breath activated and delivered into respiratory tract to treat airway diseases	albuterol MDI
Dry powder inhalers	Fine powder medications that are breath activated and delivered into respiratory tract to treat airway diseases	Advair Diskus
Nebulizer	Small micronized powders, as well as liquids, that deliver medications into a reservoir for inhalation into the respiratory tract	albuterol (Xopenex), levalbuterol (Ventolin)
Ophthalmic or otic solutions and suspensions	Sterile solutions or suspensions for use in eye (sterile) and ear; inserted using a dropper	Ophthalmic—Ocusol, Vasocon-A Otic—Cortisporin
Douches	Solutions or suspensions used in body orifices such as vagina or rectum	Vaginal douche

BOX 3-3 Important Facts about Percutaneous Medications

1. Liniments should not be used with heating pads or external heat because the patient may be burned by the combination.
2. Drug molecules in transdermal patches and disks are present for absorption over a period of time. The drug flow persists over a longer time and provides a more constant blood level than the up-and-down level found with oral and parenteral medications.
3. Some patches consist of a backing, a drug reservoir, a protective strip, and an adhesive layer, whereas others have medications embedded within the adhesive layers. The drug moves by osmosis through the patch's controlled membranes to the skin for systemic absorption. In some patches the absorption rate is controlled by the size of the openings in the membrane; in others, control comes from the skin itself. Body temperature and climate affect absorption rates depending on the size of the pores.
4. Sites of application for patches or disks should be rotated with each application to ensure proper absorption and to prevent damage to the skin and blood vessels over a period of time.
5. Patches should be wrapped before disposal to prevent accidental overdose by a child or pet that may come into contact with the discarded patch.
6. The person applying the patch should wear gloves or wash hands immediately after application to avoid unintended absorption of medication from application contact.
7. Vaginal, rectal, and urethral suppositories are made to melt at body temperature for medication release and come in a variety of shapes, depending on the site of administration and age and gender of patient (see Figure 3-6).
8. Because of the large number of blood vessels in the rectum, suppositories are often used in comatose patients or those with nausea and vomiting. Suppositories with a local rectal effect are used to stimulate defecation or administration of medications for effect in the rectum. Vaginal suppositories are used as antiinfectants and contraceptives.
9. If a suppository is wrapped, the patient should be educated to remove the outer wrapper before administration.
10. Handling of suppositories should be kept to a minimum to prevent melting before insertion into the body orifice.
11. Suppositories may have to be stored in a refrigerator during warm weather so the medication remains solid for insertion.
12. Inhalants are being increasingly used to treat systemic conditions, as well as for their local effects.
13. Placing pressure on the inner canthus of the eye, blocking ducts and reducing drainage for a few minutes after instilling eye drops can diminish systemic absorption of eye preparations.
14. Ophthalmic preparations must remain sterile and should be used by only one person. Care should be taken not to touch body surfaces with applicator's tip.
15. An ophthalmic preparation may be used in the ear in an emergency situation, but an otic preparation may never be used in the eye. The sterility of an ophthalmic preparation may be necessary if tubes have been inserted into the eardrum.
16. Sports creams should be used only as recommended by manufacturer. Overuse may lead to severe toxic effects, even death, as the active ingredient (salicylates) may be systemically absorbed.

Parenteral Medications

Parenteral medications, or those given by injection, are sterile solutions or sterile powders for reconstitution to liquid preparations. These drugs, stored in vials, ampules, or premeasured cartridges (Figure 3-5), are in small glass or plastic containers holding drugs. If the drug is in powder form, it must be mixed with a sterile liquid before administration. When drugs are unstable as liquids, they are packaged in powder form to provide a longer shelf life. After reconstitution, most powdered medications have a limited shelf life.

Water-Based Parenteral Medications

Sterile normal (isotonic) saline, a water-based solution of salt in water with approximately the same concentration as found in body tissue, is usually used to reconstitute or dilute drugs for injection and to replace lost body fluids when given IV. Sterile distilled water is used similarly to saline but tends to be more irritating because it is not isotonic with the body fluids. When powders are

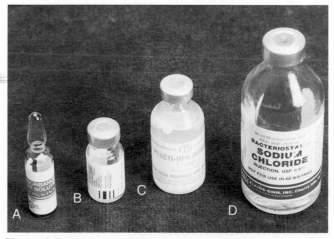

Figure 3-5 Typical containers for injectable medications. *A,* Ampule. *B,* Single-dose vial. *C* and *D,* Multidose vials.

reconstituted, a solution or suspension will be formed. If a suspension precipitates after reconstitution, before administration the medication will always need to be placed back in suspension until no precipitate is observed.

Some manufactured injectable suspensions, such as insulin, consist of small, undissolved particles in a water base. These suspensions need to be rotated in the hand (not shaken) before administration to ensure the redistribution of the particles.

Oil-Based Parenteral Medications

Some parenteral medications also come in an oil base, which provides slow release and prolongs absorption time and duration of action. Because of the oily nature of the medication, these drugs are thick, or viscous, in appearance and are given by intramuscular injection for less irritation of body tissue. Oil bases are used for many hormones that are used in replacement therapy and for treatment of certain cancers.

Other Forms of Medications

Implants or pellets are dosage forms that are placed ID, or under the skin, by means of minor surgery or special injections. This drug form is used for long-term controlled release of medications, especially hormones and radioactive isotopes, used in treatment of cancer. Tampons are drug-impregnated packs, pads, or plugs made of cotton or sponges that are inserted into body orifices for release of medication. Douches are water-based solutions used to irrigate any part of the body—topically, otically, ophthalmically, intracavitarily—or to cleanse surgical wounds. Many vaginal douches are available OTC. Medicated enemas may be ordered to administer a medication either locally or through systemic absorption. The medication is suspended in a solution for administration in the rectum and is often used with patients in whom oral consumption is restricted or who cannot swallow. Oil-retention enemas to soften feces are another type of medicated enema. Suppositories are used in body orifices for release of medication from a matrix such as cocoa butter or glycerin that will melt at body temperature (Figure 3-6).

Packaging Medications for Patient Compliance

Some medications are packaged for easy use and compliance, such as the compacts used for oral contraceptives. The container is designed to remind the user to take medication as prescribed. Automatic delivery systems are used for administering insulin for ease of compliance. An example is the Novolin-Pen, by Squibb-Nova, which

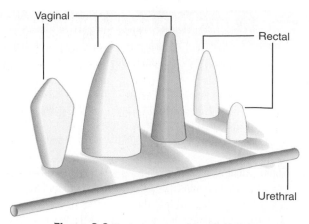

Figure 3-6 Typical shapes of suppositories.

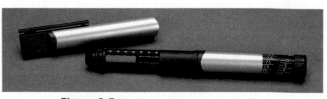

Figure 3-7 Pen for administration of insulin.

delivers either regular insulin, NPH insulin, or the combination Novolin 70/30. A cartridge containing insulin is placed into the insulin pen and remains attached until it is empty, and then it should be properly disposed. After the empty cartridge is disposed of, a new cartridge is loaded and set to maintain the desired dose. This method of administration has a mechanism for presetting the dose of insulin to reduce errors in dose and contamination, which is especially helpful for patients with visual problems or arthritis (Figure 3-7).

Important Facts

- Drugs come in solids and liquids and are administered orally, parenterally, and topically, depending on the form.
- The rate of absorption of medications varies with drug form and route of administration. Solid medications must be dissolved before absorption. Liquid medications given parenterally are absorbed faster. Inhalation and translingual sprays have fast absorption. Topical medications tend to have a longer absorption time but also a longer action time.
- Topical medications can have systemic as well as local effects, although most are applied for local action.
- Some medications are packaged for ease of compliance.
- Drug forms used must be adjusted to a patient's lifestyle and physical condition.

SUMMARY

Drugs are classified in several complex ways. In this book drugs are grouped by their effects on body systems, and icons are used to indicate the body system where the drug has its usual effect. The allied health professional should acquire general knowledge of drug classifications and their indications for use relative to medical diagnoses.

Drug nomenclature refers to various ways in which drugs are named. The chemical name describes the chemicals involved in the drug production. For the allied health professional, the generic, or official, name and the trade name are the important names to know, especially for medications used in the employment setting. When a new drug is proposed to the FDA, the manufacturer assigns it a trade name and has the right to sole production of the drug for 20 years after a patent is filed. Thereafter, other companies may manufacture the drug and use either the generic name or a trade name of their own devising for the same compound. Other terms applied to medications are *over-the-counter* and *legend drugs,* as well as *controlled substances.*

With so many medications used today, various drug references, such as drug handbooks, are used by health care workers, depending on their specialty, to distinguish among drugs and ensure accurate administration. The USP–NF is the official government source used to ensure that the drug meets FDA regulations. The drug inserts supplied with all marketed products are an excellent source of information on all aspects of the drug. The PDR provides a compilation of drug inserts, with many cross-referencing abilities. Drug cards provide health care professionals with a quick reference on medications routinely administered in the health care setting. The knowledge of medications ensures that checks and balances are in place for accurate drug administration.

Medications come in many forms. Solid drugs are given orally in tablet, capsule, and powder form. Liquids may be in a water base or in other bases such as alcohol and may be given orally (enterally), by injection (parenterally), or topically (percutaneously). The health care professional should know drug forms and how they affect administration techniques. Disease conditions, such as alcoholism or diabetes mellitus, are important factors in deciding the form of medication to use. More often the form of medication administered relies on the ability of the patient to take oral medications, such as with nausea and vomiting, or children and older adults who require a liquid because of the inability to swallow solid drugs. When a severe illness occurs, oral medications may not be appropriate, and intravenous medications may be administered because of the rapidity of medication absorption. Patient compliance may also be considered when a medication needs sustained periods of time for administration. Sustained-release or transdermal patches may be used when daily administration is not desired or necessary. Finally, topical preparations may be used when only local effects are required.

Before administering medications or performing patient education about prescribed medications, the allied health professional should be aware that many factors affect the choice of medication and should be sure that contraindications have been documented.

CRITICAL THINKING EXERCISES

Scenario

Mrs. Smith, 75, has difficulty swallowing an enteric-coated tablet. While you are taking Mrs. Smith's history, her daughter tells you that she has been crushing this tablet and mixing it with her food. The daughter is concerned that her mother may not be receiving all the medicine, as the food now tastes bitter (from the medication) and she may not be eating all of it.

1. What is your response to Mrs. Smith's daughter?
2. Is it safe to crush an enteric-coated tablet? Explain your answer.

REVIEW QUESTIONS

1. What is the importance of the USP–NF? What does the abbreviation mean? _____

_____

_____

2. Explain why oral medications are absorbed more slowly than injectables. Why are sublingual medications faster acting than swallowed oral medications? _____

_____

_____

_____

3. What are the advantages of injectable medications when rapid action is desired? What are the dangers of giving medications by injection? Why do drugs take longer to be absorbed after oral administration? _____

_____

_____

_____

_____

4. If you wanted to find a medication for smoking cessation, in what part of the PDR would you look? A manufacturer's address? Identification of a medication brought to the office but not found in the medical record? A trade name for a generic drug? The telephone number of the local Poison Control Center _____

_____

_____

_____

_____

5. Why are oral medications more often prescribed than other forms of medication? _____

_____

_____

6. What is meant by using a medication "off-label"? _____

_____

_____

7. What is the difference between liquids that are solutions and those that are suspensions? What are the implications of each for the allied health professional? What patient teaching is needed for correct dosage with suspensions? _____

_____

_____

_____

8. What is the base of a cream? An ointment? Which would you suggest to keep a dressing from sticking to a wound? Which would you suggest if you wanted the medication to be absorbed into the skin? _____

_____

_____

_____

_____

CHAPTER 4

Understanding Drug Dosages for Special Populations

OBJECTIVES

After studying this chapter, you should be capable of doing the following:

- Discussing variables that affect dosages of medications.
- Providing general patient education about contraindications and precautions for medication use.
- Identifying populations in which special understanding of medication administration may be required, such as pregnant and lactating women, older patients, and children.
- Identifying medication indications, dosages, and special precautions or contraindications with older patients, children, and pregnant or lactating women.
- Providing essential information about medications to promote patient compliance.

Mary, a 29-year-old patient, calls the gynecologic office in November thinking that she may be 6 weeks pregnant for the first time. She has been waiting to have a child because of employment opportunities. Mary says she has been taking herbal supplements and over-the-counter (OTC) medications for headaches during the past 4 months and wants to know if it will be safe to continue. She states that she has read about the dangers of herbal supplements and pregnancy. Her other concern is that she has allergic rhinitis during the spring, for which she takes OTC antihistamines. She wants to know what medications she can take at that time, and when the danger from medications during pregnancy is the greatest.

What answer would be appropriate for the allied health professional to give regarding the taking of herbal supplements?

Why is it important for her to not take medications before seeing the physician if she thinks she might be pregnant?

Why would it be safer for Mary to take OTC medications for allergic rhinitis in the spring rather than during the early months of pregnancy?

What advice should the allied health professional give Mary about medications for headaches?

KEY TERMS

Body surface area (BSA)	Contraindication	Polypharmacy	Teratogen
	Dentition	Precaution	

The effects of medications on the body are related to drug dosages and forms of medications used. No one method of determining dosages will guarantee safety because individual differences in drug effects and tolerances must be considered, especially in children. Variables such as gender, age, weight, height, genetics, and diseases affect how the patient responds to medication. As patients are examined by more than one physician, chances of polypharmacy and drug interactions increase. The system of checks and balances among the physician, pharmacist, and allied health professional becomes more important for patient safety where dosage is concerned.

In January 1997, the U.S. Food and Drug Administration (FDA) was concerned that lack of information was available to patients concerning possible reactions to prescription medications, leading to improper use of drugs. The FDA appropriations bill required the pharmaceutical industry to develop a plan to provide useful consumer medication information to 95% of people receiving prescriptions. A plan was developed for voluntary compliance by health professionals to provide accurate, unbiased, understandable, timely, and useful information to patients. It was determined that by empowering patients with the knowledge of how a drug works, when to take it, why they are taking it, what results are expected, and what the risks or side effects might be, preventable drug-related illnesses could be drastically reduced (Box 4-1). In response, the United States Pharmacopeial Convention copyrighted 81 standardized pictograms in 1997—graphic images showing patients how a medication is intended to be taken, as well as any warnings or precautions the patient should know. The U.S. Pharmacopeia Pictogram Library is available for use and can be downloaded on the Internet from www.usp.org. In order to meet the goal of providing needed consumer information to patients, the National Council on Patient Information and Education has developed a website, www.talkaboutrx.org, to provide patients with accurate information.

Today written patient instructions are provided by the pharmacy with each prescription dispensed (see Figure 3-2). These printed materials include common uses for the medication; when the medication should or should not be used; what to do if a dose is missed; how to store and dispense the medication; drug-nutrient, drug-disease, and drug-drug interactions; warnings; and possible side effects. Verbal instructions should be provided to the patient in the physician's office and then should be reinforced at the pharmacy. A pharmacist's responsibility is to counsel patients regarding medications to be taken.

Of importance to allied health professionals is the liability risk if a problem occurs with the medication and if the information provided was either incomplete or inaccurate. Information provided to patients in the medical office when sample medications are distributed is subject to the same requirements as if a pharmacist were dispensing the medication. Labeling, record keeping, and providing written information to meet FDA requirements are required.

Cultural influences on how medications are taken and interactions of medications that are not prescribed, such as over-the-counter (OTC) herbal supplements with prescription drugs, influence the way the patient takes and responds to medications. Basic cultural and ethnic beliefs may even interfere with prescribed care, placing the patient in danger. The need to gain information concerning patient compliance is a necessity for patient safety with each medical encounter.

BOX 4-1 QUESTIONS TO ASSIST WITH MEDICATION COMPLIANCE

To assist with medication compliance, patients should know the answers to the following eight questions:

1. What is the medication I have been prescribed?
2. What is this prescription for?
3. How long should I take this medication?
4. What side effects can I expect while taking the medicine?
5. Do any special instructions apply to taking this medication?
6. Are there any foods, other prescription medications, or OTC drugs (including herbals, vitamins, and natural products) that I should not take with this medication?
7. Is an equally effective generic form of the medication available at a lower price?
8. If I am taking several medications, should I be aware of any potential interactions?

VARIABLES AFFECTING DRUG DOSAGE AND ACTIONS

No two persons respond exactly alike to drugs, which is why there is no ideal drug. Even the same person may not respond in the same way to the same dose of a drug given on different occasions. Several factors influence responses to medication (Figure 4-1).

Age

Safe dosages for infants, children, adults, and older individuals have been established for some drugs, but appropriate dosage strength also depends on the person's metabolism. Many drugs do not have dosages established for all age groups because children are rarely studied and differing dosages for geriatric patients have only lately become an area of interest. The very young

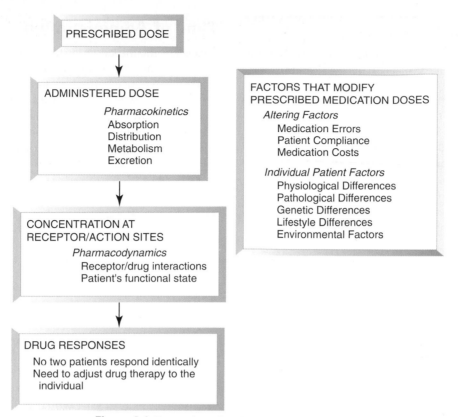

Figure 4-1 Factors that affect drug responses in the body.

may be more sensitive to medications because of immature body organs. Older adults are more sensitive than younger adults because of organ degeneration or increased sensitivity.

Weight

Whether the person is thin, "average," or obese will have a bearing on drug effects. What is wanted in drug therapy is the certain concentration of a drug that provides desired therapeutic effects. Adult doses are based on an average age and body weight (usually 18 to 65 years of age and a weight of approximately 150 lb). Therefore doses may seem to need adjustment for patients who do not fall within "normal" weight and age limits, but because the therapeutic effects may be adequate, these dose adjustments may not be necessary. Heavier individuals may need higher doses, and those with little body fat may need lower doses. For example, highly fat-soluble medications that act on the central nervous system, such as *fentanyl,* require larger initial doses for obese adults, but maintenance doses may be the same as for "normal" adults. The dosage may be determined on the basis of body surface area (BSA) rather than just body size for highly toxic medications such as chemotherapeutic drugs. This method accounts not only

for the patient's weight but also for the relationship of weight to height (see Chapter 9 for calculation methodology).

Because the correct drug dosage can vary on the basis of patient's height and weight, the allied health professional in medical facilities should accurately measure weight and height, especially of children and the older adult, at each office visit.

Diet

Effects of certain drugs are altered by diet. Diets that promote health will help to elicit a therapeutic effect of a medication, whereas poor nutrition will promote adverse effects—for example, a high-fat diet may slow the metabolism of some drugs. Starvation produces a more intense response to medicinal therapy. Even foods eaten in a therapeutic diet may affect the potency, availability, metabolism, absorption, and therapeutic effect of the medications. See Chapter 2 for drug-food interactions.

The patient's diet should be discussed as part of the medical history to ascertain if dietary considerations are significant for drug selections.

Gender

Women may react more strongly than men to some medications because of their smaller size and higher proportion of body fat. Remember that body fat can be a reservoir for lipid-soluble medications, slowing the drugs' excretion.

Genetics

Slight differences in the body's metabolic processes caused by genetic predisposition make some people more sensitive or resistant to certain medications, and pharmacokinetics are affected.

Diseases

Some diseases, especially renal and hepatic disorders, impair body functions, including metabolism and excretion of medications. Renal diseases reduce excretion of some drugs. If dosage is not adjusted in a person with renal insufficiency, toxic levels may be reached even with low doses of medication. The same is true of hepatic diseases because the liver is the major organ for metabolism of most drugs (see Chapter 2).

Mental State

The patient with a positive attitude is more likely to respond positively and potentiate the effects of medications. The patient who is depressed or despondent may not take medication and may not respond to some drugs. Strong emotions such as anger, fear, jealousy, or extreme worry will have an effect on metabolism and other physiologic processes. A strong belief that a drug will be helpful may influence results positively; conversely, patients with negative feelings and mistrust may have decreased medicinal effects.

History of Previous Medications

Long-term use of a drug can result in increased effects because of accumulation of the drug or alternatively can result in a reduced response because the individual has developed a tolerance. In either case the dosage may need to be adjusted for continuing effectiveness.

Time of Administration

Drugs should be taken at the time ordered by the physician. Some drugs need to be taken on an empty stomach, whereas others require food in the gastrointestinal tract. Stimulants should not be taken just before sleep. Body functions change with the time of day and as the body adjusts to periods of work and rest. People who work at night and sleep in the day probably will take medications differently than those with daytime work hours.

Route of Administration

The nearer the drug is administered to the blood supply or mucous membranes, the faster the drug is absorbed and distributed (see Table 2-4).

Environment

Because local weather conditions affect the size of blood vessels, with heat causing dilation of blood vessels and cold causing constriction of vessels, environmental temperature influences drug effects. At high altitudes less oxygen is available, which affects drug distribution in blood. For the patient with respiratory disorders, a smoking environment may be of importance in medication effectiveness; the patient with employment requiring prolonged standing may have the need for increased medications for arthritis. One of the greatest environmental factors is economic: patients living in poverty often cannot afford medications and must choose between medications and food. Also, many of these patients do not eat an adequate diet for safe medication administration.

Drug Dependence

Physical or psychologic drug dependence leads to increased drug use. The patient consumes more medication to achieve the same effects, causing an increased danger of overdosage or underdosage.

Patient Compliance

Patient compliance in taking medications as prescribed affects medication response. Doses missed or extra doses taken result in variations in intended response. Patient cooperation with medical therapy is needed, but such variables as manual dexterity, vision, intellectual capacity, mental state, attitude toward medications, and socioeconomic factors (such as ability to pay for drugs) play a major role in compliance. Location—whether close to or far from pharmacies and public transportation—can be a major factor in compliance for economically deprived people. In rural areas, transportation problems, medical availability, and other socioeconomic issues can be exaggerated by great travel distances for medical care; patient compliance may be an important reason for the success or failure of medicinal care. Poor educational background or inability to follow directions can result in life-threatening situations from underdosage or overdosage.

PRECAUTIONS AND CONTRAINDICATIONS TO MEDICATION USE IN CERTAIN POPULATIONS

Any medication prescribed has an undesired effect on some person. "No two people are alike" is a familiar saying but one especially true with medications; one person may exhibit an intense response, whereas another person exhibits no response. Several factors cause contraindications to use of medications in certain populations, such as tetracyclines in pregnant women because the medication is a teratogen in the fetus. Manufacturers evaluate drugs for contraindications and provide this information to the FDA for publication. Information resources list contraindications and precautions—specific warnings that should be considered when administering drugs to patients with specific conditions or diseases, such as the use of cough syrup in the person with diabetes. Even with a possible warning, the medication may still be prescribed if benefits of use outweigh possible harm.

Did You Know?

Current research is focusing on genetic differences that predispose people to adverse reactions and affect how metabolism occurs. Some people are poor metabolizers of drugs from birth, whereas others metabolize medications very rapidly. Of course, most people metabolize drugs at the rate expected.

Medication Use during Pregnancy and Lactation

The use of any medication—prescription, OTC, or "natural"(such as herbals)—during pregnancy or lactation could carry a risk for causing birth defects to the developing fetus or a risk that the drug will be transferred to the baby in breast milk. Such factors as drug route, dosage, and pharmacokinetic activities determine the amount of drug that will circulate in the blood of the mother and its potential effect on the baby or fetus—either therapeutic or harmful.

Did You Know?

No drug can be considered totally safe because problems may arise later in life or in subsequent generations. This occurred with *diethylstilbestrol* (DES), used in the 1930s through early 1960s to prevent miscarriages. The drug was later linked to an increased risk of cervical and vaginal cancer in female offspring of DES users.

The first trimester is when the developing embryo and fetus are at greatest risk for fetal defects or abnormalities if exposed to teratogens. Medications should be avoided at this stage if at all possible and certainly limited to only those absolutely necessary and approved by the physician before use.

Using **cocaine** and other recreational drugs, drinking **alcohol,** and smoking are causes for teratogenic effects today; many states have passed legislation concerning these activities during pregnancy due to the resultant effects found at birth. Because of its vasoconstrictive effects, cocaine can cause the placenta to malfunction and lead to intrauterine death. Excessive alcohol use can cause fetal alcohol syndrome. Smoking can cause pregnancy complications, preterm delivery, or a low infant birth weight in addition to serious chronic health problems for the baby. Certain drugs such as the **measles-mumps-rubella** (MMR) vaccine should not be given during the first trimester of pregnancy because of possible teratogenicity caused by the live virus in the vaccine. Even use of **tetracycline** (an antibiotic) by a pregnant woman may cause stained teeth in her baby later.

As a precaution, in 1983 the FDA established a system for classifying drugs into one of five pregnancy categories (Box 4-2) according to their potential for fetal risks. Because the law does not require manufacturers to classify drugs used before 1983, many drugs have not been assigned an FDA pregnancy category. When making a decision about drug use in pregnancy, the physician's decision should be based on the least toxic drug related to fetal gestational age at the time of the drug's administration, how long the therapy will be necessary, and what other medications are being taken (Boxes 4-3 and 4-4).

Unlike medications that cross the placenta to the fetus, drugs during lactation are not transferred directly to the breast-feeding infant because the mother metabolizes drugs, reducing the dose before passage to the infant (Box 4-5). The amount of medication transferred to the baby is based on the age of the infant, as well as how much and when breast milk was consumed in relation to the time of the drug's administration. At times breast-feeding may be temporarily interrupted for a mother's medicinal therapy. Increased or decreased changes in the activity level of a nursing infant may signal effects from drugs in the milk. Mothers should be made aware of signs of potential problems.

Important Facts about Drugs during Pregnancy and Lactation

- No pregnant woman should take any unnecessary drugs, prescription or OTC, without the knowledge of a physician. Three percent of birth defects are caused by drug-related incidences. The danger is directly related to the trimester of pregnancy and rate of fetal growth at time of drug administration. Drugs should be administered during the first trimester of pregnancy *only* when absolutely necessary and with physician's approval.
- All drugs cross the placenta to some degree. The solubility of the drug affects speed and degree of placental crossing.
- Drug use in pregnancy must balance risks involved and need for treatment—a blind decision because medicinal risks are often unknown.
- For most drugs there is no reliable information about their use in pregnancy because medications are not safety tested on pregnant women. Medications introduced after 1983 have been assigned to a pregnancy category by the FDA based on their potential for teratogenicity.
- Some drugs, such as *thalidomide*, are teratogenic after only one exposure, whereas other drugs, such as alcohol, cocaine and other recreational drugs, and tobacco require regular, frequent use during pregnancy to produce teratogenic effects.
- Fat-soluble drugs are more readily found in breast milk. All drugs are present in breast milk to some degree, but they may be present in such small amounts that they will not harm a nursing infant.
- If possible, the lactating mother who needs to take medications should take them immediately after a feeding so the milk will have a lower drug concentration by the next feeding. Administration intervals should remain relatively consistent to ensure a therapeutic medication blood level in the mother.

BOX 4-2 FOOD AND DRUG ADMINISTRATION PREGNANCY CATEGORIES

Category	Description
A	Remote risk of fetal harm—Studies have not demonstrated risk to fetus in first trimester, and there is no risk in the second and third trimesters.
B	Slightly more risk than category A—Two groups of drugs exist. One is that animal studies have not demonstrated risk to fetus, but studies are inadequate in pregnant women. The other is that animal studies have demonstrated adverse effects, but studies in pregnant women have not demonstrated a risk during any of the trimesters of pregnancy.
C	Greater risk than category B—One category is that animal studies have shown adverse effects in fetus, but there are no adequate studies in pregnant women. The other group is that there are no animal reproduction studies and no studies in humans.
D	Proven risk of fetal harm—Studies in women have shown proof of fetal damage, but potential benefits of use during pregnancy may make administration acceptable despite the risk.
X	Proven fetal risk—One category is that studies show a definite risk of fetal abnormalities in either humans or animals. Another category is that adverse reaction reports indicate evidence of fetal risk. The risks clearly outweigh any possible benefit.

Medication Use in Children

Children are not miniature adults. Their ability to absorb, metabolize, and excrete medications is very different from that of adults, resulting in differences in the medication amount needed to produce either a therapeutic or a toxic effect. An approved standard medication dosage for children is nearly nonexistent, and drugs are ordered according to body weight or BSA.

Age is no longer considered a reliable guide for administering medications to infants and small children. Medication dosage supplied to children should be recalculated regularly. As children grow, physiologic changes in the fast-growing body affect pharmacodynamics or how the drug acts in the body. Evaluation of skin hydration in infants is important when using topical water-soluble drugs. Gastric acidity and gastric motility cause differences in absorption. The ability to swallow medications as well as the size and form of the oral preparation are important factors for medications with young children.

Chronologic age correlates poorly with organ system development. Height is a better correlation in children with lean body mass, whereas larger, more obese children may need higher dosages because of weight and height, or drugs need calculation according to BSA. Because pediatric patients are more sensitive to drugs and respond on an individual basis, the chance of adverse reactions and sensitivity are heightened, especially with topical medications in thin-skinned babies such as premature and newborn infants. Drug dosages are quantitative, with the increased inherent risk of medication errors caused by the need to measure or dilute oral doses and/or possible miscalculation of doses.

Premature infants and newborns have intense responses to some drugs. Because their organ systems are not developed, medications may remain in the body longer than in older children. Both prolonged drug time

BOX 4-3 SELECTED DRUGS WITH POSSIBLE TERATOGENICITY DURING PREGNANCY

ACE inhibitors—all (especially in second and
third trimesters) especially those in Category X
captopril (Capoten)
enalapril (Vasotec)
benazepril (Lotensin)

Anticancer agents, immunosuppressants
busulfan (Myleran), Busulfex
cyclophosphamide (Cytoxan)
methotrexate (Rheumatrex, Trexall)
thalidomide

Antiseizure drugs
carbamazepine (Carbatrol, Tegretol)
phenytoin (Dilantin)
trimethadione (Tridione)
valproic acid (Depakene)

Vitamin A derivatives
etretinate (Tegison)
isotretinoin (Accutane)
vitamin A (Aquasol A)

Sex hormones
estrogens, progestins (in last trimester),
androgens

lithium (Eskalith, Lithobid [Category D and should
be discontinued if possible])

tetracycline (Vibramycin, Minocin)

warfarin (Coumadin, Jantoven)
HMG-CoA reductase inhibitors or statins (Lipitor,
Zocor)

Live vaccines

Other drugs
alcohol in large or continuous doses (exact
amount not known)
cocaine in large or continuous doses (exact
amount not known)
misoprostol (Cytotec)

ACE, Angiotensin-converting enzyme.

BOX 4-4 SELECTED DRUGS CONTRAINDICATED DURING LACTATION

Controlled substances
amphetamines and amphetamine-like drugs
cocaine
heroin
marijuana
phencyclidine
nicotine

Anticancer agents, immunosuppressants
cyclophosphamide (Cytoxan)
cyclosporine (Neoral, Sandimmune)
doxorubicin (Adriamycin, Doxil)
methotrexate (Rheumatrex, Trexall)
Other drugs

bromocriptine (Parlodel, Cycloset)
ergotamine (Ergomar)

gold salts (Ridaura)

lithium (Lithobid, Eskalith)

fluoroquinolones such as *ciprofloxacin* (Cipro)
sulfa preparations

misoprostol (Cytotec)

milligram-per-kilogram basis (see Chapter 9). By 1 year of age, the liver and kidneys have matured to a point that the infant has the ability to metabolize drugs pharmaceutically close to the adult level. Children do metabolize drugs faster, especially after the second birthday and again at puberty.

Young children are also more vulnerable to adverse reactions because of the immature state of the body organs and ongoing growth and development. Effects such as suppression of growth and development by glucocorticosteroids may occur when medications are given during times of rapid growth and development. Table 4-1 lists medications that should be avoided or used with extreme caution in children.

and delayed responses may change the drug's pharmacokinetics as well as the safety and effectiveness. Of most importance is that gastric emptying times vary, and thus the impact of a drug cannot be predicted.

With the low metabolic rate of drugs in infants up to 1 year of age and the young child because of immaturity of the liver, the dosages and the time between doses may be shorter, and often doses are reduced because of rapid metabolism of drugs. Doses for healthy infants older than 1 to 2 weeks of age may be calculated on the

Important Facts about Pediatric Medications

- Pediatric patients cannot be treated with medications used for adults unless some adjustments are made to dosage. Children are not small adults; their metabolism and excretion are not well developed. Infants and very young children have immature organ systems, making them highly sensitive to medications.

Continued

Important Facts about Pediatric Medications—cont'd

- Height and weight should be measured in children at each office visit to ensure correct statistics for dosage determination.
- In the infant and small child, medications may have a more intense effect for a prolonged period as a result of gastric motility and slow biotransformation by an immature liver.
- Pediatric doses are approximations of the needed medication and should be carefully calculated. Parents should be given information regarding adverse reactions.

BOX 4-5 MEDICATIONS CONSIDERED RELATIVELY SAFE DURING LACTATION

All medications used during lactation have the potential to be passed to the infant through breast milk. Most drugs are not recommended for use during lactation and should be carefully evaluated by a health care professional before administration.

Analgesics
acetaminophen (Tylenol)
codeine

Antiinfectives
cephalosporins
cefadroxil (Duricef)
cefazolin (Ancef)
cefoxitin (Mefoxin)
ceftriaxone (Rocephin)
erythromycin (E-Mycin)
isoniazid (INAH)
azithromycin (Z-Pak)

Cardiovascular drugs
digoxin (Lanoxin) (must be monitored very closely)
guanethidine (Ismelin)

Diuretics
spironolactone (Aldactone)

Endocrine medications such as hypoglycemics (insulin)
Thyroid preparations (must be monitored more closely)

Vaccine
Immune globulins (RhoGAM)

Gastrointestinal drugs
Antacids (Maalox, Mylanta)
Laxatives (except cascara sagrada derivatives)

Medication Use in Older Patients

As adults age, the normal physiologic changes affect pharmacokinetics. Individuals with chronic disease processes are at greater risk for toxic effects, adverse reactions, or lack of therapeutic effects than patients with acute diseases. Some older adults weigh no more than an average large child, and some weigh even less, yet often these people are prescribed "normal" adult doses, leading to potential for toxic effects.

The geriatric population (those older than 65), representing approximately 12% of the U.S. population, use approximately 30% of all prescribed drugs and 50% of all OTC medications over long periods of time because of chronic diseases.

Experts now estimate that by the year 2030, at least 20% of the population will be older than 65 years of age, making seniors the fastest-growing segment of the population. The result is an increasing danger of adverse reactions and drug interactions and an increased percent of medical complications in the total population. Older adults are more sensitive to drugs than younger adults and exhibit wider variation in how medications affect their bodies. Because of the high rate of medication use, the older adult experiences more drug-related incidents.

Factors leading to possible dangerous effects caused by the accumulation of drugs include slower metabolism; poor circulation; and impaired function of the liver, lungs, kidneys, or central nervous system. Chronic or debilitating conditions with dehydration or electrolyte imbalance can affect how the aging body uses a drug

---

TABLE 4-1 MEDICATIONS TO AVOID OR USE WITH EXTREME CAUTION IN CHILDREN

MEDICATION	ADVERSE REACTION
salicylates, aspirin	Reye's syndrome following viral diseases, especially chickenpox and influenza
androgens	Premature closure of epiphyseal lines of bones
glucocorticoids (including inhalers)	Suppress growth
hexachlorophene (pHisoHex)	Central nervous system toxicity
fluoroquinolones (ciprofloxacin, levofloxacin [Levaquin])	Weaken and cause ruptured tendons
phenothiazines	Sudden infant death syndrome
sulfonamides	Kernicterus; jaundice and collection of bile in the spine and brain
tetracyclines	Stained teeth

and may interfere with expected therapeutic effects. Estimates indicate that 70% to 80% of all adverse drug reactions in the older adult are related to drug dosage. Because body pharmacokinetics are diminished, tissues retain a higher level of the medication, resulting in adverse reactions. A narrow separation between maximum drug effectiveness and drug toxicity is common in the older adult. The use of multiple drugs simultaneously and poor compliance by many older adults add to the problems associated with medication administration in this population.

Older adults who are physically active will have minimal changes, whereas those who are inactive or bedridden will exhibit dramatic changes. Slowed gastric and intestinal emptying time allows medications to remain in the stomach, increasing absorption and increasing the risk of stomach irritation. The amount of the drug's oral dose absorbed does not change with age, but delayed stomach emptying may cause another dose of drugs to be administered before total absorption of the previous dose. Distribution is different because of changes in body fat/water ratio, reduced muscle mass, slowed metabolism caused by reduced blood flow to the liver, and decreased enzymatic activity needed to metabolize a drug; and excretion is delayed by reduced blood flow to the kidneys. These changes in the body increase the drug's half-life, allowing drug accumulation and thus causing concentration of a drug to rise to a higher level. The drug effects become more intense. Dosage and monitoring for desired and undesired effects must be individualized.

Dosages and effects of medications applied topically and transdermally may also be difficult to predict in older patients. Although skin thickness decreases, drying, wrinkling, and decreased hair follicles may change the rate of absorption. Decreased cardiac output may also affect the rate at which medications are absorbed through the skin. Because of decreased salivary secretion flow, sublingual tablets may not be properly dissolved and absorbed, nor may tablets be swallowed easily.

Other considerations include dentition, which should be evaluated before giving chewable tablets, because older adults may have insufficient teeth to chew tablets. Many drugs can affect the mental status of older individuals, leading to confusion and unintentional overdosage of medications.

Polypharmacy in the Older Adult

With increasing numbers of geriatric patients and increased medications found as OTC preparations, older adults become caught in the vicious circle of polypharmacy. The era of medical specialization has only added to this problem because a person who sees multiple physicians for multiple problems is usually prescribed multiple medications without discontinuance of any of

BOX 4-6 QUESTIONS TO ASK TO PREVENT POLYPHARMACY

- What dietary supplements, vitamins, and OTC drugs do you take?
- What pharmacies have you used in the past 2 years to fill your prescriptions?
- Who are all of the physicians that you see, and what medications has each prescribed for you?
- How would you describe your ability to read medication labels?
- When do you take your medications? Of those times, at which are you most likely to forget to take the doses? How often do you forget your medications?
- Do you have any questions about your medications and how to take them?

BOX 4-7 CONDITIONS THAT MAY RESULT FROM POLYPHARMACY

- Cardiac arrhythmias
- Disturbances in balance
- Cognition changes, confusion, depression, suicidal ideation
- Constipation
- Gastric ulcers
- Hypertension or hypotension
- Rash
- Unexpected failure of treatment

the drugs previously prescribed. The problem is increased by the patient's self-medication with OTC drugs. By taking accurate medical histories (Box 4-6), including full documentation of *all* medications being taken, the allied health professional assists in the elimination of inappropriate medications and thus improves the patient's quality of life and reduces undesirable effects of polypharmacy (Box 4-7).

Some polypharmacy is apparent when the patient receives more than one drug in the same class of medications or several different medications from different medication classes to treat the same symptoms. More likely, medications are added to treat the side effects of another medication, leading to use of more and more drugs with possible negative outcomes. Negative effects include adverse drug reactions; drug-drug, drug-nutrient, and drug-disease interactions; medication errors; increased treatment costs; and increased risk of hospitalization. Because of these inherent problems, it is important to use the lowest effective dose in the geriatric patient.

The older person is in a constant state of physiologic change, and medications and dosages must change also.

The use of drugs may remain relatively safe as long as each physician maintains a total drug profile, and as long as the potential for drug interactions and the physiologic changes in the patient are evaluated each time medications are prescribed. For this reason, it is important for the patient to fill all prescriptions at the same pharmacy so his or her drug profile is current and accurate.

Assisting the Older Adult with Medication Compliance

The allied health professional should be aware that 40% or more of older individuals do not take their medications correctly. Some fail to get prescriptions filled initially, whereas others never refill the prescription. Others do not adhere to the prescribed dosage or do not follow the schedule for taking medicines. These factors can lead to toxic effects from overdosage or nontreatment from underdosage. Underdosage and failure to respond to a medication are more common by far, accounting for approximately 90% of the problem. Unintentional noncompliance may result from forgetfulness; from not understanding instructions because of poor vision, inadequate hearing, or decreased ability to understand; or from the complexity of remembering how to take multiple drugs. Sadly, however, 75% of noncompliance is intentional. The person feels medicine is not necessary or finds the side effects unpleasant. A major reason for noncompliance may be inability of people on a fixed income to pay for drugs. Because medications are necessary for good treatment, the allied health professional should listen and ask sufficient questions to obtain a full history of medicines being taken and to look for clues that may signal an unrecognized noncompliance problem.

To help older patients comply with medication orders, simplify instructions for taking medications, being sure the medication schedule is convenient for the patient. Encourage the patient to read all labels carefully and to use only one pharmacy. The patient should make a list of all medications taken, along with their strength, their dose, and the length of time each has been taken. This list should be taken to each physician with each visit so that the medical record in each office can be updated. The allied health professional should thoroughly explain the medication schedule, making the medication times fit as closely to the person's schedule as possible. The reason for administration should be explained clearly and concisely, followed with precise written instructions. Using a calendar or a weekly pill container will assist in reminding the patient to take the medicines as prescribed. Finally, providing sample medications to those who cannot afford the medicines may help with compliance and will provide small amounts of medications for trial before expensive prescriptions are dispensed and side effects prevent the medicine's use.

Important Facts about Older Patients and Drugs

- Older people are usually more sensitive to medications because of decreased metabolism and excretion; thus the danger of overdose is increased.
- Medications must be individualized for the older adult because of changes in body organ systems and in drug pharmacokinetics associated with body changes, especially in chronically ill or debilitated patients.
- Adverse reactions, more common in older persons, may be caused by polypharmacy, severe illness, presence of multiple diseases, and resultant use of multiple drugs.
- Noncompliance is common. About 75% of noncompliance is intentional and is a result of expense, side effects, or the patient's belief that the medication is not necessary.
- Unintentional noncompliance is usually caused by forgetfulness or failure to understand treatment, with at least 40% of older individuals not complying with medical treatment.
- After the age of 50, only three medications should be taken at the same time. If more than three medications are necessary, the patient should be instructed to wait 10 minutes between each dose to allow for absorption.

ASSISTING OTHER SPECIAL POPULATIONS WITH MEDICATIONS

The health care professional should spend time with each patient to ensure that he or she understands the condition, treatment prescribed, and reasons for and actions of the medication ordered to increase the likelihood that the patient will take prescribed medications routinely. Some pharmaceutical companies provide audio, video, and written materials to assist with patient education for new medications. Asking the patient to explain what he or she has heard and understood can reveal information that has not been adequately covered. Compliance will be more easily accomplished if affordable methods of procuring medications are discussed with the patient. If a trade-name medication is required, for example, the health care professional may be able to provide the patient with samples, and some pharmaceutical manufacturers have special programs for those who cannot afford their medications. Most of the paperwork needs to be completed by both the patient and health care provider, so the necessary paperwork needs to be accessible in the medical office. See www.needymeds.org for more information.

The medical office should keep a list of available local resources that can assist with medication compliance. In some communities pharmacies cooperate with other medical entities to provide low-cost prescription copayments. Some health agencies will come to the home and prepare medications for the patient or will assist with transportation to obtain medicines.

For some older patients, it may be the caregiver who needs to understand the medication administration. In these cases the caregiver should be present when medications are discussed. Conditions that involve loss of memory, vision, hearing, or movement, as well as socioeconomic and physical situations resulting in inadequate transportation or financial resources, may cause real barriers for some patients.

A patient who is illiterate and is embarrassed to ask for help in reading prescription labels or OTC labels is at risk for inadvertent double dosaging, adverse reactions to medications, and dangerous drug interactions. Because even most literate people are not medication literate, it is important to provide an increased knowledge base for reading drug ingredients. It is not commonly understood by most patients, for example, that medications such as OTC headache preparations with salicylates, such as *aspirin*, may cause excessive bleeding in the person who is taking **warfarin sodium** (an anticoagulant) and its derivatives, or that *ibuprofen* and *aspirin* should not be taken together because **ibuprofen** is an aspirin-like compound.

Taking 5 to 10 minutes to explain areas of concern can save the time that could be involved if a problem has to be corrected later after adverse effects have occurred. Convenience in taking medications and making lifestyle changes helps a person comply with treatment.

For patients who have difficulty with medication compliance, written instructions can help ensure accuracy of dosage. Some health care facilities have printed materials that provide checklists for the areas of compliance that need special attention. Written instructions provide a guide that can be followed at home. Remember that most patients are nervous in the medical office and retain only about 50% of the information discussed.

Important Facts about Compliance with Special Populations

- Because barriers such as language, hearing, vision, culture, and religion can cause noncompliance, the patient needs should be evaluated before any medications are prescribed.
- Written instructions should be provided for patients who have difficulty remembering desired schedules or who have disabilities that make compliance difficult.
- The allied health professional should be sure that patients who are illiterate or who have language barriers understand medication instructions before leaving the physician's office.
- If a patient requires a caregiver, the caregiver should be present when medication administration is discussed.

MEDICATIONS AND CULTURAL DIFFERENCES

Perceptions about medications that influence acceptance or refusal of medicinal treatment come from cultural, social, and religious beliefs and convictions. By understanding some of these cultural differences, the health care professional can assist with communication to improve patient care and compliance.

Ethnic and cultural differences seldom affect the action of medications (even though some diseases occur only in certain racial or ethnic groups), but a patient's compliance with the physician's orders can be greatly affected by the patient's understanding of the therapy and by good communication between patient and provider concerning the need for therapy. In some cultures, people may refrain from expressing views that conflict with views of others, especially those in medical communities. Through awareness of sociocultural differences, health care professionals can surmount certain obstacles to good health care. Remember, even nonverbal communication can hinder compliance.

The allied health professional must be aware of his or her attitudes because these attitudes, transmitted both verbally and nonverbally, can affect patient compliance. Self-analysis of our own beliefs, expectations, attitudes, and practices establishes the way we accept differences. An open mind and willingness to expand personal knowledge of diversity assist in establishing patient-caregiver interactions. Barriers to communication can be overcome through tone of voice, body language, and actions that convey reassurance. Exercising patience with patients and allowing time to ensure that the patient understands medication orders are important steps in promoting compliance with medical therapy.

In 1989 Albers Herberg noted that attitudes toward health and illness generally reflect one of three views: scientific-biomedical, holistic, and magicoreligious. Each perspective regards illness and health in different, culturally determined ways (Table 4-2). In the United States the scientific-biomedical paradigm predominates, with professionals undergoing extensive training in the biomedical sciences. In the scientific-biomedical domain, disease and illness have a cause, and the goal of health care is to find a cure. Scientific research is based on finding cures for diseases and illnesses.

The holistic paradigm focuses on achieving harmony of body, mind, and spirit to prevent illness. Disharmony or imbalance among these natural components leads to disease or illness. Once the person is in harmony, health is restored. Thus health requires mind, body, and spirit balance (Figure 4-2).

The magicoreligious paradigm regards humans as under the control of supernatural, mystical forces. Witchcraft, good and evil spirits, spells, voodoo, and other

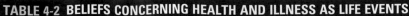

TABLE 4-2 BELIEFS CONCERNING HEALTH AND ILLNESS AS LIFE EVENTS

	SCIENTIFIC-BIOMEDICAL	HOLISTIC	MAGICORELIGIOUS
Health	Prevention activities and restorative therapy through exercise, medications, and treatment	Environment, behavior, and sociocultural factors influence and maintain health and the prevention of illness or disease; maintaining and restoring health are vital	Reward of God's blessings and good will
Illness and disease	Cause-effect relationship to life events; wear and tear happens to the body, as do accidents, injuries, diseases, and chemical imbalances; body functions as a machine; mind and body are two distinct entities	Disease, chemical or physical imbalance, and chaos occur when laws of harmony and natural balance have been disturbed; human life is only one part of cosmos; everything has its place and role to maintain order	Cause of health and illness is not organic but mystical; evil spirits, sorcery, taboos, and supernatural forces cause illness; humans are at the mercy of good and evil forces, which may initiate diseases or illnesses with or without a reason
Societies in which belief predominates	White Americans Europeans	Native Americans Various Asian groups	African Americans Persons of Hispanic culture

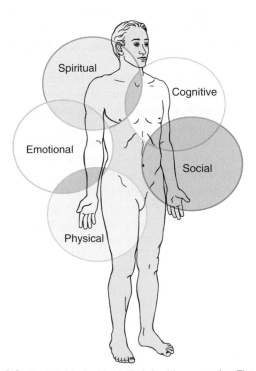

Figure 4-2 The individual with a holistic health perspective. The diagram shows the dynamic interactions among the physical, social, emotional, spiritual, and cognitive aspects of a person.

forces bring about illness and disease. Health is a blessing from God for being good, whereas illness is a sign the individual has not carried out God's will. Illness may or may not be part of God's plan, but it comes from supernatural forces.

Culture must be considered when medications are used for treatment of illnesses. One third of the U.S. population consists of individuals from racial, ethnic, or cultural subgroups that are referred to as *minorities.* Beginning in the twenty-first century, however, persons from a minority background account for more than 50% of the total population, making the need to know and understand diversity a necessity to meet the health care needs of patients. For an accurate and meaningful gathering of data, care must be sensitive to differences and respect those ideas that are in conflict with the biomedical-scientific outlook prevalent in American medical institutions. People draw on their cultural background and rely on various personal relationships in seeking assistance with decisions. In some cultures individuals seek assistance from family members, and parents or grandparents may make decisions about health matters. In other groups the patient may make decisions while assessing how the decision will affect the entire group or family. In yet other groups the individual makes his or her own health care decisions. Although family members may participate to some degree, either through influence or through participation in therapy, identifying the person who makes the decisions about medical care and including that person in teaching sessions will assist with providing successful therapy.

A number of people in the United States have a primary language that is not English. To comply with drug therapy, the patient must first understand the language of instruction. For the person who does not speak English, giving the directions in English will not lead to comprehension and compliance. Instruction sheets in the patient's language or pictographs will assist with comprehension. A person who can act as an interpreter and who will accompany the patient to the physician's office will further assist with compliance.

Individuals from certain cultural backgrounds may consider home remedies such as roots, teas, and poultices to be more effective than prescription or nonprescription medications. (Home remedies and folk medicine are discussed in Chapter 19.) The allied health professional should attempt to discover home remedies the patient is using because these remedies could interfere with prescribed medical treatment. Understanding cultural differences regarding illness and treatment is an important step toward gaining patient confidence and compliance with prescribed treatments.

Communication and Medication Compliance

Communication, both verbal and nonverbal, is vital to compliance with medication treatment. Nonverbal communication between persons of different cultures may enhance acceptance or inadvertently show disrespect for the patient. Even eye contact is interpreted differently by various cultures. Life experiences, historical and cultural backgrounds, and the patient's perception of the situation are social factors that the allied health professional must try to understand while remaining nonjudgmental and trying to clarify any information that could have been miscommunicated. In today's multicultural world, the allied health professional should adapt medical materials to meet a variety of cultural needs. Written materials may not suffice for a patient who cannot read and/or write, causing a lack understanding of why the prescribed medical therapy is important.

Important Facts

- Cultural differences in how people regard illness and health can affect compliance not only with medications but also with total medical care.
- Problems in communication can lead to noncompliance with treatment.

SUMMARY

Patient variables such as age, weight, gender, diet, genetics, concurrent diseases, and mental state must be considered when prescribing medications. Some people respond to placebos when psychologic need is more intense than physiologic response. How a medicine is given, what medicines have been previously prescribed, and the possibility of drug dependence are all important factors the physician must consider when prescribing drug treatment. Older patients and children have different rates of metabolism than the average adult, the subject for whom the average medication dosage is designed. Dosages must be adjusted in individuals with special precautions. Pregnancy and lactation may preclude the use of some drugs because of the danger to the fetus and infant.

People from different cultures have different perspectives on the role of medications in sickness and health. Their cooperation with medical treatment may be culturally biased. The allied health professional must be sure that cultural differences do not interfere with therapy and that the patient complies with the course of treatment, using and understanding education for compliance.

CRITICAL THINKING EXERCISES

Scenario

Jane, age 23 years, thinks she may be pregnant because she has missed one menstrual period. It is spring, and she has a history of allergic rhinitis that causes sinus headaches. She asks you, the medical assistant, what medications she may take for her allergies. The physician previously prescribed an antihistamine for the condition, and she wants you to call in the same prescription to the pharmacy.

1. What should you do?
2. What do you need to tell Jane about taking medicines during the first trimester of pregnancy?
3. If there were medications that could be safely given during the first trimester, in what pregnancy category would the medications be listed?

REVIEW QUESTIONS

1. What is polypharmacy? Who is at risk for polypharmacy? _____

   _____

   _____

   _____

2. What is the role of the allied health professional in polypharmacy? _____

   _____

   _____

   _____

3. How do variations in weight and the gradual decline in body functions affect dosages for the older adult? ____

   _____

   _____

4. Why is medication therapy potentially harmful in the first trimester of pregnancy? _____

   _____

   _____

   _____

5. Communication barriers and cultural differences may cause noncompliance with drug therapy. How can the allied health professional be sure that those from other cultures comply with medication therapy? _____

   _____

   _____

   _____

6. Compare the scientific-biomedical, holistic, and magicoreligious paradigms of health and illness. How can the allied health professional work with those of different cultures to promote understanding of medicinal treatment? _____

   _____

   _____

   _____

   _____

   _____

   _____

7. What variables (weight, height, and so on) affect drug dosage and actions? What does the allied health professional need to do to ensure correct dosage? _____

   _____

   _____

   _____

8. What are three of the negative outcomes of polypharmacy? _____

   _____

   _____

   _____

9. Why is it important to obtain weight and height at each medical visit? _____

    _____

    _____

10. Why is age a variable in drug dosages? _____

    _____

    _____

11. Why is it important for the person to obtain all medications from the same pharmacy? _____

    _____

    _____

12. List three reasons that patients are noncompliant with medication administration. How can allied health professionals assist with compliance with these issues? _____

    _____

    _____

    _____

    _____

CHAPTER 5

Reading and Interpreting Medication Labels and Orders and Documenting Appropriately

After studying this chapter, you should be capable of doing the following:

- Explaining the parts of a National Drug Code (NDC).
- Listing warning and caution label information and its relevance.
- Distinguishing between a prescription and a medication order.
- Using correct abbreviations when assisting with prescriptions.
- Describing parts of a prescription.
- Describing steps necessary to prepare prescriptions for a physician's signature.

- Telephoning prescriptions to pharmacies and medication orders to health facilities.
- Documenting prescriptions and medical orders in patient records.
- Safeguarding prescription pads.
- Recognizing when prescription refills might be necessary, and transferring orders for refills accurately by telephone or electronically.
- Writing a prescription for physician's signature.
- Interpreting a physician's medication orders.

Tonya, an allied health professional, knows that Mrs. Kline sees several physicians concurrently for chronic conditions. Tonya asks Mrs. Kline to give her a list of medicines that she is taking on a regular basis so that she can enter this information into the medical record. Mrs. Kline tells Tonya that she can remember some of her medicines but not all of them.

Does Tonya need to get medicines from all physicians or just those prescribed by the internist? Why or why not?

If Mrs. Kline uses the same pharmacy to fill all prescriptions, can Tonya call that pharmacy to obtain the needed information? Explain your answer.

Is that ethical? Why or why not?

Should Tonya tell Mrs. Kline to bring all of her medications or a list of medications each time she sees the physician? Why or why not?

If samples are given to Mrs. Kline, what steps does Tonya need to take to ensure patient safety?

KEY TERMS

Auxiliary labels
Compounding
Concentration
DEA number
Documentation

Dosage strength
(weight)
Inscription
Medication order
National Drug Code
(NDC)

Refill
Signature (Sig or
signa)
Standard protocol
Standing order
Subscription

Superscription
Vehicle
Verbal order
Volume

Medications may be prescribed, dispensed, or administered in a medical office but more often are administered after being ordered in health care facilities. Sample medications or other medications supplied by the health care provider and given to the patient are considered dispensed, although a pharmacist in a pharmacy setting does most of the dispensing. Being able to correctly read the label on a medication, whether prescription or over-the-counter (OTC), is a necessity for allied health professionals. Forgetting to read the label or improperly identifying the information on a label ("look-alike–sound-alike" medications or dosage difference on some medications) may result in the wrong medication or dosage form being given. If the label is not read in its entirety, undermedication or over-medication, side effects, improper usage and storage, and improper preparation of the dose may occur. Reading and comprehending labels that contain both generic and trade names and dosage strength provide an understanding of the standardized format of labels for both prescription medications and OTC purchases to ensure proper usage of medications.

Prescribing medications is a daily routine in physicians' offices. The allied health professional plays a role in prescription therapy by assisting the physician with samples, phoning or electronically delivering prescriptions to pharmacies, and documenting administration of medications to patients. This role varies with individual state laws and with protocols of the specific health care setting.

READING A LABEL FOR STOCK MEDICATIONS

The *manufacturer's label* found on stock medication bottles contains information about the quantity in the bottle, the strength of the medication, and other important facts that are necessary in providing the correct medication for patient safety. Some labels contain more detail than others, but reading the entire label is most important for quality assurance in patient care. If a patient is supplied with a new medication, patient counseling is required by law, and pharmacies provide a

patient education sheet about the drug for the patient to take home and read (see Figure 3-2).

Parts of a Medication Label

In the following section the parts of a label are indicated by a letter of the alphabet, with the figures showing each part of the label.

A. Trade (Proprietary or Brand) Name

The trade name is a copyrighted name assigned to the medication after initial patent and acceptance by the U.S. Food and Drug Administration and can be used only by the company that created the drug. Trade names are always capitalized and are usually seen first on the drug label in bold type. The symbols ® for registered trademark or ™ for trademark will follow the name. ™ is used until the U.S. Patent and Trademark Office has registered the name, and then ® is the correct symbol. In Figures 5-1 and 5-2, Dilaudid is the trade name.

B. Generic Name

Also called *official name,* the generic name is given to the medication by the *United States Pharmacopeia–National Formulary* and the manufacturer uses lowercase letters. After the patent rights have expired, the drug may be

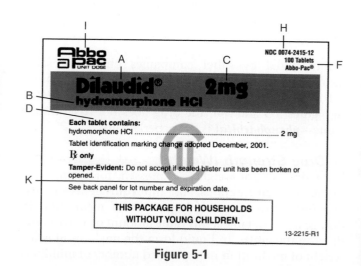

Figure 5-1

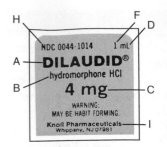

Figure 5-2

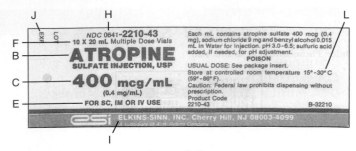

Figure 5-5

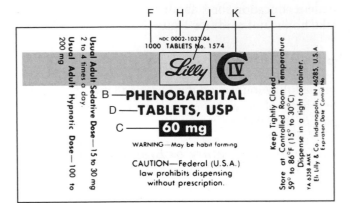

Figure 5-3

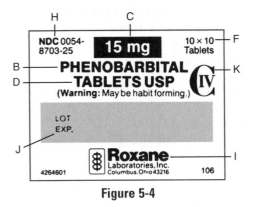

Figure 5-4

BOX 5-1 ABBREVIATIONS THAT MODIFY DRUG FORMS

Abbreviations	Example
SR = Sustained release	Calan-SR
CR = Controlled release	Sinemet CR
LA or XL = Long acting	Bicillin LA, Procardia XL
DS = Double strength	Septra DS
TR = Timed release	Gilphex TR
XR or ER = Extended release	Adderall XR

or other indication of the **volume** of medication. The dosage strength of a medication may come in various weights. The labels in Figures 5-1 and 5-2 indicate Dilaudid 2 mg per tablet and 4 mg per milliliter, respectively. In Figures 5-3 and 5-4, note that the same medication may come in different strengths, and often tablets for the same drug may even be of different colors or shapes, or both, to prevent medicinal errors.

D. Form

Form indicates whether the medication is a solid (e.g., tablets, capsules, powders), liquid (e.g., solutions, dispersions, syrups), or semisolid (e.g., creams, ointments, suppositories). (See Chapter 3 for materials related to drug release times.) Some medication labels have indications of specific dosage-release forms such as those shown in Box 5-1.

E. Route of Administration

Route of administration indicates the way the drug enters the body. Some labels, especially those for parenteral use, tell the acceptable routes for medication administration. Other labels do not provide the route to be used, but tablets, caplets, capsules, and other medications found in Table 2-4 are to be administered orally, as are the oral liquids found in Table 2-3. Note that the label for *phenobarbital* in Figure 5-3 is for a tablet and does not give the route of administration, whereas atropine (Figure 5-5) is parenteral and the label states that the medication may be given subcutaneously (SC), intramuscularly (IM), and intravenously (IV).

manufactured by other companies under the same generic name but with another trade name. In Figures 5-1 and 5-2, the generic name is ***hydromorphone HCL.*** In Figures 5-3 and 5-4, the drug does not have a trade name—***phenobarbital*** is the generic name.

C. Drug Strength (Weight)

Drug strength (or weight)—expressed, for example, in milligrams, micrograms, or milliequivalents—is the **concentration** of active ingredient of medication in dosage form. In tablets this is the amount of active ingredient in the tablet. In liquid form the medication is the weight of medication in a specified number of milliliters

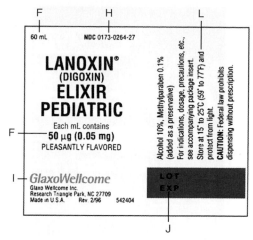

Figure 5-6

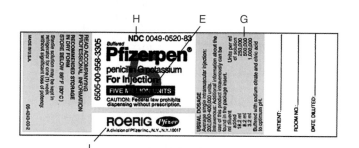

Figure 5-7

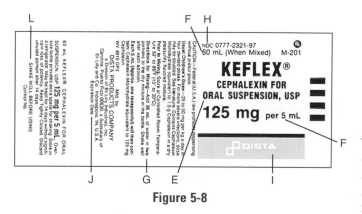

Figure 5-8

F. Total Amount of Medication in Container

The amount of medication in the container is indicated by the total number of tablets, capsules, and so on of solid oral forms of medication (see Figure 5-3). With oral liquid medications, total volume of medication in the container and weight per volume of medication are included on the label (Figure 5-6). Medications found in powdered form for reconstitution to a liquid (see Chapter 9) will provide total weight of medication, as well as concentration after reconstitution for either injectable or oral medications (Figures 5-7 and 5-8).

G. Directions for Reconstitution

Labels for medications that must be mixed with a diluent before administration will provide directions for reconstitution (see Figures 5-7 and 5-8).

H. National Drug Code

All medications are assigned **National Drug Code (NDC)** numbers to identify manufacturer, product, and size of container. The code number shown on the label, containing at least 10 digits, is preceded by the letters *NDC*.

An example of the NDC code and its meaning (related to Figure 5-4) is 0002-1037-04.

The drug manufacturer number 0002 is assigned to Eli Lilly, Inc.

The product, phenobarbital, is coded 1037.

The size of the container is designated as 04 for 1000 tablets.

I. Manufacturer's Name

The name of the manufacturer, sometimes with the address, is found on the label (see Figure 5-6).

J. Expiration Date

The expiration date is the last date for safe use of the medication. After this date, the drug should be discarded (see Figure 5-5). Lot numbers are also included with the expiration date so that if a product is recalled, the patient can be notified and the medication either discarded or returned to the manufacturer.

K. Labels for Controlled Drugs

The symbol for controlled drugs and a warning that the medication may be habit forming are found on medications that are listed in Controlled Drug Schedules (see Figures 5-1 and 5-3).

L. Auxiliary Labeling

The **auxiliary labels** placed by the pharmacy give specific additional information and advice to the patient about use or special handling of medication (see Figure 5-8). These labels include storage labels stating that the medication must be stored at a certain temperature and under certain conditions. More than one direction may be found on a single label, with instructions for patients, and precautions and cautions for use. Auxiliary labels are not seen on all containers, but those needed for patient safety with a specific medication are.

Labeling of Over-The-Counter Medications

OTC medications can be bought by anyone, but many people do not bother to read directions on the label and falsely believe that because the medication is available without a prescription the ingredients are

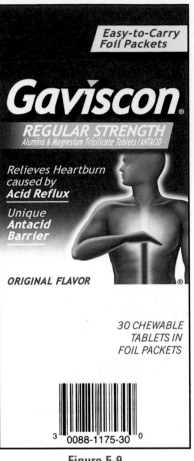

Figure 5-9

not harmful. Because the Federal Trade Commission recognized that many OTC medications were being misused, label guidelines with more specific information are now in place. Information must be in a recognizable and standardized format in a language that is understandable by most people. For information found on labels of OTC medications, refer to Box 5-2 and Figure 5-9.

ORDERING MEDICATIONS

Medications deemed needed may be ordered for the patient by means of either a prescription or a medication order. Orders may be written orders or electronic orders as prescriptions, medication orders, verbal orders, or standing orders. The safest and preferable form for ordering medications is written, such as prescriptions or electronic transmission. Standard medical abbreviations are often used as medical shorthand.

Common Abbreviations Used in Prescriptions and Medication Orders

The allied health professional must be familiar with terms and abbreviations used in writing prescriptions or medication orders. These abbreviations come from Latin or Greek words, are shorthand for directions, and are used daily in the medical field. The list of commonly used standard abbreviations, such as qid, tid, q4h, and the like, for writing prescriptions or orders can be found

TABLE 5-1 THE JOINT COMMISSION OFFICIAL "DO NOT USE" LIST

DO NOT USE (OLD ABBREVIATION)	USE INSTEAD (NEW TERMINOLOGY)
U (unit)	Unit
IU (International Unit)	International Unit
Q.D., QD, q.d., qd (daily)	Daily
Q.O.D., QOD, q.o.d., qod (every other day)	Every other day
Trailing zero (X.0 mg)	X mg
Lack of leading zero (.X mg)	0.X mg
MS, MSO_4, $MgSO_4$	morphine sulfate

inside the back cover of this text. Recently The Joint Commission (TJC) made recommendations in an official "Do Not Use" list to prevent errors in medication administration. However, these abbreviations are included in the abbreviation list of this text because use is still seen in some ambulatory medical settings and the meaning must be known (Table 5-1).

Verbal Orders

When the physician tells an allied health professional which drug or drugs to administer to a patient, the physician is giving a **verbal order (V/O).** The order is for a specific patient and designates the medication to be given, dose, form of the medication, time, and route of administration. Orders should not be routinely given verbally because of the possibility of error and confusion. However, when an order is given verbally, the person receiving the order should read it back to the person who gave it. If there is a possibility of confusion, especially if the drug name sounds like other drug names, the medication name should be spelled to reduce the chance of error. **Documentation** of all verbal orders should be accomplished as soon as possible to prevent errors in administration of the medication. "V/O" should be indicated in the written order to show that the order was verbally given. *Legally, any order not documented has not been performed.* To ensure correctness, the order should then be countersigned by the person giving the order as soon as possible. If there is a question concerning a verbal order, always get clarification before medication administration or sending the order to another health professional.

Standing Orders

Physicians may have **standing orders** that are assigned for use in specific instances. An example of a standing order might be to give a specific antipyretic, such as *acetaminophen,* to a child with a high fever who is waiting to see the physician. Physicians may also use a **standard protocol,** which is a signed set of orders to be used with specific procedures; an example is the use of a suppository, a laxative, and/or an enema before a colonoscopy. "Standard protocol" may be the documentation written in the medical record; the allied health professional knows what the physician expects and performs specific tasks exactly as they are documented in office manuals. The health care worker should ascertain the

appropriateness, dose, allergy, and weight information before administering medications in filling standing orders and standard protocols for the patient or transferring to other health facilities. That the patient has no condition that would cause adverse reactions should be ascertained. Standard protocols and standing orders should be kept in a designated place, and documents should be signed by a physician for legal purposes. After drug administration or procedures, documentation in the medical record should be performed immediately.

Medication Orders

A **medication order,** telling allied health professionals which drug or drugs to administer, should be written but may be given verbally. It is not given to the patient for filling at a pharmacy, but rather is used for administration of drugs in hospitals and ambulatory facilities. In the physician's office, medication orders may be called *standing orders* or *standard protocols.* The allied health professional has the responsibility to follow these orders within his or her legal scope of practice, which varies by state statute. The six components of medication orders are listed in Box 5-3.

BOX 5-3 SIX COMPONENTS OF MEDICATION ORDERS

1. Date
2. Patient's name
3. Medication name
4. Dosage or amount of medication
5. Route of administration (If no route is given, oral administration is appropriate. If there is doubt as to the route of administration, the allied health professional should *always* ask the physician who ordered the medication.)
6. Time or frequency of administration

Important Facts about Medication Orders

- A medication order includes date, patient's name, medication name and dosage, route of administration, and frequency of administration, much like a prescription.
- Whether an allied health professional may legally administer medications from either a written or a verbal medication order depends on the laws of the state in which he or she practices.

Prescriptions

A prescription indicates the medication needed and directions for use to meet medication needs of the patient for whom it was prescribed. Medicines are prescribed after the physician (or nurse practitioners and physician's assistants as allowed by the medical practice act of their state of practice) has evaluated the patient's symptoms and has made a diagnosis of the disease or condition that requires medication. The word *prescription* commonly refers to a slip of paper on which a physician's orders are written for **compounding,** dispensing, or administering of medicines to a particular patient. The order should always be recorded in the patient's medical record. Although only licensed health care professionals may sign prescriptions, often the allied health professional may be delegated the responsibility of completing the prescription form for signature. The physician ultimately has the responsibility of checking information for accuracy before signing.

Prescription Preparation

Any drug not available as an OTC drug requires a prescription. Prescription orders may be written on a prescription blank or submitted electronically

for a pharmacist to dispense. No matter how transmitted, prescriptions have several parts—four that are required **(superscription, inscription, signature [Sig or signa], and subscription),** with other optional information—and should always be written in permanent blue or black ink. Physicians also use computer-generated prescription forms for refills. The physician need only sign these computer-printed blanks. Some physicians prefer blanks that have space for one medication per sheet, whereas others may prefer multiple-line prescription blanks for patients whose conditions require prescribing of several medicines at the same time. If not all prescription lines on a multiple-line form are used, unused lines should be crossed through. Physicians should never sign prescription blanks that are not prepared for a specific patient.

Some states require a multiple-copy prescription program (MCPP) to deter illegal diversion of drugs. In those states the physician is required to write prescriptions for Schedule II controlled substances in triplicate—one copy for pharmacist, one for the state drug agency, and one for the physician's records. If multiple-copy prescriptions are not used, many offices make a practice of copying all prescriptions for the medical record to trace the source of possible errors if needed.

Parts of a Prescription

The following descriptions should be compared with the sample prescriptions shown in Figure 5-10.

Line A

Prescriptions are preprinted with the physician's name, address, and phone number.

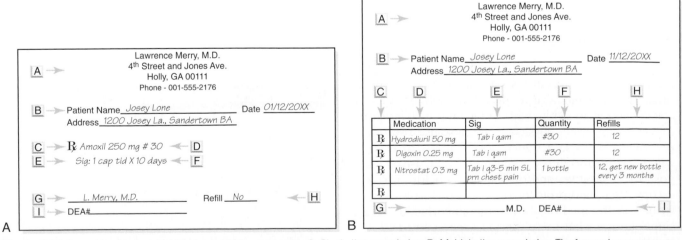

Figure 5-10 Examples of prescription blanks and their components. **A,** Single-line prescription. **B,** Multiple-line prescription. The four major components of a prescription are the superscription *(Line C);* the inscription *(Line D);* the signa, or signature *(Line E);* and the subscription *(Line F).*

Line B

The patient heading includes the patient's name and address, date the prescription was written, and patient's age, if a child. The date is important because prescriptions must be filled within 12 months of writing, and some prescriptions may be refilled for 12 months after initial filling. Prescriptions for Schedules II through V controlled substances must be filled within 6 months of original date. Variations of this may occur with individual pharmacies and state regulations.

Line C

The superscription contains the symbol ℞, meaning "take thou" or "recipe."

Line D

The inscription specifies the name and strength of the drug or ingredients and the quantity to be included in each dose. The amount (weight) of the active ingredient shown is in milligrams, or other pharmacologic weight found in each tablet, capsule, or other dosage forms. Weight usually indicates the strength of a medication, whereas a fluid measurement indicates the volume (e.g., milliliters, teaspoons, ounces) of the medication. If medicine is liquid, the concentration or weight per fluid volume such as milligrams per milliliter is used. If it is a topical medication, the strength is indicated by the percentage of the medication in the **vehicle.**

Line E

The signa or signature (Sig) gives the directions, usually in abbreviations, for the patient for taking the medication. The directions should include the route of administration and the length of time the patient is to take the medication, if applicable.

Line F

The subscription designates the number of doses, quantity to be dispensed, and form of the drug.

Line G

For the prescription to be a legal document, the physician must sign the blank. If the physician wants the patient to receive a brand-name drug, he or she must write on the prescription, "Dispense as Written," "Brand Necessary," or "Medically Necessary." Permissibility of substituting generic drugs for brand-name drugs depends on laws of each state. Many third-party insurers require use of generic medications if no medical need is documented for brand-name drugs

Line H

The **refill** line designates the number of refills permitted. This line should never be left blank. If no refills are designated, either "none" or "0" should be inserted. The use of "12" or "prn" will allow the prescription to be filled as needed for up to a year. Permitted refills expire if not used within a year of initial filling.

Line I

The line for the Drug Enforcement Administration number **(DEA number)** may be found on prescription blanks. This number is required for prescribing controlled substances. To prevent abuse of controlled drugs, the DEA number should be written only on those prescriptions that require its use; these numbers should not be preprinted. The health professional's state license number is required on the prescription pad for third-party payments in some states.

Before prescriptions are transmitted to the pharmacy, the patient's record should be reviewed by the physician and refill orders or new medication orders should be documented in the record. If the physician refuses to prescribe for the patient, this too should be documented, either by the physician or by the allied health professional, showing that the physician refused the request. When transmitting verbal prescriptions by phone, the allied health professional should ask the pharmacist to read back the prescription and confirm that the pharmacist has the correct medication and dosage before concluding the conversation. If there is a chance of misinterpretation or confusion with other medications, the pharmacist should spell the name of the drug.

The allied health professional should maintain patient confidentiality by being sure any faxed prescription is either placed in the medical record or destroyed. This prevents its improper use or the chance that it will be dispensed twice by mistake. The fax machine should be located in an area accessible only by medical personnel to provide confidentiality.

Important Facts about Prescriptions

- Prescribing medications and refilling prescriptions are major tasks in a medical office. The role of the allied health professional in the prescription process depends on the statutes of the state of practice.
- Prescriptions are written or electronically submitted orders for a drug or treatment that is usually dispensed by a pharmacist. Medication orders may be either written or verbal and are commonly used in clinical settings.
- New and refill prescriptions are legal documents and should be recorded in the medical record. Prescriptions may be written by the allied health professional but must be signed by a practitioner licensed to prescribe in the state of practice. All Schedule II medications require a physician's signature.
- Some states allow the allied health professional to relay prescription orders verbally to other health professionals such as pharmacists; other states do not. The laws of the state where the person is employed apply.

Continued

Prescription Refills

Prescription refills may be conveyed to the pharmacy either in writing or electronically, or verbally over the phone. Schedule II medications cannot be refilled except in an emergency situation—and then only a 72-hour supply may be dispensed. A new written and signed prescription must be available at the pharmacy within 72 hours of emergency dispensing. For convenience, patients may phone in a request for a prescription to the allied health professional with specific information needed by the physician (Box 5-4). Phoned requests require the physician to make decisions about refills on the basis of information obtained during the phone conversation. Pharmacists may also call with requests for refills. In either circumstance, the allied health professional should obtain the patient's medical record for the physician to use in evaluating the medication need. Verbal orders for refills should be written into the medical record immediately, and the physician should confirm all prescriptions before allied health professionals phone in refills.

Often a physician prefers to have patient messages taken and left in a designated place for evaluation at certain times of the day because he or she does not want to be disturbed while examining patients. The allied health professional should follow office protocol. To decrease confusion for patients and pharmacists who call for prescriptions, the allied health professional should give an approximate time the person can expect the prescription to be phoned in to the pharmacy for dispensing. To ensure the refill will be available when needed, patients should be instructed to call 1 or 2 days before refill is actually needed. Forty-eight–hour notice of need for a refill allows time for the office to notify the patient concerning the status of the request.

When the physician reviews the request, he or she may note approval on the request form or may document the refill in the medical record. If the physician has not documented the refill, the allied health professional who calls in the refill should document it immediately. The allied health professional should also be sure all prescriptions have been conveyed to the pharmacy before the medical record is filed and the orders have been sent before the end of the work day.

If a refill request is denied, the patient should be notified and given instructions for follow-up visits or informed of the physician's concerns. If the physician wants to see the patient, the allied health professional should call the patient and make a patient appointment.

If the patient uses mail order for prescriptions, two prescriptions will be necessary—one to be filled at a local pharmacy for use until the mail order prescription can arrive, and the other to be sent to the mail order pharmacy for long-term medication availability. If the prescription is for refills, the patient should allow sufficient time for shipment of the medication. Patients who wait until the last minute to obtain refills may find that doses are missed because of lack of medicine and the therapeutic effect is diminished. For the patient who consistently waits too long for approval of medication refills, the allied health professional should educate the patient about the timing needed for the entire process.

Important Information about Prescription Refills—cont'd

- The allied health professional should always check for allergies and adverse reactions before relaying refill requests and should monitor for therapeutic effects as appropriate.
- The pharmacist, the physician, and the allied health professional work as partners to meet prescription needs of the patient. This triangular process provides checks and balances in prescribing medications. A stenographer's pad placed near the phone for prescription refill requests will assist with compliance. One column may be used to take the patient's request in either blue or black ink, and the other column may be used for the physician's response, preferably in another color ink. With this system, refill verification is easily viewed.

Did You Know?

The U. S. Department of Health and Human Services has adopted electronic means of prescribing medications (e-prescribing) and keeping electronic health records (EHRs).

Safeguarding Prescription Pads

Prescription pads should be handled carefully and should be safeguarded at all times to prevent unauthorized use. The prescription blank should be designed so that any erasure is immediately apparent and so that it cannot be counterfeited or duplicated by photocopying. Counterfeit prevention may be accomplished by using colored paper, colored ink, or a watermark of the blank. Another way to safeguard prescription pads is to use carbonless duplicates. The original copy of the prescription is given to the patient, and the duplicate is placed in the patient's record. Finally, prescription pads should have preprinted numbers so that theft of the contents of a prescription pad can be easily detected and reported. It is good practice to keep all prescription pads locked in a safe place, with only a single pad kept on the physician's person or in a place that can only be accessed by approved office personnel.

Experienced drug abusers and drug seekers can take entire pads or sheets without being seen. Drug seekers forge prescriptions and take them to areas where the physician's handwriting and signature are not readily identified. If the pharmacist becomes suspicious of a forged prescription, a call to the physician's office for verification should occur. The allied health professional should check the medical record to verify any prescription, but should also inform the physician and verify the status of the prescription if a copy is not in the medical record.

Prescription blanks should be used only to write prescriptions. They should not be used as notepaper. Orders for anything other than medications should be written on notepaper or memo pads, and orders for laboratory tests should be written on a laboratory request form.

Prescriptions should not be used for ordering stock medicines for the office. Stock bottles should be ordered on a pharmacy order form. On delivery of these medications, the invoice should be checked against the medications received, and the invoice should be filed with the records of the office.

Important Facts about Safeguarding Prescription Pads

- A safe practice for legal protection is to add a copy of all prescriptions to the medical record. If carbonless prescription pads are not used, the allied health professional should photocopy the written prescription.
- Prescription pads must be safeguarded against theft and misuse and should be printed to prevent counterfeiting or photocopying of blank sheets.
- Prescription blanks are never to be used as notepads but are used only for writing medication prescriptions. Orders for laboratory tests should be on a laboratory request form, and instructions should be written on memo pads, not prescription pads.

SUMMARY

Allied health professionals have responsibilities for reading, interpreting, and documenting medication orders. Their duties may include writing prescriptions in preparation for a physician's signature. Allied health professionals may be allowed to relay prescriptions verbally to a pharmacist, depending on the medical statutes of the state. To relay medication orders or prescriptions correctly, the allied health professional must know medications prescribed by the physician. Medication errors can occur because of similarities in drug names; therefore allied health professionals should be careful to repeat all verbal orders to the physician as he or she gives them. In relaying the information, the health professional should ask the pharmacist or nurse (e.g., in an inpatient facility) to repeat the orders.

The allied health professional needs a working knowledge of the parts of a prescription and abbreviations used in writing a prescription. Refills of prescriptions have a major role in the medical office. Before the physician can evaluate the appropriateness of refill requests, the allied health professional needs to obtain information from the patient concerning any adverse reactions that might have occurred and whether medications prescribed were taken properly. Proper documentation of refills is an important task of the allied health professional.

CRITICAL THINKING EXERCISES

Scenario

Dr. Merry asks you to write prescriptions for J. Rex for medications for her arthritis. She takes ibuprofen 600 mg three times a day—at breakfast, in the midafternoon, and at bedtime. Ibuprofen needs to be taken with food, which may be a snack at bedtime. Dr. Merry wants J. to have a 1-month supply at a time; the prescription may be refilled three times. Also needed is Extra-Strength Tylenol, one caplet every 4 to 6 hours as needed for pain. Finally, one Norflex 100-mg tablet to be taken twice a day, at breakfast and bedtime, is prescribed. This should also be for a 1-month supply.

1. What prescriptions need to be written?
2. What documentation should be included in the medical record for these medications?
3. Is there a medication order that needs no prescription? If so, what written instructions are needed?

REVIEW QUESTIONS

Using the label shown, answer the following questions.

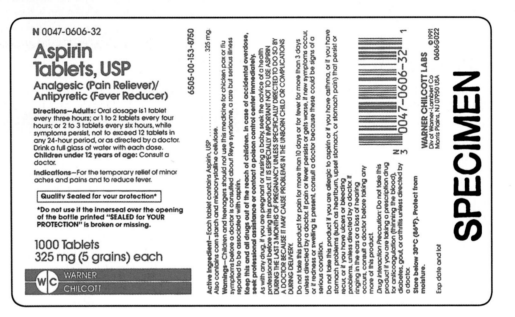

1. What is the generic name? _____
2. What is the trade name? _____
3. What are the storage requirements? _____
4. What is the manufacturer's name? _____
5. What cautions are given? _____
6. What is the expiration date? _____
7. What is the dosage strength? _____
8. What is the manufacturer's NDC code? _____
9. What is the storage container size? _____
10. What is the usual dose? _____
11. What are the warnings given? _____

Reading and Writing Prescriptions

In the following exercises, interpret the order of the physician.

12. 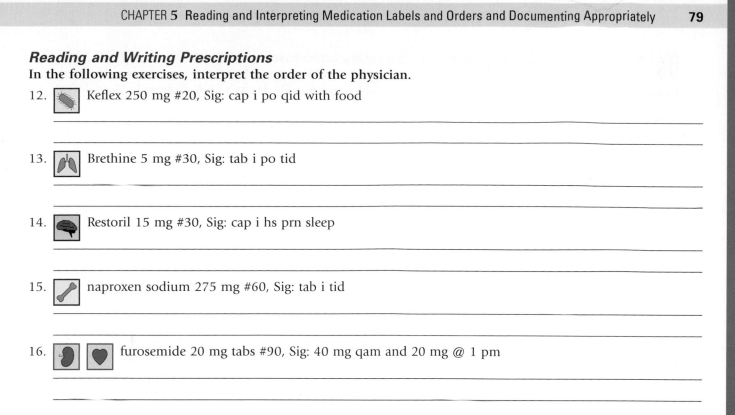 Keflex 250 mg #20, Sig: cap i po qid with food

_____

_____

13. Brethine 5 mg #30, Sig: tab i po tid

_____

_____

14. Restoril 15 mg #30, Sig: cap i hs prn sleep

_____

_____

15. naproxen sodium 275 mg #60, Sig: tab i tid

_____

_____

16. furosemide 20 mg tabs #90, Sig: 40 mg qam and 20 mg @ 1 pm

_____

_____

In the following exercises, write the prescription for signature by the physician. Check a drug reference to be sure the dosage is appropriate. If the dosage is incorrect, make note of that fact.

17. Dr. Merry wants Arthur Rice to have ibuprofen 600 mg tablets four times a day for ten days for his arthritis. Ibuprofen should be taken after meals and at bedtime with a snack. Decide on the number of tablets needed for compliance. The prescription may be refilled three times.

Lawrence Merry, M.D.
4th Street and Jones Ave.
Holly, GA 00111
Phone - 001-555-2176

Patient Name_____ Date _____

Address_____

R̵

_____ Refill _____

DEA#_____

18. **PA IN** Sara Hurt fell and fractured her leg. Dr. Merry wants her to have a prescription for Tylenol No. 3 for pain. He wants the prescription to allow her thirty tablets, and she may take one or two tablets every four to six hours as needed for pain. Tylenol No. 3 is a controlled substance. Dr. Merry's DEA number is AM0000000.

    a. Can the prescription be refilled?   Yes   No
    b. Can a generic substitute be used?   Yes   No

```
                    Lawrence Merry, M.D.
                   4th Street and Jones Ave.
                       Holly, GA 00111
                    Phone - 001-555-2176

       Patient Name_____  Date _____
       Address_____

       Rx



       _____  Refill _____
       DEA#_____
```

19. Dr. Merry has seen Susie Illy, age 3, for a bacterial upper respiratory tract infection. He wants her to have a prescription for 5 oz of amoxicillin suspension. (Write in the apothecary measure.) She is to be given one teaspoonful three times a day for ten days, or until all the medication has been taken. No refills.

```
                    Lawrence Merry, M.D.
                   4th Street and Jones Ave.
                       Holly, GA 00111
                    Phone - 001-555-2176

       Patient Name_____  Date _____
       Address_____

       Rx



       _____  Refill _____
       DEA#_____
```

20. Dr. Merry also wants Susie to have some Benadryl for her allergic rhinitis. He orders a 6-ounce bottle of Benadryl liquid for Susie, with orders for her to take half a teaspoonful every four to six hours for runny nose.

```
                    Lawrence Merry, M.D.
                   4th Street and Jones Ave.
                       Holly, GA 00111
                    Phone - 001-555-2176

       Patient Name_____  Date _____
       Address_____

       Rx



       _____  Refill _____
       DEA#_____
```

21. [♥] Dr. Merry wants Hy Tension to take Lopressor 50-mg tablets at breakfast and dinner for his high blood pressure. Dr. Merry wants 60 tablets dispensed now, with refills for three months, but he wants the label to remind Hy to get his blood pressure checked once a week and to call the office if it drops below 130/70.

```
┌─────────────────────────────────────────────────────────┐
│                    Lawrence Merry, M.D.                   │
│                  4th Street and Jones Ave.                │
│                      Holly, GA 00111                      │
│                   Phone - 001-555-2176                    │
│                                                           │
│      Patient Name_____  Date _____       │
│      Address_____                  │
│                                                           │
│      R                                                    │
│                                                           │
│                                                           │
│      _____   Refill _____             │
│      DEA#_____                              │
└─────────────────────────────────────────────────────────┘
```

Documentation

Document the following exercises as they would appear in a medical record.

22. J. Smith brings the following medicines from other physicians to the office to be included in her medical record:

a. [♥] digoxin 250 micrograms, taken daily at breakfast

_____

_____

b. [🦴] indomethacin 25 milligrams, taken three times daily with meals

_____

_____

c. [♥] nifedipine XL 30 milligrams, taken daily

_____

_____

d. [♥] Lopressor 50 milligrams, one tablet taken at breakfast and again at bedtime

_____

_____

e. [PAIN] acetaminophen 325 milligrams, one or two tablets taken every 4 to 6 hours as needed for pain

_____

_____

Mathematics for Pharmacology and Dosage Calculations

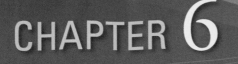
Math Review

OBJECTIVES

After studying this chapter, you should be capable of doing the following:

- Identifying proper, improper, and equivalent fractions.
- Changing improper fractions to mixed numbers.
- Reducing fractions to lowest terms.
- Finding the lowest common denominator for fractions.
- Adding, subtracting, multiplying, and dividing fractions and mixed numbers.
- Rounding decimals to whole numbers, tenths, hundredths, and thousandths.

- Converting fractions and mixed numbers to decimals.
- Adding, subtracting, multiplying, and dividing decimals.
- Changing percents to decimals.
- Changing decimals to percents.
- Multiplying and dividing percents.
- Using fractions to figure percents.
- Using proportions to figure percents.

KEY TERMS

Decimal	Improper fraction	Mixed number	Proportion
Denominator	Lowest common	Numerator	Proportional method
Dividend	denominator (LCD)	Percent	Quotient
Divisor	Lowest common	Product	Ratio
Equivalent fraction	multiple (LCM)	Proper fraction	Reciprocal

Chapter 6 PRETEST

Fractions and Mixed Numbers

Write the following as improper fractions.

1. $4\frac{3}{4} =$ _____

2. $6\frac{1}{2} =$ _____

Convert the following to mixed numbers.

3. $\frac{35}{6} =$ _____

4. $\frac{37}{4} =$ _____

5. $\frac{73}{9} =$ _____

Simplify the following fractions to the lowest terms. Answers will be whole numbers.

6. $\frac{144}{72} =$ _____

7. $\frac{32}{8} =$ _____

Chapter 6 PRETEST—cont'd

Solve. Simplify to the lowest terms.

8. $6 + 3\frac{1}{3} - 7 =$ _____

9. $8 - 2\frac{3}{4} + 4\frac{1}{7} =$ _____

10. $1 + 5\frac{1}{6} - 2\frac{2}{3} =$ _____

11. $4\frac{1}{2} \times 6\frac{1}{3} =$ _____

12. $3\frac{1}{6} \times \frac{1}{7} =$ _____

13. $2\frac{1}{3} \times 4\frac{2}{3} \times 3 =$ _____

14. $3\frac{1}{8} \div 2 =$ _____

15. $4\frac{1}{3} \div 2\frac{1}{5} =$ _____

Decimals
Round the decimal to the nearest whole number.

16. $537.64 =$ _____

17. $0.972 =$ _____

Round the decimal to the nearest hundredth.

18. $88.010 =$ _____

19. $1.0010 =$ _____

20. $5000.0016 =$ _____

Convert the fraction to a decimal.

21. $4\frac{3}{4} =$ _____

22. $2\frac{1}{2} =$ _____

Solve by adding or subtracting decimals. Round answer to the nearest tenth.

23. $80 - 54.33 + 17.21 =$ _____

24. $72.5 - 66.409 =$ _____

25. $66 + 34.667 + 91.3 =$ _____

Solve by multiplying decimals. Round answer to the nearest thousandth.

26. $7.234 \times 124.35 =$ _____

27. $27 \times 0.0001 =$ _____

28. $61.0001 \times 34.75 =$ _____

Solve by dividing decimals. Round answer to the nearest hundredth.

29. $98.5514 \div 88.58 =$ _____

30. $47.5 \div 22 =$ _____

Percents
Change the decimals to percents.

31. $0.050 =$ _____

32. $0.172 =$ _____

Change the percents to decimals.

33. $1.10\% =$ _____

34. $47.55\% =$ _____

35. $14.88\% =$ _____

Multiply percents.

36. 6% of 17 = _____

37. 25% of 34 = _____

Divide percents. Round the answer to a whole number

38. 3 is what percent of 70? _____

39. 12 is what percent of 60? _____

40. 25 is what percent of 175? _____

Continued

Chapter 6 PRETEST—cont'd

Solve for the unknown percent.

41. What is 15% of 500? _____

42. What is 90% of 90? _____

Solve for the unknown number using proportions.

43. 20 is 60% of what number? _____

44. 45 is 25% of what number? _____

45. 48 is 30% of what number? _____

Ratio and Proportion

Solve for *x* using proportions.

46. $2 : x :: 100 : 300$ _____

47. $5 : 100 :: 20 : x$ _____

48. $4 : x :: 8 : 32$ _____

49. $\dfrac{1}{4} : 500 :: \dfrac{1}{2} : x$ _____

50. $1\dfrac{1}{2} : x :: \dfrac{1}{2} : 200$ _____

FRACTIONS

Fractions, used in the apothecary and household system, are a method of writing a whole number that has been divided into parts (e.g., $\dfrac{1}{2}$, $3\dfrac{2}{5}$). Fractions are written with a **numerator** (number over the line), a *line* (meaning "divided by"), and a **denominator** (number under the line). When the number in the numerator is divided by the same number in the denominator, the equivalent is 1.

EXAMPLE 1: $\dfrac{2}{2} = 1, \dfrac{3}{3} = 1, \dfrac{12}{12} = 1$, and so forth.

Proper Fractions

With **proper fractions,** the numerator is always a lower number than the denominator.

EXAMPLE 2: In the fraction $\dfrac{1}{2}$, 1 is the numerator and 2 is the denominator. If a pizza is used as an example, the numerator states how many pieces of pizza have been taken, or a numerator of 1. The denominator of 2 states how many equal pieces the whole pizza has been divided into, or 2 equal pieces.

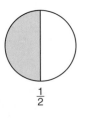

$\frac{1}{2}$

EXAMPLE 3: In the fraction $\dfrac{5}{6}$, 5 is the numerator and states how many equal pieces of the pizza have been taken. The denominator 6 states that there are six equal pieces to make one whole pizza. So $\dfrac{5}{6}$ of the pizza has been taken.

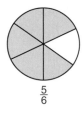

$\frac{5}{6}$

Improper Fractions

Improper fractions are fractions in which the numerator is equal to or greater than the denominator. For example, if two or more whole pizzas are equally divided and a portion is taken, an improper fraction can be formed. Improper fractions can be simplified to show how many whole pizzas + partial pizzas (pieces of pizza) exist. A whole number is formed when the numerator and denominator are the same or the numerator can be divided evenly by the denominator. A whole number plus a fraction occurs when the numerator is not divisible evenly by the denominator. The fractional portion left following division is the remainder.

EXAMPLE 4: If a pizza is cut into 8 equal pieces and we take all 8 pieces, the improper fraction to express this is $\dfrac{8}{8}$. The fraction $\dfrac{8}{8}$ is considered "improper" because a whole number can be shown instead. The whole number would be 1.

Two pizzas would be needed to increase the numerator to a number larger than 8. With two pizzas, each being equally cut into 8 pieces, there are now 16 possible pieces as numerators (8 pieces from one pizza and 8 pieces from the second pizza).

EXAMPLE 5: Two pizzas cut into 8 pieces are available, and you take 11 pieces. The improper fraction to describe the pizza taken would be $\dfrac{11}{8}$.

Equivalent Fractions

Equivalent fractions show two or more different fractions that are the same portion of the whole. Equivalent fractions (equal fractions) can be simplified to the same fraction.

The fractions have different numerical values but are equivalents, such as $\dfrac{1}{2}$ and $\dfrac{2}{4}$.

EXAMPLE 6: One pizza can be divided into any number of equal pieces, such as 6 pieces, 8 pieces, or even 12 pieces.

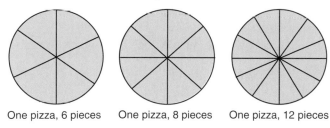

One pizza, 6 pieces   One pizza, 8 pieces   One pizza, 12 pieces

The equivalent fractions in this example are $\dfrac{6}{6}$, $\dfrac{8}{8}$, and $\dfrac{12}{12}$. If each pizza were divided into two equal halves, the equivalent fractions for each half of the pizza would then be shown as $\dfrac{3}{6}$, $\dfrac{4}{8}$, and $\dfrac{6}{12}$.

Simplifying Fractions to the Lowest Term

Fractions should be reduced to the lowest terms, or simplified. To simplify a fraction, divide the numerator and denominator by the largest number that divides evenly into both.

EXAMPLE 7: The fraction $\dfrac{3}{6}$ can be simplified to its lowest terms by dividing the numerator and denominator by 3: $\dfrac{3}{6} \div \dfrac{3}{3} = \dfrac{1}{2}$

And the largest number that will equally divide into $\dfrac{4}{8}$ is 4: $\dfrac{4}{8} \div \dfrac{4}{4} = \dfrac{1}{2}$

Finally, to simplify $\dfrac{6}{12}$, the largest number to divide by is 6: $\dfrac{6}{12} \div \dfrac{6}{6} = \dfrac{1}{2}$

In this example, the fractions $\dfrac{3}{6}$, $\dfrac{4}{8}$, and $\dfrac{6}{12}$ are also equivalent (or *equal*) fractions because when divided by the largest number possible, they are all simplified to the same final fraction of $\dfrac{1}{2}$. Therefore it can be stated that

$$\dfrac{3}{6} = \dfrac{4}{8} = \dfrac{6}{12} = \dfrac{1}{2}.$$

EXAMPLE 8:

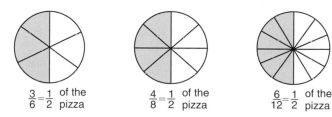

$\dfrac{3}{6} = \dfrac{1}{2}$ of the pizza $\dfrac{4}{8} = \dfrac{1}{2}$ of the pizza $\dfrac{6}{12} = \dfrac{1}{2}$ of the pizza

---

Check Your Understanding: FRACTIONS BOX 6-1

Identify each fraction; write (P) for a proper fraction, (I) for an improper fraction, or (E) for a fraction equivalent to 1.

1. $\dfrac{4}{4} =$ _____

2. $\dfrac{12}{10}$

3. $\dfrac{6}{5} =$ _____

4. $\dfrac{1}{2} =$ _____

5. $\dfrac{3}{3} =$ _____

Continued

Check Your Understanding: FRACTIONS BOX 6-1—cont'd

6. $\dfrac{11}{5} =$ _____

7. $\dfrac{3}{4} =$ _____

8. $\dfrac{20}{30} =$ _____

9. $\dfrac{1}{1} =$ _____

10. $\dfrac{2}{1} =$ _____

Change to as many equivalent fractions as possible.

11. $\dfrac{30}{90} =$ _____

12. $\dfrac{6}{24} =$ _____

13. $\dfrac{15}{60} =$ _____

14. $\dfrac{8}{32} =$ _____

15. $\dfrac{10}{40} =$ _____

Mixed Numbers

Improper fractions are those in which the numerator is greater than the denominator. When an improper fraction is simplified and written with a whole number and a fraction, the result is called a **mixed number.**

EXAMPLE 9: In Example 5, two pizzas were each cut into 8 pieces, and 11 pieces were taken. The improper fraction of $\dfrac{11}{8}$ can be simplified to $1\dfrac{3}{8}$, meaning one whole pizza plus three pieces of the second pizza were taken.

Remember to keep the 8 as the denominator because both pizzas are cut into 8 pieces.

Therefore the improper fraction is $\dfrac{11}{8}$ and the mixed number is $1\dfrac{3}{8}$.

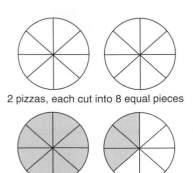

2 pizzas, each cut into 8 equal pieces

8 pieces + 3 pieces = 11 pieces

EXAMPLE 10: Always simplify the fraction to its lowest possible term. If we had taken 12 pieces of pizza from Example 5, the improper fraction would be $\dfrac{12}{8}$ and the mixed number would be $1\dfrac{4}{8}$, which can be simplified to $1\dfrac{1}{2}$.

The mixed number for $\dfrac{12}{8} = 1\dfrac{1}{2}$ (one whole pizza and $\dfrac{1}{2}$ of the second pizza).

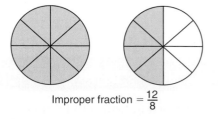

Improper fraction $= \dfrac{12}{8}$

Shortcut: When changing a mixed number to an improper fraction, multiply the whole number and denominator, then add the numerator to obtain the improper fraction.

Check Your Understanding: MIXED NUMBERS BOX 6-2

Change the improper fractions to mixed numbers.

1. $\dfrac{14}{3} =$ _____

2. $\dfrac{19}{2} =$ _____

3. $\dfrac{31}{5} =$ _____

4. $\dfrac{27}{4} =$ _____

5. $\dfrac{55}{7} =$ _____

6. $\dfrac{69}{8} =$ _____

7. $\dfrac{25}{6} =$ _____

8. $\dfrac{74}{9} =$ _____

9. $\dfrac{19}{3} =$ _____

10. $\dfrac{23}{8} =$ _____

Change the mixed numbers to improper fractions.

11. $1\dfrac{2}{5} =$ _____

12. $13\dfrac{3}{4} =$ _____

13. $6\dfrac{1}{2} =$ _____

14. $2\dfrac{5}{6} =$ _____

15. $4\dfrac{5}{6} =$ _____

16. $2\dfrac{3}{11} =$ _____

17. $17\dfrac{1}{4} =$ _____

18. $16\dfrac{3}{5} =$ _____

19. $5\dfrac{7}{10} =$ _____

20. $70\dfrac{1}{3} =$ _____

Simplify to lowest terms and show as mixed numbers.

21. $\dfrac{70}{8} =$ _____

22. $\dfrac{50}{24} =$ _____

23. $\dfrac{26}{6} =$ _____

24. $\dfrac{30}{4} =$ _____

25. $\dfrac{35}{10} =$ _____

26. $\dfrac{75}{9} =$ _____

27. $\dfrac{30}{20} =$ _____

28. $\dfrac{10}{4} =$ _____

29. $\dfrac{70}{16} =$ _____

30. $\dfrac{52}{14} =$ _____

Adding Fractions and Mixed Numbers with the Same Denominator

To add fractions with the same denominator, add the numerators of the fractions, then carry forward the denominator. Be sure to simplify improper fractions and mixed numbers to their lowest terms.

EXAMPLE 11: Solve: $\dfrac{1}{4} + \dfrac{2}{4} = ?$

The denominators are the same, so $\dfrac{1}{4} + \dfrac{2}{4} = \dfrac{3}{4}$

Before a mixed number can be used for calculations, it often has to be changed to an improper fraction. To do this, you need to know how to add fractions.

Recall that any fraction with the same numerator and denominator is equal to $1\left(\dfrac{8}{8} = 1\right)$.

EXAMPLE 12: Change $3\frac{1}{4}$ into an improper fraction.

STEP 1: Change the whole number into equivalent fractions:

$$3 = \frac{4}{4} + \frac{4}{4} + \frac{4}{4} \left(\text{same as saying } 3 = 1+1+1, \text{ because } \frac{4}{4} = 1 \right)$$

STEP 2: Add the numerators of the fractions and carry forward the denominator:

$$\frac{4}{4} + \frac{4}{4} + \frac{4}{4} + \frac{1}{4} = \frac{13}{4} \ (4+4+4+1=13)$$

Therefore the mixed number $3\frac{1}{4}$ is equivalent to the improper fraction $\frac{13}{4}$.

Adding Fractions and Mixed Numbers with Different Denominators

Often the denominators of fractions to be used are not the same, so additional steps are necessary because the lowest common denominator must be found before solving. For example, suppose there are two pizzas. The first pizza is cut into 5 equal pieces, and the second pizza is cut into 8 pieces.

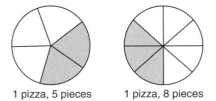

1 pizza, 5 pieces   1 pizza, 8 pieces

If 2 pieces are taken from the first pizza, the fraction is $\frac{2}{5}$. If 3 pieces are taken from the second pizza, the fraction is $\frac{3}{8}$. The total amount taken from the two pizzas can be determined by adding $\frac{2}{5} + \frac{3}{8}$.

EXAMPLE 13: Solve: $\frac{2}{5} + \frac{3}{8} = ?$

STEP 1: Make both denominators the same.

Do this by finding the smallest number that each denominator will divide into without leaving any remainder. This is called finding the **lowest common denominator (LCD)**. The number must be the same for both fractions and must be a multiple of the original denominators. Because $5 \times 8 = 40$, see if any number smaller than 40 can be divided by both 5 and 8 (the denominators). This method is also called finding the **lowest common multiple (LCM)**.

Do the math:

$5 \times 1 = 5$ $8 \times 1 = 8$
$5 \times 2 = 10$ $8 \times 2 = 16$
$5 \times 3 = 15$ $8 \times 3 = 24$
$5 \times 4 = 20$ $8 \times 4 = 32$
$5 \times 5 = 25$ $8 \times 5 = 40$
$5 \times 6 = 30$
$5 \times 7 = 35$
$5 \times 8 = 40$

By doing the math, we can verify that no number smaller than 40 divides equally into both denominators (5 and 8); therefore 40 is the LCD.

Replace each denominator with the number 40.

$$\frac{2}{5} = \frac{?}{40} \text{ and } \frac{3}{8} = \frac{?}{40}$$

STEP 1A: Write the first fraction: $\frac{2}{5} = \frac{?}{40}$

STEP 1B: Solve for ? by dividing the denominator into 40.

Do the math: $40 \div 5 = 8$

STEP 1C: Take the answer from Step 1B and multiply it by the numerator.

Do the math: $8 \times 2 = 16$

The first new equivalent fraction is $\frac{2}{5} = \frac{16}{40}$.

Recall from Example 4 that $\frac{8}{8}$ is the same as 1. Here is another way to do the math: $\frac{2}{5} \times \frac{8}{8} = \frac{16}{40}$

Continue this step by taking the second fraction and repeating Steps 1A, 1B, and 1C.

STEP 1A: Write the second fraction: $\frac{3}{8} = \frac{?}{40}$

STEP 1B: Solve for ? by dividing the denominator into 40: $40 \div 8 = 5$

STEP 1C: Take the answer from Step 1B and multiply it by the numerator.

Do the math: $3 \times 5 = 15$

The second new equivalent fraction is $\frac{3}{8} = \frac{15}{40}$.

STEP 2: Add the numerators, and carry forward the like denominators:

$$\frac{16}{40} + \frac{15}{40} = \frac{31}{40}$$

Therefore:

$$\frac{2}{5}+\frac{3}{8}=\frac{31}{40}$$

STEP 3: Simplify your final answer if possible. In this example, the answer $\frac{31}{40}$ cannot be further simplified.

EXAMPLE 14: Simplify the fraction in the following problem to the lowest form:

$$\frac{1}{5}+\frac{3}{10}=\frac{2}{10}+\frac{3}{10}=\frac{5}{10}\div\frac{5}{5}=\frac{1}{2}$$

Check Your Understanding: ADDING FRACTIONS BOX 6-3

Find the lowest common denominator for the two fractions.

1. $\frac{2}{5},\frac{3}{8}=$ _____

2. $\frac{1}{2},\frac{3}{7}=$ _____

3. $\frac{3}{4},\frac{1}{6}=$ _____

4. $\frac{1}{5},\frac{2}{3}=$ _____

5. $\frac{5}{6},\frac{4}{7}=$ _____

6. $\frac{1}{4},\frac{1}{5}=$ _____

7. $\frac{2}{3},\frac{1}{6}=$ _____

8. $\frac{1}{9},\frac{1}{10}=$ _____

9. $\frac{2}{5},\frac{5}{7}=$ _____

10. $\frac{1}{2},\frac{3}{4}=$ _____

Add the fractions. Simplify your answer if possible.

11. $\frac{1}{2}+\frac{3}{4}=$ _____

12. $\frac{5}{6}+\frac{1}{4}=$ _____

13. $\frac{1}{8}+\frac{1}{4}=$ _____

14. $\frac{2}{3}+\frac{5}{8}=$ _____

15. $\frac{1}{7}+\frac{1}{5}=$ _____

16. $\frac{2}{5}+\frac{5}{6}=$ _____

17. $\frac{1}{4}+\frac{2}{7}=$ _____

18. $\frac{4}{5}+\frac{1}{6}=$ _____

19. $\frac{1}{3}+\frac{4}{7}=$ _____

20. $\frac{6}{7}+\frac{3}{5}=$ _____

Subtracting Fractions

Subtracting fractions uses the same steps to find the LCD as adding fractions.

EXAMPLE 15: Solve: $\frac{5}{6}-\frac{1}{2}=?$

STEP 1: Make both denominators the same. The LCD for the denominators of 6 and 2 is 6. $\frac{5}{6}$ does not change; $\frac{1}{2}$ becomes $\frac{3}{6}$.

STEP 2: Subtract the numerators and carry forward the like denominators: $\frac{5}{6}-\frac{3}{6}=\frac{2}{6}$

STEP 3: Simplify the final fraction if possible. $\frac{2}{6}$ can be simplified to $\frac{1}{3}$.

Subtracting Fractions and Mixed Numbers

Subtracting fractions that use mixed numbers requires you to first change the mixed number to an improper fraction.

EXAMPLE 16: Solve: $1\frac{1}{2}-\frac{3}{4}=?$

STEP 1: Change $1\frac{1}{2}$ to an improper fraction (see Example 12): $1\frac{1}{2} = \frac{3}{2}$

STEP 2: Make the denominators the same LCD (4 in this case): $\frac{3}{2} = \frac{6}{4}$ and $\frac{3}{4}$

STEP 3: Subtract the numerators and simplify the answer if possible: $\frac{6}{4} - \frac{3}{4} = \frac{3}{4}$

Multiplying Fractions

To multiply two fractions, first multiply the two numerators, then multiply the two denominators. Simplify your answer if possible.

EXAMPLE 17: Solve: $\frac{1}{4} \times \frac{2}{5}$

STEP 1: Rewrite as $\frac{1 \times 2}{4 \times 5} = ?$

STEP 2: Multiply the numerators, then the denominators: $1 \times 2 = 2$ and $4 \times 5 = 20$, so the fraction is written as $\frac{2}{20}$

STEP 3: Simplify answer if possible: $\frac{2}{20} = \frac{1}{10}$

Use the following shortcuts to save time in obtaining the answer.

Shortcut: Cancel any numerator and denominator that can be divided equally by the same number. In this problem, the canceling would be as follows: $\frac{1}{\cancel{4}_{2}} \times \frac{\cancel{2}^{1}}{5}$. Therefore the answer will be $\frac{1}{2} \times \frac{1}{5}$ or $\frac{1}{10}$.

Check Your Understanding: SUBTRACTING FRACTIONS AND MIXED NUMBERS BOX 6-4

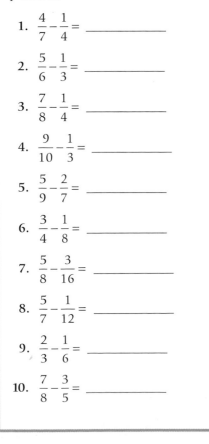

Find the LCD, then subtract. Simplify answer when possible.

1. $\frac{4}{7} - \frac{1}{4} =$ _____

2. $\frac{5}{6} - \frac{1}{3} =$ _____

3. $\frac{7}{8} - \frac{1}{4} =$ _____

4. $\frac{9}{10} - \frac{1}{3} =$ _____

5. $\frac{5}{9} - \frac{2}{7} =$ _____

6. $\frac{3}{4} - \frac{1}{8} =$ _____

7. $\frac{5}{8} - \frac{3}{16} =$ _____

8. $\frac{5}{7} - \frac{1}{12} =$ _____

9. $\frac{2}{3} - \frac{1}{6} =$ _____

10. $\frac{7}{8} - \frac{3}{5} =$ _____

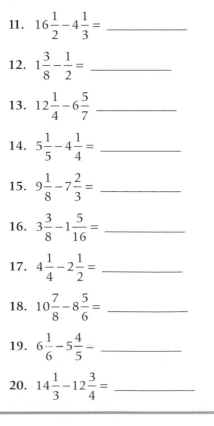

Change the mixed numbers into improper fractions, then subtract. Simplify answer to lowest terms when possible.

11. $16\frac{1}{2} - 4\frac{1}{3} =$ _____

12. $1\frac{3}{8} - \frac{1}{2} =$ _____

13. $12\frac{1}{4} - 6\frac{5}{7}$ _____

14. $5\frac{1}{5} - 4\frac{1}{4} =$ _____

15. $9\frac{1}{8} - 7\frac{2}{3} =$ _____

16. $3\frac{3}{8} - 1\frac{5}{16} =$ _____

17. $4\frac{1}{4} - 2\frac{1}{2} =$ _____

18. $10\frac{7}{8} - 8\frac{5}{6} =$ _____

19. $6\frac{1}{6} - 5\frac{4}{5} =$ _____

20. $14\frac{1}{3} - 12\frac{3}{4} =$ _____

Multiplying Mixed Numbers

EXAMPLE 18: Solve: $4\frac{1}{10} \times 5 = ?$

STEP 1: Change $4\frac{1}{10}$ to an improper fraction:

$$4\frac{1}{10} = \frac{41}{40}$$

$\left(\text{instead of } \dfrac{10}{10} + \dfrac{10}{10} + \dfrac{10}{10} + \dfrac{10}{10} + \dfrac{1}{10} = \dfrac{41}{10},\right.$

$\left. \text{multiply } 4 \times 10 + 1 = \dfrac{41}{10} \right)$

Then change 5 to an improper fraction by placing the 5 over the 1 or $\frac{5}{1}$. The problem now looks like this: $\frac{41}{10} \times \frac{5}{1} = ?$

STEP 2: Cancel (if possible) any numerators and denominators:

$$\frac{41}{10} \times \frac{5}{1} = \frac{41}{\cancel{10}_2} \times \frac{\cancel{5}^1}{1} = \frac{41}{2} \times \frac{1}{1}$$

STEP 3: Multiply across the numerator line and denominator line to solve: $\frac{41 \times 1}{2 \times 1} = \frac{41}{2}$

STEP 4: Simplify the fraction, and change it into a mixed number if possible: $\frac{41}{2} = 20\frac{1}{2}$

EXAMPLE 19: Solve: $\frac{2}{3} \times 3 \times 2\frac{3}{4} = ?$

STEP 1: Change to improper fractions:

$$\frac{2}{3} \times \frac{3}{1} \times \frac{11}{4} =$$

STEP 2: Simplify numerators and denominators:

$$\frac{\cancel{2}^1}{\cancel{3}_1} \times \frac{\cancel{3}^1}{1} \times \frac{11}{\cancel{4}_2} = \frac{1}{1} \times \frac{1}{1} \times \frac{11}{2}$$

STEP 3: Multiply across to solve:

$$\frac{1 \times 1 \times 11}{1 \times 1 \times 2} = \frac{11}{2}$$

STEP 4: Simplify the fraction, and change it into a mixed number if possible:

$$\frac{11}{2} = 5\frac{1}{2}$$

Check Your Understanding: MULTIPLYING FRACTIONS AND MIXED NUMBERS BOX 6-5

Cancel the numerator and denominator that can be divided equally by the same number, then multiply. Simplify when possible.

1. $\frac{2}{3} \times \frac{3}{4} =$ _____

2. $\frac{5}{6} \times \frac{8}{8} =$ _____

3. $\frac{1}{5} \times \frac{5}{8} =$ _____

4. $\frac{10}{12} \times \frac{1}{2} =$ _____

5. $\frac{1}{4} \times \frac{2}{7} =$ _____

Change the whole number into a fraction.

6. $17 =$ _____

7. $6 =$ _____

8. $4 =$ _____

9. $12 =$ _____

10. $3 =$ _____

Multiply, then simplify the answer when possible.

11. $\frac{1}{3} \times 2 \times \frac{5}{8} =$ _____

Continued

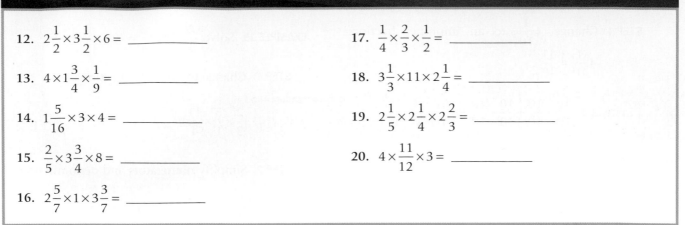

Check Your Understanding: MULTIPLYING FRACTIONS AND MIXED NUMBERS BOX 6-5—cont'd

12. $2\frac{1}{2} \times 3\frac{1}{2} \times 6 =$ _____

13. $4 \times 1\frac{3}{4} \times \frac{1}{9} =$ _____

14. $1\frac{5}{16} \times 3 \times 4 =$ _____

15. $\frac{2}{5} \times 3\frac{3}{4} \times 8 =$ _____

16. $2\frac{5}{7} \times 1 \times 3\frac{3}{7} =$ _____

17. $\frac{1}{4} \times \frac{2}{3} \times \frac{1}{2} =$ _____

18. $3\frac{1}{3} \times 11 \times 2\frac{1}{4} =$ _____

19. $2\frac{1}{5} \times 2\frac{1}{4} \times 2\frac{2}{3} =$ _____

20. $4 \times \frac{11}{12} \times 3 =$ _____

Dividing Fractions

When dividing fractions, invert the second fraction (also called the reciprocal) and then multiply the two fractions. The **reciprocal** of a fraction is the fraction "flipped" or inverted. The reciprocal of $\frac{1}{2}$ is $\frac{2}{1}$, the reciprocal of $\frac{3}{4}$ is $\frac{4}{3}$, the reciprocal of $\frac{11}{20}$ is $\frac{20}{11}$, and so forth. Simplify the answer after multiplication when possible, and write the answer as a mixed number.

EXAMPLE 20: Solve:

$$\frac{3}{4} \div \frac{1}{2} = ?$$

STEP 1: Find the reciprocal of the second fraction and change division sign to multiplication sign:

$$\frac{3}{4} \div \frac{1}{2} \text{ becomes } \frac{3}{4} \times \frac{2}{1}$$

STEP 2: Cancel the numerators and denominators that divide evenly:

$$\frac{3}{\cancel{4}_2} \times \frac{\cancel{2}^1}{1}$$

STEP 3: Multiply across to solve:

$$\frac{3}{2} \times \frac{1}{1} = \frac{3}{2}$$

STEP 4: Simplify the fraction, and change it into a mixed number if possible:

$$\frac{3}{2} = 1\frac{1}{2}$$

Dividing Mixed Numbers

To divide mixed numbers, the mixed number must first be changed to an improper fraction. Next, write whole numbers as fractions, and solve by inverting the second fraction (the reciprocal) and multiplying. Simplify if necessary.

EXAMPLE 21: Solve:

$$3\frac{5}{8} \div 2\frac{1}{2} = ?$$

STEP 1: Change to improper fractions:

$$3\frac{5}{8} = \frac{29}{8} \text{ and } 2\frac{1}{2} = \frac{5}{2}$$

The problem now looks like this:

$$\frac{29}{8} \div \frac{5}{2} = ?$$

STEP 2: Invert the second fraction, and change the sign from division to multiplication:

$$\frac{29}{8} \times \frac{2}{5} = ?$$

STEP 3: Cancel the numerators and denominators that divide evenly:

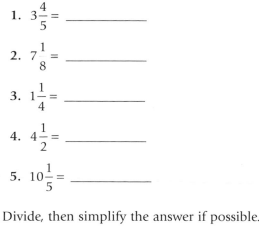

STEP 4: Multiply across to solve:

$$\frac{29}{4} \times \frac{1}{5} = \frac{29}{20}$$

STEP 5: Simplify the fraction, and change it into a mixed number if possible:

$$\frac{29}{20} = 1\frac{9}{20}$$

Check Your Understanding: DIVIDING FRACTIONS AND MIXED NUMBERS BOX 6-6

Change the mixed numbers to improper fractions.

1. $3\frac{4}{5} =$ _____

2. $7\frac{1}{8} =$ _____

3. $1\frac{1}{4} =$ _____

4. $4\frac{1}{2} =$ _____

5. $10\frac{1}{5} =$ _____

Divide, then simplify the answer if possible.

6. $4\frac{2}{5} \div \frac{1}{3} =$ _____

7. $3\frac{2}{3} \div \frac{1}{3} =$ _____

8. $7 \div 2\frac{5}{8} =$ _____

9. $5\frac{4}{9} \div 2\frac{1}{3} =$ _____

10. $2\frac{1}{2} \div 4 =$ _____

11. $4 \div \frac{5}{6} =$ _____

12. $6\frac{1}{2} \div 2\frac{3}{4} =$ _____

13. $8\frac{5}{9} \div 6\frac{1}{3} =$ _____

14. $1\frac{1}{36} \div \frac{5}{8} =$ _____

15. $10\frac{1}{5} \div 1\frac{1}{4} =$ _____

Check Your Understanding: FRACTION REVIEW BOX 6-7

Change to improper fractions.

1. $1\frac{2}{5} =$ _____

2. $2\frac{1}{3} =$ _____

Change to as many equivalent fractions as possible.

3. $\frac{4}{8} =$ _____

4. $\frac{8}{24} =$ _____

5. $\frac{17}{51} =$ _____

Change to mixed numbers.

6. $\frac{11}{8} =$ _____

7. $\frac{7}{2} =$ _____

8. $\frac{7}{4} =$ _____

Simplify to the lowest possible terms.

9. $\frac{27}{4} =$ _____

10. $\frac{18}{12} =$ _____

Continued

Check Your Understanding: FRACTION REVIEW
BOX 6-7—cont'd

11. $\dfrac{1}{3} + 1\dfrac{1}{2} =$ _____

12. $6 + 1\dfrac{3}{8} =$ _____

13. $7 - 2\dfrac{1}{3} =$ _____

14. $4\dfrac{1}{2} - 3\dfrac{2}{3} =$ _____

15. $2\dfrac{5}{8} - \dfrac{3}{4} =$ _____

16. $3\dfrac{2}{5} \times \dfrac{4}{7} \times \dfrac{1}{2} =$ _____

17. $\dfrac{2}{3} \times \dfrac{1}{2} \times \dfrac{3}{8} =$ _____

18. $4\dfrac{1}{3} \div 3 =$ _____

19. $6\dfrac{2}{5} \div 4\dfrac{1}{2} =$ _____

20. $4\dfrac{3}{4} \div 1\dfrac{1}{2} =$ _____

DECIMALS

Decimals are used to show a fractional part of a number. Metric measurements are expressed as decimals.

Decimal places appear to the right of a whole number that is followed by a decimal point to indicate a number less than 1. If no digit is to the left of the decimal point, a zero must be inserted to prevent errors (e.g., 0.5).

EXAMPLE 22: Look at this number: 432.1568

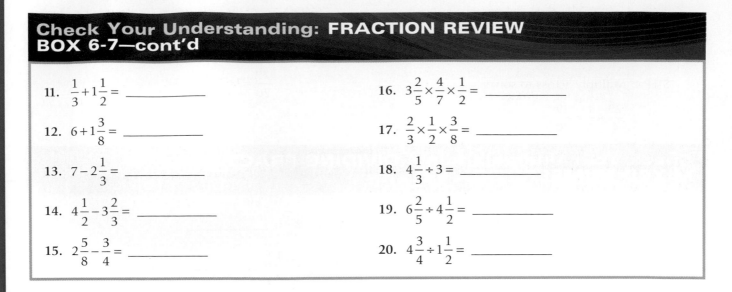

A decimal can be converted to a mixed number or fraction by dropping the decimal point, using the following rules:

- The digits to the left of the decimal point remain a whole number.
- The digits to the right of the decimal point become the numerator of the fraction.
- The denominator, when using decimals, becomes a power of 10, with one zero added for each number or decimal place to the right of the decimal point.

EXAMPLE 23: Convert 66.78 to a mixed number.

66 is the whole number.

78 becomes the numerator.

100 is the denominator because 78 is two places to the right of the decimal point, indicating hundredths.

The mixed number is $66\dfrac{78}{100}$.

LEARNING TIP

The decimal point acts as one place in the decimal.

Rounding Decimals

Decimals can be rounded to the nearest whole number or multiples of 10, usually in tenths, hundredths, or thousandths. Rounding shortens a decimal by dropping one or more digits to the right of the decimal point (e.g., 0.76 = 0.8 when rounding to tenths).

When rounding to a whole number, the digit 5 will determine how rounding will occur. If the last digit to the right of the decimal is less than 5, the whole number does not change and the digits after the decimal point are dropped. For example, to round 76.4 to a whole number, the whole number would remain 76. To round to places in the decimal, identify the desired place, such as tenth or hundredth, and follow the rule of rounding using 5 as the decision point. To round to hundredths, 16.444 would be rounded to 16.44.

When the decimal is 5 or larger, drop the decimal but increase the whole number to the next whole number. For example, to round 76.5 to a whole number, the whole number would be 77 and the .5 is dropped. If rounding to hundredths, 88.876 would be rounded to 88.88.

EXAMPLE 24: Round the following decimals to thousandths:

942.0099 ⟶ 942.010 (in this case, the final zero would be dropped, and the answer would be 942.01)

3.6666 ⟶ 3.667

0.9875 ⟶ 0.988

EXAMPLE 25: Round the following decimals to hundredths:

$$78.754 \longrightarrow 78.75$$

$$9.553 \longrightarrow 9.55$$

$$100.4893 \longrightarrow 100.49$$

EXAMPLE 26: Round the following decimals to tenths:

$$88.569 \longrightarrow 88.6$$

$$12.69 \longrightarrow 12.7$$

$$92.385 \longrightarrow 92.4$$

Check Your Understanding: ROUNDING DECIMALS BOX 6-8

Round the decimal to the nearest whole number.

1. 0.8 = _____

2. 42.35 = _____

3. 0.95 = _____

4. 100.41 = _____

5. 67.6 = _____

Round the decimals to the nearest tenth.

6. 33.67 = _____

7. 56.78 = _____

8. 54.11 = _____

9. 121.334 = _____

10. 600.707 = _____

Round the decimals to the nearest hundredth.

11. 233.332 = _____

12. 19.5726 = _____

13. 88.8883 = _____

14. 78.654 = _____

15. 100.0593 = _____

Round the decimals to the nearest thousandth.

16. 400.0099 = _____

17. 234.5574 = _____

18. 1616.1616 = _____

19. 357.9753 = _____

20. 357.9758 = _____

Converting Fractions to Decimals

To convert a proper fraction to a decimal, divide the numerator by the denominator. The answer will be a fraction of a whole number, or a decimal.

EXAMPLE 27: Convert the fraction $\frac{4}{5}$ to a decimal.

STEP 1: Divide the numerator by the denominator. Add the number 0 as many times as necessary to be able to complete the problem. (In the example, 5 will not divide into 4, but 5 will divide into 40, so one 0 is added.) Before adding a 0 in the numerator, place a decimal point after the numerator number. Then move the decimal point to the same place on the equivalent (answer) line.

$$
\begin{array}{r}
0. \\
5\overline{\smash{)}4.} \\
\end{array}
\quad \text{(5 does not go into 4, so add a zero.)}
$$

$$
\begin{array}{r}
0.8 \\
5\overline{\smash{)}4.0} \\
\underline{4.0} \\
0 \\
\end{array}
\quad \text{(Because a zero was added, the answer will have a decimal point.)}
$$

The answer is not 8, it is 0.8. Remember that any number that is only a decimal should show 0 before the decimal point to show no whole number is present before the decimal.

Therefore $\frac{4}{5} = 0.8$ (not .8)

When an improper fraction is converted to a decimal, the answer will contain a whole number and a remainder that is shown as a decimal.

EXAMPLE 28: Convert the improper fraction $\frac{21}{5}$ to a decimal.

STEP 1: The number 5 will go into 21 four times with a remainder of 1. Be sure the decimal is in the correct place.

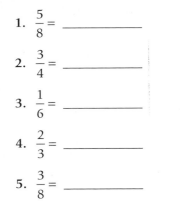

1   (5 will not go into 1, so add a zero.)

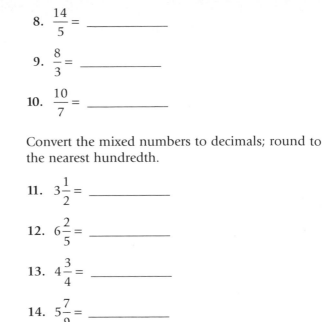

(Because a zero was added, the answer will have a decimal point.)

$$\frac{21}{5} \text{ or } 5\overline{)21} = 4.2$$

To convert a mixed number to a decimal, first change the mixed number to an improper fraction. Repeat the math in Example 27 to convert the answer to a decimal.

Check Your Understanding: CONVERTING FRACTIONS TO DECIMALS BOX 6-9

Convert the proper fractions to decimals. Round your answer to the nearest thousandth.

1. $\frac{5}{8} =$ _____

2. $\frac{3}{4} =$ _____

3. $\frac{1}{6} =$ _____

4. $\frac{2}{3} =$ _____

5. $\frac{3}{8} =$ _____

Convert the improper fractions to decimals; round answers to the nearest tenth.

6. $\frac{21}{2} =$ _____

7. $\frac{17}{9} =$ _____

8. $\frac{14}{5} =$ _____

9. $\frac{8}{3} =$ _____

10. $\frac{10}{7} =$ _____

Convert the mixed numbers to decimals; round to the nearest hundredth.

11. $3\frac{1}{2} =$ _____

12. $6\frac{2}{5} =$ _____

13. $4\frac{3}{4} =$ _____

14. $5\frac{7}{9} =$ _____

15. $2\frac{7}{11} =$ _____

Adding and Subtracting Decimals

To add or subtract numbers with decimals, the problem must be set up as a list of numbers with the decimal point of each number of the list being written directly below the decimal point in the previous number. After aligning the decimals, do the math calculation.

Place a decimal point after any whole numbers that are not followed by decimals.

Insert a decimal point and sufficient zeros after whole numbers to make all the decimals the same length as the decimal with the greatest number of places following the decimal point.

EXAMPLE 29: Find the sum of 64.3 + 18.00 + 0.33.

```
64.30
18.00
 0.33
─────
82.63
```

EXAMPLE 30: Find the difference of 69.3 − 5.94.

```
 69.30
− 5.94
──────
 63.36
```

Check Your Understanding: ADDING AND SUBTRACTING DECIMALS BOX 6-10

Add the following decimals.

1. 71.4 + 16.32 + 38 = _____

2. 53 + 14.762 + 9.3 = _____

3. 33.33 + 66.7 + 1245.121 = _____

4. 4.01 + 21.5 + 78.667 = _____

5. 0.001 + 1.34 + 654.2 = _____

6. 40.267 + 17.6 + 0.003 = _____

7. 123.5 + 688.8 + 99.99 = _____

8. 26.83 + 45.761 + 0.9 = _____

9. 9.1 + 8.23 + 765.124 = _____

10. 32 + 67.84 + 0.1 = _____

Subtract the following decimals.

11. 38.672 − 32.43 = _____

12. 142.637 − 14.263 = _____

13. 77.4 − 37.46 = _____

14. 44.62 − 14.01 = _____

15. 5.04 − 1.67 = _____

16. 374.5 − 98.44 = _____

17. 98.7 − 8.662 = _____

18. 0.4 − 0.016 = _____

19. 1.06 − 0.92 = _____

20. 246 − 0.91 = _____

Multiplying Decimals

When multiplying decimals, align the numbers without regard to the decimal points and calculate using regular multiplication rules.

To determine where to insert the decimal point after multiplication, count the number of decimal places in each line of the multiplication problem. In the answer, place the decimal point at the sum of the decimal places from each line, being sure to count from right to left.

EXAMPLE 31: Determine the product of 92.3 × 4.66.

STEP 1: Multiply without considering the decimal places:

```
    92.3
×   4.66
────────
    5538
   5538
   3692
────────
  430118
```

STEP 2: After finding an answer, find the number of decimal places in the answer by counting the one decimal place in 92.3 and two decimal places in 4.66. There are three decimal places total. Show the answer with three decimal places: 430.118.

Drop zeros that are not followed by any other digit in the answer when they are to the right of the decimal place. Remember to count decimal places from right to left of the answer.

Check Your Understanding: MULTIPLYING DECIMALS BOX 6-11

Multiply the following decimals, round answer to nearest hundredth.

1. $6.34 \times 42.44 = $ _____

2. $34.33 \times 16 = $ _____

3. $43.011 \times 17.92 = $ _____

4. $0.988 \times 942.01 = $ _____

5. $31.97 \times 16.3 = $ _____

6. $0.41 \times 2.34 = $ _____

7. $1.01 \times 0.011 = $ _____

8. $4.012 \times 77 = $ _____

9. $89.98 \times 76.4 = $ _____

10. $22.73 \times 15.5 = $ _____

Dividing Decimals

To divide decimals, the **divisor** must first be changed to a whole number by moving the decimal point. For each place that the decimal point is moved to the right in the divisor, the decimal point in the **dividend** is moved the same number of places to the right. Add zeros if necessary in the dividend to handle movement if decimal places are not sufficient for the number of places needed.

EXAMPLE 32: Determine the quotient: $\frac{5.32}{8}$

```
     0.665
 8 | 5.320
   − 4 8
   ─────
      52
    − 48
    ────
      40
    − 40
    ────
       0
```

EXAMPLE 33: Determine the quotient of $48.2 \div 0.68$ to the hundredth.

$0.68\overline{)48.2}$ First, move the two decimal places in the divisor.

$68\overline{)4820.}$ Now move the two decimal places in the dividend, add a zero to accommodate the decimal move, and drop the decimal point in the divisor and place a decimal point after the "0" in the dividend.

Do the math: The **quotient** is 70.88. This can be rounded to 70.9 or, if a whole number is desired, 71.

```
            70.88
 0.68 | 48.20.00
      − 47 6
      ──────
         600     (68 will not go into 60,
       − 544      so add zero.)
       ─────
         560     (68 will not go into 56,
       − 544      so add zero.)
       ─────
          16
```

Check Your Understanding: DIVIDING DECIMALS BOX 6-12

Divide the following decimals; round answer to nearest tenth.

1. $72.6 \div 31.5 = $ _____

2. $0.63 \div 3.11 = $ _____

3. $41.37 \div 6.777 = $ _____

4. $27.9 \div 3.33 = $ _____

5. $2.3 \div 0.76 = $ _____

6. $76.5 \div 41.5 = $ _____

7. $39.7 \div 18.4 = $ _____

8. $40.6 \div 5.12 = $ _____

9. $99.8 \div 16.22 = $ _____

10. $73.2 \div 37.8 = $ _____

Check Your Understanding: DECIMAL REVIEW BOX 6-13

Convert to mixed numbers. Do not simplify answer.

1. 32.84 = _____

2. 432.67 = _____

Round to the nearest whole number.

3. 33.333 = _____

4. 18.99 = _____

5. 0.88 = _____

Round to the nearest tenth.

6. 0.476 = _____

7. 3.717 = _____

Round to the nearest hundredth.

8. 99.8599 = _____

9. 0.3826 = _____

10. 345.678 = _____

Round to the nearest thousandth.

11. 68.2467 = _____

12. 4.2468 = _____

13. 1047.3218 = _____

Convert to decimals.

14. $\dfrac{7}{8}$ = _____

15. $17\dfrac{2}{5}$ = _____

Add; then round to the nearest hundredth.

16. 34.75 + 16.333 + 8 + 16.479 = _____

17. 16.334 + 31.6 + 34.567 + 17.889 = _____

18. 91.25 + 44.337 + 16.4 + 88 + 391.24 = _____

Subtract; then round to the nearest tenth.

19. 598.7 − 394.621 = _____

20. 34.5 − 1.047 = _____

Multiply; then simplify to the nearest whole number.

21. 91.47 × 16.3 = _____

22. 19 × 18.2 × 66.234 = _____

Divide; then simplify to the nearest thousandth.

23. 7.49 ÷ 6.33 = _____

24. 35.92 ÷ 14.64 = _____

25. 97 ÷ 33.66 = _____

PERCENTS

Percent (%) means "hundredths" or "parts per 100." Percents may be seen as a fraction (such as $\dfrac{1}{4}$%), a decimal (such as 0.25%), a whole number (such as 25%), or a mixed number (such as $1\dfrac{1}{4}$%).

Important step: When changing a percent that is expressed as a fraction, to a percent that is expressed as a decimal, remember that the result or number is still a percentage that must be changed to a decimal number for further calculations.

LEARNING TIP

Remember to change a fraction to a decimal by dividing the numerator by the denominator.

EXAMPLE 34: $\dfrac{1}{4}\% = 0.25\%$

and $1\dfrac{1}{4}\% = 1.25\%$

$2\dfrac{1}{2}\% = 2.5\%$, then divide by 100, so

$\dfrac{2.5}{100} = 0.025$

Changing Percents to Decimals

Drop the % sign. Then divide by 100 because the word "percent" means "part of a hundred." The division causes the decimal to move two places to the *left*.

EXAMPLE 35: 4% becomes $\dfrac{4}{100}$ or 0.04

1.8% becomes $\dfrac{1.8}{100}$ or 0.018

Hint: Remember to carry the decimal point from the percent problem to the fractional problem.

Percents that contain a fraction must first be changed to decimal percents before dividing by 100.

EXAMPLE 36: $\dfrac{1}{4}\% = 0.25\%$ then divide by 100, so

$\dfrac{.25}{100} = 0.0025$

Hint: Be sure to keep the decimal point in the correct place in the numerator when dividing by 100.

Changing Decimals to Percents

First, multiply the decimal by 100. This causes the decimal to be moved two places to the right. Second, add a % sign.

EXAMPLE 37: 2.64 becomes 264%

$2.64 \times 100 = 264.0$

264 becomes 264%

EXAMPLE 38: 0.022 becomes 2.2%

$0.022 \times 100 = 2.2$

2.2 becomes 2.2%

Check Your Understanding: CHANGING PERCENTS TO DECIMALS BOX 6-14

Change the percents to decimals. Round your answers to the nearest hundredth.

1. $\dfrac{2}{3}\% =$ _____

2. 8% = _____

3. $4\dfrac{1}{2}\% =$ _____

4. $64\dfrac{3}{4}\% =$ _____

5. 31% = _____

6. 5.5% = _____

7. $7\dfrac{7}{8}\% =$ _____

8. $3\dfrac{1}{3}\% =$ _____

9. $17\dfrac{7}{10}\% =$ _____

10. $98\dfrac{7}{10}\% =$ _____

Check Your Understanding: CHANGING DECIMALS TO PERCENTS BOX 6-15

Change the decimals to percents; simplify answers to nearest tenth.

1. 3.59 = _____

2. 44.2 = _____

3. 0.06 = _____

4. 7.34 = _____

5. 0.047 = _____

Check Your Understanding: CHANGING DECIMALS TO PERCENTS BOX 6-15—cont'd

6. 0.0352 = _____

7. 1.17 = _____

8. 78.421 = _____

9. 0.055 = _____

10. 3.672 = _____

Multiplying Percents

In the statement "Find 5% of 20," the term "of" means to multiply a number by a percent. The first step is to change the percent to a decimal: 5% becomes 0.05. Next, multiply the number found in the problem by the decimal: $20 \times 0.05 = 100$ (before correct decimal placement). The final step is to input the correct number of decimal places. In the example, 0.05 has two decimal places, so the answer, 100, would need two decimal places. The answer is 1 (1.00).

Hint: Remember to move decimal places from right to left, and always drop zeros that appear after the decimal point (called trailing zeros).

EXAMPLE 39: Find 3% of 42.

STEP 1: Change % to a decimal: 3% = 0.03

STEP 2: Multiply: $42 \times 0.03 = 126$

STEP 3: Input decimal places as needed. Two decimals in step 1 (0.03) means the answer has two decimal places. Answer = 1.26

In the next example, an additional step must be performed because the mixed number must be changed to decimal form. Change the mixed number to an improper fraction, then (as in Example 28) convert the improper fraction to a decimal before attempting to find the percent.

EXAMPLE 40: Find $3\frac{1}{2}$% of 90

STEP 1: $3\frac{1}{2}$ is the same as $\frac{7}{2}$, which in decimal form is 3.5 ($\frac{1}{2}$ can be changed to 0.5% by dividing 2 into 1 to obtain 3.5%)

STEP 2: Change % to a decimal: 3.5% = 0.035

STEP 3: Multiply $90 \times 0.035 = 3150$

STEP 4: Input decimal places as needed. Three decimals in step 2 (0.035) means the answer has three decimal places. Answer = 3.150 (same as 3.15 because the last zero should be deleted because it is not necessary, as 15 hundredths is equivalent to 150 thousandths, drop the trailing zero)

Check Your Understanding: MULTIPLYING PERCENTS BOX 6-16

Multiply by a percent; round answers to nearest hundredth.

1. 14% of 28 = _____

2. $3\frac{1}{2}$% of 17 = _____

3. $6\frac{2}{3}$% of 80 = _____

4. $5\frac{1}{4}$% of 14 = _____

5. 19% of 75 = _____

6. 27% of 10 = _____

7. 48% of 100 = _____

8. 11% of 20 = _____

9. 82% of 19 = _____

10. $\frac{41}{2}$% of 11 = _____

Dividing Percents

Dividing percents answers the question of "what." To find "what" percentage one number is of another number, use these steps:

STEP 1: Set up the problem as a fraction.

STEP 2: Simplify the fraction (if possible).

STEP 3: Divide the fraction's denominator into its numerator to obtain a decimal.

STEP 4: Change the decimal to a percent.

EXAMPLE 41: 15 is what percent of 45?

STEP 1: Write as a fraction: $\dfrac{15}{45}$

STEP 2: Simplify the fraction: $\dfrac{15}{45} = \dfrac{1}{3}$

STEP 3: Divide $3\overline{)1.00} = 0.33$

STEP 4: Change step 3 answer to a percent: $0.33 = 33\%$

Check Your Understanding: DIVIDING PERCENTS BOX 6-17

Divide by a percent. Round your answer to tenths.

1. 70 is what percent of 84? _____

2. 32 is what percent of 50? _____

3. 14 is what percent of 77? _____

4. 11 is what percent of 15? _____

5. 3 is what percent of 7? _____

6. 15 is what percent of 19? _____

7. 2 is what percent of 13? _____

8. 44 is what percent of 63? _____

9. 7 is what percent of 77? _____

10. 4 is what percent of 9? _____

Using Fractions to Figure Percentages

With this method, two fractions will be determined. The first fraction will show the numbers given in the problem. The second fraction will show a number as a percentage of 100. The unknown number in either fraction is labeled x. Set up the two fractions as shown in the following example. Then solve for x—identified by "what." Use an equals sign (=), identified by "is," to indicate equality when showing the relationship between two equal fractions. Always round the answer to the nearest whole number.

Formula for fractions: $\dfrac{a}{b} = \dfrac{c}{d}$

a—Numerator for fraction one is the amount or part of a whole portion being compared to the base. May be a number found in the problem or may be the unknown.

b—Denominator for fraction one is the base or the whole in the problem or standard used for comparison. The base often follows the word "of." This may be a number found in the problem or may be the unknown.

c—Numerator for fraction two will be a percent of 100 (the number or unknown followed by %) and may be the unknown.

d—Denominator for fraction two will always be 100 when solving for percents.

The letters a, b, or c can be the unknown, so any one of these letters can be labeled x in a given problem. When percents are being found, the letter d is always 100 because it signifies 100%.

For example: What is 20% of 200?

$$\downarrow \quad \downarrow \quad \downarrow \quad \downarrow \quad \downarrow$$
$$a \;=\; c \;\times\; b$$

Note: The 20% is c because the % sign is attached; d is always 100; what is unknown; 200 is base.

$$\frac{x(a)}{200(b)} = \frac{20(c)}{100(d)}$$

A problem can be stated three different ways when fractions are used. The following three examples show each way the question can be asked, followed by the solution. The most difficult part of the problem is understanding what is unknown and then correctly placing the understood x into either the a, b, or c part of the fraction.

EXAMPLE 42: 15 is what percent of 45?

When a problem is asked like Example 42, the unknown "what" is the percentage. The number beside the word "is" becomes the numerator of fraction one. The number beside the word "of" becomes the denominator of fraction one. In the second fraction, x is used for the percentage over 100. Using the formula shown earlier, the letter $a = 15$, $b = 45$, $c = x$, and $d = 100$.

STEP 1: Set up the problem as two equivalent fractions:

$$\frac{15 \ \text{(portion of base)}}{45 \ \text{(base)}} = \frac{x \ \text{(percent)}}{100}$$

STEP 2: Cross-multiply:

$$45 \times (x) = 15 \times 100$$
$$45x = 1500$$

STEP 3: Isolate the x so that it is by itself (by dividing both sides by 45):

$$x = \frac{1500}{45}$$
$$x = 3333$$

STEP 4: Remember that you must still move the decimal two places to the left and add a percent sign to obtain an answer shown as a percent. Show final answer in whole percentage number only:

$$x = 33.33 \text{ will be written as } 33\%.$$

The fractions in this problem could have been simplified. $\frac{15}{45}$ is the same as $\frac{1}{3}$. The answer would still be the same: $x = 33\%$.

EXAMPLE 43: 15 is 33% of what number?

In Example 43, the unknown "what" is a number. Therefore the unknown x is in the first fraction, and the second fraction is $\frac{33}{100}$. The number beside the word "is" becomes the numerator of fraction one. The denominator of fraction one is the unknown.

STEP 1: Set up the problem as two equivalent fractions:

$$\frac{15 \ \text{(portion of base)}}{x \ \text{(base)}} = \frac{33 \ \text{(percent)}}{100}$$

STEP 2: Cross-multiply:

$$33x = 1500$$

STEP 3: Isolate x:

$$x = \frac{1500}{33}$$
$$x = 45.45$$

STEP 4: Show the answer as a whole number only. Hint: Always remember what you are solving for. You may be solving for a percent or a number. In this problem, you are looking for a number, so:

$$x = 45$$

EXAMPLE 44: What number is 33% of 45?

In Example 44, the unknown "what" is a number; therefore the unknown x is in the first fraction, and the second fraction is $\frac{33}{100}$. Because there is no number beside the word "is," the numerator in fraction one is x. The denominator in fraction one is 45. Use the formula shown previously.

STEP 1: Set up the problem as two equivalent fractions:

$$\frac{x \ \text{(portion of base)}}{45 \ \text{(base)}} = \frac{33 \ \text{(percent)}}{100}$$

STEP 2: Cross-multiply:

$$100x = 1485$$

STEP 3: Isolate x:

$$\frac{100x}{100} = \frac{1485}{100}$$
$$x = 14.85$$

STEP 4: Show the answer as a whole number:
$$x = 15$$

Check Your Understanding: USING FRACTIONS TO FIGURE PERCENTS BOX 6-18

Using the equation method, translate the following and solve. Round to whole numbers.

1. What number is 25% of 40? _____

2. 16 is what % of 64? _____

3. 15 is 60% of what number? _____

4. 30 is what % of 90? _____

5. 5 is 10% of what number? _____

6. What number is 3% of 90? _____

7. What number is 25% of 500? _____

8. 4 is what % of 80? _____

9. 12 is 40% of what number? _____

10. 13 is 5% of what number? _____

Using an Equation to Figure a Percentage

To solve percentage problems using an equation, the parts of the problem are translated to the equivalent parts. Remember "of" translates to "times"; "what" translates to the unknown or "x"; "is" translates to "=."

For example, what (x) is (=) 20% of ($\times$) 200?

$x = 0.2 \times 200$

Note: 20% has been changed to a decimal for calculation.

$x = 40$

The following are the same as Examples 42 to 44, placed in the equation method.

EXAMPLE 45: 15 is what percent of 45?

$$15 = x \quad \times 45$$
$$45x = 15$$
$$x = 33.33\% \text{ or } 33\%$$

EXAMPLE 46: 15 is 33% of what number?

$$15 = .33 \quad \times \quad x$$
$$.33x = 15$$
$$x = 45.45 \text{ or } 45$$

EXAMPLE 47: What number is 33% of 45?

$$x \quad = .33 \times 45$$
$$x = 14.85 \text{ or } 15$$

Check Your Understanding: PERCENT REVIEW BOX 6-19

Change to decimals.

1. $\frac{1}{2}\% =$ _____

2. $3\frac{1}{4}\% =$ _____

3. $1.44\% =$ _____

4. $7.25\% =$ _____

5. $33\frac{1}{3}\% =$ _____

Change to percents.

6. $1.89 =$ _____

7. $72.34 =$ _____

8. $0.0631 =$ _____

9. $0.05 =$ _____

10. $0.11 =$ _____

Check Your Understanding: PERCENT REVIEW
BOX 6-19—cont'd

Solve, round answer to nearest tenth.

11. 27% of 2 = _____

12. 70% of 44 = _____

13. 66.67% of 49 = _____

14. $84\frac{1}{2}$% of 99 = _____

15. $33\frac{1}{2}$% of 50 = _____

Solve, writing as a percent. Round answer to a whole percent.

16. 20 is what percent of 80? _____

17. 67 is what percent of 200? _____

18. $\frac{1}{2}$ is what percent of 2? _____

19. 30 is what percent of 45? _____

20. $4\frac{3}{4}$ is what percent of 19? _____

Solve for the number. Round answer to a whole number.

21. 6 is 10% of what number? _____

22. 20 is 25% of what number? _____

23. 25 is 50% of what number? _____

24. 30 is 70% of what number? _____

25. 2 is 60% of what number? _____

Solve for the number. Round answer to a whole number.

26. What number is 15% of 45?

27. What number is 40% of 80?

28. What number is 5% of 55?

29. What number is 80% of 60?

30. What number is 25% of 16?

RATIO AND PROPORTION

A **ratio** shows a relationship between two numbers by using a colon to separate the numbers.

A **proportion** shows the relationship between two equal ratios or fractions.

The **proportional method** is used to find the relationships between ratios, including finding unknowns and dosage calculations.

Use two colons (::) to show a relationship between two ratios.

EXAMPLE 48: This is a ratio: 1:3
This is a ratio: 2:6
This is a proportion: 1:3 :: 2:6

Note that if you divide the second ratio by 2, the two ratios are identical.

Solving for x in a Proportion

In a proportion, the **product** of the means must equal the product of the extremes. In the following proportion,

multiply the extremes together (1×8) and then multiply the means together (4×2). Therefore $1 \times 8 = 4 \times 2$.

$$\overset{\ulcorner \quad \text{extremes} \quad \urcorner}{1:4 \quad :: \quad 2:8}$$
$$\underset{\llcorner \text{means} \lrcorner}{}$$

Knowing that proportions must be equal makes it easy to solve for an unknown part of the equation. Let x stand for the unknown.

If the problem is $x:3 :: 2:6$, solve for the unknown x by multiplying.

STEP 1: Multiply the extremes together: $x \times 6 = 6x$

STEP 2: Multiply the means together: $3 \times 2 = 6$

STEP 3: The problem would now be $6x = 6$. Isolate x by dividing each side by the number that is in front of x. In this problem, divide by 6. This will allow x to be equal to 1.

STEP 4: Prove the computation by replacing x in the original problem with your answer. The answers of the means and extremes should be equal.

EXAMPLE 49: Solve for x in this proportion: $1:x::2:8$

STEP 1: Multiply extremes: $1 \times 8 = 8$

STEP 2: Multiply means: $2 \times x = 2x$

STEP 3: Isolate x by dividing by 2:

$$\frac{2x}{2} = \frac{8}{2}$$

$$x = 4$$

STEP 4: Prove answer: $1:4::2:8$ The means and extremes are equal; therefore this is a true proportion.

Check Your Understanding: RATIO AND PROPORTION BOX 6-20

Solve for x in the proportions.

1. $5:x :: 4:20$ $x =$ _____

2. $1:3 :: 3:x$ $x =$ _____

3. $11:22 :: x:44$ $x =$ _____

4. $16:20 :: 4:x$ $x =$ _____

5. $50:x :: 3:9$ $x =$ _____

6. $4:x :: 32:16$ $x =$ _____

7. $x:14 :: 12:24$ $x =$ _____

8. $6:24 :: 1:x$ $x =$ _____

9. $8:2 :: x:4$ $x =$ _____

10. $x:30 :: 5:6$ $x =$ _____

11. $x:5 :: 12:10$ $x =$ _____

12. $64:2 :: 32:x$ $x =$ _____

13. $1:9 :: x:81$ $x =$ _____

14. $8:250 :: x:125$ $x =$ _____

15. $6:x :: 3:1$ $x =$ _____

16. $x:9 :: 3:1$ $x =$ _____

17. $2:x :: 4:250$ $x =$ _____

18. $x:325 :: 1:650$ $x =$ _____

19. $3:600 :: 2:x$ $x =$ _____

20. $10:100 :: 25:x$ $x =$ _____

USING RATIO AND PROPORTION TO FIGURE PERCENTS

The method of using ratio and proportion to figure the percent is similar to the fractional method once you have determined x. The first ratio will show the numbers in the problem, and the second ratio will show a number as a percentage of 100. The unknown number in either ratio is labeled x. Set up the two ratios as a proportion (as shown in the following example). Remember to use one colon (:) between the numbers in a ratio and two colons (::) to show a relationship between the two ratios. Round the answer to the nearest whole number.

Formula for Ratio and Proportion

$a:b::c:d$

a = One of the extremes is the amount or part of the whole portion being compared with the base, always a number or the unknown variable in the first ratio.

b = One of the means or the whole number in the problem or the standard used for comparison, always a number or the unknown variable in the first ratio.

c = One of the means; when figuring percents, "c" will always be a percent of 100. In practical applications, this number is a portion of the total of an item.

d = One of the extremes; when figuring percents, this will always be 100. When using practical applications this number is the total amount of an item.

The following three examples show each way a ratio and proportion question can be asked using percents, followed by the solution.

The letter *a*, *b*, or *c* can be the unknown, so any one of these letters can be labeled *x* in a given problem. In the following examples, letter *d* is always 100 for 100%.

EXAMPLE 50: 15 is what % of 45?

In this example, the two numbers being compared are 15 and 45. Set the first ratio up to express this comparison. The second ratio is asking "what" percent 15 is to 45, so the "unknown" is a percent. Hint: Recall that a proportion is a comparison between two equivalent ratios. Using the formula shown earlier, the letter a = 15, b = 45, c = x, and d = 100.

STEP 1: Set up the two ratios. The numbers in the first ratio are given. The "what" is the percent:

$15:45 :: x:100$

STEP 2: Multiply the means and the extremes:

$45 \times x = 15 \times 100$

$45x = 1500$

STEP 3: Isolate the *x* so that it is by itself (by dividing both sides by 45):

$$\frac{45x}{45} = \frac{1500}{45}$$

$x = 33.33$

STEP 4: Because the question is asking for a percent, round off as needed, add a percent sign, and write as a whole number:

$x = 33.33$ will be written as 33%

If you wish to prove your answer, replace the *x* with 33 in the original problem.

$15:45 :: 33:100$

The answer is correct because 1500 is approximately equal to 1485. Remember that you rounded from 33.33% to 33%.

The problem can be asked three different ways depending on what is known or given, as well as where the *x* is placed in the proportion. In Examples 50 to 53, the same numbers found in previous examples are used to show how to set up the problem using ratios and proportions.

EXAMPLE 51: 21 is what percent of 35?

STEP 1: Set up the two ratios. The numbers in the first ratio are given. The "what" is the percent:

$21:35 :: x:100$

STEP 2: Multiply the means and the extremes:

$21 \times 100 = 35 \times x$

$2100 = 35x$

STEP 3: Isolate the *x*:

$x = 60$

STEP 4: The problem is asking for a percent, so the answer will be 60%.

EXAMPLE 52: 21 is 60% of what number?

STEP 1: Set up the two ratios. Only one number in the first ratio is given. The "what" is the second number. The percents are given:

$21:x :: 60:100$

STEP 2: Multiply the means and the extremes:

$21 \times 100 = 60 \times x$

$2100 = 60x$

STEP 3: Isolate the *x*:

$x = 35$

STEP 4: The problem is asking for a number, so the answer will be 35.

EXAMPLE 53: What number is 60% of 35?

STEP 1: Set up the two ratios. Only one number in the first ratio is given. The "what" is the first number. The percents are given:

$x:35 :: 60:100$

STEP 2: Multiply the means and the extremes:

$x \times 100 = 35 \times 60$

$100x = 2100$

STEP 3: Isolate the *x*:

$x = 21$

STEP 4: The problem is asking for a number, so the answer will be 21.

Check Your Understanding: USING PROPORTIONS TO FIGURE PERCENTS BOX 6-21

Solve for the unknown number using the proportional method. Round answer to the nearest whole number.

1. What number is 12% of 500? _____

2. What number is 70% of 250? _____

3. What number is 81% of 11? _____

4. What number is 66% of 75? _____

5. What number is 34% of 60? _____

6. What number is 22% of 21? _____

7. What number is 47% of 400? _____

8. What number is 53% of 19? _____

9. What number is 38% of 70? _____

10. What number is 85% of 90? _____

Solve for the unknown number using the proportional method. Round answer to the nearest whole number.

11. 16 is 25% of what number? _____

12. 32 is 10% of what number? _____

13. 50 is 40% of what number? _____

14. 5 is $33\frac{1}{3}$% of what number? _____

15. 14 is 75% of what number? _____

16. 3 is 20% of what number? _____

17. 7 is 15% of what number? _____

18. 11 is 5% of what number? _____

19. 72 is 90% of what number? _____

20. 60 is 80% of what number? _____

PRACTICAL APPLICATIONS

Many applications in a medical facility require the practical use of basic mathematical calculations. The math problems will not be set up for you, and often setting up the problem correctly is the most difficult part of finding a solution. Always check your calculations by placing your answer into the original math problem in place of x. The following section shows a ration and proportion math calculation used in inventory replacement and in determining medication administration.

EXAMPLE 54: There are 24 ampules of Xylocaine in one box of medication. How many ampules of Xylocaine are in two boxes?

STEP 1: Set up the two ratios. The numbers in the first ratio are given:

24 ampules : 1 box :: x ampules :: 2 boxes

STEP 2: Multiply the means and the extremes:

$1 \times x = 2 \times 24$

$x = 48$

STEP 3: Normally you need to isolate the x in Step 3 but because $x \times 1 = x$, skip Step 3 in this problem.

STEP 4: Determine what the problem is asking for (ampules). Since $x = 48$, the correct answer is 48 ampules.

When working with ratios and proportions that contain unit of measure descriptions such as mg, mL, inches, and teaspoons, both ratios in the proportion must contain the same units.

EXAMPLE 55: A dose of 500 mg of amoxicillin sodium is prescribed. On hand is amoxicillin sodium 250 mg/5 mL. How many milliliters would be given for the order using the dosage strength on hand?

STEP 1: Set up the two ratios. The numbers in the first ratio are given.

$$250 \text{ mg} : 5 \text{ mL} :: 500 \text{ mg} : x$$

STEP 2: Multiply the means and the extremes:

$$250 \times x = 5 \times 500$$

$$250x = 2500$$

STEP 3: Isolate the x by multiplying both sides by 250:

$$\frac{250\,x}{250} = \frac{2500}{250}$$

$$x = 10$$

STEP 4: Determine what the problem is asking for (milliliters). Be sure to include the proper measurement in your answer. The correct answer is 10 mL.

Check Your Understanding: RATIO AND PROPORTION
REVIEW BOX 6-22

Solve for x.

1. $1 : x :: 3 : 12$ $x = $ _____

2. $x : \dfrac{1}{2} :: 7 : 3\dfrac{1}{2}$ $x = $ _____

3. $4 : 5 :: 16 : x$ $x = $ _____

4. $4 : 5 :: x : 15$ $x = $ _____

5. $0.2 : 0.8 :: x : 0.16$ $x = $ _____

Solve the following word problems. Set each one up as a ratio and a proportion.

PAIN

6. A patient has *ibuprofen* that is available in 100 mg/5 mL. The physician desires that ibuprofen 50 mg be administered. What quantity of ibuprofen should be administered to the patient? _____

7. A prescription reads "take two tablets four times a day." If the patient takes the prescription correctly, how many tablets will he or she have taken by the end of 1 week? (Hint: Figure the number of tablets needed in a day first.) _____

8. After reconstituting a medication, if a 200-mg dosage strength is prescribed, what volume of the 300 mg/0.5 mL solution would be prepared to provide a 200-mg dose? _____

9. If $2\dfrac{1}{2}$ tablets of *dextroamphetamine* contain 25 mg of medication, how many tablets equal 15 mg?

_____

Continued

Check Your Understanding: RATIO AND PROPORTION REVIEW
BOX 6-22—cont'd

10. A dose of *Prozac* 60 mg is prescribed. On hand is Prozac 20 mg/5 mL. How many milliliters of Prozac would be given for the order using the dosage strength on hand? _____

11. When *Humulin R* is 100 U/1 mL, how many milliliters would 20 units of Humulin R be? _____

12. When *Acthar Gel* 80 units/1 mL is available for an order, how many milliliters would be needed for *Acthar Gel* 60 units? _____

13. One kilogram is equivalent to 2.2 pounds. What is the kilogram equivalent for 110 pounds? _____

14. One kilogram is equivalent to 2.2 pounds. An 80 kg person would weigh how many pounds? _____

15. The patient's total daily dose of *sulfamethoxazole* is 1000 mg. The drug is available in 500 mg tablets. How many tablets would the patient take daily? _____

16. A cleaning solution is to be diluted 1 teaspoon to 64 oz of water. How much water would be added to a container containing $\frac{1}{4}$ teaspoon of cleaning solution? _____

17. One hour is 60 minutes. What fractional part of an hour is 45 minutes? _____

18. If 1 tablet of *chlorothiazide* (Diuril) is equivalent to 250 mg, how many milligrams would $2\frac{1}{2}$ tablets be? _____

19. 1000 mg is equivalent to 1 g. What is the milligram equivalent for 0.9 g? _____

20. *Amoxicillin/clavulanate potassium* (Augmentin) is supplied in the oral suspension of 200 mg/5 mL. If amoxicillin/clavulanate potassium 300 mg is ordered every 8 hours, how many milliliters would be prepared for one dose? _____

Measurement Systems and Their Equivalents

OBJECTIVES

After studying this chapter, you should be capable of doing the following:

- Identifying the basic units of measure in the metric system and their abbreviations.
- Writing metric measurements in correct notation.
- Converting within metric measurement units.
- Discussing the limited use of the apothecary system and the units of measure within the system.

- Using symbols and Roman numerals in the apothecary system.
- Identifying the basic units of measure in the household system and their abbreviations.
- Explaining units and milliequivalents in determining drug measurements.
- Identifying current trends in the use of symbols and abbreviations.

KEY TERMS

Apothecary	Grain	Liter	Milliequivalent
Apothecary system	Gram	Meter	Minim
Dram	Household system	Metric system	Unit

Chapter 7 PRETEST: MEASUREMENT SYSTEMS AND THEIR EQUIVALENTS

Answer the following questions.

1. Name the three base metric units of measure. _____

2. Provide abbreviations for the following metric terms:

    kilogram _____   microgram _____

    centimeter _____   milliliter _____

3. Write the correct metric notation for "three hundred twenty centimeters." _____

Continued

Chapter 7 PRETEST: MEASUREMENT SYSTEMS AND THEIR EQUIVALENTS—cont'd

4. Determine the answer:

   2.8 m = _____ cm   2500 mcg = _____ mg

   850 mg = _____ g   3250 cc = _____ mL

   0.78 kg = _____ g   2.8 L = _____ mL

5. Supply the equivalents using the household measurement system.

   90 gtts = _____ t

   1 qt = _____ c

   1 c = _____ T

   48 in = _____ yd

   8 oz = _____ lb

METRIC SYSTEM

The **metric system** originated in France more than 200 years ago. It is sometimes referred to as the *SI system*, from the French words, *Système International*. The metric system, used in more than 90% of developed countries, is based on the decimal system and is the international standard for scientific and industrial measurements. The United States has been slow to adopt the metric system and still relies heavily on the household method of measurement (sometimes referred to as the *English measurement system*). Today in the United States, many items are labeled in the metric and household systems. The metric system uses the decimal (or base 10) numbering system. By simply moving the decimal point, one can move within the metric system to other metric units (e.g., 12 mm = 1.2 cm).

Three basic units of measure exist in the metric system. The basic unit of weight is the **gram.** The basic unit of volume is the **liter.** The basic unit of length is the **meter.** In medical applications, weight usually references a mass (such as the weight of a pathology specimen) or a solid (such as the amount of medication in a tablet or capsule of medicine). Volume usually references a liquid or a gas, and length references distance.

A prefix may be added to each of the root words (*gram, liter,* and *meter*). Figure 7-1 shows the relationships of the common prefixes to their decimal value. As Figure 7-1 shows, deci-, centi-, milli-, and micro units are all less than one whole unit. The following should be memorized:

- *deci* = 0.1 (one tenth of one unit)
- *centi* = 0.01 (one hundredth of one unit)
- *milli* = 0.001 (one thousandth of one unit)
- *micro* = 0.000001 (one millionth of one unit)
- *kilo* =1000 (one thousand units)

To reduce medication errors, a zero is always used *before* the decimal point if the unit is less than one whole unit. For example, .78 would be written as 0.78. Trailing zeros to the right of the numbers following the decimal

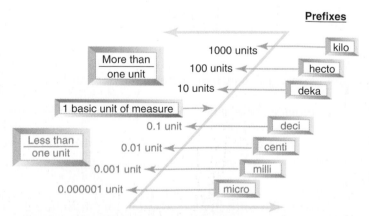

Figure 7-1 The basic units of measure—gram, liter, and meter—with prefixes indicating larger or smaller measures. Thus *deka-* ("ten") refers to 10 basic units, and *deci-* ("tenth") refers to one tenth of the basic unit.

point should be deleted. For example, 1.0100 would be 1.01.

The base units are abbreviated as follows: gram (g), liter (L), and meter (m). Common units with prefixes used in medicine for weight are kilogram (abbreviated kg; 1 kilogram = 1000 grams, or 1 kg = 1000 g); milligram (abbreviated mg; one thousandth [0.001] of a gram; 1000 mg = 1 g); and microgram (abbreviated mcg; one millionth of a gram [0.000001 g]; 1,000,000 mcg = 1 g). A common prefixed unit used for liquids is the milliliter (abbreviated mL; one thousandth of a liter [0.001 L]; 1000 mL = 1 L). Common prefixed units used for measuring length are the centimeter (abbreviated cm; one hundredth of a meter [0.01 m]; 100 cm = 1 m) and the millimeter (abbreviated mm; one thousandth of a meter [0.001 m]; 1000 mm = 1 m). Clinical applications of these different units of measure include measuring a patient's weight (in kilograms), measuring the concentration of a medication (in grams, milligrams, or micrograms), and measuring a surgical wound (in centimeters or millimeters).

In the metric system, decimals are used instead of fractions (e.g., 0.1, not $\frac{1}{10}$). Because decimals are used, it is simple to convert from one unit to another in the metric system. Moving the decimal point to the right (and adding a zero) raises the value by a power of 10. For example, 1.20 m = 120 cm = 1200 mm. Moving the decimal point to the left lowers the value by a power of 10 for each unit moved. For example, 20 mm = 2 cm = 0.02 m.

When a metric measurement is written, the Arabic number is written first, followed by the metric abbreviation for units. For example, three hundred twenty-five milligrams is written as 325 mg, one hundred sixty-five centimeters is written as 165 cm, and three liters is written as 3 L.

In 1960 the International Bureau of Weights and Measurements adopted the International System of units to reduce possible errors in drug transcriptions. A few common abbreviations may still be written the old way. For example, *gram* is often abbreviated as gm instead of g, as in the SI system. Either is appropriate. This book

TABLE 7-1 COMMON METRIC UNITS USED IN MEDICINE

METRIC TERM	UNIT VALUE	ABBREVIATION
WEIGHT OR MASS		
kilogram	1000 units or grams	kg
gram	**base unit**	**g**
milligram	0.001 of a gram	mg
microgram	0.000001 of a gram	mcg
VOLUME OR LIQUID		
liter	**base unit**	**L**
milliliter*	0.001 of a liter	mL
LENGTH		
meter	**base unit**	**m**
centimeter	0.01 of a meter	cm
millimeter	0.001 of a meter	mm

Note: Basic units are in **boldface**.
*One milliliter (mL) = 1 cubic centimeter (cc); *cc* should not be used.

uses g. *Liter* may be abbreviated as L (in the SI system) or as lowercase l; either may be used. Table 7-1 shows the metric units most often used in clinical medicine, along with their unit value and abbreviation.

The cubic centimeter (cc) is a measurement that is on The Joint Commission's (TJC's) "possible inclusion on a future Do Not Use" list. As of June 2011, "cc" is still only on the watch list. This measure is still seen on measuring devices for over-the-counter (OTC) cough syrups, syringes used for oral medications, and input measuring devices such as patient hospital cups and urine collection containers. One cubic centimeter (cc) is equivalent to one milliliter (mL). The "cc" may possibly be phased out of medical documentation in the future because "cc" may be mistaken for units when poorly written. Milliliter (mL) is the preferred abbreviation.

LEARNING TIP

Memorize the equivalency: 1 cc = 1 mL.

Check Your Understanding: METRIC SYSTEM BASICS BOX 7-1

Identify whether the prefix is "greater than" or "less than" one basic unit.

1. centi _____

2. deci _____

3. deka _____

4. hecto _____

5. kilo _____

6. micro _____

7. milli _____

Continued

Check Your Understanding: METRIC SYSTEM BASICS BOX 7-1—cont'd

Identify the three basic units of measure in the metric system.

8. Basic unit of length _____

9. Basic unit of weight _____

10. Basic unit of volume _____

Write the decimal correctly.

11. 1.00100 _____

12. .001 _____

13. 0.00110 _____

14. 1.010 _____

15. .101010 _____

Calculation Review

Two answers are required for each of the following. On the first line, identify the unit of measure as a weight, volume, or length measurement. Then write the metric notation using abbreviations.

	IDENTIFCATION OF UNIT	METRIC NOTATION
16. Four tenths of a milliliter	_____	_____
17. One hundred twenty centimeters	_____	_____
18. Six hundred twenty-four milligrams	_____	_____
19. Three thousand and seventy-five-hundredths meters	_____	_____
20. Two and three-tenths liters	_____	_____
21. One thousand micrograms	_____	_____
22. Ten grams	_____	_____
23. Five kilograms	_____	_____
24. One and one-half liters	_____	_____
25. Seven hundred fifty kilometers	_____	_____

✎ LEARNING TIP

Remember that the base metric units are gram, liter, and meter.

LENGTH MEASUREMENT AND CONVERSION IN THE METRIC SYSTEM

The basic unit of length in the metric system is the meter. A meter is 39.37 inches, or slightly longer than a yardstick (36 inches). Other than for height, a meter is too long to be useful for most measurements in medicine, so subdivisions of a meter, or smaller units, are used. The centimeter (one hundredth of a meter; 1 cm = 0.01 m and 100 cm = 1 m) is most commonly used. Approximately 2.5 cm equals 1 inch. Centimeters may be used to measure a person's height, to measure the circumference of a newborn baby's head, or to measure the length of a wound. The millimeter (one thousandth of a meter; 1 mm = 0.001 m, 1000 mm = 1 m, and 10 mm = 1 cm) is used for very small measurements such as the length of a small lesion. A millimeter is about the size of the head of a pin.

LEARNING TIP

The conversions to memorize for length include:

Meter to millimeter	1 m = 1000 mm
Meter to centimeter	1 m = 100 cm
Centimeter to millimeter	1 cm = 10 mm

Note that the conversion factor is always in multiples of 10; therefore you can simply move the decimal point in the direction needed to obtain the desired unit. Recall that the basic length unit is a meter, and both the centimeter and the millimeter are subdivisions of *one* basic unit. To convert measurements between different metric lengths, either *divide* by multiples of 10 if a *smaller* unit is given and a larger unit needs to be found, or *multiply* by multiples of 10 if a *larger* unit is given and a smaller unit needs to be found. To divide by 10, move the decimal point to the left one unit place for each unit difference in conversion of smaller units to larger units. To multiply by 10, move the decimal point to the right for each unit needed for unit conversion of larger units to smaller units. In some cases, to get the desired value in the new unit, the decimal point is moved more than one place to the right or left. In moving the decimal point to the right, we are multiplying by 10 for each space the decimal point moves. Because a millimeter is very small, only one thousandth of a meter, we need many millimeters (1000) to equal 1 meter (length). When converting from millimeters to centimeters, moving the decimal point to the left, or dividing by 10, gives the larger value wanted for the millimeter measurement quickly. And, of course, the same thing works in

reverse. If we start with 50.2 millimeters and want to know the amount in meters, we move the decimal place three places to the left (divide), bypassing centimeters and decimeters:

EXAMPLE 1: 50.2 mm = _____ m

$$50.2 \text{ mm} = 0.0502 \text{ m}$$

Because a meter is large in relation to a millimeter, the value for the meter measurement will be a smaller decimal number. Remember that length problems have three conversions that could be multiplied or divided, using numbers: 10, 100, or 1000. Be careful to use the correct conversion.

LEARNING TIP

When solving a problem, if you are:
  GIVEN the *smaller* unit, *divide* to find the answer.
  GIVEN the *larger* unit, *multiply* to find the answer.

EXAMPLE 2: _____ cm = 75 mm

GIVEN: Smaller unit, divide to find your answer. (Hint: 1 cm = 10 mm.)

75 ÷ 10 = 7.5, so 75 mm = 7.5 cm

EXAMPLE 3: _____ mm = 2.5 m

GIVEN: Larger unit, multiply to find your answer. (Hint: 1 m = 1000 mm.)

2.5 × 1000 = 2500, so 2.5 m = 2500 mm

Check Your Understanding: METRIC LENGTH CONVERSIONS
BOX 7-2

Determine whether to multiply or divide based on unit GIVEN in the problem.

1. 6900 mm = _____ m

2. 4.3 cm = _____ mm

3. 4.3 cm = _____ m

4. 5 m = _____ mm

5. 90 mm = _____ cm

6. 3 m = _____ cm

7. 8.8 cm = _____ mm

8. 1.7 cm = _____ m

9. 1200 mm = _____ cm

10. 12 mm = _____ cm

Continued

Check Your Understanding: METRIC LENGTH CONVERSIONS
BOX 7-2—cont'd

Practical Application
Answer the following questions.

11. A 1-month-old child has a head circumference of 42.5 cm. What is the child's head circumference in millimeters? _____

12. An emergency room patient needs sutures to close a wound that is 8 cm long. How many millimeters long is the wound? _____

13. An infant is measured from head to foot. The measurement is 500 mm. What is the height in centimeters? _____

14. A premature baby has a head circumference of 13 cm. How many millimeters is the circumference? _____

15. A child stands 1 meter tall. Calculate the height in centimeters. _____

VOLUME MEASUREMENT AND CONVERSION IN THE METRIC SYSTEM

The basic unit of volume in the metric system is the liter. In medicine, liquid volumes are expressed in liters or units of liters. Gas volumes, such as volume of oxygen, are also measured in liters. For comparison, many soft drinks are now sold in 1-, 2-, or 3-liter bottles. The 1-liter bottle is approximately equivalent to (slightly more than) 32 ounces or 1 quart in the household system. A gallon of milk is approximately equivalent to 4 liters (3.78 liters). Many OTC cough medicines now come with a medicine cup calibrated in milliliters (mL), cubic centimeters (cc), and teaspoons (t) or tablespoons (T). Many students find the volume measurement easiest to learn because there is only one conversion to remember—always multiply or divide by 1000.

This section explores the volume (liquid or gas) measurements of the milliliter and liter, which in medicine measure a patient's liquid intake and output. Intravenous solutions are usually measured in liters, with the drip volume measured in drops per milliliter.

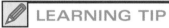 **LEARNING TIP**

The conversions to be remembered for volume include the following:

Liter to milliliter	1 L = 1000 mL

The same procedure used for converting meters is used for converting liters. If given the larger unit and converting to a smaller unit, multiply by 1000. The same prefixes are used with volume as found with weight.

EXAMPLE 4: _____ mL = 4 L

GIVEN: Larger unit, multiply to find your answer. (Hint: 1 L = 1000 mL.)

1000 × 4 = 4000, so 4000 mL = 4 L

EXAMPLE 5: _____ L = 200 mL

GIVEN: Smaller unit, divide to find your answer. (Hint: 1 L = 1000 mL).

200 ÷ 1000 = 0.2, so 0.2 L = 200 mL

Always remember to place a 0 to the left of the decimal (.2 is written as 0.2).

Check Your Understanding: METRIC VOLUME CONVERSIONS
BOX 7-3

Determine whether to multiply or divide based on unit GIVEN in the problem.

1. 1 mL = _____ L

2. 0.5 L = _____ mL

3. 6.4 L = _____ mL

4. 14 mL = _____ L

5. 500 mL = _____ L

6. 2500 mL = _____ L

7. 1450 mL = _____ L

8. 4 L = _____ mL

9. 100 mL = _____ L

10. 3000 mL = _____ L

Practical Application
Supply answers to the following questions.

11. A patient is instructed to drink 2 L of water every day to replace body fluids. How many milliliters is this? _____

12. You are instructed to measure the urine output of a patient with a Foley catheter. If the urine collection bag contains 1.5 L of urine, what volume in milliliters will you record when emptying the bag? _____

13. A standard intravenous bag contains 1000 mL of liquid. How many liters is that? _____

14. A patient is to receive 250 mL of fluids. How many liters will the patient receive? _____

15. A patient is to receive 3000 mL of intravenous fluids. How many liters should be ordered from the pharmacy? _____

WEIGHT MEASUREMENT AND CONVERSION IN THE METRIC SYSTEM

The base unit used to measure weight (mass) in the metric system is the gram. Other units of interest are the kilogram (kg; 1000 g), milligram (mg; one thousandth of a gram [0.001 g]), and microgram (mcg; one millionth of a gram [0.000001 g]). Newborn babies are weighed in kilograms unless they are premature, in which case they may be so small that their weight must be expressed in grams. A gram is about the weight of one large paper clip. Drug weights are usually expressed in grams, milligrams and micrograms.

LEARNING TIP

The conversions to be remembered for weight include the following:

Kilogram to gram	1 kg = 1000 g
Gram to milligram	1 g = 1000 mg
Milligram to microgram	1 mg = 1000 mcg

These weight units are commonly used in medicine, and they have an interesting relationship: each is one thousandth of the next higher (used) weight. The same ratio of 1:1000 exists between the kilogram and the gram, between the gram and the milligram, and between the milligram and the microgram (thus a microgram is a thousandth of a milligram or a millionth of a gram). Memorizing this feature of weights should help you remember the conversions. (Other units such as the deci-gram, centigram, dekagram, and so on exist but are used infrequently in the medical field.) As with length and volume, to convert from a larger unit to a smaller unit, multiply. If the smaller unit is given and the value of the larger unit is wanted, divide.

EXAMPLE 6: _____ mg = 8 g

GIVEN: Larger unit, multiply to find the answer. (Hint: 1 g = 1000 mg.)

$8 \times 1000 = 8000$, so 8000 mg = 8 g

EXAMPLE 7: _____ mg = 635 mcg

GIVEN: Smaller unit, divide to find the unit. (Hint: 1 mg = 1000 mcg.)

$635 \div 1000 = 0.635$, so 0.635 mg = 635 mcg

Remember: Add the zero in front of the decimal.

EXAMPLE 8: _____ g = 4.5 kg

GIVEN: Larger unit, multiply to find the answer. (Hint: 1 kg = 1000 g.)

$4.5 \times 1000 = 4500$, so 4500 g = 4.5 kg

EXAMPLE 9: _____ g = 3250 mg

GIVEN: Smaller unit, divide to get answer. (Hint: 1 g = 1000 mg.)

$3250 \div 1000 = 3.25$, so 3.25 g = 3250 mg

Note that the zero following 3.25 is a trailing zero and has therefore been dropped.

Check Your Understanding: METRIC WEIGHT CONVERSIONS
BOX 7-4

Determine whether to multiply or divide based on unit GIVEN in the problem. Drop or add zeros as appropriate.

1. 1500 mcg = _____ mg

2. 400 mg = _____ g

3. 6.5 g = _____ mg

4. 4800 mcg = _____ mg

5. 0.34 kg = _____ g

6. 500 g = _____ kg

7. 0.09 g = _____ mg

8. 2.75 mg = _____ mcg

9. 0.03 kg = _____ g

10. 225 mg = _____ g

Practical Application
Answer the following questions.

11. A premature baby weighs 2.2 kg. How many grams does the baby weigh? _____

12. A laboratory specimen weighs 1850 g. Convert the gram weight into kilograms. _____

13. The dosage strength of _Lanoxin_ is 500 mcg. The drug is prescribed in milligrams. Convert the 500 mcg available to the prescribed dosage. _____

14. The dosage strength of _Xanax_ is 0.25 mg. The drug is prescribed in micrograms. Convert 0.25 mg to micro-grams. _____

15. A medication comes in a tablet with dosage strength of 88 mcg. The medication bottle reads milligrams. What would you expect the dosage to read in milligrams? _____

TABLE 7-2 UNITS OF MEASURE IN THE APOTHECARY SYSTEM

LIQUID VOLUME	SOLID WEIGHT
60 minims = 1 fluid dram (fʒ)	60 grains = 1 dram
8 fluid drams (fʒ viii)= 1 fluid ounce (f ʒ i)	

TABLE 7-3 HOUSEHOLD MEASUREMENT SYSTEM

HOUSEHOLD TERM	UNIT VALUE	ABBREVIATION
WEIGHT OR MASS		
ounce		oz
pound	16 oz	lb
VOLUME OR LIQUID		
drop		gtt
teaspoon	60-75 gtts	tsp; t
tablespoon	3 t	Tbsp; T
ounce	2 T	oz
cup	8 oz	c
pint	2 c; 16 oz	pt
quart	2 pt; 4 c; 32 oz	qt
gallon	4 qt; 8 pt; 16 c; 128 oz	gal
LENGTH		
inch		In
foot	12 in	Ft
yard	3 ft; 36 in	yd

APOTHECARY SYSTEM

The **apothecary system** is one of the oldest systems for indicating drug mass or volume but is nearly obsolete today because it has been gradually replaced by the metric system. The **apothecary** basic unit of measure for solid weight is the **grain** (gr).

1 grain = approximately the weight of 1 grain of wheat or rice

When liquids are measured, the volume may be expressed in minim, drams, or ounces. A **minim** (ꝳ) is still found on some syringes, especially tuberculin syringes. The most commonly used apothecary unit for a liquid is a **dram** (ʒ). This unit is most often found on a prescription for the household measure of the teaspoon. Some physicians still use the ounce symbol (ʒ) on prescriptions. See Table 7-2 for the commonly used apothecary measures.

Numbers and symbols in the apothecary system are written in reverse order from the metric system. In the metric system, quantity is written first, followed by the unit (e.g., 3 liters, 3L). In the apothecary system, the symbol or abbreviation comes first, followed by the quantity, which is expressed in lowercase Roman numerals. An example is gr iv, which means 4 grains. Usually only the digits 1 through 10, 20 and 30 are expressed in Roman numerals. Most other quantities are expressed in Arabic numbers. However, all numerals are written in Arabic if the entire unit measurement is written in full. For example, 8 grains would not be written viii grain because the word "grain" is written out; it is either "8 grains" or "gr viii".

Another difference between the metric system and the apothecary system is that fractions are used in the apothecary system when necessary. (Remember the metric quantities are expressed in decimals.) For example, the fraction three-quarters is noted as ¾ in the apothecary system but as 0.75 in the metric system.

HOUSEHOLD MEASUREMENT SYSTEM

Consumers who measure drugs at home may use the household measurement system because of ease of availability of the utensils. However, today most medications are dispensed with the appropriate utensil for accurate measurement of the dose. The **household system** is also called the *U.S. Customary System of Measurement*. This system is used in patient education in pharmacology for home administration of medications, especially liquids and with diabetic and weight control management. It is also used to increase patient compliance when comparing amounts of food and liquids that make up one serving of a food or liquid. The household measurement system is usually based on the number of ounces in a measuring device when quantities of weight or volume are measured. The most commonly used household system of measuring volume (liquids) are the dropper, teaspoon, tablespoon, ounce, and cup as units of measure. The pint, quart, and gallon are also household measurements, but these measurements are not often associated with medical use because the metric measurements are becoming better known and are more frequently used. Although the household system is applicable primarily to liquid medications, the ounce and pound could also be used to measure a patient's solid food intake or a patient's weight. The common household measures of length include the inch, the foot, and the yard. Table 7-3 shows the household measurement units most often used. Note that the table identifies the smallest measure first. When discussing food intake with a patient, the health professional should clearly define the content amount of a "cup," because there are teacups, coffee cups, measuring cups, and other sized cups, all with different capacities.

The household system is not recommended for medical measurements in a medical facility because of the different sizes of the measuring devices. For example, a dropper may have a large or small hole (aperture) for the medicine to pass through, and the medication itself could be either viscous or aqueous, which would change the amount contained in a drop unless an appropriate dropper is provided with the medication. To instruct the patient to use a few drops would not be appropriate without specifying exactly what dropper the person needs to use. Another problem with droppers is that different patients using the same dropper may exert a different amount of force when pinching the plunger of the dropper, thus dispensing different amounts of medication. For OTC and prescription drugs that are to be administered by a teaspoonful of medicine, most pharmaceutical companies are now packaging the medicine with a graduated medication cup, a calibrated hollow-handle spoon, or a calibrated dropper.

Check Your Understanding: HOUSEHOLD SYSTEM BOX 7-5

Identify the household abbreviation.

1. T _____

2. gtt _____

3. c _____

4. t _____

5. Tbsp _____

Write "greater than," "less than," or "equal" to make each household measurement a true statement.

6. t _____ Tbsp

7. tsp _____ gtt

8. T _____ t

9. T _____ c

10. gtt _____ Tbsp

Practical Application
Instruct the patient on how to use the following OTC remedies.

11. For the relief of occasional constipation, dissolve 2 level tsp of *magnesium sulfate*, USP, into 1 c of H_2O and take PO. _____

12. Add 1-2 c of Epsom salts to warm bath to soothe and refresh your entire body. _____

13. For temporary relief of cough caused by bronchial irritation, take elix *Benylin*, 1 tsp of q4h not to exceed 6 doses daily. _____

14. Take Milk of Magnesia, 1 ounce PO after meals prn. _____

15. To increase moisture, instill *Liquifilm tears*, 2 gtts in each eye prn. _____

Unlike in the metric system, which uses the movement of decimals to identify equivalents, the unit values must be memorized to find household equivalents. For example, to determine how many ounces are found in a gallon, you must first remember how many ounces are in a cup, how many cups are in a pint, how many pints are in a quart, and how many quarts are in a gallon or memorize all the conversions found in this system.

UNITS

Some drugs are measured in **units.** Units may be expressed as IUs (International units) or USP (*United States Pharmaceutical*) units and are expressed as Arabic numbers followed by the unit designation. Drugs measured in units may be derived from plant or animal sources or manufactured in a laboratory (synthetic drugs). Most insulin drugs today are synthetically produced to prevent variations in the insulin. Insulins from animal sources are basically nonexistent in today's market as most are DNA produced.

Common drugs dispensed in units include *heparin* (a powerful anticoagulant that prevents blood clots), *insulin* (for people with inadequate insulin production, such as those with diabetes mellitus), and *penicillin G* and *penicillin V* (antibiotics). Some fat-soluble vitamins such as *vitamins A, D,* and *E* are also dispensed in units.

CLINICAL TIP

Always read the label carefully to obtain the correct dosage strength desired.

Milliequivalents

The term **milliequivalent** pertains to the amount of a solute contained in a solution. Milliequivalent is abbreviated mEq and is usually expressed as milliequivalent per volume, mEq/L or mEq/mL, mEq/tab, or mEq/cap.

To express drugs in milliequivalents, the Arabic numbers (numerals 0 through 9) are written first, followed by the milliequivalent indicator. For example, if the physician orders 100 units of insulin, this is written as 100 units; and 2 milliequivalents is written as 2 mEq.

CLINICAL TIP

Weight = strength or mass
Volume = amount or liquid

CURRENT TRENDS FOR SYMBOLS AND ABBREVIATIONS

In 2004 it was determined that in order to meet the National Patient Safety Goal (NPSG), an official list of "Do Not Use" abbreviations would be developed (see Table 5-1). In May 2005, TJC mandated that all medical facilities adhere to the changes on the "Do Not Use" list. It was also determined that each year TJC would review the list and possibly implement further changes in additional abbreviations, acronyms, and symbols. For the most current information on any new changes, please refer to TJC's website (www.jointcommission.org) under the tab of Patient Safety. A second website, from the Institute for Safe Medication Practices (www.ismp.org), includes not only the abbreviations and symbols, but also dose designations and drug abbreviations that should be avoided.

SUMMARY

Several systems of measurement are encountered in clinical medicine for measuring mass, volume, and length. The metric system is most common and is accepted worldwide. OTC drug instructions frequently refer to household measures such as a drop or cup. Certain medications, such as insulin and penicillin, are measured in units. Finally, the apothecary system, one of the oldest systems of measurement devised, is discussed. Because it is important for allied health professionals to know and be able to use all systems, the next chapter introduces conversions among the commonly used metric system and the less frequently used household and apothecary systems.

Abbreviations are important in most of the measurement systems. Being able to recognize the differences among the various systems will help the student to understand how to read and interpret medication orders, prepare drug inventory records and Material Safety Data Sheets, and assist in patient education when reading and interpreting patient charts. The "Do Not Use" list assists in preventing medication errors by reducing misinterpretation of abbreviations.

CRITICAL THINKING EXERCISES

Supply the missing information in the following table of metric terms and abbreviations. The first row is completed as an example. (NA, not applicable.)

METRIC TERM	UNIT VALUE	PREFIX	ROOT WORD	ABBREVIATION	TYPE OF UNIT
kilogram	1000 units	kilo	gram	kg	weight (solid)
_____	_____	micro	_____	mcg	weight (solid)
_____	1 unit	NA	_____	_____	length
_____	0.001 of a unit	milli	_____	_____	volume (liquid)
_____	1 unit	NA	_____	g	_____
_____	_____	_____	meter	cm	length
milligram	_____	milli	gram	_____	_____
_____	1 unit	NA	liter	_____	volume (liquid)
millimeter	_____	milli	_____	mm	_____

REVIEW QUESTIONS

Fill in the blank.

1. A drug derived from an animal source, such as insulin, is measured in _____.

2. The term _____ refers to the weight of a drug contained in a normal solution.

3. Consumers who measure drugs at home most often use the _____ measurement system.

4. A microgram is abbreviated _____.

5. _____ (system) quantities are expressed in decimals.

6. One cubic centimeter is equivalent to _____ _____.

7. The three basic units in the metric system are the _____, _____, and _____.

Circle the correct notation.

8. 100 U or 100 units

9. ii milliequivalents or 2 mEq

Match the correct prefix with the unit given.

10. 1000 _____ centi

11. 0.1 _____ deci

12. 0.01 _____ kilo

13. 0.001 _____ micro

14. 0.000001 _____ milli

All of the following statements are *false*. Determine the errors, and then write the correct answers in a complete sentence. (Answers can vary.)

15. A milliliter is equal to a cubic millimeter. _____

_____

_____

16. Consumers who measure drugs at home most often use the apothecary system. _____

_____

_____

17. The household system is considered the international standard of measurement systems. _____

_____

_____

18. Micrograms are larger than milligrams. _____

_____

_____

19. The metric system sometimes has a conversion factor that is a power of 10. _____

_____

_____

20. Medications prescribed in the metric system are measured in teaspoons and tablespoons. _____

_____

_____

21. Milliliters are used to measure solids. _____

_____

_____

22. All measurement systems discussed in this chapter are still in use today. _____

_____

_____

23. The meter and the yard are the same length. _____

_____

_____

24. Premature babies are often weighed in metric pounds. _____

_____

_____

25. When referring to insulin, the term *milliequivalent* identifies the weight of the solution. _____

_____

_____

Converting Between Measurement Systems

OBJECTIVES

After studying this chapter, you should be capable of doing the following:

- Reading the time of day on the international standard 24-hour clock and the 12-hour clock and converting time between the two time standards.
- Converting between Fahrenheit and Celsius scales.
- Computing and converting approximate volume equivalents within and between metric, household, and apothecary systems.
- Computing and converting approximate weight equivalents within and between the metric system and the household system or the metric system and the apothecary system.
- Computing and converting from one length unit to another within and between the metric and household systems.

KEY TERMS

Celsius
Conversion factor

Convert
Dimensional analysis

Fahrenheit

International Standard
ISO 8601

Chapter 8 PRETEST—CONVERTING BETWEEN MEASUREMENT SYSTEMS

Answer the following questions.

1. Convert the following English standard times into international standard notation.

10:15 PM = _____   5:47 PM = _____

9:20 AM = _____   1:25 AM = _____

2. Convert the following temperatures between Fahrenheit and Celsius. Round to the nearest tenth.

18° C = _____ ° F   80° C = _____ ° F

104° F = _____ ° C   100° F = _____ ° C

Chapter 8 PRETEST—CONVERTING BETWEEN MEASUREMENT SYSTEMS—cont'd

3. Convert the following volume units between systems.

10 mL = _____ tsp   32 oz = _____ mL

$\frac{1}{2}$ qt = _____ mL   3 Tbsp = _____ mL

4. Convert the following weight units between systems.

30 g = _____ oz   5 lb = _____ kg

gr $\overline{\text{iss}}$ = _____ mg

5. Convert the following length units.

35 cm = _____ ft _____ in

150 mm = _____ in

17.5 cm = _____ in

To **convert** means to change from one system to another system. In the medical field, it is often necessary to change between measurement systems because there is currently no world standard for drug measurement. Many of the measurement systems that are commonly used in the United States are not used by scientists or medical professionals in other parts of the world. Because of this, health care providers must become familiar with all the systems currently in use. This chapter begins by discussing the system of time used in most of the world; followed by temperature conversions (**Fahrenheit** and **Celsius**); and methods of converting measurements among metric, apothecary, and household volumes, weights, and lengths. With the exception of time values, when numbers are converted from one system to another, they will be approximately equal. *Conversions that are approximately equal may differ by as much as 10%.*

TIME CONVERSIONS

International Standard ISO 8601 has been recognized in most countries of the world as the universal standard for interpreting time and writing the date. The United States has not widely adopted this standard except in the military, in the computer industry, in scientific publications, and in hospitals. The international standard notation for the time of day is *hhmmss*.

Did You Know

Because digital watches did not become widely available in the United States until 1971, health care providers have been trained to take vital signs using the second hand of the analog watch.

The *hh* signifies the total complete hours that have passed since midnight; the *mm* states the total minutes that have passed since the start of the hour; and the *ss* identifies the total seconds that have passed since the start of the minute. For example, 25 seconds after 10:20 AM would be written as 102025. (In most cases, seconds are not included in the conversion, so only the hour and minutes would be documented—e.g., 1020 would be 10:20 AM.) Most countries do not use the abbreviations "AM" and "PM" because they do not recognize the 12-hour notation that is used in the United States. The history of the 12-hour clock dates back to the dark ages when Roman numerals were used and there was no symbol for the digit "zero." A good example of how the 12-hour clock is still used is the analog watch, which displays the numbers 1 through 12. The 12-hour clock has only the numbers 1 through 12, so to differentiate between morning and evening, the time from midnight to noon is followed by the letters AM. The hours from noon to midnight are written with the letters PM after the numbers. To understand how to convert from the 12-hour (AM-PM) format to the 24-hour format, refer to Box 8-1 (for the hour designated). Note that midnight starts the 24-hour clock at 0000. Each hour is shown by the first two digits, which are numbered from 00 to 24. When you get to noon (1200),

BOX 8-1 THE 12-HOUR CLOCK AND THE 24-HOUR CLOCK

12-Hour Clock	24-Hour Clock
12 midnight	0000 (2400)
1 AM	0100
2 AM	0200
3 AM	0300
4 AM	0400
5 AM	0500
6 AM	0600
7 AM	0700
8 AM	0800
9 AM	0900
10 AM	1000
11 AM	1100
12 noon	1200
1 PM	1300
2 PM	1400
3 PM	1500
4 PM	1600
5 PM	1700
6 PM	1800
7 PM	1900
8 PM	2000
9 PM	2100
10 PM	2200
11 PM	2300
12 midnight	2400 (0000)

keep increasing by one digit for each hour. On the 24-hour clock, "AM" and "PM" are not used because one o'clock in the afternoon is written "1300," two o'clock is written "1400," and so on. Minutes are written as the two digits following the hour and are numbered from 00 to 59, just as in the familiar 12-hour system. (Seconds do not vary between the systems either.) The clock in Figure 8-1 shows the comparison of hours between the two systems.

EXAMPLE 1: 8:20 AM = _____ international time

The AM symbol tells you that this is in 12-hour format, so change the format to 24-hour notation by dropping the AM, adding a zero before the 8, and deleting the colon.

So, 8:20 AM is 0820 in 24-hour notation.

EXAMPLE 2: 11:55 PM = _____ international time

The PM symbol tells you that this is in the 12-hour format and that it is in the evening, so add one digit for each hour after noon, drop the PM symbol, and delete the colon.

12 + 11 = 23. Therefore the time is 2355.

Several valid reasons to use the international standard time in the medical field instead of the old English 12-hour clock exist. With the 24-hour clock there is less chance for human error because there is no duplication in the hours of the day. With the 12-hour clock, if the symbols AM and PM are not used, mistakes can be made, especially when medications are meant to be given only once every 24 hours.

Another way to remember how to change from the English 12-hour clock to the 2400 international clock is described as follows (see Figure 8-1).

Standard clock

International standard clock

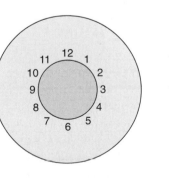

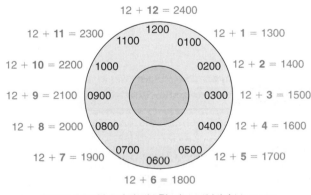

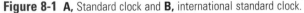

A 12-hour English clock, AM and PM

B 2400 international clock. Black = midnight to noon; green = noon to midnight

Figure 8-1 A, Standard clock and **B,** international standard clock.

Draw two circles.

On the first circle, draw a second circle inside the larger circle and label the 12-hour clock.

On the second circle using the number 12, add each number from the 12-hour English clock to obtain the 2400 clock. 2400 is midnight on the international clock, and 0001 is 1 minute after midnight. The first 12 hours after midnight are written the same on both clocks; however, the English clock will identify AM and the international clock is always written using four digits.

Check Your Understanding: TIME CONVERSION 8-1

Convert the time shown into international standard time.

1. 4:40 AM = _____

2. 6:25 PM = _____

3. 11:02 AM = _____

4. 2:56 AM = _____

5. 10:45 PM = _____

6. 8:10 PM = _____

7. 12:33 AM = _____

8. 10:00 AM = _____

9. 3:33 PM = _____

10. 7:17 AM = _____

Convert the international time to the 12-hour English time.

11. 2121 = _____

12. 1615 = _____

13. 0045 = _____

14. 1234 = _____

15. 2400 = _____

16. 1830 = _____

17. 0210 = _____

18. 1605 = _____

19. 1515 = _____

20. 1357 = _____

MEASURING TEMPERATURE

In Chapter 7 the metric system was introduced as the international standard for scientific and industrial measurements. Most of the world measures temperature in the metric system, so temperature is measured using the Celsius scale. In the United States the Fahrenheit scale is predominant. The Celsius scale was introduced in the mid-1700s and is often referred to as the *centigrade scale*. Because the metric system is the predominant mathematical system used in much of the rest of the world, it is important to be able to convert from the Fahrenheit scale to the Celsius scale.

The Celsius temperature is always the lower number when a temperature is shown with the equivalent degrees on the Fahrenheit scale. Both Celsius and Fahrenheit temperatures are always measured in degrees. For example, 0° Celsius is equivalent to 32° on the Fahrenheit scale. (The small ° symbol stands for "degrees.") Table 8-1 shows a comparison of some common equivalents between the Celsius and Fahrenheit scales.

TABLE 8-1 COMMON BASELINES FOR FAHRENHEIT AND CELSIUS TEMPERATURES

	CELSIUS	FAHRENHEIT
Water boils	100°	212°
Normal body temperature	37°	98.6°
Room temperature	20°	68°
Water freezes	0°	32°

Some special considerations should be remembered when placing a decimal in the answer when converting temperatures. The decimal place is used in tenths only and may need to be rounded off. For example, if the answer is 35.55° the answer would be written as 35.6° C.

TEMPERATURE CONVERSIONS

There are two ways to convert between Celsius and Fahrenheit. Although both methods can be used to obtain the correct results, you should memorize only one of them and consistently use that method to avoid confusion when converting between Celsius and Fahrenheit. Both methods are explained, and you should choose the one that works best for you. Always round your answer to the nearest tenth.

Method 1

To change from Fahrenheit to Celsius, use this formula:

$$C° = \frac{5}{9}(F° - 32)$$

EXAMPLE 3: _____° C = 104° F

Using the formula, the first step would be to do the calculation in parentheses by subtracting 104° F − 32 = 72. The second step is to multiply 72 × 5 = 360. The final step would be to divide 360 by 9 = 40.

Therefore 40° C = 104° F.

To change from Celsius to Fahrenheit, use this formula:

$$F° = \left(\frac{9}{5}C°\right) + 32$$

EXAMPLE 4: _____° F = 38.3° C

Using the formula, the first step would be to do the calculation in parentheses by multiplying 38.3 × 9 = 344.7. The second step would be to divide: 344.7 ÷ 5 = 68.94.

The final step is to add: 68.94 + 32 = 100.94. Round to 100.9° F, so 100.9° F = 38.3° C.

Review the two formulas:

From °F to °C	From °C to °F
$C° = \frac{5}{9}(F° - 32)$	$F° = \left(\frac{9}{5}C°\right) + 32$

Method 2

Use the formula °C = (°F − 32) ÷ 1.8 to change from Fahrenheit to Celsius. (In this formula, 1.8 is the decimal equivalent of ⅝.)

EXAMPLE 5: _____° C = 99.8° F

Using the formula °C = (°F − 32) ÷ 1.8, the first step would be to subtract (99.8° F − 32) = 67.8. The second and final step is to divide 67.8 ÷ 1.8 = 37.67. Remember to round your answer to tenths.

Therefore 37.7° C = 99.8° F.

Some students find that Method 2 is easier because only two steps instead of three are necessary to find the correct answer.

Method 2 can also be used to convert from Fahrenheit to Celsius using the formula °F = 1.8 (°C) + 32.

EXAMPLE 6: _____° F = 22° C

Using the formula °F = 1.8(°C) + 32, the first step would be to multiply (1.8 × 22° C) = 39.6. Then just add 32 to your answer: 39.6 + 32 = 71.6.

Therefore 22° C = 71.6° F.

When changing _from_ Fahrenheit _to_ Celsius, you must remember to do what is in parentheses first (°F − 32) before attempting to divide by 1.8. When changing _from_ Celsius _to_ Fahrenheit, remember to multiply 1.8 × °C before adding the 32.

Review the two formulas again.

From °C to °F	From °F to °C
Multiply °C by 1.8	_Subtract_ 32 from °F
Add 32	_Divide_ by 1.8

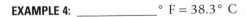 **LEARNING TIP**

When performing temperature calculations, remember to first complete the operation in parenthesis.

Check Your Understanding: TEMPERATURE CONVERSIONS 8-2

Practice Problems

Convert the temperatures and round to the nearest tenth. Use the one method that is most comfortable for you.

1. _____° C = 99.6° F

2. _____° C = 76° F

3. _____° C = 103° F

4. _____° C = 100.8° F

5. _____° C = 80° F

6. _____° C = 98.6° F

7. _____° C = 212° F

8. _____° C = 68° F

9. _____° C = 0° F

10. _____° C = 97.2° F

11. _____° F = 14° C

12. _____° F = 30° C

13. _____° F = 5° C

14. _____° F = 21° C

15. _____° F = 96° C

16. _____° F = 50° C

17. _____° F = 42.3° C

18. _____° F = 18.8° C

19. _____° F = 11° C

20. _____° F = 83° C

CONVERTING BETWEEN MEASUREMENT SYSTEMS USING RATIO AND PROPORTION

Sometimes a medication will be ordered in an amount that is not in the same measurement system as the medication on hand. When this occurs, you must be able to convert between the systems to obtain the correct amount of medication for administration.

Several methods are used to convert between measurement units. The easiest conversion method is using ratio and proportion. To solve for an unknown variable, a comparison of ratios will provide an answer for solving for x. Be sure that the unit values in both ratios are identified. The numerators must be in the same units and the denominators must be in the same units for ratio and proportion to be used. For example: 1 mL is equal to 15 gtts, so 2 mL is equal to 30 gtts. (Note that both mL values are in the same place in the ratios and the gtt values are in the same place.) This can be written with both numerators in fractional units being in mL and both denominators being in gtts: $\left(\dfrac{1\,\text{mL}}{15\,\text{gtts}} = \dfrac{2\,\text{mL}}{30\,\text{gtts}} \right)$.

This can also be written as a linear proportion as follows: 1 mL : 15 gtts :: 2 mL : 30 gtts. When the proportion contains an unknown measurement, the unknown should be identified with an x. After determining the unknown measurement, a proportion, either fractional or linear, may be formed. In the proportion, use the first ratios for the known element that corresponds to the unknown desired and the second ratio for the identified unknown. To solve for x in the second ratio, cross-multiply the fractions or multiply the means and extremes.

EXAMPLE 7:

$$\frac{1\,\text{g}}{2\,\text{mL}} \diagtimes \frac{x\,\text{g}}{4\,\text{mL}} \quad or \quad 1\text{g} : 2\,\text{mL} :: x\,\text{g} : 4\,\text{mL}$$

$2x = 4 \qquad\qquad (2\,\text{mL} \times x\,\text{g} = 4\,\text{mL} \times 1\,\text{g})$

$x = 4 \div 2$

$x = 2\,\text{g}$

Check Your Understanding: RATIO AND PROPORTION 8-3

Calculation Review

Replace the following ratios with the fractional equivalent.

1. 1:5 = _____

2. 3:6 = _____

3. 2:5 = _____

4. 4:5 = _____

5. 9:10 = _____

Replace the following fractions with the ratio equivalent.

6. $\dfrac{3}{4}$ = _____

7. $\dfrac{1}{2}$ = _____

8. $\dfrac{1}{10}$ = _____

9. $\dfrac{1}{100}$ = _____

10. $\dfrac{4}{9}$ = _____

LEARNING TIP

When setting up both ratios, be sure to label all of the terms, including the x, with the correct measurement to ensure that the equations are equivalents.

SYSTEM CONVERSIONS

This section compares approximate equivalents among three different systems—metric, apothecary, and household—commonly used to find weight, length, and volume in the medical field. The metric system is the most often used system of measurement for drug labels in the United States. It is important that you are able to convert these units among the systems. The first two measurements, volume and weight, are used primarily in the field of medicine for dosage calculations. Volume, measured in milliliters or liters, is usually associated with oral liquid medications, contents of a syringe, intake and output of a patient, and intravenous (IV) medications. Weight, used to measure solid mass, is usually associated with medications measured in milligrams, grams, or micrograms, whereas body weight is usually measured in kilograms or pounds. Except in a few cases, such as with *nitroglycerin* ointment, length measurements are not usually associated with dosage calculations. Length is primarily used for measuring body surface areas and medical equipment such as needles or suture thicknesses and to measure medical appliances for specific patients. Understanding that there will be as much as a 10% variation in dosage calculations when converting among the systems is *very important*.

TABLE 8-2 VOLUME MEASUREMENTS

METRIC SYSTEM	HOUSEHOLD SYSTEM	APOTHECARY SYSTEM
0.06 mL	1 drop (gtt)	℥ i
1 mL	15 or 16* drops	℥ 15-16
4 mL (5 mL)*	1 teaspoon (t, tsp)	℥ i
15 mL	1 tablespoon (T, Tbsp, tbsp)	℥ss
30 mL	2 tablespoons, 1 oz	℥ i
240 mL (250 mL)*	1 cup (c), 8 oz	
480 mL (500 mL)*	1 pint (pt), 16 oz	
960 mL (1000 mL)*, 1 L	1 quart (qt), 32 oz	
3480 mL (3.48 L)	1 gallon, 4 qt	

*Remember that conversions are approximate measurements.

Also, do not forget that the 10% variance is considered equivalent when comparing the equivalents among systems.

Volume

Table 8-2 compares the *approximate* equivalents found between the metric, household, and apothecary systems to calculate different units of liquid volume. Equivalents are known as **conversion factors.** Although it is best to memorize the equivalents, some facilities will have equivalency tables available, usually in the medication room.

As previously stated, this table shows approximate equivalents. The four generally accepted amounts in the metric system (5 mL = 1 t; 250 mL = 1 c, or 8 oz; 500 mL = 1 pt, or 16 oz; and 1000 mL or 1 L = 1 qt, or 32 oz) are usually rounded for ease of calculations. For example, regarding the equivalents between metric and household systems, 4 or 5 mL in the metric system is usually accepted as being equivalent to a teaspoon in the household system and 1 dram in the apothecary system. Similarly, when converting between the metric and household system, 480 mL is usually rounded up to 500 mL and is considered equivalent to a pint; and 960 mL is usually rounded up to 1000 mL and is considered equivalent to a quart. Examples in this text use the rounded equivalents (5 mL, 250 mL, 500 mL, and 1000 mL). Remember to use the correct expression (such as decimals or fractions) in your answer when converting between systems. In the metric system, answers are shown in decimal format, whereas the household system usually uses fractions but can also use decimals. The apothecary system uses fractions with Arabic numerals but also uses Roman numerals for the digits 1 through 10, 20, 30, and $\overline{ss}$ for $\frac{1}{2}$.

Converting Volume Measurement Units between Systems

Use the information provided in this section for ratios, proportions, and conversions to determine the volume measurements between the metric, household, and apothecary systems.

EXAMPLE 8: 24 oz = _____ mL

Set up the known ratio: 30 mL = 1 oz.

Write as either a fraction or a linear ratio: $\dfrac{30\text{ mL}}{1\text{ oz}}$ *or*

30 mL : 1 oz.

Next, set up the second ratio with the unknown information so the proportion will look as follows:

$\dfrac{30\text{ mL}}{1\text{ oz}} = \dfrac{x\text{ mL}}{24\text{ oz}}$ *or* 30 mL : 1 oz :: x mL : 24 oz

Now cross-multiply; the answer will be in milliliters.

$\dfrac{30\text{ mL}}{1\text{ oz}} \diagup\!\!\!\!\diagdown \dfrac{x\text{ mL}}{24\text{ oz}}$ *or* 30 mL : 1 oz :: x mL : 24 oz

30 mL × 24 = 1 × x

720 mL = x

The answer is 24 oz = 720 mL.

EXAMPLE 9: 750 mL = _____ pint(s)

Set up the known ratio first. Known ratio: 500 mL = 1 pint. Next, set up the second ratio with the given and unknown information. Your problem now looks like these linear or fractional proportions:

$\dfrac{500\text{ mL}}{1\text{ pint}} = \dfrac{750\text{ mL}}{x\text{ pints}}$

or

500 mL : 1 pint :: 750 mL : x pint

Cross-multiply:

$\dfrac{500\text{ mL}}{1\text{ pint}} \diagup\!\!\!\!\diagdown \dfrac{750\text{ mL}}{x\text{ pint}}$

or

500 mL : 1 pint :: 750 mL : x

The problem now looks like this:

500 x = 750

Next, solve for x by dividing both sides by 500.

$\dfrac{500x}{500} = \dfrac{750}{500}$

We now have $x = \dfrac{750}{500}$.

Simplifying, the answer is x = 1.5.

x was expressed in pints, so the answer remains in pints.

750 mL = 1.5 pints or 1½ pints.

✎ **LEARNING TIP**

- Remember the answer may be written as 750 mL = 1½ pints or 750 mL = 1.5 pints because pints are household measurements and either fractions or decimals may be used.
- Also note that if you try to use the exact equivalent of 480 mL = 1 pint, instead of the approximation that 500 mL = 1 pint, your final answer becomes more difficult to calculate.

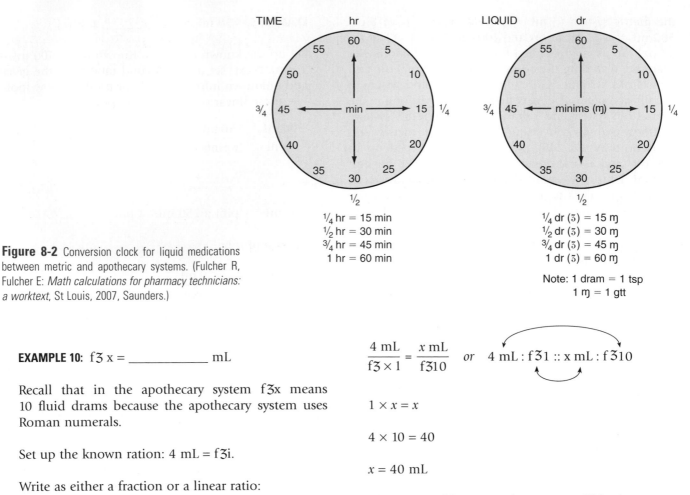

Figure 8-2 Conversion clock for liquid medications between metric and apothecary systems. (Fulcher R, Fulcher E: *Math calculations for pharmacy technicians: a worktext*, St Louis, 2007, Saunders.)

TIME   hr

¼ hr = 15 min
½ hr = 30 min
¾ hr = 45 min
1 hr = 60 min

LIQUID   dr

¼ dr (ℨ) = 15 ♏
½ dr (ℨ) = 30 ♏
¾ dr (ℨ) = 45 ♏
1 dr (ℨ) = 60 ♏

Note: 1 dram = 1 tsp
1 ♏ = 1 gtt

EXAMPLE 10: fℨ x = _____ mL

Recall that in the apothecary system fℨx means 10 fluid drams because the apothecary system uses Roman numerals.

Set up the known ration: 4 mL = fℨi.

Write as either a fraction or a linear ratio:

$\dfrac{4\ mL}{fℨi}$ or   4 mL : fℨi

Next, set up the second ratio with the unknown information so the proportion will look as follows:

$\dfrac{4\ mL}{fℨi} = \dfrac{x\ mL}{fℨx}$ or   4 mL : fℨi :: x mL : fℨx

Now cross multiply, changing the apothecary Roman numerals to Arabic numbers.

$\dfrac{4\ mL}{fℨ \times 1} = \dfrac{x\ mL}{fℨ10}$ or   4 mL : fℨ1 :: x mL : fℨ10

$1 \times x = x$

$4 \times 10 = 40$

$x = 40\ mL$

x is expressed in mL so the answer will be in mL.

Although not used often, a conversion of liquids in the apothecary system includes 60 minims (♏ 60) to a fluid dram (fℨ). Think of a clock with 60 minutes to an hour. A fourth of a dram is 15 minims just as 15 minutes is a fourth of an hour (Figure 8-2). Please notice that HR and DR (abbreviations with "r") are on the outside of the clock with minims and minutes (abbreviations with "m") are in the center of the clock. This may assist you in remembering the known elements needed for changing minims to drams.

Check Your Understanding: VOLUME CONVERSION 8-4

Calculation Review
Convert the following volume units to the requested equivalent measurements.

1. 45 mL = _____ Tbsp

2. 2 pt = _____ c

3. 1 mL = _____ gtt

4. 30 mL = _____ oz

5. 3 oz = _____ mL

6. 1000 mL = _____ pt

Check Your Understanding: VOLUME CONVERSION 8-4—cont'd

7. 250 mL = _____ c

8. 4 tsp = _____ mL

9. 1 pt = _____ mL

10. 30 gtts = _____ mL

Practical Application
Determine the following conversions.

11. A patient calls stating that he misplaced the medicine cup for his nighttime medicine. The directions say to take 30 mL before bedtime. How many tablespoons would you direct the patient to take? _____
_____

12. A physician tells the patient that he needs to drink two pints of *GoLYTELY*. Record this amount in his chart, using the metric system. _____

13. Dr. Haus wants his patient to force fluids. He requests that you convert 2000 mL into a household equivalent for the patient's information. _____

14. A patient is instructed to instill 2 drops of medication into each eye. How many minums would be equivalent to the dropper measured in the apothecary system? _____

15. You are directed to give a patient 30 mL of medication, but the medicine cup is calibrated in ounces. How many ounces are equivalent to 30 mL? _____

Weight

Most of the conversions done in the medical field are for converting different weights or solid measurements. The same rules apply for converting weights as for volume. Remember to always *first convert the quantities to be used into the same unit of measure within the same measurement system.* If you are converting among the metric, household, or apothecary systems, you will need to set up a ratio and proportion problem to obtain the equivalent weights within the same systems first. Then do the math conversion. The most common weight conversion between the metric and household systems is from kilograms to pounds. However, in the administration of medications, often the amount of prescribed medication and the dosage available may be converted between the apothecary and metric systems such as grains to milligrams or grams.

Another important fact to remember is that drug companies sometimes use different equivalents for a measure. In weight, the most common source of discrepancy is the grain, the apothecary system's basic unit of solid measure. Some tables will show 65 mg equal to 1 gr; other tables show 60 mg equal to 1 gr. Both measures are considered correct. In this text, we will use the most commonly used equivalence of 60 mg equals 1 gr. Remember that when converting between different measurement systems, the measurement obtained is only approximate, not an exact measurement. Table 8-3 identifies the most common weight equivalencies. The table may look difficult to remember, but there are basically only two conversions to memorize, and all other measurements can be derived from these conversions, using the information on ratio and proportion provided in Chapter 7. The conversion needed for converting between the apothecary and metric systems is 1 gr = 60 mg, or 1 g = 15 gr.

TABLE 8-3 WEIGHT MEASUREMENTS

METRIC SYSTEM	APOTHECARY SYSTEM	HOUSEHOLD
0.008 gram (g) = 8 milligrams (mg)	gr $\frac{1}{8}$	—
0.01 g = 10 mg	gr $\frac{1}{6}$	—
0.015 g = 15 mg	gr $\frac{1}{4}$	—
0.06 g = 60 mg	gr 1	—
0.1 g = 100 mg	gr $1\frac{1}{2}$	—
1 g = 1000 mg	gr 15	—
30 g	—	1 ounce (oz)
0.45 kilogram (kg)	—	1 pound (lb)
1 kg = 1000 g	—	2.2 lb

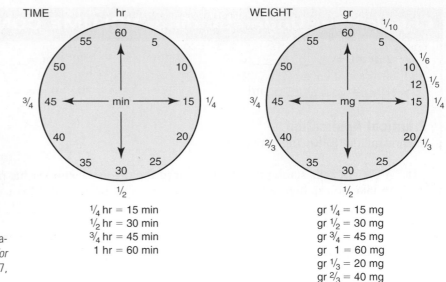

Figure 8-3 Conversion clock for weight or solid measurements. (Fulcher R, Fulcher E: *Math calculations for pharmacy technicians: a worktext,* St Louis, 2007, Saunders.)

¼ hr = 15 min
½ hr = 30 min
¾ hr = 45 min
1 hr = 60 min

gr ¼ = 15 mg
gr ½ = 30 mg
gr ¾ = 45 mg
gr 1 = 60 mg
gr ⅓ = 20 mg
gr ⅔ = 40 mg

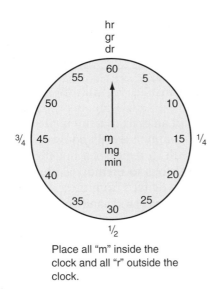

Place all "m" inside the clock and all "r" outside the clock.

Figure 8-4 Conversion clock for liquid and solid measurements. (Fulcher R, Fulcher E: *Math calculations for pharmacy technicians: a worktext,* St Louis, 2007, Saunders.)

LEARNING TIP

Weight measurement comparisons are easier to remember using the conversion clock shown. Think of 1 hour = 60 minutes (1 hr = 60 min), just as 1 grain = 60 milligrams (1 gr = 60 mg). Use Figure 8-3 to make the conversion easier. Finally you may place all three clocks together to assist with conversion of liquid to solid measurement found with the apothecary system. Remember that the abbreviations containing "r" remain outside the clock while the abbreviations containing "m" remain inside the clock (Figure 8-4).

Converting Weight Measurement Units between Systems

Converting weight units among systems is similar to converting volume units among systems. The safest way is by setting up a ratio and proportion equation. Then solve the problem using basic math.

LEARNING TIP

Always use the correct notation in your answer when converting between systems. For example, in the apothecary system the abbreviation "gr" is written first, followed by the quantity, which is written in lowercase Roman numerals, if the number used is $\overline{ss}$ or ½, 1 to 10, 15, 20, or 30. In the metric and household systems, the quantity is written first using an Arabic digit (0 to 9), followed by the abbreviation. The following examples illustrate this.

EXAMPLE 11: 300 mg = gr _____

Set up the known ratio first.
Known ratio: 60 mg = gr i.

Write as a fraction or ratio:

$\dfrac{60 \text{ mg}}{\text{gr i}}$ OR 60 mg : gr i

Next, set up the second ratio as a fraction with the given and unknown information. The problem now looks like this proportion:

$\dfrac{60 \text{ mg}}{\text{gr i}} = \dfrac{300 \text{ mg}}{x \text{ gr}}$ OR   60 mg : gr i :: 300 mg : x gr

Cross-multiply, cancelling the abbreviations, as appropriate, and change apothecary Roman numerals to Arabic numbers used in the metric system.

$$\frac{60 \text{ mg}}{\text{gr } 1} \diagdown \frac{300 \text{ mg}}{x \text{ gr}} \quad or$$

60 mg : gr 1 :: 300 mg : x gr

$60 \times x = 60x$

$300 \times 1 \text{ gr} = 300 \text{ gr}$

Rewrite the equation as:

$60x = 300 \text{ gr}$

Solve for x by dividing both sides by 60.

$$\frac{60x}{60} = \frac{300 \text{ gr}}{60}$$

Be sure to remember that the unknown for x was gr; therefore your answer will be expressed in grains. When completing the math, $x = 5$. Therefore 300 mg = gr v. The answer is expressed in Roman numerals because the answer is in the apothecary system.

EXAMPLE 12: 206 lb = _____ kg

Set up the known ratio first. Known ratio: 2.2 lb = 1 kg. Write as a fraction or ratio:

$$\frac{2.2 \text{ lb}}{1 \text{ kg}} \quad OR \quad 2.2 \text{ lb} : 1 \text{ kg}$$

Next, set up the second ratio as a fraction with the given and unknown information. Your problem now looks like this proportion:

$$\frac{2.2 \text{ lb}}{1 \text{ kg}} = \frac{206 \text{ lb}}{x \text{ kg}} \quad OR \quad 2.2 \text{ lb} : 1 \text{ kg} :: 206 \text{ lb} : x \text{ kg}$$

Cross-multiply, leaving off the abbreviations:

$$\frac{2.2 \text{ lb}}{1 \text{ kg}} \diagdown \frac{206 \text{ lb}}{x \text{ kg}} \quad or$$

2.2 lb : 1 kg :: 206 lb : x kg

$206 \times 1 \text{ kg} = 206 \text{ kg}$

$2.2 \times x = 2.2x$

Rewrite the equation as 2.2 x = 206 kg.
Solve for x by dividing each side by 2.2:

$$\frac{2.2x}{2.2} = \frac{206 \text{ kg}}{2.2}$$

Remember x was in kg; therefore your answer will be expressed in kilograms.

$x = 93.6$; therefore 206 lb = 93.6 kg. In most cases, kilograms can be rounded to a whole number so that dosage calculations will be easier, so 93.6 kg would be rounded to 94 kg.

Sometimes the conversion cannot be immediately calculated because you may need to determine the correct unit conversions before solving the problem. This occurs if you are given a problem where you must first change the measurement units, such as changing ounces to pounds or milligrams to grams or micrograms to milligrams, so the units you are seeking are the same. After you find the same units, then set up the proportion. Study the following example. Note that the requested answer is not in the same unit as the given information, so an extra step is made at the beginning of the problem to convert the numerators and denominators to the same units. After making the units the same, proceed to solve the problem by setting up the proportions as previously shown.

EXAMPLE 13: A physician orders nitroglycerin 600 mcg to be given to a patient with angina.

The medicine label reads "gr $\frac{1}{100}$ per tablet."
To convert, you must first change micrograms to milligrams; then convert to grains. First change mcg to mg.

600 mcg = 0.6 mg
Known: 60 mg = 1 gr
Set up the problem like this:

$$\frac{60 \text{ mg}}{1 \text{ gr}} = \frac{0.6 \text{ mg}}{x \text{ gr}} \quad or \quad 60 \text{ mg} : 1 \text{ gr} :: 0.6 \text{ mg} : x \text{ gr}$$

Cross-multiply, leaving off the measurement abbreviations:

$$\frac{60 \text{ mg}}{1 \text{ gr}} \diagdown \frac{0.6 \text{ mg}}{x \text{ gr}} \quad or$$

60 mg : 1 gr :: 0.6 mg : x gr

$60\,x = 0.6$

$$x = \frac{0.6}{60} \quad \text{or} \quad \frac{6}{600}$$

$$x = \frac{1}{100} \text{ gr}$$

The dose of medication would be one tablet because each tablet is gr $\frac{1}{100}$.

LEARNING TIP

Always make the conversion to the label of dosage on available medication.

Another method of completing this example is to calculate the entire problem using **dimensional analysis.** Dimensional analysis is a mathematical means of canceling unwanted units (called factors) in conversion of unit equivalency or an extended ratio and proportion. In Example 13, instead of two calculations of micrograms to milligrams and then the conversion to the apothecary system, the calculation may be performed using several ratios in the proportional equation. Each factor is written as a fraction, and the factors must be related to each other for the problem to be solved. If the units are not in the same measurement system, the conversion may be made within the one proportional equation. The following steps are needed to solve using dimensional analysis. These have been related to the problem given in Example 13.

♥ **EXAMPLE 14:** A physician orders *nitroglycerin* 600 mcg to be given to a patient with angina. The available medication is nitroglycerin gr 1/100 tablets.

There are six distinct steps in setting up dimensional or fractional analysis here and with all dimensional analysis problems.
1. Find the known quantity: gr $\frac{1}{100}$
2. What is the desired amount? 600 mcg
3. What is the conversion factor? gr i = 60 mg and; 1000 mcg = 1 mg
4. Set up the problem with the available conversion factors, placing the desired amount in the first fraction over 1.

$$x = \frac{600 \text{ mcg}}{1} \times \frac{1 \text{ mg}}{1000 \text{ mcg}} \times \frac{1 \text{ gr}}{60 \text{ mg}}$$

5. Cross out unwanted units that are in both the numerator and the denominator.

$$x = \frac{600 \text{ mcg}}{1} \times \frac{1 \text{ mg}}{1000 \text{ mcg}} \times \frac{1 \text{ gr}}{60 \text{ mg}}$$

6. Multiply the numerators and denominators and solve the calculation.

$$x = \frac{600}{1} \times \frac{1}{1000} \times \frac{1 \text{ gr}}{60}$$

$$x = \frac{600 \text{ gr}}{60000}$$

$$x = \frac{600 \text{ gr}}{60000}$$

$$x = \text{gr} \frac{1}{100}$$

Since the available medication is nitroglycerin gr 1/100 tablet, one tablet should be administered because gr $\dfrac{1}{100} = 600 \text{ mcg}$.

LEARNING TIP

Dimensional analysis is helpful when more than one conversion is needed to complete a calculation. This will be discussed again in Chapter 9.

The physician desires the weight of a premature baby to be converted to kilograms to be able to calculate the needed dosage for a medication. The physician asks you to convert the pounds and ounces to kilograms.

EXAMPLE 15: A premature baby weighs 4 lb 3 oz. Convert this weight to kilograms.

Household System:
Known: 16 oz = 1 lb
To solve, first change the 4 lb to ounces, then add 3 oz.

$$4 \times 16 = 64 + 3 = 67 \text{ oz}$$

You want to convert ounces to kilograms.

Metric System:
Known: 1 kg = 2.2 lb or 0.45 kg = 1 lb
Now you can set up the proportion, and solve.

$$\frac{16 \text{ oz}}{0.45 \text{ kg}} = \frac{67 \text{ oz}}{x \text{ kg}} \quad \text{OR} \quad 16 \text{ oz} : 0.45 \text{ kg} :: 67 \text{ oz} : x \text{ kg}$$

Cross-multiply, leaving off the abbreviations:

$$\frac{16 \text{ oz}}{0.45 \text{ kg}} \times \frac{67 \text{ oz}}{x \text{ kg}} \quad or$$

16 o̶z̶ : 0.45 kg :: 67 o̶z̶ : x kg

$16 \times x = 16 \; x$

$0.45 \text{ kg} \times 67 = 30.15 \text{ kg}$

Write as an equation: $16x = 30.15 \text{ kg}$
Divide each side by 16 to find x.

$$\frac{16x}{16} = \frac{30.15 \text{ kg}}{16}$$
$$x = 1.88 \text{ kg}$$

Finally, round the answer to a whole number for easier dosage calculation: $1.88 \cong 2$. So the final answer is 4 lb 3 oz = 2 kg.

Remember that x was expressed in kg so your answer will be in kilograms.

To compute using dimensional analysis:

$$x = \frac{67 \text{ oz}}{1} \times \frac{1 \text{ lb}}{16 \text{ oz}} \times \frac{1 \text{ kg}}{2.2 \text{ lb}}$$

$$x = \frac{67 \text{ o̶z̶}}{1} \times \frac{1 \text{ l̶b̶}}{16 \text{ o̶z̶}} \times \frac{1 \text{ kg}}{2.2 \text{ l̶b̶}}$$

$$x = \frac{67}{1} \times \frac{1}{16} \times \frac{1 \text{ kg}}{2.2}$$

$$x = \frac{67 \text{ kg}}{35.2}$$

$$x = 1.88 \text{ or } 2 \text{ kg}$$

Check Your Understanding: WEIGHT CONVERSIONS 8-5

Calculation Review

Convert the following weight units to the requested equivalent measures. Round decimals to the nearest tenth.

1. gr $\dfrac{3}{4}$ = _____ mg

2. 12 lb = _____ kg

3. gr xv = _____ mg

4. 0.015 g = _____ mg

5. gr v = _____ g

6. 2.45 kg = _____ g

7. 360 mg = _____ gr

8. gr $\dfrac{1}{60}$ = _____ mg

9. gr vi = _____ mg

10. 15 kg = _____ g

Practical Application

Solve the following conversions.

11. A premature infant weighs 1426 g. How many pounds does the baby weigh? (Round to the nearest pound.)
_____

12. A patient weighs 45 lb. What is the patient's weight in kilograms? _____

13. How many milligrams of **penicillin** are left in a vial containing penicillin 5 g after 750 mg are removed?
_____

14. A physician writes an order for **aspirin** gr v. How many grams would this be? _____

15. A biopsy sample weighs $2\frac{1}{2}$ ounces. Record this in grams._____

TABLE 8-4 LENGTH MEASUREMENTS	
METRIC	**HOUSEHOLD**
10 millimeter (mm) = 1 cm	0.4 or $\frac{4}{10}$ inch (in)
2.5 centimeters (cm)	1 inch
30 cm	1 foot (ft) = 12 inches
90 cm	1 yard
100 cm = 1 meter (m)	39.4 or 39$\frac{4}{10}$ inches

Length

The unit measurement of length is the most versatile of the basic conversions we study because length can be measured for many different reasons and in many different ways. For example, patient supplies such as medical garments, elastic stockings, Ace bandages, and even gauze pads are all made to specified sizes that could be measured in terms of a body area circumference, length, or height. Linear measurements are recorded in medical records for lengths of surgical incisions; lengths of wounds being sutured; baseline areas for tests such as the *purified protein derivative* (PPD) test for tuberculosis (TB); and even the diameter of moles and other lesions. The newborn's length, chest, and head circumference are measured. Orthopedic appliances are measured to fit a specific patient usually by girth, length, or both. Table 8-4 shows the length measurement conversions practitioners must know. As with the other conversions, these are approximations.

Converting Length Measurement Units between Systems

With medical measurements, many of the instruments used are calibrated in metric and household units, but you may occasionally need to convert between those two measurement systems using Table 8-4. The metric units are used in measuring lesions and lacerations for insurance coding, whereas household measurements are used to measure height and hypodermic needle lengths.

> **EXAMPLE 16:** An abdominal cavity was opened using a 14-inch incision. Convert this measurement into a metric length.

Set this problem up as a proportion. Known ratio: 2.5 cm = 1 in. Set up a proportion with the known and unknown information to look like this:

$$\frac{2.5\ cm}{1\ in} = \frac{x\ cm}{14\ in} \quad OR \quad 2.5\ cm : 1\ in :: x\ cm : 14\ in$$

Cross-multiply, dropping the abbreviations.

$$\frac{2.5\ cm}{1\ in} \diagup\!\!\!\!\diagdown \frac{x\ cm}{14\ in} \quad or$$

2.5 cm : 1 in :: x cm : 14 in

$$2.5 \times 14 = 35$$

$$1 \times x = x\ cm$$

$x = 35$. Therefore 14 inches = 35 cm. Remember x was expressed in cm therefore the answer is in centimeters.

> **EXAMPLE 17:** A patient is 185 cm tall. Record this using the household measurement of feet and inches.

This problem can also be set up as a proportion. Known ratio: 30 cm = 12 in *or* 2.5 cm = 1 in. Either ratio can be used; both are shown in this example.

Set up a proportion with the known and unknown information, using the conversion that you most easily remember. Your problem will look like either of these:

A) $\dfrac{30\ cm}{12\ in} = \dfrac{185\ cm}{x\ in}$ or   30 cm : 12 in :: 185 cm : x in

or

B) $\dfrac{2.5\ cm}{1\ in} = \dfrac{185\ cm}{x\ in}$ or   2.5 cm : 1 in :: 185 cm : x in

Cross-multiply, dropping the abbreviations.

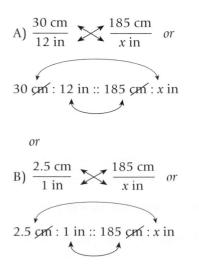

A) $\dfrac{30\ cm}{12\ in} \diagup\!\!\!\!\diagdown \dfrac{185\ cm}{x\ in}$ or

30 cm : 12 in :: 185 cm : x in

or

B) $\dfrac{2.5\ cm}{1\ in} \diagup\!\!\!\!\diagdown \dfrac{185\ cm}{x\ in}$ or

2.5 cm : 1 in :: 185 cm : x in

A) $30 \times x = 30\,x$ or   B) $2.5 \times x = 2.5\,x$

A) $12 \times 185 = 2220$ or   B) $1 \times 185 = 185$

Solve for x by dividing both sides by 30 or 2.5 as shown.

A) $\dfrac{30\,x}{30} = \dfrac{2220}{30}$

or

B) $\dfrac{2.5\,x}{2.5} = \dfrac{185}{2.5}$

By either method, $x = 74$ inches, but remember that this measurement is in inches because x was in inches. Because the problem asks you to identify feet and inches, the next step is necessary.
Known equivalent: 12 in = 1 ft.
Set up the problem to determine how many feet are in 74 inches.

$\dfrac{1\,ft}{12\,in} = \dfrac{x\,ft}{74\,in}$ OR $1\,ft : 12\,in :: x\,ft : 74\,in$

Cross-multiply.

$\dfrac{1\,ft}{12\,in} \;\times\; \dfrac{x\,ft}{74\,in}$ or

$1\,ft : 12\,in :: x\,ft : 74\,in$

$12 \times x = 12x$

$74 \times 1 = 74$

Solve for x by dividing both sides by 12.

$\dfrac{12x}{12} = \dfrac{74}{12}$

$x = 6$ feet with 2 inches left over.

Remember this must be in feet, as x was expressed in feet.

185 cm = 6 ft 2 in

Using dimensional analysis the equation would be as follows:

$x = \dfrac{185\,cm}{1} \times \dfrac{1\,in}{2.5\,cm} \times \dfrac{1\,ft}{12\,in}$

$x = \dfrac{185\,cm}{1} \times \dfrac{1\,in}{2.5\,cm} \times \dfrac{1\,ft}{12\,in}$

$x = \dfrac{185}{30}$

$x = 6.16$ ft   or   6 ft 2 in

Check Your Understanding: LENGTH CONVERSIONS 8-6

Calculation Review
Solve these length conversions. Round answers to nearest whole number.

1. 8 in = _____ cm

2. 5 ft 6 in = _____ cm

3. 3 m = _____ ft

4. 28 mm = _____ cm

5. 60 cm = _____ ft

6. 80 cm = _____ m

7. 75 in = _____ m

8. 2 in = _____ mm

9. $3\frac{1}{2}$ ft = _____ m

10. 13 mm = _____ cm

Practical Application
Determine the following conversions.

11. A patient needs a dressing changed when her wound drainage on the bandage measures 2.5 cm. The current bandage drainage measures 50 mm. What is the difference in millimeters between the measurements? _____Does the dressing need to be changed? _____

Continued

Check Your Understanding: LENGTH CONVERSIONS 8-6—cont'd

12. A physician needs 75 cm of suture material to close a long laceration. What is the minimum number of feet of suture material you would need to place on the suture tray? (Round to whole number.) _____

13. A small newborn is 18 inches long. Record this in centimeters. _____

14. A pediatric chart to measure height measures up to 120 cm. How many inches is this? _____

15. A physician orders **nirtoglycerin** ointment 1.5 cm. The measurement paper for the ointment is in inches. How many inches of ointment should be applied to the paper for administration? _____

SUMMARY

This chapter begins by introducing the international standard for time, the 24-hour clock. Temperature conversions between Fahrenheit and Celsius are then discussed. The majority of the chapter focuses on conversions among the metric, household, and apothecary measurement systems for units of volume, weight, and length. The conversion methods shown in this chapter are ratio and proportion and dimensional analysis. Although most Americans are most familiar with household measurements, the metric system is the predominant method used by health care providers and in other parts of the world. A general knowledge of all three measurement systems is necessary in order to work accurately with patients, to complete accurate medical documentation, and to read medical information.

The next chapter introduces calculating dosages of nonparenteral medications. The information learned in this chapter will be used to understand how nonparenteral dosages can be calculated using actual drug dosages and drug names.

CRITICAL THINKING EXERCISES

Study each case independently. The icon for the body system in which the drug is used is shown. Determine each answer by solving for the missing information. Be sure to show your calculations on a separate sheet of paper.

1. CA **Cyclophosphamide** (Cytoxan) is used intravenously in chemotherapy to inhibit the growth of neoplasms. The vial of medication contains Cytoxan 1 g. Could you prepare a dose of 750 mg from this container? Explain your answer. _____

2. The physician orders **phenobarbital** 100 mg. Available are phenobarbital gr $\overline{ss}$ tablets. Can you administer this medication with the tablets supplied? Show your work. _____

3. A patient is prescribed **fexofenadine** (Allegra) for seasonal allergic rhinitis. If the patient is to take two tablets a day, half of the dose in the morning and the other half 12 hours later, give the international standard time for the second dose if the first one was taken at 10:30 AM. _____

4. PA IN For juvenile arthritis, the physician might prescribe **ibuporofen** (Motrin). If the usual dosage for a child is based on weight in kilograms and the child weighs 66 pounds, how many kilograms does the child weigh? _____

5. The physician's office has scales that weigh in kilograms. The patient asks you how much weight he has lost when the scale shows 22 kg of weight loss. _____

6. **Testosterone** (Depo-Testosterone) is a hormone used for replacement in the hypogonadal male. This medication is administered by injection with vials that need to be stored at 20° C to 25° C. Convert this temperature to Fahrenheit. Would this medication be stored in a refrigerator? Show your work. _____

REVIEW QUESTIONS

Practical Application

Solve by using the method of calculation you feel most comfortable using.

1. If a dosage strength is 2 g in 10 mL, what is the correct amount of liquid when 4 g are ordered? _____

2. When preparing surgical packs for autoclaving, you need one Allis tissue forceps and three hemostats for each pack you prepare. What are your proportions for six packs? _____

3. A medication contains 1 part pure drug to 25 parts of solute. What is the ratio and what is the fraction? _____

   How many parts of pure drug are in 150 parts of solute? _____

4. The dosage of phenobarbital ordered is gr ¼. The tablets available are phenobarbital gr $\overline{ss}$ in a scored tablet. How many tablets would you administer to the patient? _____

All of the following statements are *false*. Determine the error(s) and rewrite the statement, giving completely correct information in the space provided.

5. A medication that is to be given once a day before bedtime (10:00 PM) is given at 2000. _____

6. The approximate value of 500 mL is 1 quart. _____

7. In the metric system, the primary measurements used for dosage calculations are volume and length. _____

8. In the apothecary system, 16 oz are equal to 1 lb. _____

9. A scar that measures 14 cm is approximately 2 inches long. _____

10. A biopsy specimen weighs 45 g. This would be approximately a half pound in the household system. _____

11. A ratio is a comparison of two fractions that are considered equivalent. _____

12. Conversions can be immediately calculated because you do not need to determine unit proportions before solving. _____

13. A metric-sized orthopedic appliance measures 6 inches in length. _____

14. A medication weighing gr v would be equivalent to 200 g. _____

15. The 24-hour clock is often used in the United States. _____

16. When converting between measurement systems, answers will usually vary by ±1%. _____

17. *Volume* refers to weight. _____

18. 50° Celsius would be a comfortable room temperature. _____

_____

19. When converting from Celsius to Fahrenheit, remember to multiply first because Fahrenheit is the smaller number. _____

_____

20. In the apothecary system, 15 drops are the equivalent of 1 metric mL. _____

_____

21. Forty-five kg are equivalent to 1 lb. _____

_____

22. The acceptable metric equivalency of one-half teaspoon is 2 mL. _____

_____

23. A centimeter is smaller than a millimeter, and a centimeter is smaller than an inch. _____

_____

24. A medication is ordered for gr ¾, and the available amount is 30 mg. The proper amount to administer is one tablet. _____

_____

Calculating Doses of Nonparenteral Medications

After studying this chapter, you should be capable of doing the following:

- Determining the correct dose of medication to be administered, based on a physician's order.
- Calculating the doses of nonparenteral drugs administered in solid form, using ratio and proportion, formula, or the dimensional analysis method.
- Calculating the doses of nonparenteral drugs administered in liquid form, using ratios and proportions, formulas, or the dimensional analysis method.
- Calculating doses on the basis of body surface area and weight in kilograms.

KEY WORDS

Body surface area (BSA) calculation
Factors

Formula method
Nomogram

Nonparenteral medications

Reconstitution
Unit

Chapter 9 PRETEST—CALCULATING DOSES OF NONPARENTERAL MEDICATIONS

Calculate the following doses.

1. Fill in 1 teaspoon.

2 TBS	30 mL
	25 mL
	20 mL
1 TBS	15 mL
2 TSP	10 mL
1 TSP	5 mL

2. Fill in 25 mL.

2 TBS	30 mL
	25 mL
	20 mL
1 TBS	15 mL
2 TSP	10 mL
1 TSP	5 mL

Continued

Chapter 9 PRETEST—CALCULATING DOSES OF NONPARENTERAL MEDICATIONS—cont'd

On the provided lines, explain exactly what quantity of medication and the number of doses of medications should be taken.

3. Ordered: hydrochlorothiazide 50 mg PO bid with morning and early afternoon meal.
   Available: hydrochlorothiazide 25 mg tablets.
   Dose to be given: _____
   How often? _____

4. Ordered: allopurinol 300 mg PO daily.
   Available: allopurinol 100 mg tablets.
   Dose to be given: _____
   How often? _____

5. Ordered: Zyrtec 10 mg PO daily.
   Available: Zyrtec 1 mg/1 mL syrup. Please give the dose in metric and household measures.
   Dose to be given: _____
   How often? _____

6. Ordered: warfarin sodium 6 mg PO daily.
   Available: warfarin sodium 4 mg scored tablets.
   Dose to be given: _____
   How often? _____

7. Ordered: Amoxil chewable 400 mg tablets q12h.
   Available: Amoxil 200 mg chewable tablets.
   Dose to be given: _____
   How often? _____

8. Tina has an infection with moderate pain and was prescribed Lortab Elixir 15 mg/1000 mg tid prn. Using the following label, calculate the desired dose to be given:
   Dose to be given: _____
   How often? _____

INTRODUCTION TO METHODS OF DOSAGE CALCULATION

Nonparenteral medications are usually drugs taken orally or by inhalation. In this chapter, a comparison of three different methods for calculating dosages for nonparenteral medications is shown. It is not important that you memorize all three methods. It is more important that you choose *one* method and use that method to prevent potential medication errors that could result from switching among the methods. With the first two methods (ratio and proportion and the **formula method**), the most important concept is *always* to be sure that the **units** ordered and the units on hand are measured in the same system and the same weight or volume measurement. For example, if the drug requested is given in grams but you only have milligrams, the first step must be to convert milligrams to grams or vice versa. In another example, the physician may write the medication in the apothecary system for a drug that is available in the metric system. Then grains (apothecary measure) must be converted to milligrams, micrograms, or a measure of the metric system. *As a rule of thumb, when deciding which measurement to find in the final conversion, the final dose or unit of measure should match the unit found on the container of available medication. The conversion should be to that measurement.*

In a perfect world, all drugs would come in the same measurement system and would be found in a unit-dose system. Then no calculations would be necessary to find a specific dose. Administration errors would be decreased to a minimum. Sometimes the health care provider will need to determine and prepare the proper doses using conversions between systems when the amount of medication ordered does not match the medication on hand. By reviewing a few basic guidelines about the various medications, you can make sure that administration of drugs is still safe. Box 9-1 covers the basic guidelines.

BOX 9-1 NONPARENTERAL DOSAGE GUIDELINES

- Do not open or divide a capsule.
- Tablets that are not scored are not intended to be divided.
- A tablet that is scored may be divided or broken.
- An enteric-coated tablet or caplet should not be broken or crushed.
- Buccal and sublingual tablets should not be broken, crushed, or swallowed.
- Sustained- or extended-release tablets should not be broken or crushed.
- Before crushing or breaking any tablet or caplet, always check to be sure this action will not affect the drug's purpose and physician's permission has been obtained.

It is important to avoid math errors when calculating the drug dose. A few basic rules can help you remember to calculate with confidence. First, always be sure to use the same units of measure when setting up the problem unless conversion is needed. If a conversion to the same units of measure is needed, the conversion will be the first step, unless dimensional analysis is being used. Make the needed conversion only when using the ratio and proportion or the formula method. Next, even if the problem seems easy, work the math on paper to find a solution. Although it is always important to take the time to do the calculations, thinking ahead can prevent errors. *If your calculations do not result in the solution you anticipated or do not seem sensible, recheck all calculations.* After calculating the dosage, always be sure to check and recheck decimals or fractions. If the dose is calculated according to body surface area (BSA), insert the appropriate factors into the formula and then make the calculations; use a calculator with these measurements to determine the appropriate dose, as many of these may be long and complicated. Finally, read the health care provider's order one more time to ensure you are calculating for the dose ordered before administering the medication. Most medications are designed to be administered as a whole tablet or capsule, so if you are dividing the medication form, it should be available as a scored tablet or a pourable liquid.

A few additional words of warning about combining different dosages to substitute for the strength on hand. Different dosage strengths must be considered before starting dose calculations. With some oral medication orders, using combinations of dosage strengths of the desired medication is appropriate. However, be careful with delayed-release and sustained-release medications. With these types of medications, administering two 5 mg tablets to make a 10 mg dose is not equivalent because the release time is not the same as when taking one 10 mg tablet. Therefore, as a rule of thumb, timed-release medications—whether delayed or sustained—are not interchangeable; the dose should be given only in the dosage strength and in the medication form prescribed.

Remember, for conversions between measurement systems, the answer will only be *approximate*. In reality, today most physicians prescribe medications in the manufactured dosage strength and form. However, you will have to convert from grains to grams or milligrams on some occasions. With prescriptions from ambulatory care facilities, the pharmacist will usually make the calculation per the physician's order. However, the allied health professional may be expected to make the conversion when administering medications in the ambulatory care setting or when providing physician ordered samples that are not in a strength that has been ordered. If you have any doubts about the medication calculation, always ask that someone verify your calculations before you administer the medication. This may mean that you verify the calculation with a fellow employee or that you verify the medication order and the calculation of the dose with the physician.

Each drug calculation problem will have two parts. The first part of the problem tells you what the physician has ordered and is sometimes referred to as "dose desired" or "dose ordered" (DO). The second part of the problem tells you the medication you have on hand and is usually referred to as "dose available" (DA). Regardless of the method you choose to use, remember that this basic method applies to all dose calculations.

The following steps are necessary to calculate a dose of medication:

1. Note the information provided on the medication bottle on hand, or what the *available* medication is (DA). This is also referred to as *what you have.*
2. Determine what is asked for on the physician's order, or what dose is *ordered* (DO). This is also referred to as *what you want.*
3. Identify the available unit of measure for the form that will be used to supply the desired dose (DO), or dose to be given, such as tablets, capsules, milliliters, and ounces.

4. Be sure all units are in the same measurement system. The conversion should be to the units found on the available medication bottle. Conversion between systems must be done before the calculation of the dose except with dimensional analysis.
5. Calculate the desired dose.
6. Verify the dose calculation with the medication order using the correct measurement system for your answer.

DOSAGE FORMS FOR NONPARENTERAL MEDICATIONS

Dosage forms are presented in Chapter 3. This section is added as a short review of medication forms and the calculation of doses given orally. Solid medications are designated as the weight of medication per dosage form, such as milligrams per tablet or milligrams per milliliter for liquids. Because most people do not have utensils for measuring in the metric system, conversion to the household systems of teaspoons and tablespoons is appropriate. Always be sure that patients understand exactly how to measure a dose for administration.

Check Your Understanding: DOSAGE MEASUREMENTS BOX 9-1

Calculation Review
Identify the amount of solution in each calibrated medication container.

1. _____ tsp

2. _____ tsp

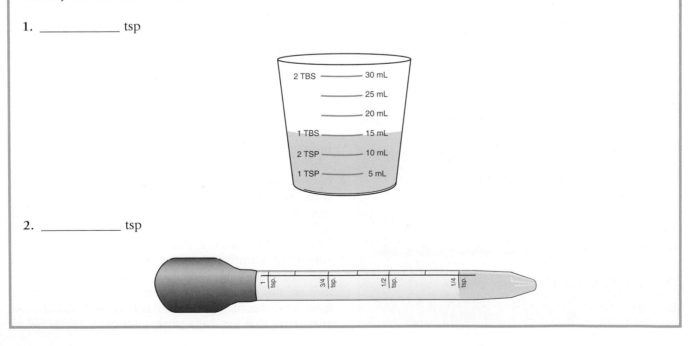

Check Your Understanding: DOSAGE MEASUREMENTS
BOX 9-1—cont'd

3. _____ mL

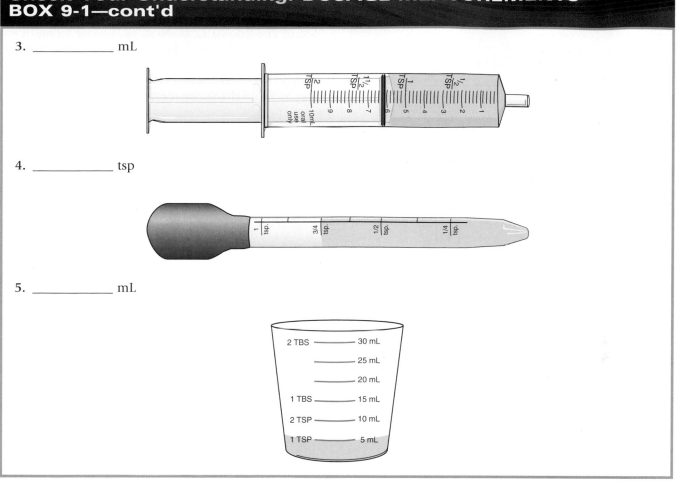

4. _____ tsp

5. _____ mL

THREE METHODS OF CALCULATING DOSES

The next three sections will show you how to calculate drug doses by using different methods of calculation. It is important to review each method independently, then choose the method that is easiest for you to use for calculations. To help prevent calculation errors, use *only one* of the three methods. Always keep in mind that if the answer you computed does not seem logical, you should redo the math.

The first method uses *ratio and proportion* and requires the preparer to first convert the problem so that the measurements in the problem are in the same measurement system. The second method is called the *formula method,* which also requires conversion so that factors are converted to equivalent measurements in the same measurement system. The third method of drug calculations is called *dimensional analysis.* In this method the problem does *not* convert measurements into equivalent units as a separate step. To solve a problem using dimensional analysis, one extended fractional equation is necessary, and units are cancelled. The following sections explain the three methods further.

Calculating Doses Using Ratio and Proportion

When a physician requests that a drug be given to a patient, sometimes the dosage available (dosage on hand) will not be in the same measurement unit as the physician prescribed. When this occurs, you must be able to convert, or change, measurement systems to provide the patient with the correct dose. To understand the ratio and proportion method, first analyze the terms "ratio" and "proportion." See Box 9-2 for the terminology used with this method.

BOX 9-2 UNDERSTANDING THE TERMINOLOGY OF RATIO AND PROPORTION

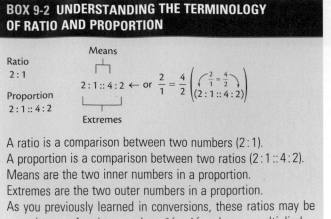

A ratio is a comparison between two numbers (2:1).
A proportion is a comparison between two ratios (2:1::4:2).
Means are the two inner numbers in a proportion.
Extremes are the two outer numbers in a proportion.
As you previously learned in conversions, these ratios may be
  written as fractions, such as $\frac{2}{1} = \frac{4}{2}$ and cross-multiplied.

If you did not know one of the parts of the ratio, you could find it by using a symbol such as x to stand for the unknown number. Suppose you know only the first complete ratio: 3:1. In the second ratio you know the first number is 6. You can find the second ratio by replacing the second number with x. It would look like this: 3:1::6:x. Now multiply the means and the extremes to solve for x. You should have the results of $3x = 6$, so x is equal to 2. Put the number 2 into the second ratio and you have 3:1::6:2, or $\frac{3}{1} = \frac{6}{2}$, which shows an equivalency when you multiply means and extremes. Be sure to identify the unit values of both of the ratios. *The numerators and denominators must be of the same measurement units, respectively.* For example, 1 mL:15 gtts is the same as 2 mL:30 gtts and would be written with both numerators expressed in "mL" and both denominators expressed in "gtts," or

$$\frac{1\ mL}{15\ gtts} = \frac{2\ mL}{30\ gtts} \text{ or } 1\ mL:15\ gtts::2\ mL:30\ gtts$$

Use the following formula to find medication doses using ratios or proportions.

Dosage Available (DA):Dosage Form (DF)::Dosage
  Ordered (DO):Dose to be Given (DG)

If using fractions, the formula would be as follows:

$$\frac{DA}{DF} = \frac{DO}{DG}$$

 PROBLEM: Sulfamethoxazole oral suspension is supplied as 1 g/10 mL. The physician orders sulfamethoxazole 2 g. How many milliliters would be administered? How many teaspoons would be given?

The easiest way to show proportion between measurement systems is by comparing the known ratio (available) to the unknown ratio. To set up the problem, first identify the known ratio. Next, set up the second ratio using x to signify the unknown unit. Be careful to use the same order for the units in setting up the second ratio as used in the first ratio. Then solve for x in the second ratio by multiplying the means and extremes, reducing when appropriate.

EXAMPLE 1:

$$\frac{1\ g}{10\ mL} \bowtie \frac{2\ g}{x\ mL} \text{ or } 1\ g : 10\ mL :: 2\ g : x\ mL$$

$$1 \times x = 2 \times 10$$

$$x = 20$$

In this problem, x is stated in milliliters because milliliters were the unknown.

Therefore sulfamethoxazole oral suspension 20 mL is the dose to be given.

Now solve for the teaspoons in household measuremnets.

$$\frac{1\ tsp}{5\ mL} = \frac{x\ tsp}{20\ mL} \text{ or } 1\ tsp:5\ mL::x\ tsp:20\ mL$$

$5 \times x = 1 \times 20$ (Note that the appropriate abbreviations for measurement systems have been dropped.)

$$5x = 20$$

$$x = 4$$

Remember that the x represents teaspoons.

In household measurements the dose to be given is 4 tsp.

🖉 LEARNING TIP

When setting up both ratios, be sure to *label all* of the terms including the x with the correct measurement unit to be sure equations are equivalents.

Check Your Understanding: RATIO AND PROPORTION
BOX 9-2

Calculation Review
Replace the following ratios with the correct fractional equivalent. Do not simplify.

1. 2:3 = _____

2. 1:50 = _____

3. 1:150 = _____

4. 2:800 = _____

5. 2:7 = _____

Replace the following fractions with the correct ratio equivalent. Do not simplify.

6. $\dfrac{2}{500}$ = _____

7. $\dfrac{1}{250}$ = _____

8. $\dfrac{1}{3}$ = _____

9. $\dfrac{1}{1000}$ = _____

10. $\dfrac{2}{7}$ = _____

Practical Application
Set up the following problems using the ratio and proportion method. Be sure to use a conversion ratio if necessary. Then solve.

11. Zoloft 75 mg PO is ordered. The strength available is Zoloft 50 mg scored tablet. How many tablet(s) would provide the desired amount? _____

12. Metformin 750 mg PO is ordered. The strength available is Metformin 0.5 g tablet. How many tablet(s) would be necessary to fill the desired order? _____

13. K-Cl 40 mEq PO is ordered. The strength available is K-Cl 20 mEq tablet. How many tablet(s) would be necessary for the desired order? _____

14. Amoxicillin oral suspension 500 mg PO is ordered. Available is amoxicillin 125 mg/5 mL. How many milliliters would be administered for the desired order? _____
How many teaspoons would be administered? _____

15. Levothyroxine 0.5 mg PO is ordered. Strength available is 125 mcg tablet. How many tablet(s) would be necessary for the desired order? _____

Calculating Doses Using the Formula Method

The first step to calculating drug dosage when using the formula method is to check that the strength of the drug ordered and the strength of the drug available are in the same unit of measure. For example, if the drug is ordered as 0.5 g and the available drug is in milligrams, the first step would be to change the grams to milligrams. Then set up the formula. However, if the drug ordered is in grams and the available drug is in grams, then skip the first step and go directly to the formula.

The formula is as follows:

$$\frac{\text{Dosage Order (DO)}}{\text{Dosage Available (DA)}} \times \text{Quantity (form or unit of measure)(DF)} = \text{Dose to be Given (DG)}$$

The formula can be abbreviated as:

$$\frac{\text{DO}}{\text{DA}} \times \text{DF} = \text{DG}$$

Here is how the formula method can be analyzed:

(DO) To find the desired part of the formula, answer this question, "What did the physician order?"

(DA) The *dosage available* part of the formula answers the question, "What dosage strength of medication is available?"

(DF) The *dosage form* identifies the physical characteristics of an available medication. For example, solid medications may come in tablets or capsules; liquid medications may be syrups or solutions; while other medication forms might include suppositories, transdermal patches, or an aerosol mist.

(DG) The amount to give represents the unknown dose of the drug that you will want to administer. Like the quantity, the *dose given* will be stated in the volume or dosage form of the available drug.

> ### ✎ LEARNING TIP
>
> Always remember to perform dosage calculations in writing and not in your head. Written calculations reduce the chance of error and thus increase patient safety. It is always important to check calculations with a calculator.

PROBLEM: Sulfamethoxazole oral suspension 1 g/10 mL is the available medication. The physician orders 2 g. How many milliliters would be prepared for administration? How many teaspoons should be administered?

Determine the dosage ordered, dosage on hand, dosage form, and dose to be given:

DO = 2 g; DA = 1 g; DF = 10 mL; DG = x mL

Now set up the formula.

EXAMPLE 2:

$$\frac{2\,g\,(DO)}{1\,g\,(DA)} \times 10\,mL\,(Qty\,or\,DF) = x\,mL\,(DG)$$

$$\frac{2\cancel{g}}{1\cancel{g}} \times 10\,mL = x\,mL$$

$$\frac{2}{1} \times 10 = x\,mL$$

$$\frac{20}{1} = x\,mL$$

$$x = 20\,mL$$

Now solve for the teaspoons:

$$\frac{5\,mL}{1\,tsp} \bowtie \frac{20\,mL}{x}$$

$$5x = 20\,tsp$$

$$x = 4\,tsp$$

> ### ✎ LEARNING TIP
>
> Remember that the medication on hand and the medication ordered must be in the same unit measurement before solving using the formula method.

Here are some additional examples using the guidelines provided.

EXAMPLE 3: Ordered: Glucophage 850 mg PO daily with meal

Available: Glucophage 850 mg tablet

Are the units the same measurement? (Yes)

What is the desired unit? 850 mg tablet daily

$$\frac{850\,mg\,(DO)}{850\,mg\,(DA)} \times 1\,tablet\,(DF) = x\,tablet\,(DG)$$

$$\frac{850\,\cancel{mg}\,(DO)}{850\,\cancel{mg}\,(DA)} \times 1\,tab\,(DF) = x\,tablet\,(DG)$$

$$\frac{1}{1} \times 1\,tablet = x$$

$$x = 1\,tablet$$

Because the amount of medication desired and the amount available are equal to 1 tablet, the dose to be given is 1 tablet.

 EXAMPLE 4: Ordered: phenobarbital gr iii PO daily hs

Available: phenobarbital 100 mg scored tablets

Are the units in the same measurement? (No)

What is the equivalency for conversion? gr i = 60 mg or gr iss = approximately 100 mg (see Table 8-3).

First convert to the same measurement system using one of the following conversions. Using gr iss as the conversion factor:

$$\frac{\text{gr } 1\frac{1}{2}}{100 \text{ mg}} = \frac{\text{gr } 3}{x \text{ mg}} \text{ or gr } 1\frac{1}{2}:100 \text{ mg}::\text{gr } 3:x \text{ mg}$$

$$\frac{\cancel{\text{gr }} 1\frac{1}{2}}{100 \text{ mg}} = \frac{\cancel{\text{gr }} 3}{x \text{ mg}} \text{ or } \cancel{\text{gr }} 1\frac{1}{2}:100 \text{ mg} :: \cancel{\text{gr }} 3 : x \text{ mg}$$

$$1\frac{1}{2}x = 300 \text{ mg}$$

Next, change 1½ to an improper fraction (³⁄₂) and solve for x (cross-multiply).

$$\frac{3}{2} \times x \text{ mg} = 3 \times 100 \text{ mg } or \frac{3}{2}:100::3:x$$

$$x = \frac{300}{1} \diagdown\diagup \frac{2}{3}$$

$$x = \frac{\overset{100}{\cancel{300}}}{1} \times \frac{2}{\underset{1}{\cancel{3}}}$$

$$x = 200 \text{ mg}$$

Therefore the dose to be given is 200 mg.

Using gr i = 60 mg as the conversion factor:

$$\frac{\text{gr i}}{60 \text{ mg}} = \frac{\text{gr iii}}{x \text{ mg}} \text{ or 1 gr}:60 \text{ mg}::3:x \text{ mg}$$

$$x = 3 \times 60 \text{ mg}$$

$$x = 180 \text{ mg}$$

gr iii = 180 mg or rounded to 200 mg
(Recall conversions are only approximate; in this example round answer to 200 mg.)

Now solve the problem by the formula method.

$$\frac{200 \text{ mg (DO)}}{100 \text{ mg (DA)}} \times 1 \text{ tablet (DF)} = x \text{ (DG)}$$

$$\frac{200 \text{ mg}}{100 \text{ mg}} \times 1 \text{ tab} = x$$

$$\frac{2}{1} \times \text{tab} = x$$

$$2 \text{ tab} = x$$

The dose to be given is 2 tablets.

 EXAMPLE 5: Ordered: oxybutynin HCl 10 mg PO bid

Available: oxybutynin HCl 5 mg scored tablets
Are the units in the same measurement? (Yes)

$$\frac{10 \text{ mg (DO)}}{5 \text{ mg (DA)}} \times 1 \text{ tablet (DF)} = x \text{ (DG)}$$

$$\frac{10 \text{ mg}}{5 \text{ mg}} \times 1 \text{ tab} = x$$

$$\frac{\overset{2}{\cancel{10 \text{ mg}}}}{\underset{1}{\cancel{5 \text{ mg}}}} \times 1 \text{ tab} = x$$

$$2 \times 1 \text{ tab} = x \text{ (DG)}$$

$$2 \text{ tab} = x$$

The dose to be given is 2 tablets twice daily.

Check Your Understanding: FORMULA METHOD BOX 9-3

Show your work on a separate sheet of paper. Save your worksheet.

1. Using the formula equation $\dfrac{\text{Keflex 500 mg}}{\text{Keflex 1000 mg}} \times 5 \text{ mL} = 2.5 \text{ mL}$, identify:
   a. What the physician ordered _____
   b. What streng th is on the shelf _____
   c. What is the unit of measure _____
   d. How much of the drug will be administered _____

2. Using the formula equation $\dfrac{\text{warfarin sodium 10 mg}}{\text{warfarin sodium 20 mg}} \times 1 \text{ tab} = \dfrac{1}{2} \text{ tab}$, identify:
   a. What the physician ordered _____
   b. What strength is on the shelf _____
   c. What is the unit of measure _____
   d. How much of the drug will be administered _____

Continued

Check Your Understanding: FORMULA METHOD
BOX 9-3—cont'd

3. Using the formula equation $\dfrac{\text{Diovan 160 mg}}{\text{Diovan 320 mg}} \times 1\ \text{tab} = \dfrac{1}{2}\ \text{tab}$, identify:

   a. What the physician ordered _____
   b. What strength is on the shelf _____
   c. What is the unit of measure _____
   d. How much of the drug will be administered _____

4. Using the formula equation $\dfrac{\text{dimenhydrinate 22.5 mg}}{\text{dimenhydrinate 15 mg}} \times 5\ \text{mL} = 7.5\ \text{mL}$, identify:

   a. What the physician ordered _____
   b. What strength is on the shelf _____
   c. What is the unit of measure _____
   d. How much of the drug will be administered _____

5. Using the formula equation $\dfrac{\text{guaifenesin 400 mg}}{\text{guaifenesin 200 mg}} \times 5\ \text{mL} = 10\ \text{mL}$, identify:

   a. What the physician ordered _____
   b. What strength is on the shelf _____
   c. What is the unit of measure _____
   d. How much of the drug will be administered _____

Practical Application

Using the same set of problems found in the ratio and proportion method, set up the problems this time using the formula method. Be sure to use a conversion ratio if necessary, then solve.

6. Zoloft 75 mg PO is ordered. The strength available is Zoloft 50 mg scored tablet. How many tablet(s) would provide the desired amount? _____

7. Metformin 750 mg PO is ordered. The strength available is Metformin 0.5 g tablet. How many tablet(s) would be necessary to fill the desired order? _____

8. K-Cl 40 mEq PO is ordered. The strength available is K-Cl 20 mEq tablet. How many tablet(s) would be necessary for the desired order? _____

9. Amoxicillin oral suspension 500 mg PO is ordered. Available is amoxicillin 125 mg/5 mL. How many milliliters would be administered for the desired order? _____
   How many teaspoons would be administered? _____

10. Levothyroxine 0.5 mg PO is ordered. Strength available is 125 mcg tablet. How many tablet(s) of the drug would be necessary for the desired order? _____

Calculating Doses Using Dimensional Analysis

The dimensional analysis method of dose calculation is different from the previous two methods discussed because this method does not require the conversion between units in order to solve the problem. Recall in the ratio and proportion method and in the formula method, the first step is to change the strength of the drug ordered and the strength of the drug available to the same unit of measure, and then the problem can be

solved. In the dimensional analysis method, only one *linear equation* is used. Linear equations have a right side and a left side separated by an equals sign. A simple example of a linear equation is $x = 2$. The x in this linear equation represents the measurement you are looking for (typically milliliters, capsules, or tablets). Always begin the dimensional analysis problem by determining what unit of measure your answer should be in, and place this unit of measure on the left side of the equals sign.

Next, in dimensional analysis there will be a series of fractions (or ratios) in which the numerator and denominator contain related conversion factors. A **factor** is a common fraction that shows a relationship between two numbers such as 60 mg = 1 gr or 1 tsp = 5 mL. Using the dimensional analysis method avoids the need to perform multiple calculations to solve drug dosages because the process involves writing fractional factors that include the conversion factors that are needed to solve the calculation. The starting factor (first fraction *after* the equals sign on the linear equation) will always be the measurement you are looking for in your answer as the numerator and the number 1 as the denominator. Next, determine the conversion factors needed to make the starting factor cancel out. Remember that the numerator abbreviation in the starting factor will be the denominator in the next conversion factor, with the same happening throughout the equation.

The most difficult task in computing problems using dimensional analysis is to set up the original linear equation correctly. To set up the common fraction correctly, remember that the numerator will show the name or abbreviation of the ordered medication. Then continue to add factors (as fractions), one at a time as needed so that the linear equation can be cancelled out and the answer becomes obvious. Most of the time the wrong answer for the dose ordered (DO) can be recognized because the answer does not make sense.

EXAMPLE 6: Ordered: phenobarbital gr iii tab PO hs

Available medication: phenobarbital 100 mg scored tablets

Write down what you know.

First, the x will be "tablets."

Next, the starting factor is gr iii.

Conversion factors needed to solve this problem include: 60 mg = gr i or 100 mg = gr iss

$$DA = \frac{100\ mg}{tab}$$

Using 60 mg = gr i as conversion, set up the linear equation:

$$x = \frac{gr\ iii}{1}$$

The above step shows just the starting factor; remember, x will be "tablets."

Add the first known conversion factor, which will put the grains as the denominator.

$$x = \frac{gr\ iii}{1} \times \frac{60\ mg}{gr\ i}$$

Now you want to use the math equation that will give you a denominator of milligrams.

The problem looks like this:

$$x = \frac{gr\ iii}{1} \times \frac{60\ mg}{gr\ i} \times \frac{1\ tab}{100\ mg}$$

Take off all abbreviations so that only the numbers remain:

$$x = \frac{3}{1} \times \frac{60}{1} \times \frac{1}{100}$$

$$x = \frac{180}{100}$$

When you finish the math, you have the *approximate* answer, but to make sense you need to round the answer from $^{180}/_{100}$ to $^{200}/_{100}$ to get the number of tablets to administer.

So $x = 2$ tablets

or using 100 mg = gr iss as a conversion, again start by setting up your linear equation:

$$x = \frac{gr\ iii}{1}$$

Add the known conversion to your starting factor:

$$x = \frac{gr\ iii}{1} \times \frac{100\ mg}{gr\ iss}$$

Add the final factor:

$$x = \frac{gr\ iii}{1} \times \frac{100\ mg}{gr\ iss} \times \frac{1\ tab}{100\ mg}$$

Take off all abbreviations and do the math:

$$x = \frac{3}{1} \times \frac{1}{1.5} \times \frac{1}{1}$$

$$x = \frac{3}{1.5}$$

$$x = 2$$

In the above example, because you used an approximate equivalent (100 mg = gr iss) at the beginning of the problem, the answer came out without the need to estimate the number of tablets.

LEARNING TIP

For each factor added, the numerator should match the previous factor's denominator so that you can cancel the unnecessary units.

EXAMPLE 7: Sulfamethoxazole oral suspension is supplied as 1 g/10 mL. The physician orders 2 g. How many milliliters would be prepared, and how many teaspoons would be administered?

Using dimensional analysis to solve this problem, first set up the linear equation. On the left side of the equation place an x. Remember, the problem is looking for teaspoons. The starting factor is $\frac{2\,g}{1}$, and the other factors necessary to solve this using DA are: 10 mL = 1 g and 1 tsp = 5 mL.

Now show your work:

The starting factor: $x = \dfrac{2\,g}{1}$

Place your next conversion in the problem:

$$x = \frac{2\,g}{1} \times \frac{10\,mL}{1\,g}$$

Now include the last conversion so the problem looks like this:

$$x = \frac{2\,g}{1} \times \frac{10\,mL}{1\,g} \times \frac{1\,tsp}{5\,mL}$$

Take out all the abbreviations, leaving only the numbers, cancel numbers appropriately, and cross multiply.

$$x = \frac{2}{1} \times \frac{\overset{2}{\cancel{10}}}{1} \times \frac{1}{\cancel{5}_1}$$

$$x = \frac{4}{1}$$

$$x = 4$$

Since you are looking for teaspoons $x = 4$ tsp.

Note that when the second factor was added, grams became the denominator so that the starting factor numerator grams could cancel out. Repeat this method of adding factors and canceling the previous factor until you can solve the problem because all of the measurement factors except the desired measurement have been cancelled out. Remember, in dimensional analysis, do not convert between measurement units, but rather make the measurement units factors in the equation.

CHOOSING A CALCULATION METHOD

Three methods of dosage calculation have been identified in this chapter. The example problem under each method is the same so that you will be able to see how each method differs. It is strongly suggested that you choose only *one* of the three methods and always use that method to avoid confusion and reduce math errors.

Check Your Understanding: DIMENSIONAL ANALYSIS BOX 9-4

Show your work on a separate sheet of paper. Save your worksheet.

The starting factor is given first. Using the guidelines for dimensional analysis, circle the correct second factor.

1. x mL $= \dfrac{10\,mL}{250\,mg}$ $\dfrac{1\,g}{1000\,mg}$ *or* $\dfrac{1000\,mg}{1\,g}$

2. x cap $= \dfrac{1\,cap}{600\,mcg}$ $\dfrac{1000\,mcg}{1\,mg}$ *or* $\dfrac{1\,mg}{1000\,mcg}$

3. x tsp $= \dfrac{2\,tsp}{20\,mL}$ $\dfrac{1\,tsp}{10\,mL}$ *or* $\dfrac{10\,mL}{200\,mg}$

4. x mg $= \dfrac{187\,mg}{5\,mL}$ $\dfrac{1000\,mg}{1\,g}$ *or* $\dfrac{1\,g}{1000\,mg}$

5. x tab $= \dfrac{1\,tab}{0.25\,g}$ $\dfrac{1000\,mg}{1\,g}$ *or* $\dfrac{1\,g}{1000\,mg}$

Check Your Understanding: DIMENSIONAL ANALYSIS
BOX 9-4—cont'd

Practical Application

Using the same set of problems found in the ratio and proportion method and in the formula method, solve using dimensional analysis. Show your work on a separate sheet of paper. Save your worksheet.

6. Zoloft 75 mg PO is ordered. The strength available is Zoloft 50 mg scored tablet. How many tablet(s) would provide the desired amount? _____

7. Metformin 750 mg PO is ordered. The strength available is Metformin 0.5 g tablet. How many tablet(s) would be necessary to fill the desired order? _____

8. K-Cl 40 mEq PO is ordered. The strength available is K-Cl 20 mEq tablet. How many tablet(s) would be necessary for the desired order? _____

9. Amoxicillin oral suspension 500 mg PO is ordered. Available is amoxicillin 125 mg/5 mL. How many milliliters would be administered for the desired order? _____
How many teaspoons would be administered? _____

10. Levothyroxine 0.5 mg PO is ordered. Strength available is 125 mcg tablet. How many tablet(s) would be necessary for the desired order? _____

Check Your Understanding: DOSAGE CALCULATIONS
BOX 9-5

Show your work on a separate sheet of paper. Identify the method you use. Save your worksheet.

Calculation Review

Using only *one* of the calculating methods, calculate the following solid drug doses. Then write in the number of tablets or capsules for each dose. Interpret the orders to show the number of times the dose is taken each day.

1. Ordered: Glucophage 1 g PO bid with meals. Available: 500 mg tablets.
   Dose to be given: _____

2. Ordered: theophylline, 300 mg PO 1 h pc q6h. Available: 100 mg tablets.
   Dose to be given: _____

3. Ordered: dipyridamole 100 mg PO qid. Available: 50 mg tablets.
   Dose to be given: _____

4. Ordered: phenytoin sodium 300 mg cap PO daily. Available: 100 mg capsules.
   Dose to be given: _____

5. Ordered: griseofulvin 1 g PO daily. Available: 250 mg tablets.
   Dose to be given: _____

Continued

Check Your Understanding: DOSAGE CALCULATIONS BOX 9-5—cont'd

6. Ordered: furosemide 40 mg PO daily. Available: 20 mg tablets.
   Dose to be given: _____

7. Ordered: levothyroxine sodium 0.025 mg PO daily. Available: 0.05 mg tablets.
   Dose to be given: _____

8. Ordered: bupropion hydrochloride 200 mg PO q12h. Available: 100 mg tablets.
   Dose to be given: _____

9. Ordered: allopurinol 600 mg PO daily in divided doses to be given bid. Available: 300 mg tablets.
   Dose to be given: _____

10. Ordered: cimetidine 300 mg PO q8h. Available: 100 mg tablets.
    Dose to be given: _____

RECONSTITUTING A POWDER

Some medications must be reconstituted from powder to liquid form before administration. The label on these medications will give the total strength of the medication in the bottle and the strength per volume of the medication after it has been reconstituted with the required diluents (Figure 9-1). Zithromax suspension will contain azithromycin 200 mg in every 5 mL when the medication has been properly reconstituted. The label on Zithromax shows the total strength of medication, the volume of solute to be used, and the strength of medication per volume when the solute has been added.

Table 9-1 shows the **reconstitution** of Zithromax by total strength and volume of medication in the bottle. The weight (amount) of drug is measured in milligrams, so the azithromycin is available with the contents per bottle being either 300 mg, 600 mg, 900 mg, or 1200 mg. The amount of solute (water) added to the

TABLE 9-1 RECONSTITUTING INSTRUCTIONS FOR ZITHROMAX

TOTAL AMOUNT OF ZITHROMAX	AMOUNT OF WATER TO BE ADDED	TOTAL VOLUME AFTER RECONSTITUTION (AZITHROMYCIN CONTENT)	AZITHROMYCIN CONCENTRATION AFTER RECONSTITUTION
300 mg of drug	9 mL	15 mL	100 mg/5 mL
600 mg of drug	9 mL	15 mL	200 mg/5 mL
900 mg of drug	12 mL	22.5 mL	200 mg/5 mL
1200 mg of drug	15 mL	30 mL	200 mg/5 mL

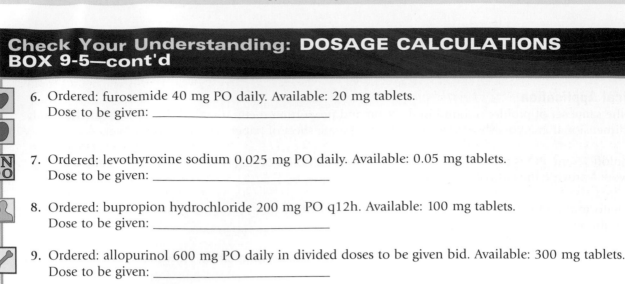

Figure 9-1 Label for Zithromax.

available drug makes the solution a dosage strength. If 9 mL of water is added to either the 300 mg or 600 mg bottle, the total volume after reconstitution will be 15 mL of suspension. The difference between the two bottles with 15 mL of oral suspension is that the dosage strength in the azithromycin 300-mg bottle is 100 mg/5 mL, and in the azithromycin 600-mg bottle, the oral suspension is 200 mg/5 mL after reconstitution. A powder can be reconstituted from a vial into only one dosage strength. If a different dosage strength is ordered, do *not* add additional solution, instead start over with a new vial so the powder is at full strength. Many multi-vial reconstituted medications do not have a long shelf life. The medication must be used or discarded usually within a timeframe of as little as an hour to as much as 2 weeks. Often the medication must be refrigerated after reconstitution. Read all manufacture labels carefully. Finally, always be sure to properly label reconstituted medication with the prepared dosage strength, the date and time of reconstitution, and your initials. More information on reconstituting guidelines can be found in Chapter 10 on parenteral routes.

Check Your Understanding: RECONSTITUTING A POWDER
BOX 9-6

Practical Application

Using the label in Figure 9-1 and the information in Table 9-1, assuming the medication is properly reconstituted, answer the following questions.

1. According to the label, how much azithromycin is available in the bottle if it is properly reconstituted? _____

2. According to the label, what dosage strength is available if properly reconstituted? _____

3. According to the label, what is the total volume of the bottle after reconstitution? _____

4. Does this medication expire as soon as the suggested dosage of "once daily for 5 days" is over? _____

5. Would you instruct a patient to use a teaspoon for the 5-mL dose? Explain your answer. _____
_____
_____

6. What specific instructions would you give to the patient? (Give two answers.)_____
_____
_____

Using the label in Figure 9-1 and assuming the medication is properly reconstituted, answer the following questions.

7. If the physician instructs the patient to take a teaspoon a day, how many milligrams would the patient be taking per day? _____

8. How many milliliters of water were added to the drug powder? _____

9. How many days would this medication last if the patient were to take 5 mL a day? _____

10. Could you add less fluid to make a stronger dose? Why or why not? _____
_____

Continued

Check Your Understanding: RECONSTITUTING A POWDER BOX 9-6—cont'd

Using the following reconstituting instructions for Augmentin suspension 400 mg/5 mL, answer questions 11 and 12.

BOTTLE SIZE	AMOUNT OF WATER REQUIRED FOR SUSPENSION TO OBTAIN 400 mg/5 mL
50 mL	44 mL
75 mL	66 mL
100 mL	87 mL

11. How much water would you need to add to a 100-mL bottle in order to have the Augmentin suspension of 400 mg/5 mL? _____

12. What size bottle would you need to use if you were adding only 66 mL of water to obtain an Augmentin suspension of 400 mg/5 mL? _____

SPECIAL CALCULATIONS

Not every patient will be able to tolerate the "dosage for the average adult" so special calculations are used. Infants and children, because of their small size and percentage of fluids in their body makeup, cannot tolerate adult medications that are simply reduced in volume or amount of drug. In pediatric patients, this is referred to as "immature body systems," meaning that the body systems may not tolerate adult medications. Infants' body systems are not fully developed, and they lack the enzymes necessary to metabolize drugs. Also, the child's volume of total body water, when compared with that of an adult, is much greater, so the medication will be distributed differently, thus altering the effects of the drugs. The geriatric patient may require more specific calculation of medication dosage because of the potential toxicity resulting from the decrease in body functions. Finally, because of the toxicity of chemotherapeutic agents, the patient's height and weight become factors in the safe administration of chemotherapy drugs.

Calculations Using the Body Surface Area Method

Infants and children can receive medications via the same routes as adults—parenteral and nonparenteral—but **body surface area (BSA) calculation** for determining the correct dosage is used for calculating special dosages for children and geriatric patients, especially with toxic drugs such as antineoplastics. There are both children's and adult's nomograms. The nomogram pictured in this book was developed for children.

BSA is found by placing the patient's height and weight on a nomogram that calculates the body surface area, rather than prescribing medications based on "normal adult" size. If a child is of normal height for weight, the BSA can be determined by weight alone, as is calculated in the box found in the center of the nomogram (Figure 9-2). However, if the height and weight of the child are not proportional, the nomogram may be used. The purpose of the **nomogram** is to measure the total surface area in square meters (m^2). Note that height is measured in both cm (centimeters) and in (inches) and weight is in lb (pounds) and kg (kilograms). When using the nomogram, be careful that you read the appropriate calibration for both height and weight. To read a nomogram, use a ruler to line up the height (extreme left) and weight (extreme right) to obtain the BSA in square meters (m^2), that is found between these two columns. (All patients who require the use of a nomogram should be weighed and measured for height before calculations with the nomogram are performed.) Read the BSA at the point where the ruler intersects the graph. The number found in the BSA column is the BSA you will record. Note that the calibrations between designated numbers on BSA are not consistent from the top to the bottom of the graph. Some of the calibrations are in 0.01 increments, others are in 0.1 increments and some are even in 0.2 increments. The nomogram measurements are in both metric and English measures. The use of the measurements are interchangeable. Now try a few examples to calculate BSA.

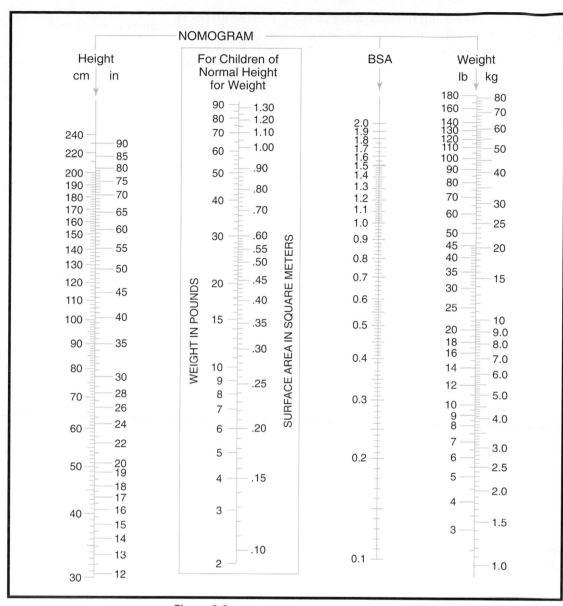

Figure 9-2 West body surface area nomogram.

EXAMPLE 8: A child weighs 55 lb and is 85 cm tall. Determine this child's BSA using the nomogram.

Using the nomogram in Figure 9-2, do the following:

STEP 1: Find and mark the child's height in the first column. Be sure to find the height in centimeters, not inches.

STEP 2: Find and mark the child's weight in pounds (not kilograms) in the last column.

STEP 3: Use a ruler to align the marks. Then look on the column marked BSA at the top, and read the BSA from that column.

The answer is 0.82 m².

EXAMPLE 9: A child is of normal height for weight and weighs 32 lb. Determine this child's BSA using the nomogram.

Using the nomogram in Figure 9-2, do the following:

STEP 1: Find the middle column, headed "Children of Normal Height and Weight," which is enclosed within a box.

STEP 2: Find and mark the child's weight on the left side of the centerline.

STEP 3: Use a ruler to read the corresponding number on the right side of the centerline. This is the BSA.

The answer is 0.62 m².

Using Body Surface Area

After determining the BSA of the patient, the dosage calculation is completed by entering this information into a given formula. In the metric system, square meters (m²) are used for the size of the body in height and weight. The assumption is that the BSA of an average adult weighing 140 lb is 1.7 m². Because most medications are based on average adult dosage, this dose must be adjusted for the person who needs a special amount of medication, such as an infant or child, an older person who no longer has the average weight for height, or a person taking very toxic medications such as antineoplastics.

The formula for calculating the dose is:

$$\frac{BSA \ m^2}{1.7} \times Adult \ dose = Desired \ dose$$

EXAMPLE 10: A child weighs 55 lb and is 85 cm tall. The physician orders amoxicillin based on BSA for the child. BSA for this child on the nomogram is 0.82 m². The adult dose of amoxicillin is 500 mg. What is the dose for the child?

$$\frac{0.82 \ m^2 (BSA)}{1.7} \times 500 \ mg = 241 \ mg$$

Now calculate the dose of amoxicillin that is to be given using the formula or the ratio and proportion method. The example below uses the formula method.

The child's dose would be 241 mg. Amoxicillin suspension is available in 250 mg/5 mL.

$$\frac{241 \ mg \ (DO)}{250 \ mg \ (DA)} \times 5 \ mL \ (DF) = 4.8 \ mL, \ or \ 5 \ mL \ (DG)$$

This child would receive 1 teaspoon of amoxicillin.

EXAMPLE 11: A child weighs 70 lb and is 45 inches tall. The physician orders albuterol for the child based on the BSA. The BSA is 1.2 m². The normal adult dose is albuterol 4 mg. What is the dose for the child?

$$\frac{1.2 \ m^2 \ (BSA)}{1.7 \ m^2 \ (DA)} \times 4 \ mg \ (adult \ dose) = 2.8 \ mg, \ or \ 3 \ mg$$

The child's dose would be albuterol 3 mg. Albuterol syrup available is 2 mg/5 mL.

$$\frac{3 \ mg \ (DO)}{2 \ mg \ (DA)} \times 5 \ mL \ (DF) = 7.5 \ mL \ (DG)$$

The child would be administered 7.5 mL or 1½ tsp of albuterol.

Check Your Understanding: USING A NOMOGRAM BOX 9-7

Calculation Review

Use the nomogram in Figure 9-2 to calculate the BSA in m².

1. A child is 60 cm and weighs 7 kg. _____

2. A child is 35 lb and 72 cm. _____

3. A child is 45 inches and weighs 70 lb. _____

4. A child is 20 kg and 90 cm. _____

5. A child is of normal weight and height and weighs 75 lb. _____

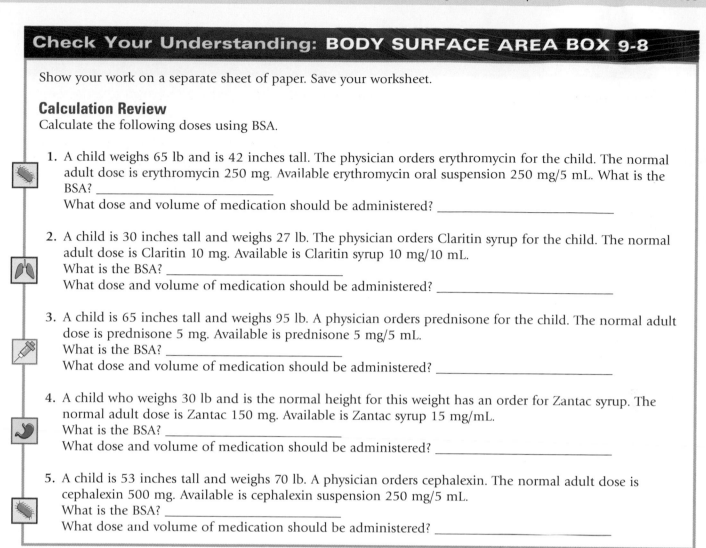

Check Your Understanding: BODY SURFACE AREA BOX 9-8

Show your work on a separate sheet of paper. Save your worksheet.

Calculation Review
Calculate the following doses using BSA.

1. A child weighs 65 lb and is 42 inches tall. The physician orders erythromycin for the child. The normal adult dose is erythromycin 250 mg. Available erythromycin oral suspension 250 mg/5 mL. What is the BSA? _____
   What dose and volume of medication should be administered? _____

2. A child is 30 inches tall and weighs 27 lb. The physician orders Claritin syrup for the child. The normal adult dose is Claritin 10 mg. Available is Claritin syrup 10 mg/10 mL.
   What is the BSA? _____
   What dose and volume of medication should be administered? _____

3. A child is 65 inches tall and weighs 95 lb. A physician orders prednisone for the child. The normal adult dose is prednisone 5 mg. Available is prednisone 5 mg/5 mL.
   What is the BSA? _____
   What dose and volume of medication should be administered? _____

4. A child who weighs 30 lb and is the normal height for this weight has an order for Zantac syrup. The normal adult dose is Zantac 150 mg. Available is Zantac syrup 15 mg/mL.
   What is the BSA? _____
   What dose and volume of medication should be administered? _____

5. A child is 53 inches tall and weighs 70 lb. A physician orders cephalexin. The normal adult dose is cephalexin 500 mg. Available is cephalexin suspension 250 mg/5 mL.
   What is the BSA? _____
   What dose and volume of medication should be administered? _____

Calculating Dose Using Milligrams per Kilogram

In many pediatric settings the use of milligrams per kilograms (mg/kg) is used to express a standard dose. For example, in the Health Maintenance Organization (HMO) formulary, the dose information for amoxicillin is given as 30 to 50 mg/kg/day for a standard dose and 80 to 100 mg/kg/day for a high dose.

To calculate a dosage using milligrams per kilogram, the first step is to change pounds to kilograms if the weight has been obtained in pounds. Remember that 2.2 lb = 1 kg. The easiest method for converting these measurements is by using ratio and proportion.

✏ LEARNING TIP

The "/" in mg/kg means to multiply the numbers. Therefore the equation actually reads mg × kg × frequency of administration or dose.

EXAMPLE 12: 2.2 lb : 1 kg :: 22 lb : x kg

2.2 x = 22 kg
x = 10 kg

Medication ordered: amoxicillin 50 mg/kg/day in three divided doses

The child weighs 10 kg.

Calculation: 10 × 50 mg × 1 day = 500 mg per day

Now divide the total amount by three doses so that each dose will be 167 mg (500 mg : 3 doses [3 times a day] :: x : 1 dose) of amoxicillin.

Check Your Understanding: MILLIGRAMS PER KILOGRAM BOX 9-9

Show your work on a separate sheet of paper. Save your worksheet.

1. Ordered: Veetids 10 mg/kg/q8h for a child who weighs 55 lb.
   Available medication: Veetids 250 mg/5 mL
   What is the strength of medication for one dose? _____
   What is the volume of medication to be given with that dose? _____

2. Ordered: Dilantin 2.5 mg/kg per dose for a child who weighs 44 lb.
   Available medication: Dilantin chewable tablet(s) 30 mg
   What is the strength of medication for one dose? _____
   How many chewable tablet(s) should be given with each dose? _____

3. Ordered: amoxicillin suspension 20 mg/kg/day in three divided doses for a child who weighs 42 lb.
   Available: amoxicillin suspension 125 mg/5 mL
   What is the strength of the medication for a day? _____
   What is the strength of the medication for a dose? _____
   What is the volume of medication for a dose? _____
   What is the volume of the dose in household measurement? _____

4. Ordered: Zyrtec syrup 0.1 mg/kg daily for a child weighing 55 lb.
   Available medication: Zyrtec syrup 5 mg/5 mL
   What is the strength of medication to be administered for a day? _____
   What is the volume of medication to be administered daily? _____

5. Ordered: Zarontin syrup 20 mg/kg bid for a child who weighs 54 lb.
   Available medication: Zarontin syrup 250 mg/5 mL
   What is the strength of the medication to be given with each dose? _____
   What is the volume of medication to be given with each dose? _____
   What is the volume of medication to be given in household measurements? _____

OTHER NONPARENTERAL MEDICATIONS

Medications used for nonparenteral routes come in several dosage forms other than the oral liquid and solid forms. Examples include ophthalmic and otic drops, which are almost always prescribed with a dropper because they are instilled into a body orifice; nasal sprays, inhalation solutions, and aerosols, which are prescribed in metered doses; aerosol powders, lotions, creams, ointments, and transdermal patches, which are applied topically; and chewable tablets for children, which are prescribed like other tablets, except that the patient is instructed to chew the medication. The importance of patient education cannot be stressed enough, especially with a drug form that the patient may be unfamiliar with, leading to the chance that the patient may use it incorrectly. For example, the patient instruction sheet for the nasal spray *triamcinolone acetonide* tells the patient to "prime" the medication and then goes into detail about how the patient should do this. However, most patients do not take the time to read the accompanying literature. The allied health care professional should explain and demonstrate the correct procedure and allow the patient to ask open-ended questions to confirm understanding of the correct administration of the medication.

SUMMARY

Medication is most frequently administered orally because of the ease of administration and dosage calculation. Nonparenteral medications are drugs that usually are taken orally or by inhalation and come in solid or liquid form. Some medications, such as lotions and sprays, are prescribed for use on the skin and will be prescribed by the number of doses to the area per day.

This chapter shows three methods to calculate doses. The first two methods, called the *ratio and proportion method* and the *formula method*, require you to first convert to like measurement systems when necessary in order to solve the drug calculation. The third method, called *dimensional analysis*, uses common fractions that include the conversion for measurement systems as factors to allow cancellation of unnecessary units to solve the calculation using only one linear fraction. It is recommended that you choose only one of the three methods and that the method chosen be the one with which you are the most comfortable, to decrease math errors.

Solid medications such as tablets may be prescribed in either partial or whole tablets per dose. Capsules cannot be divided, and timed-release medications should be given in the prescribed dosage only. Liquid medications can easily be administered in the incorrect dosage if proper measuring devices are not used.

Some patients are not what is considered "normal adults" and may not tolerate adult medications that have not been clinically approved for their body systems. Sometimes the BSA is measured to determine the amount of medication to administer to children, older adults, and persons taking highly toxic medications used in chemotherapy. The BSA method for calculating doses is based on the weight and height of the patient. This calculation is then compared with the normal adult BSA of 1.7 m², so the normal adult dose may be modified.

CRITICAL THINKING EXERCISES

Using the medication label provided, calculate the oral dosage of each medication. Show your work. On the dosage line, explain exactly how much medication is taken and how often the medication is taken.

1. Mr. Walters is taking an antiulcer medication in an effort to manage an acute duodenal ulcer. He is currently taking ranitidine 150 mg PO bid.

   Dose to be given: _____

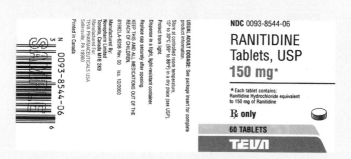

2. Ms. Lechuga has type 2 diabetes mellitus and has been prescribed Prandin 2 mg by mouth bid, with a meal, to regulate her blood glucose level.

   Dose to be given: _____

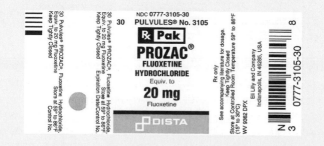

3. Mr. Bates has been prescribed the antidepressant drug fluoxetine and is instructed to take fluoxetine 20 mg every morning.

   Dose to be given: _____

Continued

CRITICAL THINKING EXERCISES—cont'd

4. Ms. Allison is on a trip, and her purse with her heart medication in it has been stolen. She is taking the anticoagulant Coumadin 5 mg daily.

Dose to be given: _____

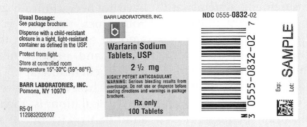

5. Mr. Davis is being treated for Paget's disease with risedronate 30 mg daily at least 30 minutes before the first food or drink of the day, for the next 2 months.

Dose to be given: _____

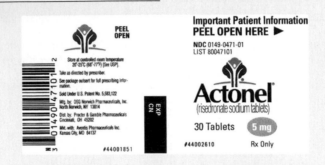

6. After her thyroidectomy, Bernadette was instructed to take levothyroxine tablets once a day for the rest of her life. She currently takes levothyroxine 100 mcg daily.

Dose to be given: _____

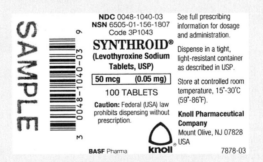

7. Mr. Rockwell has been diagnosed with congestive heart failure and will be prescribed lisinopril 10 mg daily to control his hypertension.

Dose to be given: _____

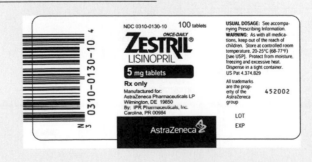

CRITICAL THINKING EXERCISES—cont'd

8. Mark White experienced constant muscle hyperactivity after his car accident, and Dr. Merry prescribed metaxalone 800 mg tid.

Dose to be given: _____

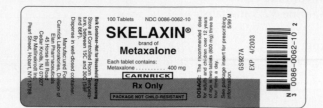

9. Ms. Marta had bacterial pneumonia and was prescribed azithromycin 400 mg the first day and 200 mg for days 2 through 5.

Dose to be given on first day: _____

Dose to be given on days 2 through 5: _____

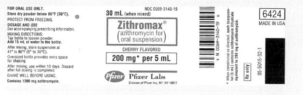

Calculation Review

Calculate the following problems using *only* one method. Be sure that the dose is in the correct dosage form. Show your work on a separate sheet of paper. Save your worksheet.

DOSE TO BE GIVEN

1. Ordered: Benadryl 50 mg
   Available: Benadryl 25 mg caps
   _____

2. Ordered: chlorpromazine HCl 20 mg
   Available: Thorazine 10 mg tabs
   _____

3. Ordered: warfarin sodium 10 mg
   Available: warfarin sodium 5 mg tabs
   _____

4. Ordered: Proventil syrup 4 mg
   Available: Proventil syrup 2 mg/5 mL
   How would you give this in household measure?
   _____
   _____

5. Ordered: Captopril 25 mg
   Available: Captopril 12.5 mg tabs
   _____

6. Ordered: amoxicillin 500 mg
   Available: Amoxil 250 mg caps
   _____

7. Ordered: Biaxin 150 mg
   Available: Biaxin 250 mg/tsp
   What is the dose in mL?
   _____
   _____

DOSE TO BE GIVEN

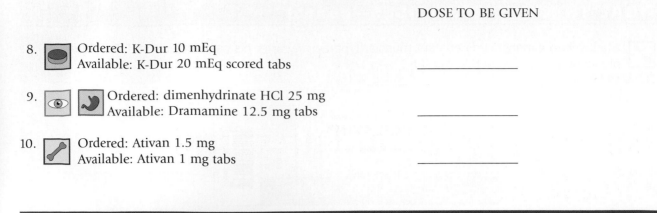

8. Ordered: K-Dur 10 mEq
   Available: K-Dur 20 mEq scored tabs   _____

9. Ordered: dimenhydrinate HCl 25 mg
   Available: Dramamine 12.5 mg tabs   _____

10. Ordered: Ativan 1.5 mg
    Available: Ativan 1 mg tabs   _____

REVIEW QUESTIONS

All of the following statements are *false.* **Determine the error(s) and rewrite the answer, giving complete and correct information in the space provided.**

1. BSA is calculated by measuring weight alone. _____

   _____

2. A comparison of the relationship between two ratios is called the *formula method* of dosage calculation. _____

   _____

   _____

3. One household teaspoon is approximately equal to 15 milliliters. _____

   _____

   _____

4. A value in a measurement system is called a *nomogram.* _____

   _____

5. When a medication needs to be reconstituted, adding more fluid than required will give you a better dosage unit.

   _____

   _____

Calculating Doses of Parenteral Medications

OBJECTIVES

After studying this chapter, you should be capable of doing the following:

- Determining the correct syringe for administration of parenteral doses.
- Calculating doses of parenteral medications in the metric system.

- Calculating doses of parenteral medications in units.

KEY TERMS

Agitate
Parenteral
Unit

Chapter 10 PRETEST—CALCULATING DOSES OF PARENTERAL MEDICATIONS

Identify the most appropriate syringe size to use to administer the medication given in Column A. Use the choices in Column B as many times as necessary, but use only one answer per question.

COLUMN A

1. _____ 1.1 mL
2. _____ 86 units of U-100
3. _____ 2.4 mL
4. _____ 0.22 mL
5. _____ 0.86 mL
6. _____ 0.25 units
7. _____ 0.25 units of U-100

COLUMN B

A. insulin syringe
B. tuberculin syringe
C. 3-mL syringe

Calculate the answers to the following problems, then shade in the syringe with the exact dose you would administer.

Continued

Chapter 10 PRETEST—CALCULATING DOSES OF PARENTERAL MEDICATIONS—cont'd

8. A patient comes to Dr. Merry complaining of shortness of breath after ingesting mushrooms found near his home. The physician diagnoses mushroom poisoning and prescribes *atropine* 0.5 mg SC, as an antidote. The available atropine vial is labeled 0.4 mg/mL.

   Volume of dose to be administered: _____

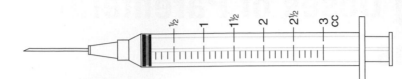

9. After confirming that the patient has no known allergies, Dr. Merry prescribes *V-Cillin K* 400,000 units IM to combat the patient's pneumococcal infection. Available: a vial of V-Cillin K powder 1 million units. Directions for reconstitution state: Add 4.5 mL normal saline solution to the powder to provide a dosage of 1 million units/5 mL.

   Volume of medication to be administered: _____

PARENTERAL MEDICATIONS

Parenteral medications can be injected, infused, implanted, or are administered to provide quick absorption of the drug into the bloodstream or when a patient cannot take oral medications, such as when the patient is uncooperative or unconscious. Also, some medications cannot be administered orally because the gastrointestinal tract enzymes and acids do not allow for proper absorption of the medication. This chapter concentrates on calculating doses for parenteral medications in the metric system or in **units.** Also included is an introduction of the proper syringe size to choose when preparing parenteral medications based on the results of your calculations and the amount of fluid necessary to administer the injection. Some calculations will use reconstituted powders. Finally, calculations for medications found in units per volume and reading percentages of solutions that are also indicated in the metric system are presented. Drugs may be labeled in both percentage strengths and in metric system units. For example, the label for *lidocaine HCl* inj. 1% USP will also indicate the amount of medication (drug) per milliliter, and is written as 10 mg/mL, thus for every one milliliter of fluid drawn into a syringe, there will be 10 milligrams of the drug also being drawn into the syringe.

Many drugs, such as some antibiotics, come in a powdered form and must be reconstituted to a liquid for parenteral administration. These drugs are packaged in dry form because they are unstable for prolonged periods of time in liquid form. After reconstitution the shelf life is short, with rapid loss of potency and effectiveness. When reconstituting medications, it is extremely important to read and understand the vial label or package insert because in some cases different dosage strengths are determined by the amount of diluent added to the vial; in other vials a specific volume of liquid must be added to provide only one dosage strength. A medication can have only one dosage strength per vial once it has been reconstituted. In other words, more fluid cannot be added to the vial to make the dose weaker after the powder has been reconstituted if any amount of the medication has been withdrawn from the vial. During reconstitution, the directions will specifically instruct the allied health professional either to roll the medication to dissolve the powder or to shake **(agitate)** the vial to modify the dry ingredients into the needed liquid state for injection. Some medications, when found as a suspension, will have to have the precipitate placed back into the liquid before preparing the medication for injection; in other cases, the medication becomes a solution that does not need agitation with each administration.

Drugs are usually reconstituted with sterile water or 0.9% sodium chloride (normal saline [NS] solution). If a drug comes packaged with a specific solution to be used in reconstituting the medication, never substitute another liquid. Some medications for reconstitution will come in single-dose vials that are reconstituted for immediate use. Single-dose vials should never be reconstituted before the time for use. When multiple-dose vials are prepared, the reconstituted medication should be labeled with the reconstituted dosage strength, the reconstitution date and time, and the expiration date. The person doing the reconstitution should initial the vial for patient safety. Labeling of medication should be done consistently by all personnel. It is important when administering reconstituted medications to check the expiration date of the original vial and the expiration date after reconstitution.

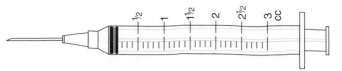

Figure 10-1 Typical 3-mL syringe.

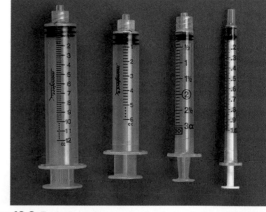

Figure 10-2 Typical metric measured syringes. *Left to right,* 12-mL, 6-mL, 3-mL, and 1-mL tuberculin syringes.

READING SYRINGES FOR PARENTERAL DRUG ADMINISTRATION

Intramuscular (IM) medications are administered directly into a muscle for rapid absorption. Antibiotics, antihistamines, steroidal antiinflammatory drugs, pain medications, and immunizations are all examples of types of medications that are administered intramuscularly. Intramuscular injections are typically administered in volumes up to 3 milliliters depending on the site of the injection. In most cases, syringes used for IM injections are calibrated in tenths of a milliliter (mL) with the 3-mL syringe being the typical choice (Figure 10-1).

Subcutaneous (SC) injections are administered into the subcutaneous layer of tissue, which is between the muscle and epidermal layer of skin. The volume of a subcutaneous injection is usually 0.5 to 1 mL; the maximum amount of fluid that can be injected SC is 2 mL, depending on the size of the person. The 3-mL syringe may be used for SC injections, but in specific instances tuberculin syringes may be used when small amounts of medication are ordered. Insulin syringes are used only for the administration of insulin (Figures 10-2 and 10-3).

Intradermal (ID) injections are used to administer medications into the dermis layer of the skin. The dermis area is located just above the subcutaneous layer. The volume of drug administered is usually 0.1 mL or less

but is always less than 0.2 mL. The syringe used is the 1-mL tuberculin syringe, which is calibrated in 0.01 increments from 0.01 mL to 1 mL. The calculations of the medications for ID injection use are performed in the same manner as for other parenteral medications.

Calculations to find doses of parenteral medications are performed in a manner similar to that introduced in Chapter 9 for nonparenteral medications. However, instead of calculating how many tablets, capsules, teaspoons, or even milliliters to administer orally, you will be calculating the number of milliliters, or the volume of medication (liquid), to be drawn into a syringe. To calculate the dosage using the 3-mL syringe, first observe that the numbers on the syringe start with ½ and are in increments of ½, so they include the numbers ½, 1, 1½, 2, 2½, and 3. Between each number are markings that signify one tenth of 1 mL. Therefore the syringe has four short markings for tenths between the longer markings that show ½-mL increments. Medication dose would not typically be written as ½; it would be written as 0.5 mL because the designation is in the metric system. Recall that when no number appears before the decimal point, a zero should be placed in front of the decimal place to aid in reducing calculation errors. To calculate a dose in a syringe, read the fluid level from the tip of the plunger just even with the calibration mark.

EXAMPLE 1: 2.2 mL is shown here:

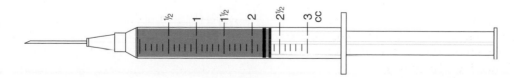

Some medications such as penicillin are given in units per milliliter. When you see units per mL, always check to see how many units of medication are equivalent to 1 mL. Then work the problem by calculating units per volume or milliliters to provide the needed dose.

If a medication has to be reconstituted, the calculation is performed in the same manner as for other medications in strength per volume or milligrams per milliliter after reconstitution.

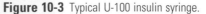

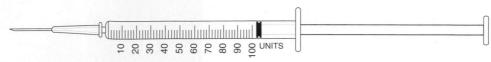

Figure 10-3 Typical U-100 insulin syringe.

Check Your Understanding: READING SYRINGES BOX 10-1

Calculation Review
Read each syringe and write the amount of medication that is indicated.

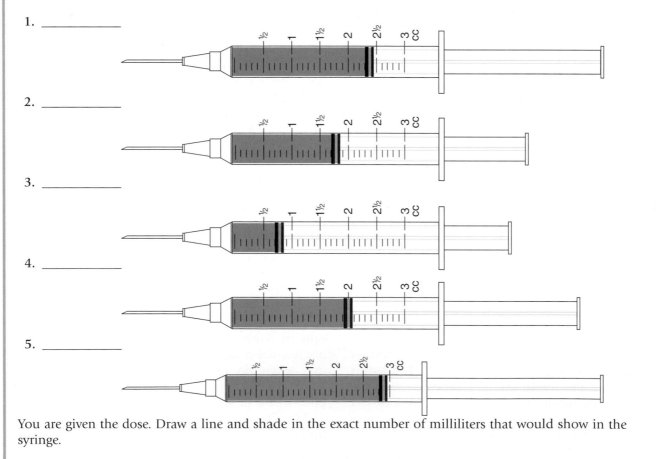

1. _____

2. _____

3. _____

4. _____

5. _____

You are given the dose. Draw a line and shade in the exact number of milliliters that would show in the syringe.

6. 1.4 mL

Check Your Understanding: READING SYRINGES BOX 10-1—cont'd

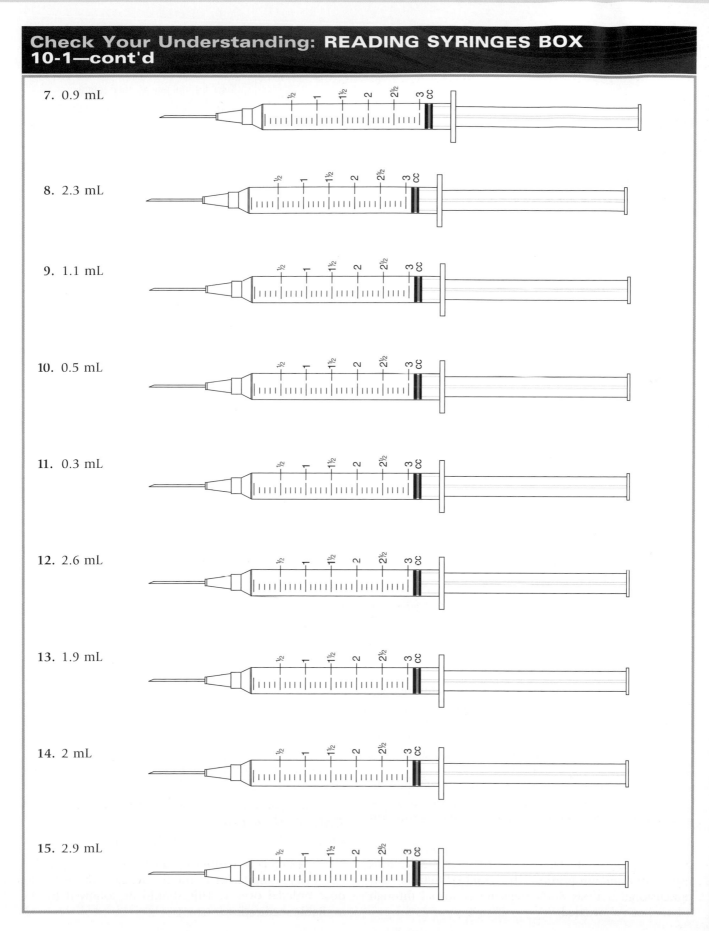

7. 0.9 mL

8. 2.3 mL

9. 1.1 mL

10. 0.5 mL

11. 0.3 mL

12. 2.6 mL

13. 1.9 mL

14. 2 mL

15. 2.9 mL

TABLE 10-1 SYRINGE AND DOSAGE VOLUME COMPARISON			
SYRINGE SIZE	**TYPICAL VOLUME**	**CALIBRATION**	**ROUND CALCULATIONS TO:**
3 mL	1-3 mL	Tenths	Two decimal places, then tenths.
Tuberculin	0.01-1.0 mL	Hundredths	Three decimal places, then hundredths.
Insulin	1-100 units (0.01 mL = 1 unit)	May be in 1- or 2-unit calibration	If medication ordered in even units, either syringe may be used. If ordered in odd unit amounts, the syringe used must be calibrated in one-unit increments.

Insulin is manufactured in units per milliliter; therefore insulin should always be administered using an insulin syringe that is calibrated in units, not milliliters.

When finding the answer to dosage calculations, a few points should be remembered. First, all calculations in milliliters requiring the use of a 3-mL syringe are carried out two decimal places and then rounded to the nearest tenth if necessary. For example, 1.25 mL would be rounded to 1.3 mL, and 1.24 mL would be rounded to 1.2 mL. For tuberculin syringes, when calculating milliliters, carry calculations out to three decimal places and round to the nearest hundredth, because the tuberculin syringe is marked in hundredths (0.01) of a milliliter. For example, 0.836 mL would be rounded to 0.84. Table 10-1 shows the comparison between syringes and dosage volumes.

CALCULATING PARENTERAL MEDICATIONS USING THE METRIC SYSTEM

Unlike calculating a dose of oral medication that can be in several solid and liquid forms, parenteral medications will always be in a liquid form—in most cases, milliliters or units. The basic strength unit for parenteral medications is usually the milligram, although units, grams, or milliequivalents may be used. When using any of the weight designations, the cancellation of the designation during calculation will allow the final dose to be in a liquid form.

Once you have practiced reading the volume in syringes, the next step is to calculate the dose using one of the methods learned in Chapter 9. If the medication requires conversions between measurement systems, use the conversion information found in Chapter 8, which includes the actual steps for calculating medications using ratio and proportion, the formula method, and dimensional analysis. Some steps in Examples 2 through 4 have been shortened.

 EXAMPLE 2: Ordered: *meperidine* (Demerol) 100 mg IM every 3-4 hours for pain management

Dose Available: 50 mg/1 mL

Calculating Dose Using the Ratio and Proportion Method

Compare the dose available ratio to the dose ordered ratio.

Dose Available (DA): 50 mg : 1 mL

Dose Ordered (DO): 100 mg

Use the formula: DA : DF :: DO : DG

Set up the proportional equation: 50 (DA) : 1 (DF) :: 100 (DO) : x (DG)

$50x = 100$, so $x = 2$. Recall that the drug form is in milliliters, so draw 2 mL into a 3-mL syringe.

Administer Demerol 2 mL IM every 3 to 4 hours.

Calculating Dose Using the Formula Method

Set up the formula:

$$\frac{DO}{DA} \times DF = DG$$
$$\frac{100 \text{ mg (DO)}}{50 \text{ mg (DA)}} \times 1 \text{ mL (DF)} = x \text{(DG)}$$
$$DG = \text{Demerol 2 mL q3-4 h}$$

The volume of the drug to draw into a 3-mL syringe is 2 mL.

Calculating Dose Using the Dimensional Analysis Method

The first step is to set up the equation with x on the left and the starting factor in the linear equation being the dose ordered over 1. This should be followed by the available medication.

The problem looks like this:

$$x = \frac{100 \text{ mg}}{1}$$

Recall that the second factor must cancel the numerator of the starting factor (100 mg), so the denominator of the second factor must be in milligrams.

The problem now looks like this:

$$x = \frac{100 \text{ mg}}{1} \times \frac{1 \text{ mL}}{50 \text{ mg}}$$

Cancel when appropriate.
The dose to be given is Demerol 2 mL IM q3-4h.

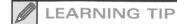 **LEARNING TIP**

Regardless of the method of calculation, the dose to be drawn into the syringe must be a liquid volume, so the answer must be expressed as a liquid as designated on the container. Additionally, always be thinking ahead to what syringe size you will need.

Check Your Understanding: CALCULATING DOSES IN THE METRIC SYSTEM BOX 10-2

Calculation Review

Calculate the following parenteral doses. Then show the correct amount of fluid in the syringe. Show your work on a separate sheet of paper. Save your worksheet. (Label your answer on the syringe with the correct number of milliliters.)

1. Ordered: **hydrocortisone sodium phosphate** 125 mg IM. Available: hydrocortisone sodium phosphate 50 mg/mL.
   Desired dose: _____
   Show this amount on the syringe.

2. Ordered: **furosemide** 25 mg IM. Available: furosemide 10 mg/mL.
   Desired dose: _____
   Show this amount on the syringe.

3. Ordered: **atropine sulfate** 0.5 mg IM. Available: atropine sulfate 1 mg/mL.
   Desired dose: _____
   Show this amount on the syringe.

4. Ordered: **diazepam** 2 mg IM every 3-4 hours. Available: diazepam 5 mg/mL.
   Desired dose: _____
   Show this amount on the syringe.

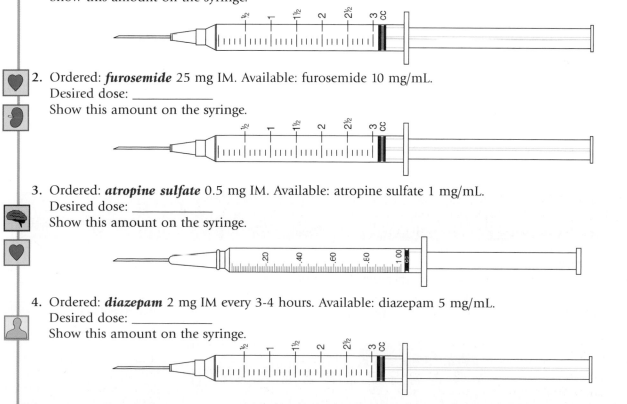

Continued

Check Your Understanding: CALCULATING DOSES IN THE METRIC SYSTEM BOX 10-2—cont'd

5. Ordered: *digoxin* 375 mcg IM stat. Available: digoxin 0.125 mg/mL.
   Desired dose: _____
   Show this amount on the syringe.

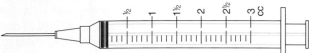

6. Ordered: *methylprednisolone* (Solu-Medrol) 125 mg. Available: methylprednisolone reconstituted to 62.5 mg/mL.
   Desired dose: _____
   Show this amount on the syringe.

CALCULATING DOSES OF PARENTERAL DRUGS IN UNITS

Aqueous-based medications such as analgesics (opioids), vitamin B_{12}, epinephrine, certain vaccines, insulin, heparin, and anticoagulants, of less than 2 milliliter may be given subcutaneously. Medications that are injected intradermally or are less than 1 milliliter, including those in units (except for insulin), are prepared in a tuberculin syringe. Insulin, however, should always be prepared in an insulin syringe that is marked in units. Heparin is designated in units, but the doses are indicated in milliliters, so the medication is prepared in a tuberculin syringe for doses less than 1 milliliter.

The tuberculin syringe has a capacity of 1 mL and is calculated in hundredths of a milliliter (0.01). The U-100 insulin syringe holds 100 units (1 mL) of medication and is calibrated in units. The number of units of insulin indicates the amount of insulin being given. The standard insulin syringe used today is the U-100 1 mL (100 units), but insulin syringes also come in a 0.5-mL (50-unit) size and a 0.3-mL (30-unit) size. The U-50 insulin syringes are marked off in "ones" and are therefore more precise when insulin is ordered in an odd number of less than 50 units. The syringes holding the smaller volume are for use by people with visual impairment and are using only small doses.

Check Your Understanding: READING INSULIN AND NONINSULIN DOSES IN UNITS BOX 10-3

Calculation Review
Read the syringe and write the amount of medication that is indicated.

1. _____

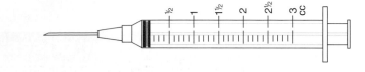

Check Your Understanding: READING INSULIN AND NONINSULIN DOSES IN UNITS BOX 10-3—cont'd

2. _____

3. _____

4. _____

5. _____

You are given the dose. Draw a line and shade in the exact amount (volume) that would show in the syringe.

6. 80 units insulin

7. 46 units insulin

8. 36 units insulin

9. 5000 units heparin (10,000 units/mL)

10. 2500 units heparin (5000 units/mL)

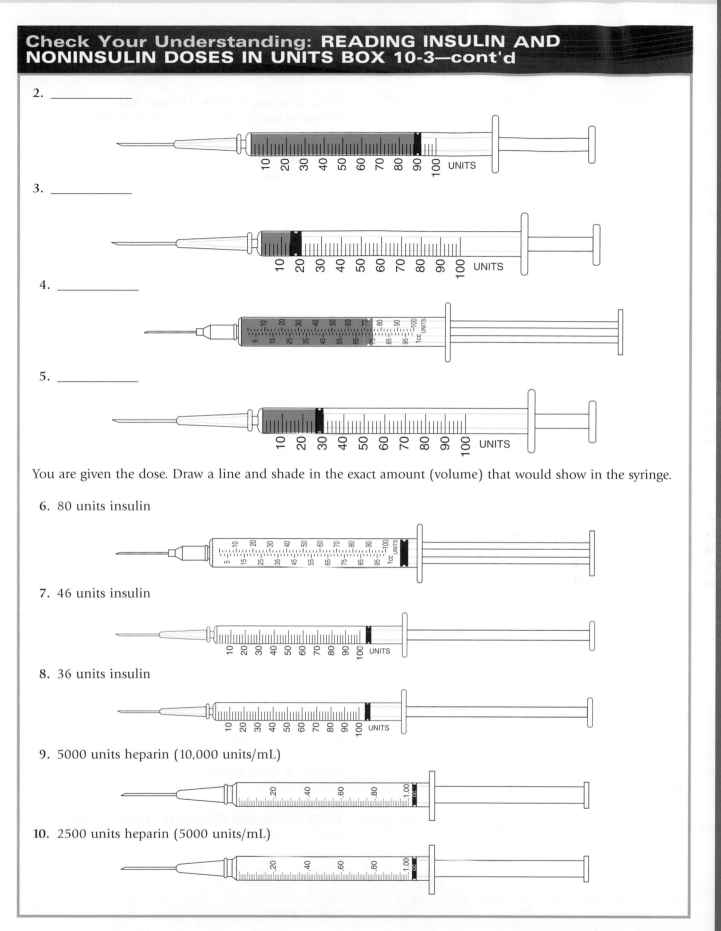

CALCULATING A PARENTERAL MEDICATION AVAILABLE IN UNITS

To calculate units, set up the problem as shown previously using one of the three methods of calculation.

 LEARNING TIP

When calculating with numbers with multiple zeros at the end, such as 200,000, cancel as many zeros as possible to make the calculations easier.

 EXAMPLE 3: Ordered: penicillin G 200,000 units IM

Dose Available: penicillin G 250,000 units/mL

Calculating Units Using the Ratio and Proportion Method

Dose Available (DA): 250,000 units/mL
Dose Ordered (DO): 200,000 units
Use the formula: DA : DF :: DO : DG
Cancel out as many zeros from the DO and DA as possible. The proportional equation looks like this:

25 units : 1 mL :: 20 units : x mL

$$20 = 25x$$

$$x = \frac{4}{5}$$

The answer must be changed to the metric system: $\frac{4}{5} = 0.8$

$$x = 0.8 \text{ mL}$$

The drug form is in milliliters, so draw 0.8 mL into a 1-mL syringe or 3-mL syringe.
Administer penicillin G 0.8 mL IM.

Calculating Units Using the Formula Method

$$\frac{DO}{DA} \times DF = DG$$

Cancel out as many zeros from the DO and DA as possible. The equation looks like this:

$$\frac{20}{25} \times 1 = x$$

$$x = \frac{4}{5}$$

Change the answer to the metric system: $\frac{4}{5} = 0.8$, so $x = 0.8$ mL.

The drug form is in milliliters so draw 0.8 mL into a 1-mL syringe or 3-mL syringe.
Administer penicillin G 0.8 mL IM.

Calculating Units Using the Dimensional Analysis Method

x is on the left of the linear equation (left side of the equal sign), and the drug ordered over 1 is the starting factor (on the right side of the equal sign). Cancel out as many zeros as possible so your problem setup looks like this:

$$x = \frac{20 \text{ units}}{1}$$

Cancel the starting factor by adding a second factor (dose available) with "units" as the denominator. The problem now looks like this:

$$x = \frac{20 \text{ units}}{1} \times \frac{1 \text{ mL}}{25 \text{ units}}$$

$$x = \frac{4}{5}$$

This answer must be shown in the metric system: $\frac{4}{5} = 0.8$
The drug form is in milliliters, so draw 0.8 mL into a 1-mL syringe or 3-mL syringe.
Administer penicillin G 0.8 mL IM.

Remember to complete the additional steps for parenteral doses:

What size syringe would you choose? (1-mL tuberculin or 3-mL syringe)
How much penicillin G would you draw into this syringe? (0.8 mL)
What parenteral route is used? (Intramuscular [IM])

Calculating Heparin Doses in Units

Heparin is available in units/mL. Orders for heparin are written in units but the dose to be given will be in milliliters. If the dose is less than 1 mL, the medication should be prepared in a tuberculin syringe for accuracy. If the dose is larger than 1 mL, the medication will be prepared in a 3-mL syringe.

EXAMPLE 4: Dose Ordered: heparin 2500 units
Dose Available: heparin 10000 units/mL

Calculating Heparin Units Using Ratio and Proportion

DA: $10{,}000 \text{ units}/\text{mL}$

DO: 2500 units
Use the formula: DA : DF :: DO : DG
Cancel zeros.

100 units : 1 mL :: 25 units : x mL
100 x = 25

x = ¼ units, which must be changed to metrics: ¼ = 0.25 mL
Dose to be given is heparin 0.25 mL.
Use the 1-mL syringe for the most accurate measurement.

Calculating Heparin Units Using the Formula Method

Set up the formula:

$$\frac{DO}{DA} \times DF = DG$$

Cancel zeros from original example.
Problem is set up like this:

$$\frac{25}{100} \times 1 = x$$

$$x = \frac{1}{4}$$

Change to metrics: ¼ = 0.25
Dose to be given: heparin 0.25 mL SC
Use the 1-mL syringe.

Calculating Heparin Units Using Dimensional Analysis

x is on the left of the linear equation, and the drug ordered over 1 is the starting factor (on the right of the equal sign).

Cancel zeros from original example; the problem would look like this:

$$x = \frac{25}{1}$$

Multiply a second factor (dose available) to cancel the starting factor numerator.

$$x = \frac{25}{1} \times \frac{1}{100}$$

x = ¼ , which must be changed to the metric system: ¼ = 0.25
Dose to be given: heparin 0.25 mL
Because this is a small dose volume, a 1-mL tuberculin syringe should be used.

Measuring Insulin in Units

Insulin is measured in units, and some forms of insulin may be mixed for administration.

Insulin is *always* prepared and administered using *only* an insulin syringe. *Do not use a tuberculin syringe for insulin except as directed by a physician in an emergency!* Parenteral routes (Chapter 14) will describe the correct method of combining two types of insulin, along with the proper procedure to inject a parenteral medication. This chapter introduces how to calculate the *total* amount of medication. When calculating the total amount of insulin to be drawn into the syringe, individual dose units of each insulin type must be added together to find the total dose unit volume to be administered.

 EXAMPLE 5: Ordered: Humulin R 22 units and Humulin N 26 units

Available: 10-mL vials of Humulin R U-100 and Humulin N U-100
How much insulin would you draw into a U-100 syringe?
To do the math, add the number of units for each type of insulin.
22 units + 26 units = 48 total units
The insulin syringe would have a total of 48 units of insulin. Because 48 units is close to full capacity of the 50-unit syringe, a 100-unit syringe would be preferred.

Check Your Understanding: CALCULATING INSULIN AND NONINSULIN DOSES IN UNITS BOX 10-4

Calculation Review

Compute the following doses in units. Then draw in the correct amount of fluid on the syringe. Show your work on a separate sheet of paper. Save your worksheet.

1. Ordered: Humulin R 35 units SC
   Available: Humulin R U-100 10 mL vial
   Desired dose: _____

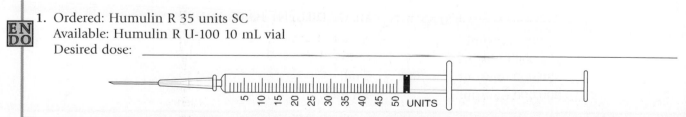

Continued

Check Your Understanding: CALCULATING INSULIN AND NONINSULIN DOSES IN UNITS BOX 10-4—cont'd

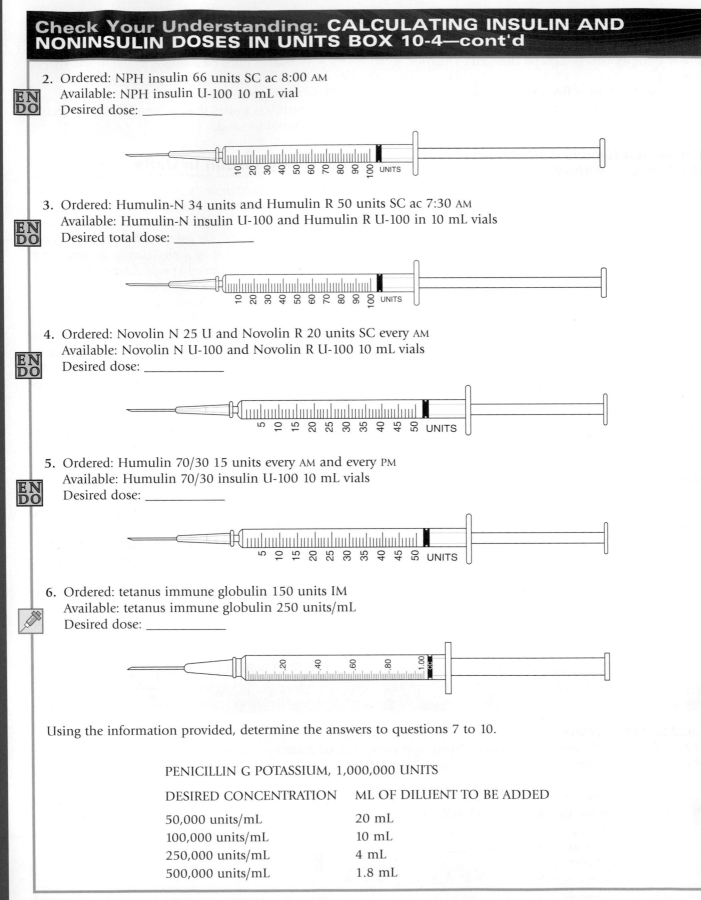

2. Ordered: NPH insulin 66 units SC ac 8:00 AM
   Available: NPH insulin U-100 10 mL vial
   Desired dose: _____

3. Ordered: Humulin-N 34 units and Humulin R 50 units SC ac 7:30 AM
   Available: Humulin-N insulin U-100 and Humulin R U-100 in 10 mL vials
   Desired total dose: _____

4. Ordered: Novolin N 25 U and Novolin R 20 units SC every AM
   Available: Novolin N U-100 and Novolin R U-100 10 mL vials
   Desired dose: _____

5. Ordered: Humulin 70/30 15 units every AM and every PM
   Available: Humulin 70/30 insulin U-100 10 mL vials
   Desired dose: _____

6. Ordered: tetanus immune globulin 150 units IM
   Available: tetanus immune globulin 250 units/mL
   Desired dose: _____

Using the information provided, determine the answers to questions 7 to 10.

PENICILLIN G POTASSIUM, 1,000,000 UNITS

DESIRED CONCENTRATION	ML OF DILUENT TO BE ADDED
50,000 units/mL	20 mL
100,000 units/mL	10 mL
250,000 units/mL	4 mL
500,000 units/mL	1.8 mL

Check Your Understanding: CALCULATING INSULIN AND NONINSULIN DOSES IN UNITS BOX 10-4—cont'd

7. Calculate the number of milliliters to be given per dose for a patient who was prescribed penicillin G potassium 400,000 units daily IM in four divided doses when the volume of diluent added was 10 mL.
   Desired dose: _____
   Show this amount on the syringe.

8. The physician prescribed penicillin G potassium 400,000 units to be administered IM bid. Diluent added: 4 mL to obtain the desired dosage strength. Identify the dosage strength per milliliter and calculate the volume per dose to be administered.
   Dosage strength: _____
   Volume per dose: _____

9. How much diluent should be added to the penicillin G potassium to make a concentration of 500,000 units/mL dosage strength? _____

10. Explain how so many dosage strengths are possible with just one vial of medication. _____
_____

SUMMARY

This chapter concludes the calculation of medications section of this textbook. At this point, the successful student should feel comfortable with calculating doses for parenteral and nonparenteral medication delivery. This chapter emphasizes the importance of always knowing the dosage available on hand before attempting to compute the desired dose (dosage ordered). This chapter also covers an introduction to the selection of the correct syringe size when preparing medication. Throughout this section, all math calculation examples are shown using ratio and proportion, the formula method, and dimensional analysis. If a review of the exact steps necessary in these calculations is needed, the student should go back to Chapters 8 and 9 for the information. Students should find the method with

which they are most comfortable, that produces the correct results, and then use that method with consistency. Dose calculation errors are less likely to occur if the student consistently computes dose calculations using only one method.

Three basic syringes are used to administer most parenteral medications in ambulatory care facilities. Choosing the correct syringe for the amount of medication to be administered is extremely important. Insulin and heparin are both calibrated in units and must be administered in exact doses. Insulin units should be administered with an insulin syringe that is standard at U-100/mL, whereas heparin units should be administered with a tuberculin syringe. Most other medications are administered in calibrated syringes using milliliters. The syringe size that is most frequently used is a 3 mL (3 cc) syringe.

Check Your Understanding: REVIEW BOX 10-5

Calculation Review
Calculate the following problems. Show your work on a separate sheet of paper. Save your worksheet.

Ordered: conjugated estrogens 2.5 mg SC
Available: conjugated estrogens 5 mg/mL
   1. Desired dose: _____
   2. What size syringe would you use? _____

Continued

Check Your Understanding: REVIEW BOX 10-5—cont'd

Ordered: Demerol 75 mg IM
Available: Demerol 50 mg/mL
  3. Desired dose: _____
  4. What size syringe would you use? _____

Ordered: procaine penicillin G 1,200,000 units IM
Available: procaine penicillin G 600,000 units/mL
  5. Desired dose: _____
  6. What size syringe would you use? _____

Ordered: ampicillin 1 g IM
Available: ampicillin reconstituted 2 g/1.8 mL
  7. Desired dose: _____
  8. What size syringe would you use? _____

Ordered: furosemide 2 mg IM
Available: furosemide 10 mg/mL
  9. Desired dose: _____
  10. What size syringe would you use? _____

CRITICAL THINKING EXERCISES

Name each of the syringes shown, and then identify the characteristics of each. Then circle the appropriate injection route(s) for each.

1. Type of syringe: _____
   Volume capacity: _____
   Calibration: _____
   Typically used for: Intradermal   Subcutaneous   Intramuscular

2. Type of syringe: _____
   Volume capacity: _____
   Calibration: _____
   Typically used for: Intradermal   Subcutaneous   Intramuscular

3. Type of syringe: _____
   Volume capacity: _____
   Calibration: _____
   Typically used for: Intradermal   Subcutaneous   Intramuscular

REVIEW QUESTIONS

All of the following statements are *false*. Determine the error(s) and rewrite the answer giving completely correct information in the space provided.

1. To calculate a syringe dose, read the fluid level from the tip of the plunger just above the calibration mark. ___

_____

_____

2. A tuberculin syringe is calibrated in units only. _____

_____

3. Usually only solutions of 2 to 3 mL are given subcutaneously. _____

_____

4. The most common insulin syringe is called the *U-50*. _____

_____

5. Heparin is normally given using an insulin syringe. _____

_____

6. The typical intramuscular syringe holds 100 units of medication. _____

_____

7. The strength of a reconstituted medication can be changed by adding more powder. _____

_____

8. Typically, a tuberculin syringe is used to administer an antibiotic. _____

_____

9. Many medications given SC are irritating to the tissues. _____

_____

10. Insulin may be administered in a 3 cc syringe if it is calibrated in units. _____

_____

11. When using a 2 or 3 mL syringe, always round calculations to the nearest whole number. _____

_____

Calculate the following problems. Show your work on a separate sheet of paper. Save your worksheet. Determine the correct amount of medication to draw into the syringe (Desired Dose), then determine which syringe to use from the following choices: 3 mL syringe, 1 mL syringe, 100 unit insulin syringe, or 50 unit insulin syringe.

12. 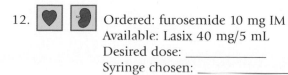 Ordered: furosemide 10 mg IM
     Available: Lasix 40 mg/5 mL
     Desired dose: _____
     Syringe chosen: _____

13. Ordered: procaine penicillin G 500,000 units IM
    Available: procaine penicillin G 250,000 units/mL
    Desired dose: _____
    Syringe chosen: _____

14. Ordered: Benadryl 25 mg IM
    Available: Benadryl 50 mg/mL
    Desired dose: _____
    Syringe chosen: _____

15. Ordered: Phenergan 75 mg IM
    Available: Phenergan 50 mg/mL
    Desired dose: _____
    Syringe chosen: _____

16. Ordered: heparin 4000 units SC
    Available: heparin 10,000 units/mL
    Desired dose: _____
    Syringe chosen: _____

17. Ordered: Humulin R 35 units
    Available: Humulin R U-100
    Desired dose: _____
    Syringe chosen: _____

18. Ordered: Rocephin 500 mg IM
    Available: Rocephin 1000 mg/4 mL
    Desired dose: _____
    Syringe chosen: _____

Medication Administration

Safety and Quality Assurance

After studying this chapter, you should be capable of doing the following:

- Explaining the importance of safety when using over-the-counter (OTC) medications.
- Describing legal, ethical, and other measures to protect health care personnel during medication administration.
- Describing quality assurance in medication administration.
- Explaining the relationship of the medical office and Occupational Safety and Health
- Administration (OSHA) regulations related to pharmacology.
- Discussing three "befores" and seven "rights" of administering medications.
- Explaining procedures necessary to prevent medication errors and documentation required in the event an error occurs.
- Describing routes by which medications are delivered to the body.

Betty, an allied health professional in a physician's office, is asked by a co-worker to administer a physician-ordered dose of Decadron to Joseph, in Room 5, who has arthritis. Betty picks up a bottle that appears to be Decadron from the shelf. She draws the dose and administers it to the patient in Room 2 without asking the patient his name because she thinks she knows the patient. Actually, Betty has drawn an estrogen preparation and given it to Mac. The other allied health professional working in the area later realizes that Betty has given the wrong medication to the wrong patient.

What rules of medication administration has Betty failed to follow?
What information does Betty need to document?
Does she need to notify the physician? Why or why not?

KEY TERMS

Medication administration

Medication error
Quality assurance (QA)

Remember, safety with medications, whether the medication is an over-the-counter (OTC) or a prescription agent, is an important factor in therapeutic patient care. Allied health professionals have the responsibility to obtain a list of all medications—prescription, herbal, and OTC—that a patient is taking so that safety in drug usage occurs. A complete list of medications includes both drugs taken regularly and those taken as needed (or prn).

When teaching patients about OTC drugs, the allied health professional should be sure the patient realizes these preparations are actually drugs and need to be taken with the same precaution as prescription medicines. This means taking OTC drugs as they are meant to be taken, with the patient reading all instructions and following the manufacturer-recommended dosages for age and weight. The safe dose in a 24-hour period as noted on the label on the container should not be exceeded. All ingredients in an OTC medication should be evaluated by the patient, or person administering the medication, before these preparations are used, to be sure that harmful ingredients that have caused drug intolerances, allergies, and adverse reactions are not found in the drug. An important fact is that OTC medications may have changes in inert ingredients between purchases, so the label should be read each time before buying to ensure allergic reactions and intolerances will not occur because of changes.

SAFETY WITH MEDICATIONS TAKEN BY PATIENTS

Self-medication may delay needed medical care because OTC drugs can mask important symptoms. When OTC medications are taken, printouts supplying drug interactions are not provided, and the patient is therefore not aware of possible dangers. Box 11-1 lists safety tips

for patient administration of medications. Furthermore, with self-medication, chemical ingredients of all OTC substances including drugs and herbals must be evaluated for their potential detrimental effects related to the patient's physical condition and the potential for life-threatening effects. The following are important factors regarding use of OTC preparations for self-treatment:

- For safety, document excessive use of drugs such as alcohol or caffeine (found in coffee, soft drinks, energy drinks, and tea) and nicotine (tobacco products).
- OTC and herbal drugs may be obtained without a prescription, and use should be completely documented in the medical record.
- Spend extra time with the patient who takes OTC medications to be sure the patient is aware of possible dangers of self-treatment in conjunction with the use of prescription drugs. Remind the patient that OTC preparations should be used only as

---

BOX 11-1 TIPS TO ENSURE SAFETY IN MEDICATION ADMINISTRATION

1. For safe and effective therapy, explain how and why the drug is to be taken.
2. Specify a time for the medication to be taken. Some medications need to be taken with meals, whereas others need to be taken on an empty stomach. Some drugs need to be taken at a specific time each day; others may need to be taken several times a day with no relationship to a specific time.
3. If the patient is elderly or has difficulty remembering the schedule, suggest making a chart or calendar to remember when to take medications. A large calendar may be used to check off medications throughout the day. Medications that are dispensed for more than one dose per day may be dispensed in containers with reminder mechanisms such as individual slots for daily medications or different-colored containers for different times of day.
4. Be sure the patient knows how long the medication is to be taken. Some drugs are prescribed for short-term therapy and others for long-term, even lifetime, use. If short-time medications such as antibiotics are prescribed, the patient should be instructed to complete the entire course of treatment. For chronic conditions, the patient should be instructed to continue taking medication as directed until physician stops the medication, if that is the physician's protocol.
5. Be sure the patient knows that some medications such as antihypertensives may make him or her feel worse while the body is adjusting closer toward homeostasis. Also, the patient should be taught symptoms of dangerous side effects. Medications should be discontinued only on advice of the physician.
6. The patient should be instructed that some medications (e.g., *prednisone*, tranquilizers) cannot be stopped abruptly but must be tapered off as instructed by the physician.
7. The patient should be taught the side effects of the medication (e.g., drowsiness from antihistamines) and safety

measures to follow while taking the medicine (e.g., avoid driving or operating machinery with narcotic analgesics).
8. Inform the patient that all adverse reactions should be reported so they can be noted in the medical record and adjustments to medications can be made as needed.
9. The patient should be told that misuse of any medication might lead to dangerous side effects, such as bleeding ulcers with aspirin or drug dependence with pain relievers.
10. Proper storage of medications should be discussed with the pharmacist. Warmth and dampness of bathrooms and sunny windowsills make these places inappropriate storage sites.
11. Old medicines should be discarded by removing drugs from their original container and mixing with an undesirable substance (i.e., coffee grounds or kitty litter), and place in an impermeable, non-destructive container to prevent ingestion by children or pets. Then place in trash or incinerate. See federal acceptable government guidelines for disposal of medications at www.WhiteHouseDrugPolicy.gov.
12. Expired medications lose efficacy, and their effects are unpredictable, even toxic.
13. Medications are prescribed for a certain person with a specific condition and should not be shared with others. A person who takes drugs prescribed for someone else might experience severe adverse reactions.
14. The patient should always check with the pharmacist or physician before mixing medications with alcohol, tobacco, or other medications, including OTC drugs and herbals.
15. Medications should be taken in well-lighted areas so the label can be safely read. Never assume a bottle of medicine is the correct bottle; always read the label. For a person with poor eyesight, print on the bottle label should be large, or the patient should have someone else prepare the medications. Ask the pharmacist to assist in providing aids for safe administration with low-vision individuals.

directed on the labels after always reading the label carefully.

- Inform the patient that dosages of many OTC drugs are low, so the dose may not supply the patient with adequate medication to have a sufficient therapeutic effect—for example, Aleve (200 mg) one or two tablets twice daily for arthritis compared with the prescription strength of **naproxen** of 375 to 500 mg twice to three times a day. The amount of OTC medication used may even mask the true severity of symptoms.
- OTC medications often contain more than one active ingredient, allowing drug interactions to occur. Remember that only one of the active ingredients may be needed to cause an interaction, such as **guaifenesin** (for coughs) and antihypertensive medications.
- Any adverse or allergic reactions the patient has experienced with any medication should be documented in the medical record.
- Finally, patients may not be aware that ingestion of the same medication under different names such as Advil, Motrin, and **ibuprofen** may cause an overdose. Some persons may also take multiple doses of the same prescription medication if the appearance of the generic drug has changed (e.g., because the manufacturer is different).

MEDICATION ADMINISTRATION

Many laypeople think that administering medications is the main thrust of pharmacology. In reality, pharmacology is the knowledge necessary to give medicines safely. **Medication administration** means giving a dose of medication to a person. (If the medication has been dispensed, the patient self-administers the drug in most conditions.) All three persons in the professional medical triangle (physician, pharmacist, allied health professional) are necessary for safe drug therapy.

Proper techniques in giving medications using seven "rights" (right patient, medication, dose, route, time, technique, and documentation) and three "befores" (before removing from storage, before preparing medication, and before returning to storage) and proper safety precautions as determined by regulatory agencies cannot be overemphasized to ensure high-quality patient care.

OCCUPATIONAL SAFETY AND HEALTH ADMINISTRATION STANDARDS IN MEDICATION ADMINISTRATION

In July 1992 the Occupational Safety and Health Administration (OSHA) started to enforce workplace controls concerning bloodborne pathogens. Body fluids may contain pathogenic microorganisms capable of causing disease. Each medical facility must have its own exposure control plan dictating how the facility will comply with OSHA standards.

Standards that are specific to giving medications include the following:

- Barrier equipment should be worn if a chance of splashing or spraying of body fluids during medication administration is possible.
- When performing injections, health care personnel should wear gloves to protect against possible cross contamination.
- Used needles and other single-use equipment such as vaginal applicators or inhalation devices that have contact with potentially infectious body secretions must be properly disposed of in puncture-resistant containers.
- All disposable syringes and needles should have retractable safety caps and should be placed in a puncture-resistant container located close to the area of use (Figures 11-1 and 11-2).
- If the needle must be recapped after use, place one hand behind your back and "scoop" the cover over the needle (Figure 11-3). Sterile needles are not contaminated by body fluids and may be recapped after they have been used to withdraw medications from vials.
- A needle should never be directed toward any part of the allied health professional's body.

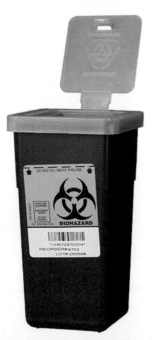

Figure 11-1 Disposable syringes and sharps should be disposed of in a puncture-proof container. (From Young AP, Proctor DB: *Kinn's the medical assistant*, ed 11, St Louis, 2011, Elsevier.)

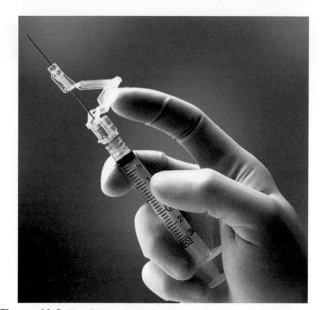

Figure 11-2 The Occupational Safety and Health Administration suggests using syringes with retractable needle covers. (From Young AP, Proctor DB: *Kinn's the medical assistant*, ed 11, St Louis, 2011, Elsevier.)

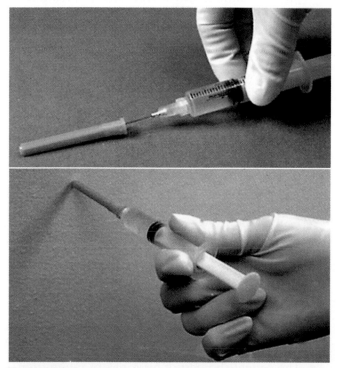

Figure 11-3 To recap needles, use one hand and a scooping technique. (From Young AP, Proctor DB: *Kinn's the medical assistant*, ed 10, St Louis, 2007, Elsevier.)

- Contaminated waste must be disposed of in accordance with federal, state, and local regulations.
- Any exposure must be evaluated, and a postexposure follow-up plan for the facility completed, including an incident report and confidential medical evaluation.

In subsequent chapters the icons shown are used for procedures, to illustrate their need for different routes of medication administration.

> ## Important Facts about Medication Administration and Occupational Safety and Health Administration (OSHA) Standards
>
> When medications are administered, the latest appropriate OSHA standards relating to splashes and possible contact with body fluids should be followed.

QUALITY ASSURANCE IN MEDICATION DELIVERY

Quality assurance (QA)—establishing standards of excellence in patient care and tailoring professional practice to those standards—is the core of applied medicine. Quality assurance is prescribed by a set of policies and procedures found in each office and by various federal regulations that affect medical practice. When followed, these rules provide a safety net for patients and practitioners alike. If they are not followed, a multitude of problems can result: medication errors, personnel exposure to dangerous pathogens, and costly litigation. QA ensures that practices result in the highest possible level of patient care and that services are consistent with high principles of professional conduct. The allied health professional should monitor all aspects of patient care for quality assurance.

To provide quality assurance, the following steps are necessary:

- When medication shipments arrive, the health professional should check that medications have been maintained at appropriate temperature during transport.

> ### Did You Know?
>
> A study on medications concluded that only 8% of drugs shipped were arriving within the temperature and humidity limits developed by manufacturers. More than 26% were subjected to excessive heat, and 65% of these drugs were subjected to temperatures of 86° F to 104° F, making drug effectiveness less than optimum and in some cases dangerous.

- When ordering medications, the facility should avoid having items in transit during weekends or holidays when timely delivery cannot be made.

- Medications that require special considerations should be stored in accordance with relevant controls.
- As medications are stocked, strength, size of container, and drug itself should be checked against inventory and packing slip and stored in the appropriate location.
- Medications should be placed in exact storage locations, with the label facing toward the front, with same medications of the same strength being stocked as previously found.
- Drugs should be separated by route of administration, especially ophthalmic and otic preparations.
- Drugs with specific uses (e.g., estrogen preparations) should be stocked together.
- Check expiration dates. Possible loss of stock because of expiration or use of more than one container at a time may occur if stocking is done in an inconsistent manner.
- As new medications arrive at the office, expiration date—the indicator of shelf life—should be carefully observed. Those with an expiration date that is soon may need to be returned to the purchase source immediately.
- Supplies should be placed where they are most accessible yet protected from damage and exposure to such elements as heat, light, moisture, and air.
- Check storage requirements with each order, as the manufacturer may make changes. Most drugs should be stored in a cool, dark area away from direct light to avoid deterioration.
- Medications for external use should be stored separately from those for internal use.
- Poisons and chemicals, including disinfectants and other cleaning agents, that may cause harm to a patient if used in error should not be stored with drugs and chemicals used as drugs, either internally or topically.
- Labels should be carefully preserved, and all medications must be stored in their original containers.
- A container without a label or with a label so damaged that it is difficult to know what is in the container should be destroyed. Never relabel a medication.

Important Facts about Quality Assurance

- Quality assurance in medication administration ensures that the patient receives high-quality drugs given safely using the correct manner.
- Quality assurance ensures that a medication has been properly transported and stored, has not expired, and is safe for administration.

MEDICATION ADMINISTRATION FOR PATIENT SAFETY

Medications may be given only under direct order and supervision of a health care provider. However, the allied health professional has a responsibility to assess a situation and to address problems related to administering drugs. The physician performs a physical assessment of the patient, but the allied health professional should again assess the patient and environment before giving a drug. If changes have occurred that would make administration of the drug undesirable or improper, the allied health professional should notify the health care provider for advice before giving the medication.

Some factors that might cause variance in drug use include the following:

- Size and age of the patient
- Changes in vital signs
- Changes in organ system function
- Possible contraindications to the drug (e.g., previous illness, concurrent use of medications such as heparin or OTC medications) or drug interactions
- Food or animal allergies that may prohibit the use of a medication (e.g., allergies to eggs, animal dander)
- Possible drug dependency
- The patient's medical status might make use of the usual route of administration undesirable (e.g., oral administration for a person who has difficulty swallowing, injuries at the site of appropriate parenteral or topical administration)
- The proper dose or dosage of the medication. If in doubt, the allied health professional should ask the health care provider to confirm the order. Never hesitate to question the possibility of a mistake in interpreting a medication order.
- The presence of an appropriate person in the event that an allergic reaction occurs. Do not give medications without a physician present (even if the drug has been ordered or given on multiple occasions) in case a situation requiring emergency care should occur.
- The patient should not be at risk of injury from a fall or from inappropriate behavior. Safe surroundings are especially important after pain medications have been administered.
- Medications should always be stored in the same place during cleaning or during replacement of drugs. Potential for errors may occur when medications are moved from the usual place.
- When a drug is administered, certain rules must be followed to ensure safety. Box 11-2 lists these important rules.

BOX 11-2 RULES TO FOLLOW WHEN ADMINISTERING MEDICATIONS

- Give only medications that have been ordered by the health care provider, either in writing or verbally. If there is no order, do not give medication.
- Know the drug you are giving. If you are not familiar with a certain medication, consult a drug reference before administration. Calculate the needed dose in a quiet area where you will not be interrupted. If you are unsure of the dose, ask someone else to check the medication order and any calculations.
- Always wash your hands before administering medications. Do not handle drugs directly.
- All prepared medications should be given immediately or safely stored until administered. Do not give any medications that you did not personally prepare unless prepared in a pharmacy for that patient, then check for proper patient identification.
- Identify the patient and ask about possible allergies even if you think you know the person and his or her medical history.
- Never return medications that have been prepared to their original containers. Any medication not given should be properly disposed. Proper documentation of disposal of Drug Enforcement Administration (DEA) scheduled medications is required.

- Never document administration of any medica giving it. All documentation should be done immed administration.
- Observe the patient for adverse reactions after administration of drugs.
- Give specific information concerning the signs of adverse reactions that need to be reported to the health care provider.
- Patients taking medications such as penicillin or immunotherapeutic drugs that might cause allergic reactions should be carefully monitored for a specified time in standard protocol to be sure an allergic reaction does not occur.
- Allergic reactions, no matter how small, should be documented so that careful evaluation can occur before administration of future doses of the medication.
- If you make an error when administering medications, immediately report the error to the health care provider and document the error and any treatment required in the medical record.
- Medical drug references, including those for pediatric and geriatric doses, should be used for calculating doses, with the calculation double-checked and compared with the available drug. Doses may be rounded to an easily administered amount with permission from the health care provider.

Important Facts about Patient Safety with Medication Administration

- Labels should be present on all drugs and chemicals.
- The health care professional should be sure that he or she understands the drug order. If there is doubt concerning the order, the allied health professional should ask for clarification.

REDUCING MEDICATION ERRORS USING 3 + 7

Administration of drugs should never become routine; it should be an organized, concise procedure to ensure safety for the patient and provision of high-quality care by the allied health professional. Medication administration requires 10 steps to ensure a high-quality process. Throughout this text, these steps are not repeated when each route of administration is discussed. Therefore these rules will be indicated by the icon **3+7**. When this icon appears, these rules should be followed.

Three Befores

Before administering any drug, the professional—whether the allied health professional or health care provider—should use the three befores for checking

labels. If medications are consistently stored according to medicinal use and preference, the befores will be more easily processed.

The three befores in preparing a drug for medication administration follow:

1. Read label on medication *before* removing drug from shelf. Be sure correct medication and dosage strength are obtained from storage for administration.
2. Read label on medication *before* preparing medication for administration. Double-check to be sure correct drug is being used.
3. Read label on medication before returning drug to storage after drug preparation for administration. *Remember, never give medications that you have not personally prepared.*

Seven Rights

Seven rights of medication administration should be adhered to without deviation. Before administering medication, ask yourself whether you have followed the seven rights (Figure 11-4).

1. *Right patient*—Even if you believe you know the patient, address the patient by name to identify any discrepancy in identification. Verify the name on the medical record. If the person is not known,

ask the patient to provide his or her name by asking, "What is your name?"

2. *Right drug*—Using three befores, be sure the medication is the one ordered. Compare the order with the medicine on shelf. When checking the label, always check the expiration date. *Never use an expired drug* when preparing a dose. Always "palm the label" to protect it; this is especially important with liquid medications.

3. *Right dose*—Compare the medication order with the dose prepared for administration. This requires reading the label carefully and ensuring the dose and order are in the same measurement system. Be sure the dose is within the acceptable dose range for the patient, and double-check any necessary calculations. Use the proper administration device that will give the most accurate measurement of the dose.

4. *Right time*—Be sure the medication is being given at the proper time, especially with medications that are given in a series such as allergy injections and immunizations. The time factor is important in maintaining consistent blood levels of the drug, in maximizing effectiveness of the drug, and in ensuring proper absorption of the medication.

5. *Right route*—Be sure the form of medication being prepared matches the route of administration ordered and is appropriate for person receiving the medication.

6. *Right technique*—After a final review of the medical record and an assessment of the patient, select an appropriate site and route and use appropriate delivery techniques. Be sure to use aseptic technique.

7. *Right documentation*—For medicolegal reasons, precisely and accurately enter the documentation in the patient's record *immediately after* giving medication to avoid **medication errors** (Figure 11-5). If adverse reactions occur, record any adverse symptoms and any actions taken as a result. If the administration is documented before it is performed and the patient then refuses the medication, an error in charting will have occurred. If you wait to document later, you may forget what was given, or even worse, someone else may repeat the administration (Box 11-3).

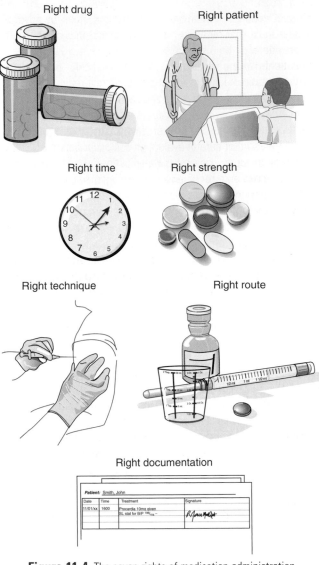

Figure 11-4 The seven rights of medication administration.

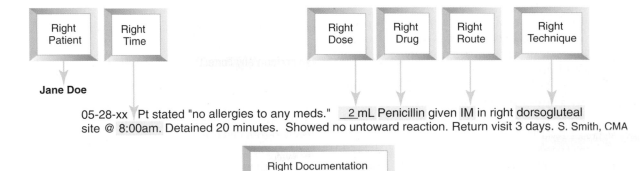

Figure 11-5 Documentation of the seven rights of medication administration.

BOX 11-3 CHECKLIST FOR DOCUMENTING MEDICATION ADMINISTRATION

- Record in the medical record any patient assessments that were done before and after the medication was administered.
- Record the date, time, and name of the medicine and the dose administered.
- If the treatment was an immunization, record the name of the manufacturer, expiration date, site of injection, and lot number of the vaccine.
- If a parenteral or percutaneous route of administration was used, record the route and site of administration.
- Record any patient reactions that may have occurred. If the medication is associated with possible reactions (such as penicillins), record the waiting time of the patient and whether reactions occurred.
- If patient education was provided, record the education given and the time required to give it.
- If the patient refused medication, record the reason for the refusal (see Figure 11-5).

If these seven rights are followed, the allied health professional will be using the "right knowledge" base for giving drugs safely. To ensure safe medication administration, the health care professional must comply with the 3 + 7 steps.

Important Facts for Reducing Medication Errors

- Use the three "befores" and seven "rights" when preparing medications. **3+7**
- To reduce the possibility of error, prepare medications in a quiet, well-lit, controlled environment.
- Always administer only medications that you prepare.
- Know the drug you are administering and the condition for which it is being prescribed.
- After administering a medication, observe the patient for possible unexpected reactions.
- Never return medications that have been prepared to their original containers. If not used, discard these medications properly.
- Always check for possible medication allergies before administering a drug. Check the medical record and ask the patient about allergies.
- Identify the patient before giving medicine.
- Medication errors occur even with the utmost of care. If an error is made, assess the patient, notify the health care provider, proceed with needed therapy as directed, and document what has happened. Assess the cause of the situation and make needed adjustments so the same error does not occur in the future.

SOURCES OF MEDICATION ERRORS

A medication error is at best an inconvenience and at worst a tragedy. Each error is potentially tragic and costly for patients and professionals alike. The goal of medication administration is to correctly give medication on each and every occasion (use the three befores and seven rights.) If this is done, no error in medication administration should occur. However, mistakes are sometimes made, and adverse drug events and medication errors do occur. For example, Celebrex is a medication for arthritis, Celexa is an antidepressant, and Cerebyx is an antiepilepsy drug; these names sound alike and are spelled similarly, leading to the potential for errors.

Medication errors are not trivial. Preventable medication errors cause approximately 2% of all hospitalizations, at a cost of $17 billion to $29 billion per year. The need for extreme care in medication administration is obvious. An inquiring attitude by the patient and professional may make the difference between a medication error and safety. Reporting any mistake to the proper supervisor will initiate the needed measures to counteract the effect of the drug as warranted. Appropriate documentation after an error is essential (Box 11-4).

DELIVERY OF MEDICATIONS

The method of administration depends partly on the purpose of the drug. Some drugs can be given in a variety of ways, whereas others must be administered in specific ways to be effective. Generally, drugs are given either through enteral or parenteral routes to produce systemic or general effects. Percutaneous administration occurs when the drug is placed in direct contact with and is absorbed through the skin, tissue, or mucous membranes. Drugs given for systemic effect are absorbed and circulate in the bloodstream to produce effects on body cells and tissues, whereas those for local effect are given

BOX 11-4 IF A MEDICATION ERROR OCCURS

- Observe the patient and evaluate his or her reaction.
- Notify the health care provider of the error and the patient's apparent reaction.
- Perform any corrective steps as directed by the health care provider.
- Document the error, including filing an incident report if that is the policy of the facility. If a report form is not available, document the incident completely. Use the guidelines of the liability insurance carrier for proper placement of documentation.
- Evaluate the circumstances and make any necessary changes in policy or procedure to prevent the same error from occurring in the future.

locally to remain at the site of administration and to prevent systemic dosage.

Medication administration denotes the introduction of a drug into or its application to the body. The goal is to deliver a precise, reliable dose with desired effects to the desired site. When the route of medication administration is being chosen, five factors are considered:

- Chemical properties of the drug
- Physical properties of the drug
- Desired site of action
- How rapidly the drug response is wanted
- Physical and mental health of the person receiving the drug

Routes of administration discussed in this text are gastrointestinal system, or enteral, routes (medications swallowed by mouth or given through rectal suppository or enema); parenteral routes of administration (subcutaneous, intramuscular, Z-track, intradermal, and intravenous routes of administration); and percutaneous routes (through skin; by vaginal applications; through mucous membranes such as eye, ear, mouth, or nose instillations; and by inhalation).

The most commonly used route for ambulatory care medications is the enteral route. Medicines given by this route have advantages of being safe, convenient for most patients, relatively economical, and, in most cases, readily available. Disadvantages include slowness of action and low dependability of absorption. Some medicines such as insulin are destroyed by digestive fluids and cannot be administered through the gastrointestinal tract.

Generally, the parenteral route is considered to be administration of medications by injection, or under the skin. With parenteral route administration, drug action is more rapid than with the enteral route, but the duration of action is shorter in most instances. Dosage with this route tends to be smaller because absorption is more rapidly accomplished. Disadvantages include greater cost of supplies, an increased chance of adverse patient reaction, and such complications as infections and abscesses, which may occur because skin has been broken.

The percutaneous routes are those in which absorption occurs through skin or mucous membranes. In most cases the drug action is confined to the site of application; in some cases, however, medication may be applied transdermally for systemic use, such as **fentanyl** transdermal patches for pain. Chances of a systemic reaction are reduced because the medication's action is usually confined to the place of application. Disadvantages include a slow rate of absorption (although this may also be a reason to use this route), irritation at the application site, difficulty in applying the drug, or messy residue occurring from the drug base. Because the duration of action is decreased in most instances, these medications may require more frequent application. However, some of these medications remain in place for several days depending on rate of absorption.

SUMMARY

Medication administration requires knowledge of the drug being given and proper route of administration, following the three befores and seven rights. All health care workers must follow OSHA guidelines for personal and patient safety.

To give medications safely, the professional should demonstrate the ability to follow the health care provider's orders, calculate doses correctly, and assess the patient, drug, and environment before administering the medicine. Following administration of medicine, patient observation for possible adverse reactions is necessary, including documentation of any adverse reaction.

When medication errors occur, the person administering the medication must take responsibility for the mistake and report and document the error, the treatment (if any) used to reverse the error, and any subsequent adverse effects. The goal is error-free administration of a precise, reliable drug dose to target tissues with fewest side effects, but in reality errors do occur.

CRITICAL THINKING EXERCISES

Scenario

Judy, an allied health care professional, is to administer a dose of penicillin to Jim for an upper respiratory tract infection. The physician has ordered a dose that Judy thinks is excessive for Jim, but this is her opinion based on her background, not on actual dosage charts.

1. What should Judy do first?
2. Judy finds that the dose is actually at the high end of the acceptable dosage range. What should Judy do next?
3. After Judy talks with the health care provider and is assured the dose is acceptable, Jim tells her that in the past, he might have had a rash after taking penicillin, but he guesses it does not matter. Should Judy give the penicillin?
4. If not, what should she do? If so, what reaction should she look for?

REVIEW EXERCISES

Documentation of Medications

Document the following as it should appear in the medical record. All entries will be the date and time the exercise is performed. Sign the documentation as a student in the field of study.

1. Sara Medici, age 2, has come to Dr. Merry for a measles-mumps-rubella (MMR) vaccination. Dr. Merry orders the vaccine to be given to Sara in the vastus lateralis muscle. The lot number is No. 12356, manufactured by Sohol Drugs. The expiration date is 10/04/xx. The dose for MMR is one vial (or 1 mL) after reconstitution. You informed the patient's parent of the side effects to expect and possible reactions, including the possibility of a rash and low-grade fever in 2 to 3 days. _____

2. Mary Alleri has come to the office to receive her allergy injections. She has a standing order from Dr. Merry to receive the next ordered dose unless she had a reaction to the previous dose. Ms. Alleri tells you that she had no problems with the last dose. Today's dose comes from Allergy Extract Bottle No. 4, 0.2 mL of extract. You give the injection in the right deltoid area subcutaneously as ordered. Ms. Alleri always waits 20 minutes after receiving the injection to be sure no reactions occur. When you check on her, there is no redness or swelling at the site of injection, and she has no signs of an allergic reaction. _____

REVIEW QUESTIONS

1. What is quality assurance? _____

2. What does "properly storing medications" mean? Where does an allied health professional obtain the needed instructions for this task? _____

3. The physician must order and supervise any medication administration in a medical office setting. Why is this important? _____

4. When should an allied health professional question an order from a health care provider? Why? _____

5. What are the three befores of medication administration? _____

6. What are the seven rights of medication administration? _____

7. Why is it important for a health care provider to be readily available when medications are administered, especially by parenteral route? _____

CHAPTER 12

Enteral Routes

OBJECTIVES

After studying this chapter, you should be capable of doing the following:

- Explaining what is meant by enteral route of medication administration.
- Describing forms of medications that are administered orally.
- Describing the role of the allied health professional in administration of oral medications.
- Demonstrating procedures for administering oral medications.
- Preparing a solid form of medication.
- Preparing liquid medications using a medicine cup, dose spoon, and graduated-dose syringe.

- Discussing indications for use of a rectal suppository.
- Administering medications using a rectal suppository for absorption in rectal mucosa.
- Discussing indications for and contraindications to a rectal enema.
- Discussing how to administer a rectal enema.
- Explaining to a patient how to self-administer medications rectally.
- Providing patient education for safety and compliance with enteral route.

Billy, a 2-year-old with a cough and runny nose, is brought to Dr. Merry's office by his mother. Dr. Merry examines Billy and prescribes liquid medication for his symptoms. Billy's mother tells you that Billy always wants to drink water after taking cough syrup.
Is this a matter that requires patient education? Why or why not?
Should Billy take cough syrup with meals? Why or why not?
What kind of measuring equipment would you tell Billy's mother to use for accurate administration of medicine?
Billy's mother also tells you she has to call medicine "candy" to get Billy to take it. Is this a safe practice? Why or why not?

KEY TERMS

Dose spoon
Dose syringe

Enema
Meniscus

The general rules for drug administration were discussed in Chapter 11 and should be followed when administering medications by any route, but techniques differ for each route of administration. Although the icon ⟨3+7⟩ is present, such common practices as the three "befores" and seven "rights" and basic procedures in medication administration are not included but are shown as an icon in each procedure. It is expected that you, the allied health professional, are now aware of the necessity of these steps for personal and patient safety.

This chapter considers medications that are absorbed by the gastrointestinal (GI) tract (or enterally) through the mouth or rectum through the mucous membranes. *Oral medications* are administered by having a patient swallow a drug. Drugs are absorbed in the GI tract, usually in the intestines—thus the name *enteral* medications. *Rectal medications* are administered into the rectum, either by a suppository or by an enema, and are included in this chapter because of absorption in the GI tract. Medications may also be administered into the GI tract through nasogastric or gastric tubes. These are not as common as oral and rectal administration and are more commonly found in inpatient settings.

With the oral route of administration, Occupational Safety and Health Administration (OSHA) standards may not include any personal protective equipment or special disposal of products used for administration because body fluids are not expected to be present for cross-contamination. However, with rectal administration of enemas or suppository medications, depending on the condition of patient, a higher level of protective equipment such as a gown may be necessary, and gloves will always be necessary. Icons for OSHA standards are also included with the procedures. One OSHA standard necessary for administration of any medication is hand sanitization, and this icon 🖐 appears with procedure guidelines.

ORAL ADMINISTRATION OF MEDICATIONS

Even with possible side effects from oral administration and length of time for absorption, it is the route of choice for most drug therapy (Procedures 12-1 to 12-3). Most people can self-administer medications with few problems when drugs are prescribed for oral use. Occasionally the oral route is not desirable, such as in the following situations:

- When the drug may be irritating to the stomach when taken by mouth
- When the effect of the drug may be altered by GI juices
- In the presence of vomiting, poor GI absorption, and inability to swallow food or fluids (or drugs)

The important precaution with oral administration is to avoid aspiration of medications. Aspiration occurs when medications intended for the GI tract are drawn into the respiratory tract. The risk can be reduced by first assessing the patient's ability to swallow.

When forms of medicine for oral consumption—tablets, capsules, powders, elixirs, syrups, solutions, and suspensions—enter the mouth, the medication must be swallowed to reach the stomach and then small intestine for absorption (forms of medication for oral administration are found in Chapter 3). F... tive disorders will change the rate of a... flow of medicine through the GI tract... tions cannot be given orally because digestive... make the drug ineffective or slow absorption into... bloodstream. Solid forms (tablets, capsules, and so on) should be taken with fluids. Many liquid preparations such as cough syrups should not be taken with another fluid to avoid diluting the medication. Be sure to read patient education materials and follow directions when administering any medication (Box 12-1). Finally, in some instances food may be required for absorption, whereas in others it is contraindicated (see Chapter 2). Always follow safety rules found in Chapter 11 for medications.

Important Facts about Administering Oral Medications

- All medications should be given according to the general rules of medication administration discussed in Chapter 11.
- The easiest, most desirable, safest, and most frequently used route of drug administration is the oral route because most people can self-administer medications effectively.
- Persons who cannot swallow should not be given oral medications.
- Aspiration of medications into the respiratory tract is the main danger of the oral route.
- Oral medications may be administered in solid or liquid form.
- The presence or absence of food in the GI tract and digestive disorders affect the rate of absorption of oral medications.
- Adequate fluids must be administered with medication so that the patient can swallow solid preparations, whereas fluids are rarely given after liquid preparations. Extra fluids should be given with sulfa medications to prevent crystallization.
- Some medications may be crushed or chewed for ease of administration, whereas enteric-coated or timed-release forms should not be altered before they are swallowed. With permission of the physician, scored tablets may be divided to give a partial dose of the medication; other medications may be used by dividing them as directed.

RECTAL ADMINISTRATION OF MEDICATIONS

Rectal medications are usually given as suppositories or ointments or by enema. Because the rectal mucosa has an excellent blood supply in the relatively small area, these medications are rapidly absorbed into the bloodstream. Medications inserted into the rectum are not changed by the digestive juices and do not irritate the lining of the GI tract except possibly at the site of insertion. Many rectal medications relieve discomfort locally

PROCEDURE 12-1 Administering Solid Medications Orally

Objective: To safely administer solid medications orally.

Guidelines

Equipment Needed

- Medication order
- Container of ordered medication
- Cup for measuring or holding medication
- Liquid for swallowing medication
- Tablet splitter if applicable

Methodology 3+7

1 If giving tablets or capsules, open container and tap correct number into bottle cap.
2. If the tablet is scored and needs dividing, break on the score line using a tablet splitter as appropriate to provide equal parts for the dose needed.
3. Do not touch medicine or inside of cap or bottle because these areas are considered clean, whereas the countertop is considered contaminated. To prevent further contamination, inside of the medication bottle cap should not be placed on the countertop; the cap should be turned with the inside up to place on counter if necessary.
4. After dispensing drug into bottle cap, transfer drug to a medicine cup.
5. After identifying and assessing patient, give medicine to patient with sufficient liquid for swallowing.
6. Watch patient take medicine.
7. Document the medication administered, your assessment, and observation of patient after administration. Answer patient questions and supply patient education as appropriate.

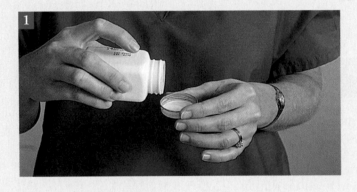

TYPICAL DOCUMENTATION

3/15/xx 9:10 AM acetaminophen 650 mg PO given with no apparent adverse reactions. _____G. OLSEN, CMA

(e.g., anesthetic ointments and creams used to treat rectal discomforts) or may be used to stimulate evacuation of the bowel or as a stool softener. Other suppositories have systemic action and are used for rapid absorption in patients with nausea and vomiting or fever. The rectal route is not as reliable as the oral or parenteral routes, but it is safe because, except for local irritation, side effects from administration are rare, although medication side effects remain the same as if administered by another route.

Rectal ointments and creams are usually administered by means of an applicator attached to the medication tube. Most medication orders read to apply ointment or cream to the area, with no specific dosage given.

Rectal suppositories are manufactured in a glycerin or cocoa butter base that melts on contact with the body. Most suppositories are bullet shaped (Figure 12-1) with rounded ends to prevent trauma to the rectal mucosa on insertion. Most suppositories administered in the ambulatory care facility are for the treatment of nausea and

PROCEDURE 12-2 Administering Liquid Medications Orally Using a Medicine Cup

Objective: To safely administer oral liquid medications using a medicine cup.

Guidelines

Equipment Needed
- Medication order
- Container of ordered medication
- Calibrated medicine cup for holding medication

Methodology 3+7

1. When giving a liquid medication, obtain a calibrated medicine cup and ordered medication. If necessary, shake or roll medication as appropriate for even drug distribution.
2. Locate ordered dosage on medicine cup and place a thumbnail at that line.
3. Hold cup at eye level and pour correct amount of liquid into container, reading to the **meniscus.** To keep medicine from dripping on label, always pour away from label, or "palm" label.
4. After pouring medicine, place cup on a level surface and check level of medication to meniscus for accuracy. If you have poured excess medicine, discard extra amount. Do not return poured medicine to stock container.
5. Identify patient and give medicine, watching patient to be sure all medication has been swallowed. Additional liquids are usually not given after administration of a liquid medication.
6. Discard medicine cup and observe patient for indications of adverse effects.
7. Document medication administration and any observations of patient. Answer patient questions and supply any patient education needed.

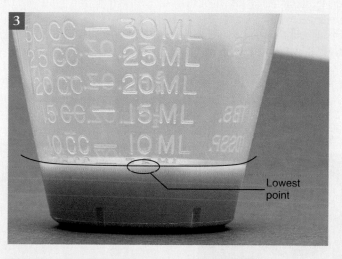

Lowest point

TYPICAL DOCUMENTATION

3/15/xx 10:00 AM ibuprofen liquid, 100 mg (1 tsp) PO given with no apparent adverse reactions. ___G. OLSEN, CMA

vomiting and to reduce fever in young children (Procedure 12-4).

Enemas are liquids instilled into the rectum; they may be used to soften hard feces, relieve fecal impactions, or evacuate the bowel, or as a means of administering medication (Procedure 12-5). Single-use enemas such as Fleet enemas may be prescribed for use before diagnostic tests (Figure 12-2). Although enemas are rarely performed in an ambulatory care setting, it may be necessary to teach the patient the technique for home use. The patient should be told to remove the cover on the container tip, lubricate the tip with water or other lubricant, and insert the enema tip into the rectum, then administer the liquid. The patient should then hold the medication in the rectum for as long as possible to obtain best possible results. The enema fluid breaks up the fecal mass, stretches the rectal wall, and induces the defecation reflex.

BOX 12-1 SAFETY IN ADMINISTRATION OF ORAL MEDICATIONS

- Tell the patient to place oral medications in solid form (tablets, caplets) on the back of tongue for ease of swallowing. Then tilt the head forward to stimulate the tongue and swallowing reflex, then tilt the head back for actual swallowing.
- The mouth should be moist to prevent solid medication from adhering to the inside of a dry mouth. A dry mouth tends to make swallowing more difficult, increasing the chance of a medication's dissolving in the mouth.
- Oral medications should not be stored in strong light, high humidity, or open air. Discard medications that have changed color, are out of date, or have an unexpected odor, such as the vinegar odor that occurs with out-of-date aspirin.
- If a medication has the potential to stain teeth (iron preparations, iodides), the liquid medication should be ingested through a straw. If the person has dentures, the dentures should be removed before ingestion of staining medications. Patients should always rinse the mouth with water after taking these medications.
- If a medication in solid form cannot be swallowed whole, some tablets may be crushed or split for ease of administration. Medications with enteric coating, sustained release, or other special release capabilities should never be crushed, chewed, or split unless they are scored. Consult a drug reference and ask the physician's permission to determine if the medicine may be crushed, split, or chewed.
- Effervescent tablets or powders should be given immediately after the solid form has dissolved in water and while desired effervescence is maintained.
- Some medications come in solid sprinkles that are dispersed on food for administration, such as **valproic acid** for seizures and **theophylline** for asthma. All food on which sprinkles are applied must be eaten for the desired dose to be administered.
- Sprinkles should not be applied to hot food because this activates the medication; the drug should be applied only to food at room temperature or colder to allow for absorption in the GI tract.
- Unless contraindicated, medications that are difficult to swallow may be placed in thick liquids such as applesauce or pudding to make swallowing easier. Products to thicken liquids and make swallowing easier may be found over the counter.
- A scored tablet is usually a sign that the tablet may be split or divided.

Oral Medication Safety with Children and the Elderly

- Young children and older adults may have difficulty swallowing. If this is the case, check to see if the solid preparation is available in a liquid form.
- To give oral medications to children, approach them as if you expect cooperation, and praise the child for cooperating and taking the medication.
- Never tell a child that medicine is "candy" because the child may take more medication than prescribed thinking it is candy.
- Never trick a child about taking medicines.
- Never try to force a child to swallow medicine or hold the child's nose or mouth shut, because this may cause choking.
- Never give medicine to a crying child, because of the chance of aspiration.

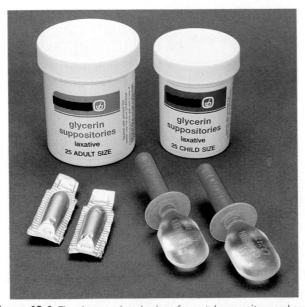

Figure 12-1 The shape and packaging of a rectal suppository and small enemas for infants. (From Perry AG, Potter PA: *Clinical nursing skills and techniques,* ed 7, St Louis, 2010, Mosby.)

Important Facts about Rectal Medications

- Be sure the wrapper covering the suppository if present, is removed before insertion. Lubricate the end of the suppository with either water-soluble lubricant or water.
- Keep a suppository cool before insertion because a soft suppository is difficult to insert. To keep medication from melting, do not hold the suppository in your hand. If the suppository is soft, place it in the freezer for a few minutes to harden, but do not let the medication freeze.
- Wear a glove on the hand used for insertion. Gently insert the rounded end of the suppository past the anal sphincter for retention.
- Remain lying down for approximately 5 to 10 minutes to allow the suppository to melt. Tell patients to resist the urge to have a bowel movement immediately so the medication can melt and be absorbed.
- Medications inserted into the rectum are not changed by digestive juices and do not irritate the GI tract, except possibly at the insertion site.

PROCEDURE 12-3 Administering Oral Liquid Medication Using a Dose Syringe or Dose Spoon

Objective: To safely administer oral liquid medications using a dose syringe or dose spoon.

Guidelines

Equipment Needed
- Medication order
- Container of ordered medication
- Dose syringe or dose spoon

Methodology 3+7

1. Placing syringe into liquid medicine, draw desired amount of medication into syringe or pour correct amount of medication to meniscus into dose spoon, holding spoon upright.
2. After identifying patient, slowly squirt medicine into the side of patient's mouth to prevent choking. If using dose spoon, allow person to slowly swallow medicine.
3. Care should be taken so the person taking medicine does not aspirate drug.
4. Immediately wash the utensil to keep medicine from drying in the syringe or dose spoon.
5. Document medication administration and any observations of patient. Answer patient questions and supply any patient education needed.

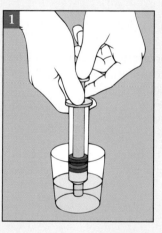

TYPICAL DOCUMENTATION
3/15/xx 9:15 AM amoxicillin 500 mg (10 mL) given PO with no apparent adverse reactions._____G. OLSEN, CMA

SUMMARY

Oral administration of medicines is the easiest, safest, and most frequently used route. The drug is placed in the mouth and swallowed for absorption in the GI tract, usually in the small intestines. Some solid forms of oral medications may be crushed or divided for administration with permission of the physician; others have specific coatings or forms that should not be altered. Medications may irritate the GI tract or may be altered by juices found in the stomach and intestines. In these cases the drug may not be given via oral administration. Danger of aspiration should be evaluated before oral medications are given. Patients who cannot swallow should not be given drugs orally.

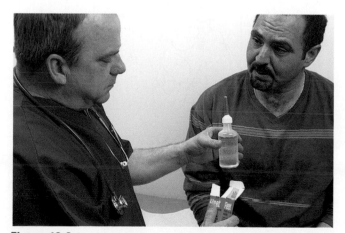

Figure 12-2 Prepackaged enemas. (From Perry AG, Potter PA: *Clinical nursing skills and techniques,* ed 7, St Louis, 2010, Mosby.)

PROCEDURE 12-4   Administering Rectal Medications by Suppository

Objective: To safely administer a rectal suppository.

Guidelines

Equipment Needed
- Medication order
- Appropriate rectal suppository for order
- Gloves
- Drape to cover body for privacy
- Water-soluble lubricant
- Tissues

Methodology 3+7

1. Identify person and place in Sims position, being sure to drape for privacy. (Children may be placed in dorsal recumbent position. Infants and small children may be placed supine so both legs can be elevated to observe rectum.)
2. Remove wrapper from suppository if necessary. Do not handle suppository more than necessary because body temperature may lead to softening of suppository, and insertion into rectum may be hindered.
3. Using water-soluble lubricant or water, lubricate rounded end of suppository and the gloved finger to be used for insertion.
4. Elevate the upper buttocks to show anal opening. Ask patient to take deep breaths through the mouth to relax rectal sphincter.
5. With a gloved hand, gently push suppository past anal sphincter into rectum (about 4 inches). Do not insert suppository into fecal matter because medication will not be absorbed.
6. Wipe excess lubricant from anal area with tissues.
7. Ask the patient to remain quiet for about 5 to 10 minutes to allow medication to be absorbed without a bowel movement occurring.
8. Remove gloves and wash hands.
9. Observe the patient for reactions, both expected and possibly adverse.
10. Document medication administration. If medication is for bowel evacuation, document results obtained.

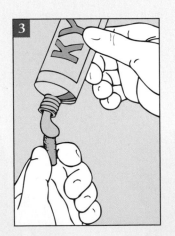

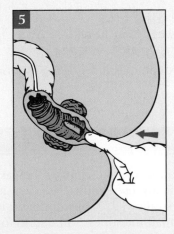

TYPICAL DOCUMENTATION

3/15/xx 3:15 PM Phenergan 25-mg suppository inserted into rectum with no apparent side effects. Suppository retained and symptoms of nausea decreased in 30 min. _____G. OLSEN, CMA

PROCEDURE 12-5 Using an Enema to Administer Rectal Medications

Objective: To safely administer a rectal enema.

Guidelines

Equipment Needed
- Medication order
- Appropriate enema for medication order
- Gloves
- Water-soluble lubricant
- Tissues
- Drape for privacy

Methodology 3+7

1. Identify patient and place in Sims position, or other appropriate position; drape for privacy.
2. Remove plastic cap and lubricate tip of the enema, if necessary. (Some enemas come prelubricated.) Clear tip of enema with fluid to prevent inserting air into rectum.
3. Locate rectum and ask patient to breathe deeply and slowly to relax rectal sphincter.
4. Gently insert fluid-filled tip into rectum. If using a prepackaged enema, roll bottle from bottom to tip until all liquid has been delivered into rectum. If using a nondisposable enema, hold enema bag 6 to 8 inches above rectum and slowly administer liquid.
5. Instruct patient to retain enema for at least 5 to 10 minutes before expelling fluid and any waste materials.
6. Remove gloves; wash hands.
7. Assist patient to bathroom at proper time.
8. Observe return from enema, if any.
9. Observe patient for any adverse effects.
10. Document procedure including return from enema, as well as any adverse effects.

TYPICAL DOCUMENTATION

3/16/xx 1:15 PM Fleet enema administered with no adverse effects. Return of enema contained large amounts of hard, constipated feces. _____ G. OLSEN, CMA

Rectal medications may be administered by either suppository or enema, with neither route being irritating to the GI tract except at the site of administration. The base for suppositories is usually either glycerin or cocoa butter for ease of melting in the rectum. Therefore suppositories should not be handled any more than necessary, to prevent changes in shape or melting before insertion. Enemas may be used for cleansing purposes or to soften hardened feces. Medications are infrequently administered rectally in the ambulatory care setting, so the allied health professional's responsibility may be focused on teaching the patient how to administer an enema at home. For a person who cannot swallow medications, rectal administration, especially in a patient with vomiting, may be the route of choice.

CRITICAL THINKING EXERCISES

Scenario

Sally is providing patient education to an older patient, Mrs. Campo, who is having difficulty swallowing the large tablets needed for her medical condition. She tells you that two of the tablets have "deep lines" through the tablet and one has a very hard coat. Mrs. Campo wants to know if there is any way she can make swallowing the medicine easier.

1. What information can Sally give her about scored tablets?
2. Can these tablets be crushed or divided for easier administration?
3. What about the tablet that seems to have an enteric coating?
4. Mrs. Campo states the tablets seem to stick to her mouth because her mouth is so dry. What instructions should Sally give Mrs. Campo that will make swallowing easier?

REVIEW QUESTIONS

1. Why is oral administration of a medication the most desirable route? _____

_____

_____

2. Why can some medications not be given orally? _____

_____

_____

3. What medications can be divided for doses? What medications should not be crushed for administration?

_____

_____

_____

4. What does it mean to "pour a medication to the meniscus"? _____

_____

_____

5. Why are medications given by rectal suppository? _____

_____

_____

6. "All medications given by rectum are for local effect." Why is this statement false? _____

_____

_____

Percutaneous Routes

OBJECTIVES

After studying this chapter, you should be capable of doing the following:

- Describing percutaneous routes of medication administration.
- Administering topical forms of medications.
- Administering nitroglycerin ointment.
- Describing patch testing for allergens.
- Explaining how to apply transdermal drugs.
- Discussing use of sublingual and buccal forms of medicine.
- Administering ophthalmic liquids and ointments.

- Administering otic medications.
- Describing how to properly use nasal medications.
- Administering inhalation medicines using a metered dose inhaler.
- Describing use of vaginal suppositories and douches.
- Providing patient education for safety and compliance with the percutaneous routes.

Allie, age 2, has an earache and no other symptoms. Dr. Merry looks in Allie's ear and sees that ear tubes are in place but the ear canal is red. He orders otic drops for use four times a day.

At what temperature should the drops be instilled to stop further pain?
How should you tell Allie's mother to hold Allie's ear to get the maximum effect from the drops?
With tubes in Allie's ears, can Allie's mother use any ear drops, or do drops need to be sterile? Explain your answer?
Why should Allie's mother massage Allie's ear after inserting drops?

KEY TERMS

Aerochamber	Excoriation	Percutaneous	Sublingual
Buccal	Metered dose inhaler	Rebound congestion	Topical
Dry powder inhaler	(MDI)	Spacer	Transdermal
(DPI)	Nebulizer		

Medications for **percutaneous** use are absorbed through skin or mucous membranes. Rectal medications are included and discussed in Chapter 12 because of the inclusion in the gastrointestinal (GI) tract, but actually rectal medications are absorbed through the mucous membranes of the rectum.

Both over-the-counter (OTC) and prescription drugs may be given percutaneously, with these medications having local or systemic effects or sometimes both. This route of administration includes **sublingual** and **buccal** medications, which are absorbed through mucous membranes of the mouth; **topical** or surface preparations such as ointments, liniments, and lotions; and **transdermal** or through-the-skin medications, including patches. Percutaneous routes of administration are used when direct contact of the medication with skin is desired because of ease of administration and low risk of systemic adverse reactions. Because of absorption rate differences of some topical agents, this route has unreliable systemic action and so is seldom used for treating systemic diseases. Drugs absorbed percutaneously, except those absorbed through mucous membranes of the mouth, rectum, and lungs, are slow acting and are used when slow and extended medication administration is desired.

TOPICAL MEDICATIONS

Medications may be applied topically for local effect, such as to relieve itching (calamine lotion) or provide warmth (Bengay), or for systemic action, such as relief of unstable angina using nitroglycerin ointment or patches. Topical medications can cause systemic adverse reactions and for safety should be applied as prescribed. Types of skin preparations range from such common forms as creams, ointments, and powders to wet dressings and soaks for wound care and patches for conditions such as hormone replacement therapy. (For discussion of forms of medication, see Chapter 3.)

The area of skin for medication application should be clean, dry, and free of infection, rashes, encrustations, open areas, and dead tissue unless a rash or wound is being treated. Before topical medications are applied, skin should be inspected for integrity and cleansed with water. The skin should be free of all soap residues before application because soap can alter medication absorption.

When applying topical medications, adequate skin hydration is necessary. The fastest site for absorption of transdermal medications is behind the ear. The back, chest, and abdomen are the next most rapid sites of absorption. Slowest sites of absorption are the thigh and forearm.

Patient Education for Compliance

If medication is indicated to reduce itching, it should be applied with gentle strokes. If the drug is rubbed vigorously, friction will heat the skin, increasing itching.

Applying Topical Medications

Powders

To use powders such as those for fungal conditions, follow these steps:

- Skin surface should be thoroughly dry to minimize crusting and caking of the powder.
- Skin surface should be fully exposed, with folds of skin spread open for powder application.
- Powder should be lightly dusted onto the surface, leaving a fine, thin layer. A thin layer of powder is more absorbent than a thick layer, reducing friction by increasing evaporation of moisture.

Soaks, Compresses, and Wet Dressings

For soaks, compresses, and wet dressings such as Betadine, the following points apply:

- Active ingredient is dissolved in water-based solution to leave a film on the skin.
- These substances contain a mild astringent, providing a soothing, cooling, and antipyretic effect when used on blistered or oozing skin areas.
- Bandages may be soaked in solution and then applied to skin. If appropriate, an extremity may be soaked in the solution. With a wet dressing, a plastic wrap may be placed over the dressing to keep it damp.

Creams, Ointments, Gels, and Lotions

Creams and ointments are semisolid preparations used for topical applications; examples include Neosporin and Triple Antibiotic Cream or Ointment.

- Active ingredients for creams are in a water base.
- Creams are used to deliver drugs directly to or into skin.
- Creams are absorbed into skin and vanish, usually having a cooling effect.
- Creams and ointments may be used to deliver antipyretics, antimicrobials, and softening compounds.
- Ointments are soft, fatty substances with the active ingredient carried in an oil, lanolin, or petroleum base.
- Ointments deliver drugs, such as antimicrobials and steriods, to the surface of the skin to remain in contact longer than a cream.

The application of an antimicrobial ointment or cream is described in Procedure 13-1.

Nitroglycerin ointment, used in treatment of angina pectoris, is applied directly to the skin on the chest, back, upper arms, or thighs. The site should be dry and relatively free of hair and scar tissue. To prevent overdose, any ointment residue should be removed before a new dose is applied. When nitroglycerin ointment is administered, care should be taken to avoid contact with the drug because a headache may occur from accidental contact. The procedure for applying nitroglycerin ointment is described in Procedure 13-2.

Gels, such as K-Y Jelly, are thick water-based substances used for lubrication or for ease of applying active drug to the skin. Some gels have an oil ingredient added for better coverage that lasts for longer periods of time.

PROCEDURE 13-1   Administering Topical Medications

Objective: To apply topical medications appropriately.

Guidelines

Equipment Needed
- Medication order
- Medication ordered
- Gloves
- Supplies for cleansing skin
- Dressing and bandages as applicable

Methodology 3+7

1. After identifying the patient, cleanse skin and pat dry, using good aseptic technique.
2. Change gloves if wet or contaminated after cleansing the skin.
3. If a topical medication is to be applied, place medication in a cleanly gloved hand. The applicator tip should not touch the glove or skin site. If medication is sterile, sterile technique using a sterile tongue blade to apply the medication to sterile gauze should be used.
4. Hold medication in your hand to allow the preparation to soften to body temperature to allow the medication to spread easily and evenly.
5. Apply medication using long, even strokes to avoid irritating hair follicles.
6. A dressing and bandage may be applied to keep the medication in contact with the skin, if applicable.
7. In some instances medication may be applied to the dressing, then the dressing is applied to the skin.
8. Document the procedure.

TYPICAL DOCUMENTATION

6/30/XX 11:25 AM Abrasion on left knee cleansed with soap and water and dried. Polymyxin B sulfate/neomycin sulfate/bacitracin ointment applied to lesion. Dry dressing applied. No apparent sign of adverse reaction.

G. OLSEN, CMA

Time/Date/when it expires.

Pastes are thick oil- or water-based compounds, such as **zinc oxide**, often used as sunblocks and to deliver medications.

Lotions are water-based compounds used to control itching (e.g., **calamine lotion**) or to relieve muscle and joint pain (e.g., BenGay), leaving the area feeling cool after evaporation of the water base. Lotions are applied lightly to the skin surface using a gauze pad and stroking in the direction of hair growth. Some lotions contain powder, leaving a thin film at the site of application. If a lotion is in the form of a suspension, the container should be shaken vigorously to mix solute in the solvent.

Patches, Disks, and Transdermal Dots
Some topical medications are prepackaged in transdermal disks, patches, or dots to provide extended effects—up to several days. An example is **scopolamine** patches for motion sickness.
- These forms are a painless, convenient method of administering medications for many medical conditions.
- Medication released from the patch passes through the skin and into circulatory system for continuous treatment without repeated dosing. Patches must be reapplied as indicated to maintain desired dosage level.
- When a patch, dot, or disk is applied, the date and time of application should be written on the application material or noted on a calendar when self-administered.
- Remove old patch before applying the new patch.
- Transdermal forms of medication should be applied by the patient and should be handled carefully to avoid contact with the medication, which may be accidently absorbed (Figure 13-1). Washing hands immediately after medication application to avoid undesirable absorption and undesired side effects is important.
- Soap should not be used at the application site because soap enhances and prolongs absorption.

See Box 13-1 for information concerning medications that typically come as transdermal patches.

PROCEDURE 13-2   Application of Nitroglycerin Ointment

Objective: To properly apply ordered quantity of nitroglycerin ointment.

Guidelines

Equipment Needed

- Medication order
- Nitroglycerin ointment with measured application papers
- Gloves
- Supplies to cleanse skin (if applicable)
- Tape as appropriate

Methodology 3+7

1. After identifying patient, cleanse skin of residual nitroglycerin ointment. Site should be dry, relatively free of hair, and without scar tissue and rotated on a daily basis.
2. The prescribed dose of **nitroglycerin** in inches should be squeezed and measured directly to the manufacturer's applicator paper.
3. Check the patient's pulse and ensure rate is greater than 60 beats/min. If below 60 beats/min, consult with physician before applying ointment.
4. Apply ointment to skin and hold in place for 10 seconds. A strip of adhesive tape may be applied to prevent slippage of paper.
5. A plastic or wax occlusive dressing that comes with the ointment may be added if the desired effect is not being achieved.
6. Document the procedure.

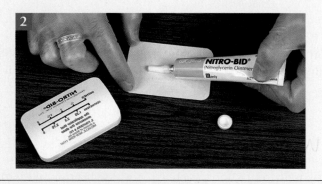

TYPICAL DOCUMENTATION

7/13/XX 9:15 AM Pulse 72. Nitroglycerin ointment 2 inches applied to left upper chest after skin cleaned of residue. Tape applied to application paper. No apparent immediate adverse reactions. _____ G. OLSEN, CMA

Sprays and Aerosols

Some medications, such as *ethyl chloride*, come in aerosol or spray applications. Before application the skin must be clean and dry. The container must be vigorously shaken to ensure medication and propellants are evenly distributed before application. The container label will specify the distance to hold the medication from skin; the usual distance is 6 to 12 inches. Spray should be fine and even, applying a thin medication coating to skin. Holding the container too close to the skin may result in a thin, watery distribution.

Special Considerations for Topical Medications in Geriatric Patients

The skin of older people is fragile, and the blood supply is close to the surface with thin skin, increasing the risk of bruising. Medication should be applied directly to the skin with minimal friction, as the elderly also have diminished sensations of pain, temperature, and itching. Skin should be observed on a regular basis to ensure that the medication is not causing irritation and breakdown of the skin itself. With dry flaky skin excoriation may occur and any skin changes should be observed and documented when applying topical medications.

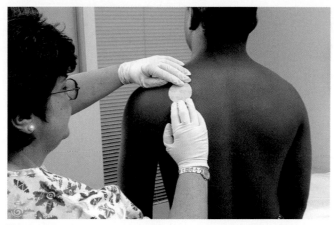

Figure 13-1 Application of a transdermal medication patch. (From Young AP, Proctor DB: *Kinn's the medical assistant,* ed 11, St Louis, 2011, WB Saunders.)

BOX 13-1 COMMON MEDICATIONS IN TRANSDERMAL PATCHES, DOTS, OR DISKS

- Nitroglycerin for angina pectoris is applied as a patch to upper chest, to be worn for 12 hours in the morning and then removed at bedtime, with site rotation on a daily basis.
- Female hormones in the form of *estradiol* dots and patches to relieve menopausal symptoms such as hot flashes, night sweats, and vaginal dryness should be applied to thighs and buttocks for slow absorption. Sites should be rotated on a prescribed schedule at the prescribed site.
- *Scopolamine*, used to prevent the nausea and vomiting of motion sickness, is applied as a dot behind the ear. For maximum effectiveness, this medication should be applied 4 hours before travel.
- *Fentanyl citrate* (Duragesic) patches are used as continuous analgesia for chronic pain. These patches remain in place for 3 days, with the site of application changed with each application to prevent skin irritation and possible lack of absorption in tissues.
- *Nicotine* patches are used to assist with smoking cessation. Prescribed as a 3-month supply, the patch is changed every 24 hours. The patient should be warned against smoking while wearing the patch because the increased nicotine may cause coronary symptoms.
- Patches are used to assist with diagnosing allergies. Patches containing small amounts of 20 to 30 suspected allergens are individually placed on forearm or back, covered with cellophane, and read 24 to 48 hours later. As with all patches, the allergen and date and time of application should be on the patch.
- Contraceptives are applied to hips every 7 days for 3 weeks. During the fourth week, no patch is applied. These patches are usually applied to buttocks, upper outer arm, or upper torso so clothing does not effect placement.
- *Methylphenidate* (Ritalin) is applied as a patch in the morning and removed midafternoon (about 9 hours).
- Patches containing *testosterone*, a male hormone, are available for daily application using two different application sites. This medication is also available in creams and gels for topical application.

Important Facts about Transdermal Medications

- Percutaneous routes of medication administration are those through skin and mucous membranes.
- The percutaneous route is used because of ease of administration; low risk of systemic adverse reactions; and to achieve a slow, steady, extended-duration drug effect.
- Because the amount of medication is not always delivered with the same absorption rate, this route of administration cannot be used when reliable amounts of medication must be absorbed.
- When a topical medication is applied in powder form, the skin should be dry to prevent caking and crusting of powder, and only a thin layer of drug should be applied.
- Creams are absorbed into the skin because of their water base, whereas ointments have an oily base and tend to remain on the surface of the skin, where absorption is prolonged.
- Nitroglycerin ointment is applied directly to the chest to maintain a slow, continuous supply of medication for angina pectoris. When nitroglycerin ointment is used, any residual ointment should be removed before applying a new dose. When nitroglycerin is administered, the medication should not touch the person applying the drug because headaches and other side effects may occur if nitroglycerin is absorbed through the fingers.
- Lotions, used to control itching and relieve joint pain, should be applied lightly to prevent increased irritation.
- Prepackaged disks and patches are used for multiple medical conditions including allergy testing. Application sites are determined by the indication for the medication. Body temperature may vary the rate of absorption.
- Topical medications should be applied gently to older persons. Their skin is fragile and the blood supply is near the surface, causing easy bruising.

BUCCAL AND SUBLINGUAL MEDICATIONS

Sublingual medication administration involves placing the medication form, such as tiny porous tablets, a liquid squeezed from a capsule, or an aerosol spray, under the tongue for rapid absorption into the bloodstream through mucous membranes (Figure 13-2, *A*). Nitroglycerin is a drug typically given in this manner.

Buccal administration of medications involves placing the drug between the cheek and gums for absorption by local mucous membranes. Buccal medications may also be absorbed systemically when absorbed in saliva and swallowed (Figure 13-2, *B*).

With these medications the patient's mouth should be damp before administration. The patient should avoid eating, drinking, or chewing while the medication

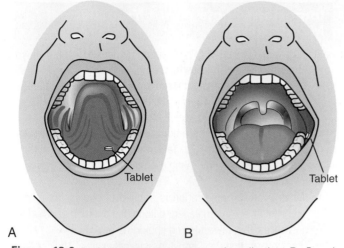

Figure 13-2 A, Sublingual administration of medication. **B,** Buccal administration of medication. (From Leahy JM, Kizilay PE: *Foundations of nursing practice: a nursing process approach,* Philadelphia, 1998, WB Saunders.)

is in place. Sublingual and buccal medications should not be swallowed but should be retained in the desired location until they have dissolved. If medications are swallowed, the time for absorption will be prolonged or the medication may be changed by gastric juices and be ineffective.

OPHTHALMIC MEDICATIONS

Common ophthalmic preparations come in the form of ointments, liquids, and intraocular disks. The disk resembles a contact lens and is placed in the conjunctival sac for a longer-lasting medication effect. After insertion by pulling the lower lid away from the eye, allowing the disk to float on the sclera, the disk remains in place for the desired period of time. The patient should be instructed to not rub the eyes, to prevent eye irritation or too-rapid absorption.

Drugs applied to the eye must be sterile, and only medications marked "ophthalmic" should be used in eyes. These drugs should not be applied directly to the cornea because the cornea has a rich supply of nerve fibers. The conjunctival sac is much less sensitive and therefore is a more appropriate site for drug administration. Eye drops should be warmed before they are instilled to prevent excessive irritation. Procedure 13-3 outlines how to instill ophthalmic medications.

OTIC MEDICATIONS

Internal ear structures are sensitive to temperature extremes, so all ear medications should be administered at room temperature. If cold drops are placed in the ear,

vertigo and nausea may occur. Drops can be warmed by holding the medication bottle between the hands for approximately 2 minutes. Although the outer ear is not sterile, sterile drops and solutions should be used if the eardrum is ruptured or if tympanic tubes are present. Nonsterile solutions that reach the middle ear may cause serious infections. *Sterile ophthalmologic drops may be used as otic medications, but otic medications cannot be used for ophthalmic use.* Never fill the ear canal with a medicine dropper because this can cause pressure in the canal and can cause further injury to the eardrum. Never force any solutions into the ear. The procedure for instilling otic medications is outlined in Procedure 13-4.

NASAL MEDICATIONS

Nasal medications, administered by atomizer, dropper, or aerosol spray for local effect, may be absorbed for systemic effects via the bloodstream but are usually considered topical or local medications. Nasal drugs are commonly used to stop nosebleeds or as decongestants for blocked nasal passages resulting from sinusitis or upper respiratory symptoms. Nasal drugs are relatively safe when administered in small doses as needed; however, these drugs may change vital signs either intentionally or accidentally. Repeated use of decongestant sprays, such as overuse of **oxymetazoline** (Afrin), can worsen nasal congestion, called **rebound congestion**.

To instill nasal drops:
- Tilt the patient's head back or place the patient in the supine position with the head tilted backward.
- After medication instillation, tilt the head forward to distribute the medication properly. Taking short, quick breaths will help spread the medication evenly.
- Any nose drops that spill into the throat should be expectorated to prevent systemic side effects.

Nasal sprays are used increasingly to administer various medications for rapid absorption into the vast capillary supply in nasal passages. Drugs for migraine headaches, smoking cessation agents, and cortisone and decongestants for sinus conditions are just a few medications administered by means of nasal spray.

Use of nasal sprays and atomizers involves the following:
- The patient should be sitting upright with the head tilted backward.
- Before application, nasal passages should be cleared as much as possible.
- To administer medication, occlude one nostril and have the patient inhale through the other.
- Be certain the spray tip is centered in the nostril and not against the nasal cavity wall.
- To deliver medication, squeeze the container while the applicator is inside the nostril.

PROCEDURE 13-3   Instillation of Ophthalmic Medications

Objective: To instill sterile ophthalmic eye medications.

Guidelines

Equipment Needed
- Medication order
- Gloves
- Ophthalmic medication as ordered
- Supplies to cleanse eye as needed

Methodology 3+7

Instilling Eye Drops

1. After identifying patient, cleanse any drainage from eye, moving from inner to outer canthus.
2. Warm eye drops by holding in hands before instillation to prevent eye irritation. Be sure medication has "ophthalmic" label.
3. Hold medication dropper approximately ½ to ¾ inch above conjunctival sac, taking extreme care not to contaminate dropper by allowing tip to touch eye.
4. Drop prescribed amount of medication into conjunctival sac to prevent irritation to cornea. If person blinks or closes the eye before administration, repeat the procedure.
5. When administering a medication that may have a systemic effect, apply gentle pressure to nasolacrimal duct for 30 to 60 seconds after administration to prevent overflow of medication into nasal and pharyngeal passages.
6. Instruct patient to close eye to help distribute medication from conjunctival sac.
7. Document the procedure.

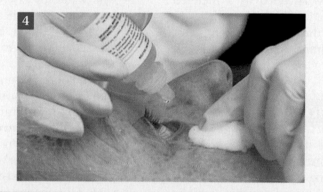

TYPICAL DOCUMENTATION
7/22/XX 3:15 PM Pilocarpine hydrochloride ophthalmic drops, gtt i both eyes, with no apparent adverse reactions.
_____ G. OLSEN, CMA

Instilling Eye Ointment

1. After identifying patient, cleanse any drainage from eye, moving from inner to outer canthus.
2. Be sure medication has an "ophthalmic" label.
3. Ask patient to look at ceiling. Hold ointment applicator ½ inch above lower lid and apply a thin stream of ointment along inner edge of lower lid from inner to outer canthus.
4. Ask the patient to close the eye slowly, then open and close the eye several times to further melt the ointment and distribute the medication across the eye.
5. If there is excess medication on the eyelid, remove with a tissue from the inner to outer canthus.
6. If an eye patch is necessary, apply clean one over eye and tape it securely without applying pressure to eye. Most ointments may blur vision for up to 30 minutes.
7. Document procedure.

Continued

PROCEDURE 13-3 Instillation of Ophthalmic Medications—cont'd

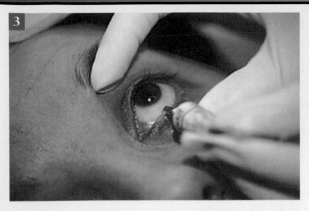

TYPICAL DOCUMENTATION

7/15/XX 4:26 PM Neosporin Opth. Oint ½″ applied to Rt eye after cleansing eye of residual matter. No apparent adverse reactions. _____G. OLSEN, CMA

• The head should remain tilted back for about 5 minutes, and the patient should not blow the nose.
• If aerosol medication is delivered as a metered dose, shake the container well and insert the tip into the nostril. Instruct the patient to hold his or her breath during the administration of the medicine (Figure 13-3).

VAGINAL MEDICATIONS

Vaginal medications take the form of suppositories, tablets, creams, or solutions and are absorbed through mucous membranes for treating local infections.
• Solutions used for irrigating, or douches, may be antiinfectants. Douches may be either prescription or OTC preparations.
• Creams and foams, available for contraception and to treat fungal infections, are inserted with applicators.

• Suppositories may require an applicator or may be hand inserted after being lubricated or moistened with water for ease of insertion.
• Most vaginal medications are prescribed for use at bedtime and are best used when lying down. Women should remain flat for at least 10 minutes after insertion of a cream or suppository.
• The medication course as prescribed by the physician should be completed because the causative condition may return if the medication is stopped early, even if improvement seems apparent.
• Vaginal medications tend to result in drainage; use of panty liners or tampons, if acceptable to the physician, will assist in keeping medication in the vagina for absorption.
• Before insertion, vaginal suppositories should not be handled more than necessary to prevent premature melting of the medication. The covering on the suppository should be removed before insertion.

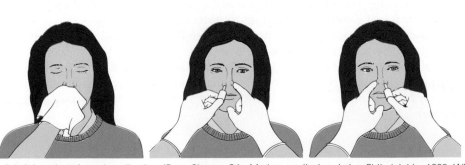

Figure 13-3 Administration of nasal medication. (From Chester GA: *Modern medical assisting*, Philadelphia, 1998, WB Saunders.)

PROCEDURE 13-4   Instilling Otic Medications

Objective: To instill ear medications.

Guidelines

Equipment Needed
- Medication order
- Otic medication
- Gloves
- Cotton to fill external auditory canal

Methodology 3+7

1. After identifying person, ask patient to lie still to prevent injury from ear dropper. Head should be turned to side with affected ear up.
2. Hold medication to warm solution.
3. For older child or adult ear, straighten ear canal by pulling external ear up and out or back. If patient is 3 years of age or younger, gently pull external ear down and back.
4. Slowly administer prescribed amount of medication, holding dropper about ½ inch above ear and aiming drops toward wall of canal rather than toward eardrum.
5. Gently massage outer ear to move medication inward.
6. Ask patient to remain in same position for 5 minutes to allow medication to be absorbed.
7. Document procedure.

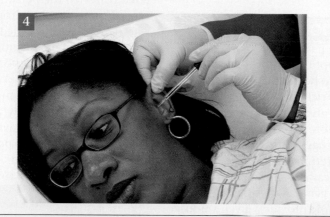

TYPICAL DOCUMENTATION

7/13/XX 2:45 PM Cortisporin Otic Solution, gtts iii Rt. ear, with no apparent adverse reaction. Patient instructed in proper method of instilling ear drops at home. _____ G. OLSEN, CMA

Did You Know?

The vagina produces its own secretions for an antiseptic effect; therefore frequent douching may change the acidity in the vaginal canal, making the woman more prone to vaginal infections from either resident body flora or invading bacteria. Advertising campaigns have caused women to believe douching is necessary; in reality, daily bathing should be sufficient for cleanliness. Excessive odor and vaginal discharge are symptoms of infection that may require medical attention.

Important Facts about Medications Absorbed through Mucous Membranes

- Buccal and sublingual medications are absorbed through mucous membranes of the mouth. Sublingual medications are absorbed rapidly because of the rich blood supply under the tongue.
- Ophthalmic medications, usually drops or ointments, are for topical administration, although some have systemic effects. Medication disks resembling contact lenses are also used to provide prolonged medication application to the eye.
- When administering ophthalmic medications, be sure the medication label reads "ophthalmic."

Continued

Important Facts about Medications Absorbed through Mucous Membranes—cont'd

- Otic medications should be at room temperature before administration. If drops are cold, nausea and dizziness may result.
- After ear medications are instilled, the patient should remain in a lying position with the affected ear facing up for at least 5 minutes.
- Before instilling nasal medications, be sure nasal passages are cleared of mucus. Although nasal preparations are considered topical medications, these medications may enter the systemic blood supply and change vital signs, especially if the medication is swallowed.
- Rebound congestion may occur if nasal preparations are used too often or inappropriately.
- Nasal preparations are now available for many types of medications, including smoking cessation agents, corticosteroids, and hormone therapy.
- Vaginal medications include suppositories, creams, tablets, and solutions; many can be purchased over the counter.

INHALED MEDICATIONS

Inhalation medications are supplied in the form of gases, sprays, powders, and liquids to be inhaled into the respiratory tract. Because of the rich blood supply of the respiratory tract through the alveolar-capillary network, medications are absorbed more rapidly than with any other mucous membrane. Drugs for inhalation may be used to liquefy bronchial secretions for expectoration or to dilate bronchi to ease breathing. Inhalation is also used for oxygen therapy and general anesthesia.

Dry powder inhalers (DPIs) provide a given amount of medication as a dry powder. Breath activated and easier to use than the metered dose inhaler, DPIs permit 20% of the medication to reach the lungs in most cases.

Metered dose inhalers (MDIs) are hand-held devices that disperse medications into airways and lungs. Each measured dose requires about 5 to 10 pounds of pressure to activate the aerosol. Older people may have insufficient hand strength to activate the application, so adapters or aerochambers are available to assist with coordination for accurate administration (Figure 13-4).

Use of an MDI also requires coordinating breathing with medication administration; if coordination is not present, the medication may be sprayed into the back of the throat only with a small amount of medication reaching the desired site. For the full amount of medicine to reach the lungs, the inhaler must be depressed just as the person breathes. Use of an MDI is outlined in Procedure 13-5.

The first inhalation of medication opens airways and reduces inflammation, whereas the second dose

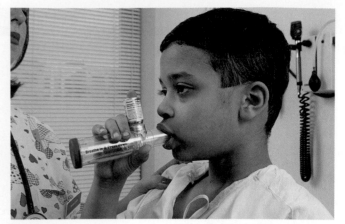

Figure 13-4 A metered dose inhaler. (From Young AP, Proctor DB: *Kinn's the medical assistant,* ed 11, St Louis, 2011, WB Saunders.)

penetrates the deeper airways. MDI medications should be administered at regular intervals throughout the day to provide constant drug levels. "Extra" doses of MDI aerosols should not be administered because of possible harmful side effects. If aerosol has not been administered correctly, the person may have a gagging sensation caused by medication droplets on the tongue or pharynx.

Nebulizers, also called *aerosols* or *atomizers*, provide a spray or mist of medication. With a nebulizer, the patient inserts a mouthpiece into the oral cavity and sprays medication while inhaling.

Rotadisk contains a medication powder. The patient should exhale as deeply as possible, insert the mouthpiece into the oral cavity, puncture the medication pouch, and inhale the powder. Each Rotadisk contains one dose of medication.

Did You Know?

Current trends in medications include introduction of antibiotics that are inhaled for treatment of lung infections. Inhaled antibiotics would provide local action in the lungs rather than systemic response found with oral or parenteral administration.

Important Facts about Inhaled Medications

- Drugs for inhalation come in the form of powders, gases, sprays, and liquids.
- Medications given by inhalation are rapidly absorbed because of the blood supply to lungs.
- Metered dose inhalers (MDIs) are hand-held inhalers that disperse inhalation medications to the lungs. Use of an MDI requires coordination and strength to push the canister and breathe at the same time. Thus elderly patients may have difficulty using an MDI. Dry powder inhalers (DPIs) administer breath-activated powdered medications into the lungs and are easier to use than MDIs.

PROCEDURE 13-5   Administration of Medication Using Metered Dose Inhaler

Objective: To effectively administer medications using MDI.

Guidelines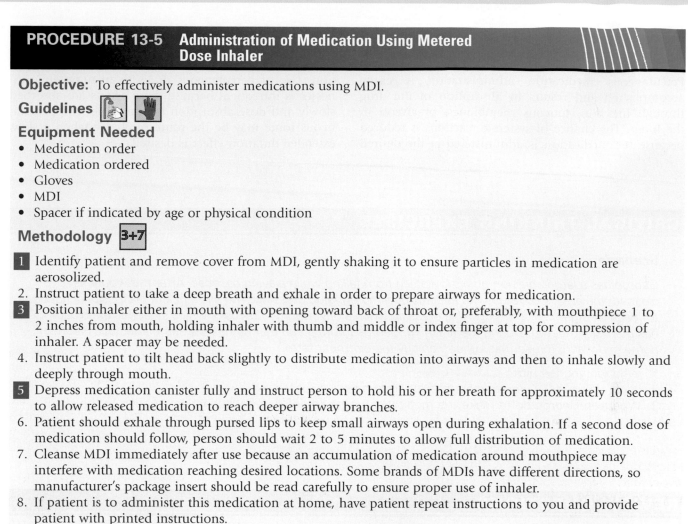

Equipment Needed

- Medication order
- Medication ordered
- Gloves
- MDI
- Spacer if indicated by age or physical condition

Methodology 3+7

1. Identify patient and remove cover from MDI, gently shaking it to ensure particles in medication are aerosolized.
2. Instruct patient to take a deep breath and exhale in order to prepare airways for medication.
3. Position inhaler either in mouth with opening toward back of throat or, preferably, with mouthpiece 1 to 2 inches from mouth, holding inhaler with thumb and middle or index finger at top for compression of inhaler. A spacer may be needed.
4. Instruct patient to tilt head back slightly to distribute medication into airways and then to inhale slowly and deeply through mouth.
5. Depress medication canister fully and instruct person to hold his or her breath for approximately 10 seconds to allow released medication to reach deeper airway branches.
6. Patient should exhale through pursed lips to keep small airways open during exhalation. If a second dose of medication should follow, person should wait 2 to 5 minutes to allow full distribution of medication.
7. Cleanse MDI immediately after use because an accumulation of medication around mouthpiece may interfere with medication reaching desired locations. Some brands of MDIs have different directions, so manufacturer's package insert should be read carefully to ensure proper use of inhaler.
8. If patient is to administer this medication at home, have patient repeat instructions to you and provide patient with printed instructions.
9. Document the procedure.

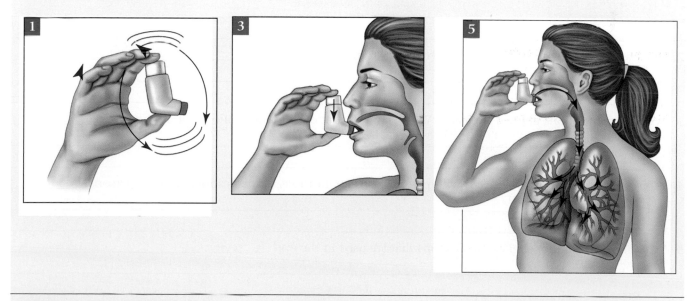

TYPICAL DOCUMENTATION

7/12/XX 9:15 AM Albuterol inhaler, two puffs as directed, with no apparent adverse reactions. Instructions given for use at home with return demonstration by patient. _____ G. OLSEN, CMA

SUMMARY

Percutaneous medication administration is easily accomplished and results in absorption of the drug through the skin, mucous membranes, or alveoli in the lungs. The chance of systemic reactions is reduced because the medication is administered at the desired site, rather than having to reach the site through systemic absorption. The site of administration should be intact and adequately hydrated to absorb the medication. Use of percutaneous drugs to treat systemic illnesses is infrequent because these agents are absorbed slowly and dose absorption is unreliable. The percutaneous route may be the route of choice when a slow, extended-duration effect is desired.

CRITICAL THINKING EXERCISES

Scenario

George has a large abrasion on his lower leg from falling while playing baseball. After the wound is cleaned, the area is covered with an antibiotic-impregnated dressing. The allied health professional needs to teach George how to change this dressing twice a day. George first asks why a systemic antibiotic has not been ordered. During the teaching, George informs you that he has the same antibiotic cream at home and wants to use that rather than buy the ointment form.

1. What do you tell him?
2. What do you tell George about residue from previous dressings?
3. What can George do to make the medication go on smoothly with little jerking motion to the skin?

REVIEW QUESTIONS

1. What is percutaneous medication administration? Why are these routes used? _____

_____

_____

2. What are the disadvantages of percutaneous medication administration? _____

_____

_____

3. Why are medications applied topically? What skin preparations and precautions should be taken? _____

_____

_____

4. What precautions should be taken with percutaneous applications of medications in older persons? _____

_____

_____

5. What must be on the label of medications that are used in the eye? _____

_____

_____

_____

6. What is the proper position of the ear when instilling drops in a young child? In an adult? _____

_____

_____

7. What are common indications for nasal medications? What are some of the newer indications for nasal sprays? _____

_____

_____

8. What are the forms of medications for vaginal administration? What documentation is necessary to show that the patient was taught how to use medication correctly? _____

_____

_____

CHAPTER 14

Parenteral Routes

OBJECTIVES

After studying this chapter, you should be capable of doing the following:

- Explaining parenteral routes of medication administration and differences among routes.
- Describing how to select the appropriate syringe and needle for administering parenteral medications.
- Preparing medications for parenteral administration from a vial and/or an ampule.
- Mixing parenteral medications for injection.

- Reconstituting powders to liquid form for parenteral administration.
- Administering medications intradermally (ID), subcutaneously (SC or SQ), and intramuscularly (IM).
- Providing patient education for safety and compliance with the parenteral route of medication administration.

Dr. Merry has ordered **cyanocobalamin** 1 mL subcutaneously once weekly, for Lynda, who has pernicious anemia. Dr. Merry has asked you to show Lynda how to give herself the injections.

What are the appropriate sites for these injections?
How often should the injection sites be rotated?
Which syringe should Lynda use?
What length needle should be used for these injections?
What gauge needle should be used with this aqueous solution?
What do you need to teach Lynda about aseptic technique?

KEY TERMS

Ampule	Diluent	Intradermal	Subcutaneous
Aqueous	Filter needle	Intramuscular	Vial
Aspirate	Gauge	Intravenous	Viscous
Bevel	Intraarticular	Lumen	Wheal
Compatible			

*P*arenteral (Greek: *para* plus *enteron,* intestine or outside the alimentary canal) administration of a substance such as a drug entails giving that substance by a route other than through the gastrointestinal (GI) tract; this route involves injections that are invasive procedures with greater risks than with the oral or percutaneous routes. Injectable medications should be given only if a designated health professional is available to intervene in case of adverse reactions. Allied health professionals may prepare and administer medications, depending on the medical practice act of the state of employment. Parenteral injections are commonly given

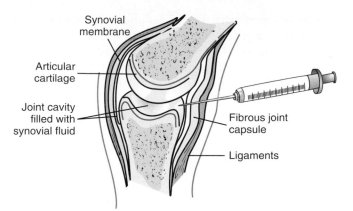

Figure 14-1 Intraarticular joint injections are performed by the physician with assistance from an allied health professional.

into the dermis of the skin, or **intradermally (ID)**; into subcutaneous tissue, or **subcutaneously (SC or SQ)**; into muscle, or **intramuscularly (IM)**; into joints, or **intraarticularly (IA)**; or into veins, or **intravenously (IV)**. Physicians may ask assistance of allied health professionals when giving intraarticular injections because giving injections into joints is beyond the scope of practice for allied health professionals (Figure 14-1).

ADVANTAGES OF PARENTERAL ADMINISTRATION

The following are reasons for using parenteral medications:

- Lower doses of medications are most often needed.
- Medicines are not initially inactivated by digestive juices and the liver.
- Availability of a drug is increased because the medication enters the circulation faster and with less inactivation from metabolism before absorption.
- The duration of action may be shorter than with enteral medications.
- Injectables may be used when a patient is unable to swallow because of physical incapacity or when patients have gastric disorders that effect swallowing or absorption of medicines.
- Agents may be added to injectable medicines to prolong desired effects.

DISADVANTAGES OF PARENTERAL ADMINISTRATION

Disadvantages include the following:

- Pain occurs on administration.
- Strict adherence to aseptic technique is necessary with parenteral administration.

- Infection is possible because the skin's protective barrier has been broken.
- Once delivered under the skin, drugs cannot be retrieved; therefore full knowledge of the drug and route of administration, and aseptic technique are necessary for patient safety.
- Improper injection of medication may result in damage to nerves, an overly rapid response to the drug, localized bleeding into the skin, sterile abscesses, and death of tissue.

SPECIAL PRECAUTIONS WITH PARENTERAL MEDICATIONS

The following special precautions are important:

- Irritating and staining medications are injected using the Z-track method for intramuscular injections.
- Parenteral medications must be in sterile liquid form, except some sterile implants that require surgical insertion.
- A parenteral drug is usually administered in a solution that is minimally irritating to tissue, such as physiologic saline or sterile water, and may contain a preservative or a small amount of antibiotic agent to prevent bacterial growth.
- *Always be sure the patient receiving injectable medications is not allergic to additives or the base for the medicine being administered, such as antibiotics found in some vaccines.*

Important Facts about Parenteral Medications

- Parenteral medications are delivered through the skin, requiring strict sterile technique and care in selecting the correct gauge of needle, syringe, and site for administration.
- Routes of medication administration most frequently seen in ambulatory care settings are ID, SC, and IM. A Z-track IM injection may be used for irritating medications or for drugs that stain skin.
- Parenteral medications are used when enteral forms of drugs cannot be used, when a more rapid rate of action is desired, or when the drug would be inactivated by digestive juices.
- Drawbacks to the parenteral administration of drugs include pain on administration, inability to retrieve medications given in error, and the possibility of infection if aseptic technique is not followed.
- Medications must be in a sterile liquid form. Additives are found in some parenteral medications, and the patient's sensitivity to additives should be checked.

EQUIPMENT SELECTION FOR INJECTABLE MEDICATIONS

Medication Containers

Injectable medicines are supplied in dated single-dose **ampules,** single-dose or multidose **vials,** or prefilled syringes. The person administering the drug should check the expiration date and that the liquid does not show deterioration from improper storage.

Syringes

Syringes, both nondisposable glass types and disposable one-use types, come in a variety of sizes, from 60 mL to insulin syringes to some holding only 0.3 mL (Figure 14-2). Some syringes are packaged with the needle attached (Figure 14-3). Most commonly used syringes in ambulatory settings are 3-mL syringes and tuberculin syringes. A 5-mL syringe may be used when larger doses of medication are required, although the usual largest acceptable amount of medication to be given to an adult IM is 4 mL. An insulin syringe is used only for administration of insulin.

Syringes consist of a cylindric barrel with a tip designed to hold the needle and a plunger for delivery of medicine (Figure 14-4). Syringe variations include the following:

- A tip may be a plain tip, in which the needle slips onto the tip, or a Luer-Lok tip, in which the needle must be twisted onto the tip and locked in place to prevent accidental removal of the needle from the syringe.
- A barrel, which holds the medication, is calibrated for measuring the dose. The inside of the barrel must remain sterile; the outside of the barrel may be touched (Figures 14-4 and 14-5).
- A flange keeps the cylindric syringe from rolling when placed on a flat surface and is used to steady the hands when administering the injection.

- A plunger, used to deliver the medication, must remain sterile within the barrel and should not be touched when outside the barrel (see Figure 14-5). The plunger fits inside the barrel and moves back and forth, forming a tight seal against interior walls.

Some syringes such as 3-mL syringe are scaled in tenths of a milliliter (mL), cubic centimeters (cc), or minims (ɱ). Those with specific applications are scaled in hundredths of a milliliter, such as tuberculin syringes

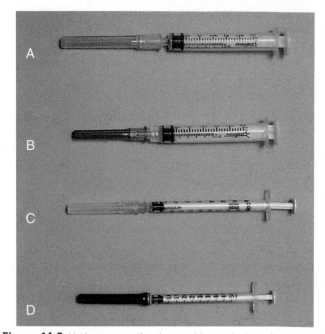

Figure 14-3 Various types of syringes with attached needles. **A,** Plain tip marked in 0.1 (tenths). **B,** Luer-Lok syringe marked in 0.1 (tenths). **C,** Tuberculin syringe marked in 0.01 (hundredths). **D,** Insulin syringe marked in units (50). (From Lilley L, Harrington S, Snyder J: *Pharmacology and the nursing process,* ed 6, St Louis, 2011, Mosby.)

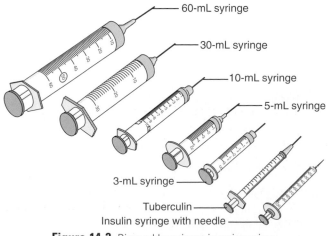

Figure 14-2 Disposable syringes in various sizes.

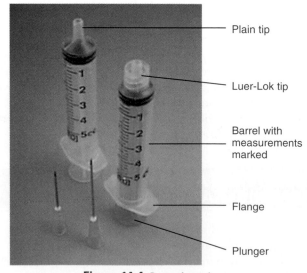

Figure 14-4 Parts of a syringe.

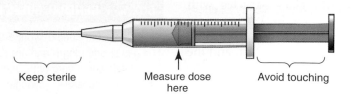

Keep sterile   Measure dose   Avoid touching
                here

Figure 14-5 Parts of a syringe that must not be touched. (From Perry A, Potter P: *Fundamentals of nursing,* ed 7, St Louis, 2009, Mosby.)

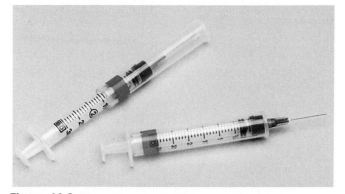

Figure 14-6 Disposable syringe with a retractable needle cover, as required by Occupational Safety and Health Administration standards.

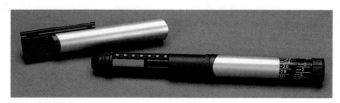

Figure 14-7 Injector pen for needleless administration of medication.

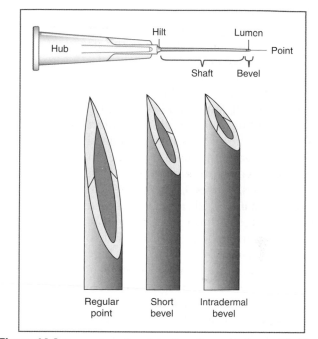

Figure 14-8 Types of needle points. (From Young AP, Proctor DB: *Kinn's the medical assistant: an applied learning approach,* ed 11, St Louis, 2011, Saunders.)

holding 1 mL and U-100 insulin syringes holding 100 units/1 mL. Insulin syringes designated as *Lo-Dose syringes* contain 50 units of insulin/0.5 mL or 30 units/0.3 mL for persons with visual difficulties. If the latter types of syringes are used, the medical record should include specific documentation of the patient's preference.

The appropriate syringe selection is the smallest syringe that will hold the prescribed amount of medication. This determination ensures the most accurate measurement because calibrations on the syringe will more accurately show the amount to be given. Specialty syringes may be found in nondisposable forms, but most syringes used in ambulatory care settings are disposable.

Safety with syringes includes the following:

- Retractable needle covers prevent needlesticks from contaminated syringes (Figure 14-6).
- Use an injector pen for insulin administration if possible (Figure 14-7). The type of pen depends on the medicine and amount dispensed with each dose.
- Use disposable syringes to prevent cross-infection. Disposable syringes do not sustain damage from

continuous use and do not require cleaning and sterilization after use.

Important Facts about Syringes

- Syringes may be disposable or nondisposable, holding from 0.3 mL to 60 mL. Syringes most commonly used in the ambulatory care setting are 3-mL and 1-ml tuberculin syringes.
- The smallest syringe that holds the amount of medication to be given should be used.
- Injector pens are available for use with ***insulin*** or the EpiPen for allergic reactions.

Needles

Needles for injection may be purchased separately or on the syringe and are available in many lengths and diameters, or **gauges.** The needle is actually a hollow metal tube with a sharp point for piercing skin.

Needles are constructed with three specific points—regular point for general injection use, short **bevel** for use with subcutaneous injections, and intradermal bevel for intradermal injections (Figure 14-8). **Filter needles** should be used when withdrawing medications from an ampule to prevent injecting glass particles with medication.

Four factors are important when selecting needles: safety, rate of medication flow, patient comfort, and the depth to which the needle must penetrate to deliver the drug at the appropriate site. The drug's *viscosity* and site of the injection are also considered in needle choice.

Needle gauges range from size 14, with the largest **lumen** (opening), to size 31, with the smallest lumen. The smallest possible needle that will administer the desired medication with the least pain is the needle of choice. Thirty-one–gauge needles are short and most frequently used on injection pens for insulin and in dermatology and plastic surgery. The higher numbered gauge (29 or 27) has a small lumen and is short ($\frac{3}{8}$ to $\frac{5}{8}$ inch) to prevent bending of the needle with injections.

The gauges from 27 to 25 are usually short needles ($\frac{5}{8}$ to $\frac{7}{8}$ inch) commonly used for **aqueous** SC injections. These needles cause minimal pain and less tissue damage. Larger needles, gauges 23 to 20, are used for IM injections of **viscous** medications administered in muscle tissue. The needle must be at least 1 inch long and of thicker gauge for the support needed to reach muscle. The patient cannot feel the difference between a 20-gauge and 22-gauge needle, and the 20-gauge needle will supply medications with less resistance when oil-based viscous medications are administered (see Figure 14-8). The general rules for selecting needles and syringes are reviewed in Box 14-1.

Important Facts about Needles

- Needles for injection come in many lengths and gauges. Choice of needle depends on site and route of injection, as well as viscosity of the medication to be given.
- Needles with retractable covers meet Occupational Health and Safety Administration (OSHA) standards.
- Four factors in needle selection are safety, patient comfort, flow rate of the medication, and depth of injection needed to deliver the drug to the proper site.
- Disposable needles are sharp and coated with silicon for ease of injection.
- Needles come with three specific points—regular point for general injection use, short bevel with SC route injection, and intradermal bevel for ID use.
- Needle gauges found in ambulatory care are from 18 (a large lumen) to 31 (smallest lumen). Lengths found in the ambulatory care setting are $\frac{3}{8}$ inch to 2 inches and are selected according to patient size, site of injection, and viscosity of medication.
- Aqueous medications require a smaller lumen, whereas drugs in oil or viscous bases are administered with a larger lumen.
- OSHA standards for needle handling should be followed at all times to prevent injury to the person giving the medication and for patient safety.

BOX 14-1 GENERAL RULES FOR INJECTIONS

- Disposable needle-syringe units are color coded for needle gauge and length and are packaged in paper wraps or rigid plastic containers with shields over the needle.
- Use disposable syringes when possible to prevent cross-contamination.
- Use aseptic technique when preparing injectable medications. If contamination occurs, discard medication being prepared and start over.
- Never swab the needle shaft.
- Always use a filter needle to withdraw medication from a glass ampule to prevent glass particles from being aspirated into fluid for injection.
- Know characteristics of medication to be administered. Give volumes of medication based on site because volumes too large will cause pain and possible destruction of involved tissue.
- Recap needles on delivery of medications to the room where the administration will take place. Do not wrap needle in a cotton ball or wipe.
- Never combine two medications in a syringe unless specifically ordered to do so.
- When preparing medications for health care provider to give, place medication container beside filled syringe.
- Choose sites of injection that are free of restrictive clothing and are not in areas where lymph nodes have been surgically removed. With a postmastectomy patient, the arm on the side of the mastectomy should be avoided, as should an area of trauma or burn.
- Use correct technique and identify correct landmarks when administering medications by injection.
- Tell patient that a little discomfort is to be expected but will last only a short time.
- Have assistance holding children to prevent injury.
- Explain to parents the need for injections for child.
- Injections should never be used as a disciplinary threat.

CONTAINERS FOR INJECTABLE MEDICATIONS

Parenteral medications must be sterile. They come in three types of containers—vials, ampules (Figure 14-9), and prefilled syringes. Before using any injectable medications, be sure to check the expiration date and for sterility.

Ampules

Ampules are small, hermetically sealed glass containers that hold a single dose of sterile medication. The neck of an ampule is thin for ease of breaking. Medications in ampules that are not used in entirety should never be

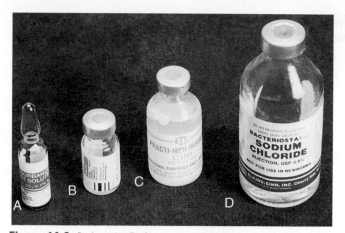

Figure 14-9 A, Ampule. **B,** Single-dose vial. **C** and **D,** Multidose vials. (From Young AP, Proctor DB: *Kinn's the medical assistant: an applied learning approach,* ed 11, St Louis, 2011, Saunders.)

kept for later use because sterility cannot be assured (for use of ampules see Procedure 14-1).

Vials

Vials, in both single-dose and multidose sizes, are labeled with the name of the medication. A single-dose vial, a small glass container with a rubber stopper on top, holds only one dose of an injectable medication or **diluent** for reconstitution.

Multidose vials contain enough medicine for multiple uses. Multidose vials may contain 1 mL to 100 mL or more. When multidose vials are used, great care must be exercised each time the vial is entered to prevent contamination. If you suspect contamination of a multidose vial has occurred or if an error has been made in preparing medication, discard the vial and start over. When medications are withdrawn from a multidose vial, the drug should be withdrawn to the exact amount, and excess waste should be avoided. Pressure within the vial must be kept equal by adding equal amounts of air to replace the amount of medication being withdrawn (Procedure 14-2).

Some single-dose vials contain a powder that must be reconstituted to liquid form. If reconstitution is required, follow directions *exactly.* Each powder vial is labeled with name of the medication and strength of medication per liquid volume (in milliliters), after reconstitution.

Prefilled Syringe

A prefilled syringe, a sterile, disposable syringe-and-needle unit, is packaged to supply a single dose. A prefilled syringe should never be used to administer an additional dose, except with new methods of insulin administration in a prefilled unit designed to be used repeatedly by the same patient.

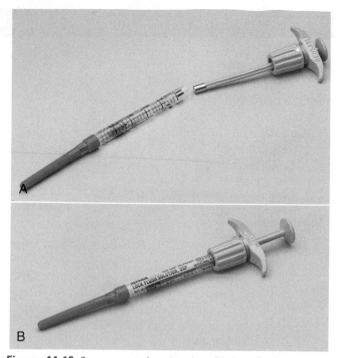

Figure 14-10 Components of a closed prefilled medication injection syringe. **A,** Unassembled. **B,** Assembled. (From Young AP, Proctor DB: *Kinn's the medical assistant: an applied learning approach,* ed 11, St Louis, 2011, Saunders.)

Disposable Injection Units

Some medications come in single-dose prefilled syringes that require use of a medication cartridge (Figure 14-10). With these units, the health professional does not need to prepare the dose except perhaps to expel a volume of medication in excess of the dose ordered by the physician. Prefilled medication injection systems use a cartridge that slips into the reusable cartridge loader (Tubex and Carpuject injection systems; Procedure 14-3).

PREPARATION OF MEDICATION FOR INJECTION

Reconstitution of Powder Forms of Medication

Some medications that are unstable in liquid form are packaged as a powder for reconstitution to a liquid at the time of administration. The vial label specifies the type and amount of diluent to be used to dissolve the powdered drug for the correct concentration of medication. After reconstitution, weight/volume of medication with the expiration and reconstitution dates and time designated on the vial (Procedure 14-4).

Text continued on p. 228

PROCEDURE 14-1   Preparing a Medication from an Ampule

Objective: To accurately prepare a medication for administration from an ampule.

Guidelines

Equipment Needed

- Medication order
- Ampule of medication to meet medication order
- Syringe and filter needle
- Alcohol swab
- Sterile gauze
- Needle of proper length for injection site and gauge for medication viscosity

Methodology 3+7

1. To open an ampule, gently tap above neck to release medication in neck into larger bottom section of container.
2. Wipe neck of ampule with an alcohol wipe to disinfect outside of container.
3. With sterile gauze around ampule, forcefully snap your wrists away from you so neck of ampule snaps to break in two. If glass does not break easily, rotate ampule a quarter turn and try again. If that does not allow opening, or if ampule does not have a scored line, score neck with a file and disinfect again. The glass of ampule is designed not to shatter or spill medication.
4. When ampule opens, you will hear a pop as the vacuum on the container is released. Discard ampule top in sharps container.
5. Uncap filter needle and insert it into ampule without touching ampule sides. Gently pull back on syringe plunger, keeping tip of needle in liquid. If necessary, turn ampule to side to obtain all available drug or amount of drug needed for desired dose. The container is designed to prevent spillage on tipping.
6. Recap filter needle and dispose in sharps container. Needle can be recapped because it is still considered sterile.
7. Replace with proper gauge and length needle for injection on the syringe.
8. Discard used supplies in biohazard container. Dispose of syringe and needle in sharps container.

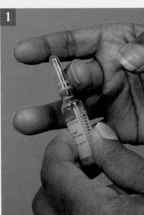
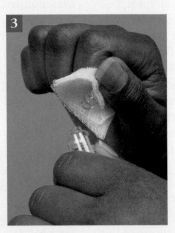
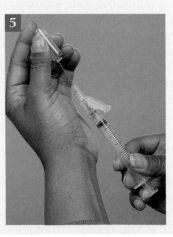

PROCEDURE 14-2   Preparing a Medication from a Vial

Objective: To accurately prepare a dose of medication for administration from a vial.

Guidelines

Equipment Needed

- Medication order
- Vial of desired medication to meet medication order
- Syringe and needle appropriate for medication and injection site
- Alcohol swab

Methodology 3+7

1. If vial is being used for first time, metal or plastic cap covering rubber stopper must be removed.
2. Cleanse stopper from center outward with an alcohol wipe to prevent contamination of fluid in vial.
3. After removing needle cover, draw volume of air into syringe to equal volume of liquid to be withdrawn from vial. Withdrawn medication must be replaced with equal amount of air, maintaining equal pressure within vial to prevent a vacuum from forming (for ease of aspiration). If too little air is injected, medication will be difficult to remove because of the vacuum. If too much air is injected, air will force medication into syringe without pulling on plunger to withdraw it.
4. Insert needle into center of rubber cap and inject air into vial.
5. Invert vial with syringe in place, being sure needle remains below liquid. If needle is out of liquid, air will be drawn into syringe.
6. Withdraw desired amount of medicine, then withdraw needle from vial. If air remains in syringe, flick outside of barrel holding needle pointing straight up. Bubbles should float into needle hub to be expelled. Draw back slightly on plunger and then gently push plunger to expel air, being careful not to expel fluid. If necessary, return needle to vial to obtain correct dose.
7. Never return unused medication to a multidose vial.

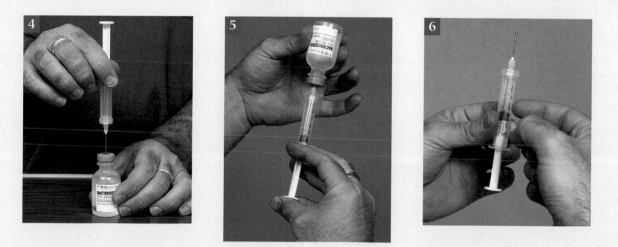

PROCEDURE 14-3 Preparing a Medication Using a Disposable Injection Unit

Objective: To accurately prepare a dose of medication for administration using a disposable injection unit.

Guidelines

Equipment Needed
- Medication order
- Prefilled disposable injection unit to meet medication order
- Appropriate injector unit

Methodology 3+7

1. To load injector, hold injector in a vertical position with plunger rod in one hand. With other hand, turn injector clockwise until it stops. This places assembly in open position for loading.
2. Insert cartridge with covered needle attached to open end.
3. Turn counterclockwise until prefilled syringe is tight and cartridge is in closed position.
4. Engage plunger rod onto threads of cartridge plunger of sterile medication cartridge.
5. Rotate plunger clockwise until resistance is felt to indicate the system is ready for use and is secure.
6. Measure ordered dose. Dispose of excess medication by pushing on plunger.
7. Inject ordered medication dose at appropriate site using proper technique (see Box 14-2).
8. After administration, remove plunger rod from cartridge.
9. The prefilled cartridge is disposed of in sharps container, holding injector with needle down. Loader is reusable and should be sanitized and saved. This system is designed to reduce risk of needlestick injuries.

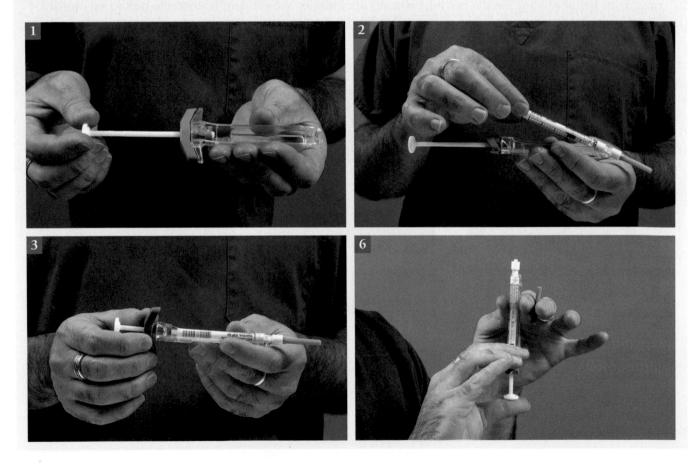

PROCEDURE 14-4   Reconstituting Medications from Powders

Objective: To accurately reconstitute powdered medications to appropriate strength.

Guidelines

Equipment Needed
- Powder for reconstitution to meet medication order
- Vial of diluent as specified by manufacturer
- Alcohol wipes
- Appropriate syringe and needle

Methodology 3+7

1. Using indicated diluent (as specified on medication packaging), withdraw correct amount (as specified on medication packaging to provide proper strength) from vial or ampule. (Note: Some medications require bacteriostatic water as a diluent, some call for sterile normal saline, and yet others have diluent provided with medication.)
2. Use same precautions to maintain sterility as when opening an ampule or vial—appropriately cleanse with alcohol and ensure sterile aseptic technique. Remember to add air to allow for withdrawal of diluent.
3. Invert vial or ampule for ease of withdrawal or slightly invert vial or ampule to withdraw diluent. After cleaning top of powder vial or ampule, insert needle into powdered medication vial or ampule and inject diluent.
4. Mix powder and diluent by gently rolling vial between your hands until mixing is complete. (Note: Some medications require shaking rather than rolling; be sure to read medication label for directions.)
5. If reconstituted medication is in a multidose vial, write reconstituted strength, date of reconstitution, and your initials on vial. Store according to label directions. (Note: Some medications must be refrigerated after reconstitution.)

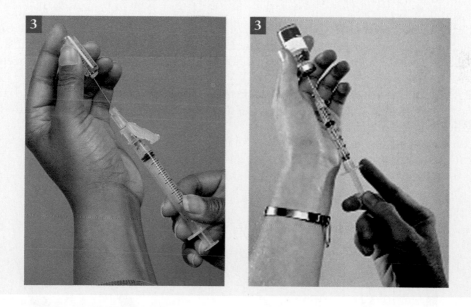

Mixing Two Medications for Administration

Occasionally two medications from vials or ampules are mixed for ease of administration and to avoid giving more than one injection. Before mixing medications, the health care professional should be sure the medications to be mixed are **compatible.** Each vial of medication must have the correct amount of air added and then medication aspirated correctly to prevent a vacuum. Care must be taken to prevent cross-contamination of medications when using multidose vials.

When medications are mixed using an ampule and vial or in two single-dose vials, the mixing is relatively easy because it is not necessary to add air to the ampule. In the case of an ampule and vial, prepare the medication from the vial first and then from the ampule. When mixing from two single-dose vials, add air to each and withdraw medications as if preparing an injection using one vial. When mixing medications from two multidose vials, follow Procedure 14-5.

PROCEDURE 14-5   Mixing Medications Using Two Multidose Vials

Objective: To accurately prepare two medications from two multidose vials for administration as one injection.

Guidelines

Equipment Needed
- Medication order
- Two medication vials to meet medication order
- Syringe with needle
- Extra needles as appropriate for medication and site of injection
- Alcohol wipes

Methodology 3+7

1. Using sterile syringe, aspirate volume of air needed to replace volume of medication to be removed from vial A.
2. Inject air into vial A. Be sure needle does not touch solution in vial A.
3. Hold plunger closed and remove syringe from vial A. Aspirate air needed to replace volume of fluid to be removed from vial B.
4. Insert syringe into vial B, injecting air and removing proper volume of medication for dose ordered. Remember: If vial is multidose of controlled substance, this medication should be drawn first.
5. Withdraw syringe and needle from vial B and check dosage to ensure proper volume has been obtained. Change needle.
6. Find point on syringe where total of both medications should measure. Insert needle into vial A, taking extreme care not to allow medication from vial B to enter vial A. Hold plunger and carefully withdraw amount of medication for ordered dose.
7. Withdraw needle and expel any excess air or fluid. Change needle as appropriate.
8. Prepare medication for administration by the proper route.

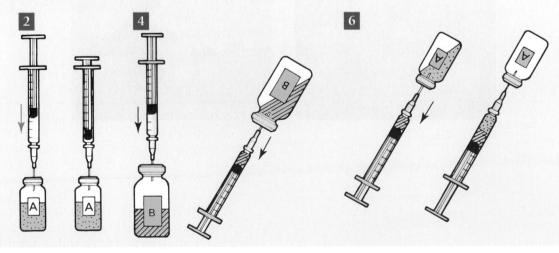

If insulin is to be prepared, special guidelines apply when mixing two types of insulin. This preparation order is necessary to prevent precipitation of insulin in the syringe barrel (Figure 14-11). When drawing two types of insulin into a syringe, the insulin preparations must be from the same manufacturer. Regular insulin should always be drawn into the syringe first (see Chapter 20 for more information on types of insulin).

Important Facts about Mixing Medications

- Occasionally two medications may be mixed for a single injection. Be sure that the medications are compatible.
- When mixing medications from an ampule and a vial, draw the medicine from the vial first. If drawing from two vials, inject the air into vial A before injecting air into vial B, followed by preparing the drug from vial B. Finally, return to vial A to withdraw the needed medicine, taking care to not contaminate multidose vials. If one vial is multidose and the other is single dose, draw from the multidose vial first.

ADMINISTERING INJECTABLE MEDICATIONS

Proper technique for administration of injectable medications is important to prevent the following:
- Injury to nerves, blood vessels, and tissues
- The possibility of infection locally or systemically
- Undue pain for the patient

See Box 14-2 for tips for administering medications by injection.

CLINICAL TIP

When injectable medications are given using incorrect methodology, legal repercussions may occur due to patient injury.

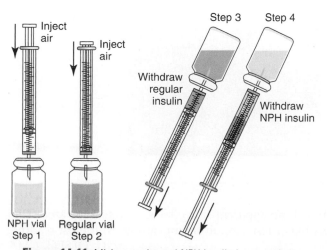

Figure 14-11 Mixing regular and NPH insulin in one syringe.

- Use smallest gauge and shortest length needle appropriate for medication to be given and injection site.
- If liquid has coated needle while medication is being prepared, change needle so the medication will not be uncomfortable going through subcutaneous tissue.
- Find injection site, position patient, and remove restrictive clothing to reduce tension at site.
- Medications should not be given near bones or blood vessels, nor should they be injected into areas where lymph nodes have been removed, such as in affected arms of postmastectomy patients.
- When giving injection, try to divert attention of the patient.
- Insert needle into tissue smoothly, quickly, and without hesitation. A jerking motion increases pain. When syringe is in tissue, hold it steady to prevent damage to tissue.
- When injecting medication, do so slowly but smoothly.
- Withdraw needle at same angle of insertion. Be sure to use proper angle for type of injection being given (see Figures 14-12 to 14-14, and 14-17 to 14-20). Wipe injection site with an alcohol pad after removing needle to reduce chance of infection. The same aseptic techniques as are used in minor surgery should be used to administer parenteral medications.
- Apply gentle pressure at injection site after administration if appropriate for the medication given. Massaging area will increase rate of absorption.
- Rotate injection sites to prevent formation of areas of induration or abscesses and to prevent thickening of skin from continuous injections.
- Follow steps necessary for preparation of medications (3 + 7). Injections require use of gloves and proper disposal of biohazardous waste. OSHA guidelines must be followed.
- Intramuscular injections in pediatric patients have faster absorption than in adults.

ROUTES OF ADMINISTRATION AND THE COMMON INDICATIONS

Certain types of medications designate the route of administration (Table 14-1).

Administering Intradermal Injections

Intradermal injections are most frequently used for tuberculin skin testing and allergy testing. The drug is injected into the top layer of skin, where many nerves are present, thus causing momentary burning or stinging (Procedure 14-6).
- The needle is inserted at a 10- to 15-degree angle in the skin's dermis (Figure 14-12).
- The injection is administered using a tuberculin syringe or a small syringe with a short (generally

TABLE 14-1 INDICATIONS FOR THE ROUTES OF ADMINISTRATION

TECHNIQUE	USE
Intradermal (ID)	Allergy, tuberculin skin testing
Subcutaneous (SC)	Immunizations, insulin, some nonirritating medications
Intramuscular (IM)	Immunizations, analgesics, antibiotics, hormones, corticosteroids
Intramuscular Z-Track	To prevent leakage of medications into subcutaneous tissue, especially when medications will discolor skin

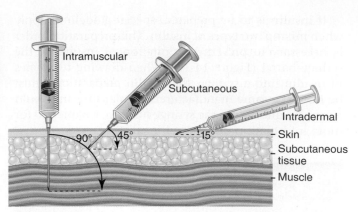

Figure 14-12 Needle angles for injecting medications. (From Hunt SA: *Saunders fundamentals of medical assisting*, St Louis, 2007, Saunders.)

PROCEDURE 14-6   Administering an Intradermal Injection

Objective: To give an intradermal injection that produces a wheal.

Guidelines

Equipment Needed
- Medication order
- Medication appropriate to meet medication order
- Tuberculin or allergy syringe as appropriate
- Short, small-gauge, intradermal beveled needle
- Alcohol wipe

Methodology 3+7

1. Prepare medication dose to physician's order.
2. Identify patient, locate proper site for injection, and wipe site in a circular motion with alcohol pad, from center of injection site outward. If injecting in forearm, choose a nonhairy area.
3. Stretch skin taut with your nondominant thumb and index finger to facilitate injecting just under skin.
4. Insert needle, with bevel up, into outermost layer of skin at a 10- to 15-degree angle.
5. Slowly inject medication just under skin to form a wheal.
6. Withdraw needle and wipe skin with an alcohol swab. Do not massage area because this will affect final reading of test. Do not apply pressure because this may force medication to leak from under skin.
7. Discard syringe and needle in sharps container. Discard gloves in biohazard waste container. Sanitize hands.
8. Document procedure. Tell patient to return in designated time to have the results read.

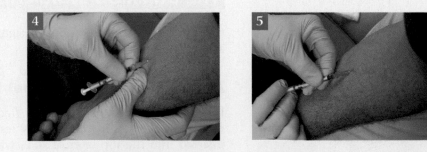

TYPICAL DOCUMENTATION

3/18/XX 10:15 AM PPD 0.1 mL administered ID, Rt forearm with no apparent side effects. Told to keep area clean and not to massage. Instructed to return in 72 hours for reading of test. Appointment card given for test reading.

G. OLSEN, CMA

$\frac{3}{8}$ inch), fine-gauge needle (26 to 28 gauge or possibly smaller) with an intradermal bevel.
- Use only small amounts of the medication (usually ≤0.1 mL) to form a **wheal** (Figure 14-13).
- The sites for intradermal injection are the forearm, upper back, upper dorsal aspect of the arm, and upper chest (Figure 14-14).
- Avoid scarred, blemished, or hairy areas.

Administering Medications Subcutaneously

Subcutaneous or adipose tissue is not as richly supplied with blood vessels as muscle, so drugs administered SC are not as rapidly absorbed (Procedure 14-7). Connective tissue under the skin is sensitive to irritating solutions and may form abscesses, as medication collects under the skin if absorption does not occur.

Use the following guidelines for administering SC injections:
- Smaller doses (≤2 mL) of nonirritating, nonviscous medications, usually in an aqueous base, are appropriate for SC administration.

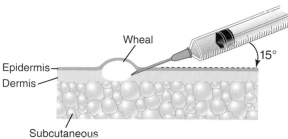

Figure 14-13 A wheal is formed by an intradermal injection. (From Hunt SA: *Saunders fundamentals of medical assisting,* St Louis, 2007, Saunders.)

- Best sites for subcutaneous injection include the posterior upper arm (in the fatty tissue over the triceps), abdomen, and anterior aspects of the thigh. The upper back and upper ventral or dorsal gluteal areas may also be used (Figure 14-15). These areas, except for the upper back, are convenient for the person who self-injects insulin.
- Injection sites should be free of infection, lesions, and scars and be away from bony prominences and large underlying muscle or nerves.
- The injection site should be rotated on a regular basis to prevent tissue damage.
- The amount of adipose tissue determines choice of needle length and insertion angle; generally the needle is 25 gauge, $\frac{5}{8}$ inch long, with a regular or short bevel, and the angle of insertion is 30 to 45 degrees (see Figure 14-12). If the patient is obese, a longer needle may be necessary to reach subcutaneous tissue.

Administering Medications Intramuscularly

Intramuscular injections (rather than injection into subcutaneous tissue) are used to provide medication for more rapid absorption because of the abundance of blood vessels in muscle tissue, if medication would be irritating, or if the volume of medication is too great for the subcutaneous tissue.
- Aqueous solutions are absorbed in 10 to 30 minutes.
- Increased danger of injecting the medication into a blood vessel exists because of increased vascularity.
- Viscous medications should be injected into muscle; however, muscle tissue that has lost muscle mass should be avoided if at all possible.

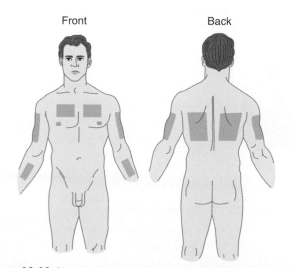

Figure 14-14 Sites for intradermal injections. (From Hunt SA: *Saunders fundamentals of medical assisting,* St Louis, 2007, Saunders.)

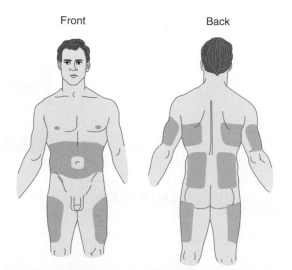

Figure 14-15 Sites for subcutaneous injections. (From Hunt SA: *Saunders fundamentals of medical assisting,* St Louis, 2007, Saunders.)

PROCEDURE 14-7   Administering a Subcutaneous Injection

Objective: To give an SC injection safely.

Guidelines

Equipment Needed

- Medication order
- Appropriate syringe (3-mL, tuberculin, or insulin syringe)
- Needle of appropriate gauge and length (usually 25 to 27 gauge, ⅝-inch length [insulin 29 to 31 gauge with ½-inch length])
- Medication appropriate for medication order
- Alcohol wipe
- Adhesive bandage

Methodology 3+7

1. Prepare medication dose according to medication order.
2. Identify patient and locate proper injection site (see Figure 14-16). Wipe area in circular motion from injection site outward using alcohol wipe.
3. Grasp skin firmly with nondominant hand, gently pinching subcutaneous tissue between thumb and index finger to minimize discomfort.
4. Insert needle at 45-degree angle. Angle may increase to 90 degrees in an obese person and decrease to 15 to 45 degrees for thin or pediatric persons.
5. Release skin and aspirate on plunger to be sure no blood enters hub. If no blood appears, slowly and steadily inject medication. If blood enters hub, immediately withdraw syringe and compress site. If blood has mixed with medication, discard and prepare medication again. If needle is removed from site and medication is not contaminated with blood, change needle before injecting in another site.
6. Withdraw needle at same angle of insertion.
7. Apply pressure with alcohol wipe to keep site from bleeding. Gently massage site if appropriate for medication administered. Apply adhesive bandage as indicated.
8. Discard syringe and needle in sharps container. Discard gloves in biohazard waste container. Sanitize hands.
9. Document procedure. If injection given was desensitization for allergies or other medication with increased possibility for allergic reactions, patient should stay for 20 minutes after injection, depending on office policy.

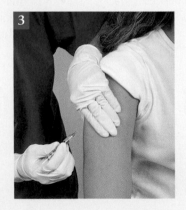

TYPICAL DOCUMENTATION

3/18/XX 11:00 AM cyanocobalamin 0.5 mL SC in the Rt upper arm with no apparent adverse reactions._____
_____G. OLSEN, CMA

- The maximum safe dose for a well-developed adult is routinely 3 mL, although tolerance up to 4 mL of medication is possible in larger muscles such as the gluteus medius. Thin adults should receive a maximum of 2 mL. Small children, especially those younger than 2 years of age, should receive no more than 1 mL per IM injection site.
- When giving an IM injection, the appropriate needle must penetrate beyond the fat layer.
- A longer heavier-gauge needle is necessary to pass into muscle tissue. Generally for an adult, a 20- to 23-gauge, 1- to 1½-inch needle is used to enter deeper tissue at a 90-degree angle (see Figure 14-13).
- Pediatric, geriatric, or thin, emaciated persons may require a smaller-gauge, shorter needle because of less muscle mass.
- Always **aspirate** before injecting medication to be sure the needle is not in a blood vessel.

A special type of IM injection is the Z-track technique, which is recommended for irritating or staining medications such as iron dextran. A zigzag path of insertion seals the needle track to prevent leakage back into subcutaneous tissue and to minimize pain. After medicine to be given by the Z-track technique has been prepared, the needle on the syringe should be changed to prevent irritation to the tissue as the needle passes to the muscle.

The tissue is displaced downward or laterally for about 1 to 1½ inches by holding it to the side of the injection site (Figure 14-16). Before releasing the skin, inject the drug slowly and remove the needle.

Sites for Intramuscular Injections

The common sites for IM injections are the deltoid area of the upper arm; dorsogluteal or upper outer portion of the hip; ventrogluteal or lateral outside portion of the hip; and vastus lateralis or midportion of the thigh. When administering IM injections, patient positioning for observation of landmarks of the entire site is of utmost importance.

Deltoid Site. The deltoid area of the arm should be used only in adult IM injections of up to 2 mL and is often used because of easy accessibility (Figure 14-17). The ideal amount of medication given in the deltoid area is 0.5 to 1 mL. Preferably, for landmarks to be visible, the person is seated with the upper arm and shoulder exposed. When locating the deltoid muscle, care is necessary because the radial and ulnar nerves and the brachial artery lie within the same area. Relax the arm at the side and then flex the elbow to find the triangular area formed by the deltoid muscle. The injection site is in the center of the triangle, or about 1 to 2 inches below the acromion process.

Dorsogluteal Site. Traditionally, IM injections have been given in dorsogluteal muscle. Extreme caution is necessary when using this area because of the underlying sciatic nerve and major blood vessels of the gluteal trunk. Penetrating the sciatic nerve with a needle may cause

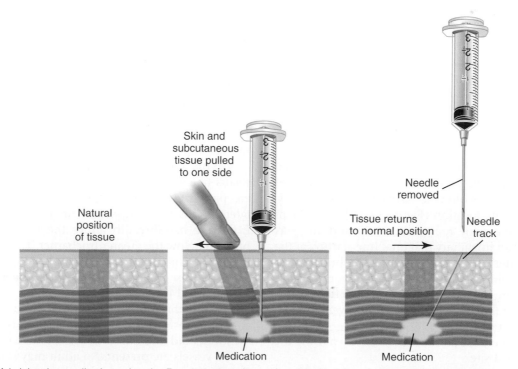

Figure 14-16 Administering medication using the Z-track method. (From Hunt SA: *Saunders fundamentals of medical assisting*, St Louis, 2007, Saunders.)

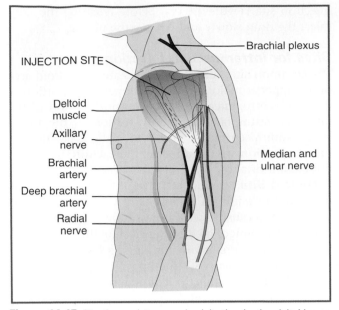

Figure 14-17 Site for an intramuscular injection in the deltoid area. (From Young AP, Proctor DB: *Kinn's the medical assistant: an applied learning approach,* ed 11, St Louis, 2011, Saunders.)

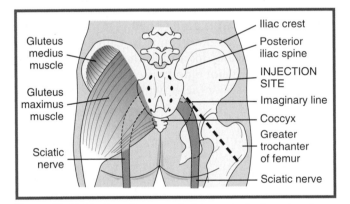

Figure 14-18 Site for an intramuscular injection in the dorsogluteal area. (From Young AP, Proctor DB: *Kinn's the medical assistant: an applied learning approach,* ed 11, St Louis, 2011, Saunders.)

permanent or partial paralysis of the involved leg. Therefore the current recommendation is that this site should not be used routinely, especially in infants or children younger than 12 years old who have small muscle mass.

For the exact site location (Figure 14-18), the patient should be prone with toes pointed inward to relax muscles. Draw an imaginary diagonal line starting at the greater trochanter of the femur, across the buttocks, to the posterior spine of the ilium. Locate bony prominences to be sure you have the correct site. Injection is made into the gluteus medius muscle several inches below the iliac crest.

- Always protect the patient's privacy when using the dorsogluteal site.
- Be sure the person receiving the injection can move his or her leg after administration.

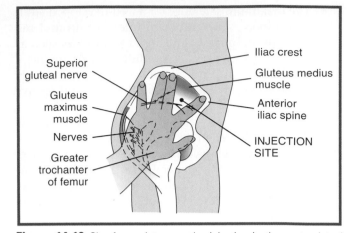

Figure 14-19 Site for an intramuscular injection in the ventrogluteal area. (From Young AP, Proctor DB: *Kinn's the medical assistant: an applied learning approach,* ed 11, St Louis, 2011, Saunders.)

Ventrogluteal Site. Although it is not used as often as other muscle tissue, the gluteus medius and minimus muscles are considered safe for all ages because the site has a relatively large muscle mass and is free of major nerves and blood vessels. All IM medications may be injected here, including viscous medications, because it is not associated with some of the injuries, such as fibrosis, tissue necrosis, and nerve damage, that are associated with other IM injection sites. For a child, a 1-inch needle may be used, whereas for an obese adult, the needle may need to be 2 to $2\frac{1}{2}$ inches long.

To locate this area, place the heel of the hand over the greater trochanter of the hip with the wrist almost perpendicular to the femur, using the right hand for the left hip and the left hand for the right hip. The index finger should be on the anterior iliac spine. Spread the middle finger back as far as possible from the index finger, attempting to touch the crest of the ilium (Figure 14-19). The center of the triangle formed by the index finger and middle finger is the injection site.

Vastus Lateralis and Rectus Femoris Sites. The vastus lateralis and rectus femoris muscles in the thigh are parts of the quadriceps muscle group. The vastus lateralis fills the midportion of the upper outer thigh from one handbreadth above the knee to one handbreadth below the greater trochanter. The rectus femoris is on the anterior thigh (Figure 14-20). The middle third of this group is preferred for the injection site. (Procedure 14-8).

Because these muscles are well developed at birth, they are considered safe for use in infants younger than 7 months old and adults because few major nerves and blood vessels are present. An adult may stand or sit, but the site is easier to find with the person in the supine position.

PROCEDURE 14-8   Administering an Intramuscular Injection

Objective: To administer an intramuscular injection safely in one of four acceptable sites.

Guidelines

Equipment Needed

- Physician's order
- Medication to meet medication order
- Syringe of appropriate size
- Needle of appropriate length and gauge for medication
- Alcohol wipe
- Bandage

Methodology 3+7

(Refer to Figures 14-17 through 14-20 for acceptable sites for administering IM medications.)

1. Prepare medication dose to medication order.
2. After patient identification, locate deltoid, dorsogluteal, ventrogluteal, vastus lateralis, or rectus femoris site indicated by age, size, and general physical condition of person and viscosity and volume of medication.
3. Choose needle of appropriate length to reach muscle tissue at chosen site and gauge for viscosity of medication.
4. Position person correctly to access selected injection site.
5. Wipe site with alcohol wipe in circular motion from injection site outward.
6. Hold skin at injection site for dorsogluteal or ventrogluteal injection taut with nondominant hand to prevent pulling of skin during insertion of needle. When using the vastus lateralis, rectus femoris, or deltoid sites, pinching of tissue with nondominant hand is acceptable.
7. Hold barrel of syringe like a dart in your dominant hand and insert entire needle into skin at a 90-degree angle. This depth ensures that medication is inserted into muscle and not subcutaneous tissue.
8. Aspirate plunger to ensure that blood does not appear in hub. If blood appears, a blood vessel has been entered, and entire process should be started again, replacing medication unit. If there is no blood, inject medication slowly and smoothly to minimize discomfort and distribute medication into muscle evenly.
9. Quickly withdraw needle at same angle as insertion to prevent further tissue trauma.
10. Apply pressure to site using alcohol swab to prevent seepage into subcutaneous tissue. If rapid absorption is desired, massage site for 1 to 2 minutes. Cover with bandage as needed.
11. Discard used equipment in proper biohazard containers. Sanitize hands.
12. Document procedure.
13. Watch patient for any signs of adverse reactions with IM injections because of rapid absorption of medication into bloodstream. If giving medication in dorsogluteal site, be sure patient is able to move leg on side of body used for injection as a means of evaluating any trauma to sciatic nerve. Be sure a health care provider is readily available in case of a serious adverse reaction.

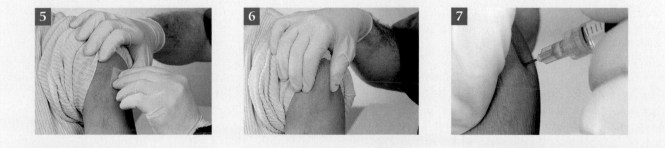

TYPICAL DOCUMENTATION

2/18/XX 11:20 AM Penicillin 300,000 units IM given in Lt upper thigh. Able to move left leg. No apparent adverse reaction after waiting 20 minutes._____G. OLSEN, CMA

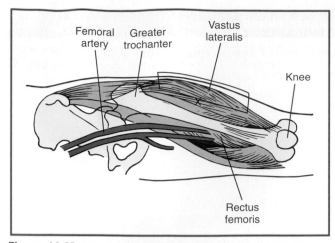

Figure 14-20 Site for intramuscular injection in the vastus lateralis. (From Perry AG, Potter PA: *Fundamentals of nursing,* ed 7, St Louis, 2009, Mosby.)

SUMMARY

Injections are invasive procedures that penetrate the skin and should be performed only if allowed by the medical practice act of the state of employment and if a physician or other health care provider is readily available in case of adverse reactions. Safety should be of utmost importance with parenteral medication administration. Parenteral administration—intradermal, subcutaneous, or intramuscular—requires special processes while maintaining sterile technique.

Drugs given by injection are absorbed and activated faster and may not have the duration of action of enteral administration. Each parenteral route requires special skills to ensure the medication reaches the desired location. The liquid is usually minimally irritating to tissue and may contain preservatives or a small amount of antibiotic. Always be sure the patient is not allergic to additives or the base fluid of the medication being administered.

Syringes are chosen according to the type and volume of medication to be given. Needles come in different lengths and gauges and are matched to injection site, depth to give drug properly, and viscosity of medication. The smallest possible needle that will produce the least pain is the needle of choice. Needles are gauged from 14 (largest lumen) to 31 (smallest lumen).

Sterile parenteral medications must be in vials, ampules, and prefilled syringes of liquid. Ampules are small sealed glass containers that hold a single medication dose. Any medication left in an ampule after administration should be discarded. When medication from an ampule is being prepared, the needle point must be kept below the meniscus of the liquid. Vials are manufactured in single-dose and multidose sizes. To prepare medication, invert the vial, keeping the needle within liquid to prevent aspirating air. Prefilled syringes and disposable injection units have medication ready for injection; however, dosages must be calculated.

Drugs unstable as a liquid come as a powder for reconstitution. To reconstitute, be sure that you have the correct diluent in the correct amount to form the correct concentration of medication. After reconstituting powders, always write the date and time of reconstitution on the multidose vial, the reconstituted strength, and your initials to prevent medication errors.

TABLE 14-2 PARENTERAL ADMINISTRATION OF MEDICATIONS

INJECTION METHOD	NEEDLE GAUGE	NEEDLE LENGTH (INCHES)	MEDICATION AMOUNT	INJECTION ANGLE (DEGREES)	SYRINGE SIZE	ADMINISTRATION SITES
Intradermal (ID)	26-29	⅜-⅝	Adult, child: 0.05-0.2 mL	10-15	Tuberculin	Forearm, back, upper chest
Subcutaneous (SC)	25-26	⅜-⅞	Adult: ↓ 2 mL or less	45	Tuberculin, insulin, 3 mL	Deltoid, thigh, abdomen
		Same as for adult	Child: 0.5-1 mL	45	Same as for adult	
Intramuscular (IM)	23-19	1-3	Small adult: 1-2 mL Large adult: 2-4 mL	90	3-5 mL	Deltoid, dorsogluteal, ventrogluteal, vastus lateralis
	Same as for adult	Same as for adult	Child: 1-2 mL	Same as for adult	Same as for adult	Ventrogluteal, vastus lateralis
Intramuscular, Z-track	Same as IM	Same as IM	Same as IM for adult and child	Same as IM	Same as IM	Dorsogluteal, ventrogluteal

Occasionally, two medications may be mixed in one syringe to avoid giving more than one injection. Always be sure the medicines to be mixed are compatible and mixing of the drugs is acceptable to the physician.

When giving injectable medications, correct technique is important to prevent trauma to nerves, blood vessels, and tissue. Given correctly, injectable medications should cause little pain; if given incorrectly, the possibility of injury to tissue increases and legal repercussions may be significant. Table 14-2 summarizes the parenteral administration of medications. These guidelines must be followed for patient safety.

CRITICAL THINKING EXERCISES

Scenario

Sally is 6 months old and needs several immunizations to be given IM as recommended by the Centers for Disease Control and Prevention.

1. In what position should Sally be placed?
2. What muscle group should the allied health professional choose for giving this medication?
3. What length needle should be chosen?
4. Should medications be mixed if the health care provider does not order mixing? Why or why not?
5. How would the allied health professional choose the size of the syringe?
6. Since these medications are to be given intramuscularly, what angle should be used for needle insertion?

REVIEW QUESTIONS

1. What does parenteral administration of medications mean? _____

2. What routes are used for administering medications parenterally? _____

3. What are three reasons for administering medications parenterally rather than orally? _____

4. What are the drawbacks to using parenteral routes of administration? _____

5. What body structures may be damaged by giving injections incorrectly? _____

6. What is the calibration on a 3-mL syringe? On an insulin syringe? On a tuberculin syringe? Give a specific use for each. _____

7. What are the factors in choosing a needle for an injection? What are the criteria for the needle of choice? _____

8. What containers are used to hold parenteral medications before preparation of injections? _____

_____

9. How much diluent is used to reconstitute powdered medications for injection? _____

_____

_____

10. Why is good aseptic technique so important when administering medications parenterally? _____

_____

_____

11. Why is it important to have a health professional available when giving medications by injection? _____

_____

_____

12. Why should medications in multidose vials be drawn first when mixing medication in a single-dose vial or ampule for injection? _____

_____

_____

Pharmacology for Multisystem Application

Analgesics and Antipyretics

After studying this chapter, you should be capable of doing the following:

- Defining analgesic, antiinflammatory, and antipyretic medications.
- Identifying analgesics that are regulated by the Controlled Substances Act of 1970.
- Describing therapeutic effects of narcotic and nonnarcotic pain relievers, nonsteroidal antiinflammatory drugs (NSAIDs), and antipyretics commonly used in ambulatory medical care.
- Classifying commonly used nonopioid analgesics and antipyretics into categories according to their therapeutic use.

- Providing patient education for safe administration of nonprescription analgesics and antipyretics and possibilities of overdose with over-the-counter (OTC) medications.
- Educating patients about drug safety by making them aware of the dangers of mixing OTC and legend (prescription) analgesics.
- Providing patient education for compliance with medications used as analgesics and antipyretics.

Jeanne has a history of headaches, for which she takes nonopioid analgesics for relief. Jeanne calls Dr. Merry to ask that the local pharmacy be called to refill her prescription. The pharmacist had informed Jeanne when she last refilled her prescription that the number of approved refills had been used.

What questions do you ask to get her to describe the pain?
Why do you need to ask Jeanne when she last refilled the prescription?
Why do you need to have the medical record available for Dr. Merry to evaluate when you know that Jeanne gets this prescription on a regular basis?

KEY TERMS

Addiction	Ceiling effect	Nonsteroidal	Pain perception
Adjuvant medication	Coanalgesia	antiinflammatory	Pain threshold
Aggregation	Drug dependence	drug (NSAID)	Pain tolerance
Analgesic	Endorphin	Opiate	Pseudoaddiction
Antiinflammatory	Narcotic	Opioid	
Antipyretic	Nonopioid medications		

EASY WORKING KNOWLEDGE OF MEDICATIONS USED AS ANALGESICS

DRUG CLASS	PRESCRIPTION	OTC	PREGNANCY CATEGORY	MAJOR INDICATIONS
Opioid (narcotic) and opiate analgesics	Yes; prescriptions for controlled substances on Schedule II must be written; prescriptions for drugs on Schedules III to V may be verbal	Yes, depending on state regulations	B, C	Control of moderate to severe pain
Combination opioid-nonopioid analgesics	Yes; prescriptions for Schedule II drugs must be written; prescriptions for Schedules III to V drugs may be verbal	Yes, depending on state regulations	B, C	Control of moderate pain; cough control; control of diarrhea
Nonopioid analgesics, antipyretics, antiinflammatories	Yes; prescriptions for Schedules III to V drugs may be verbal	Yes	B, C, D—aspirin	Control of mild to moderate pain; reduction of fever and inflammation

EASY WORKING KNOWLEDGE OF INDICATIONS AND SIDE EFFECTS

Common Signs and Symptoms of Pain
Contorted facial expressions
Fist clenching
Changes in posture
Holding breath
Increased vital signs
Irritability
Restlessness; lethargy
Guarding of body part
Self-focus
Fatigue

Common Side Effects of Analgesics
Lightheadedness, dizziness
Orthostatic hypotension
Drowsiness
Constipation
Diarrhea
Headaches
Nausea and possibly vomiting

WHAT IS PAIN?

Pain is whatever a person says it is and exists wherever and whenever the person says it exists. Pain is personal and subjective with few objective findings. Reaction to pain depends on that individual's **pain perception, pain threshold,** and **pain tolerance,** as well as physiologic changes that may cause pain.

Pain may vary in intensity in different or even similar situations such as time of day or weather conditions. Mental condition, physical stamina, and even ethnic background may affect pain because pain has both psychologic and physiologic elements; under most circumstances the person's pain threshold remains constant (Box 15-1).

The severity of pain, source or cause of pain, and physiologic and disease characteristics are factors in deciding what medication is necessary for pain relief. Response to medications is individualized, and each

person needs to know that prescribed or over-the-counter (OTC) pain medicines are safe if taken as prescribed or according to the manufacturer's directions. Fears and myths about **addiction** or tolerance to pain medications often result in the patient not receiving an adequate dosage to relieve symptoms.

When pain is being evaluated, the patient should be asked where pain is located, its duration, and the intensity of the pain on a scale of 1 to 10, with 1 being the least intense pain and 10 being the most intense. Any precipitating factors for pain or for intensification of pain should also be noted.

Pain and Emotional Responses

Pain is a stimulus to the nervous system and somatic and visceral organs. The nervous system recognizes the stimulus and carries it from pain receptors to the brain,

BOX 15-1 FACTORS THAT AFFECT THE RESPONSE TO PAIN

Factors That Increase Sensitivity	Factors That Decrease Sensitivity
Sleeplessness	Sleep
Anger	Empathy
Tiredness	Diversion
Fear	Tolerance
Anxiety	Medications
Isolation	Addiction
Depression	
Hunger	

BOX 15-2 WAYS PATIENTS COMMUNICATE PAIN LEVELS

Pain is usually evaluated on the basis of patient's subjective report of type, duration, site, and intensity. Pain medications are often prescribed on the basis of subjective symptoms. The allied health professional can evaluate pain and pain management by observing the following:

- Facial expressions
- Posture
- Patient's grasping or holding a body part
- Presence or absence of restlessness or irritability
- Vital signs and their evaluation

In the drug abuser, the allied health professional may find nonverbal expressions missing. Lack of the listed signs should be reported to the health care provider for further evaluation during the physical examination.

where stimuli are interpreted as painful. The brain continues to react until the stimulus causing pain is removed. Response of the nervous system causes a stress response to release endorphins that decrease the stimulus. Prolonged stress of pain, as well as prolonged use of pain relievers, will decrease endorphin levels and increase an individual's perception of pain (Box 15-2).

Some pain is not apparent at the physical pain site but is felt in a different body area. This pain is called *referred pain*. Figure 15-1 shows sites of referred pain.

Pain and Medications

Pain may be acute or chronic.

- Acute pain warns of tissue damage in some part of the body and is usually of short duration, responding to analgesics.
- Chronic pain has a longer duration and does not have the sole purpose of indicating body tissue damage.

- In most cases the body adjusts to chronic pain over a prolonged period of time because nerve endings have decreased sensitivity. The patient may not even report chronic pain because it has become a way of life. An example is the patient with arthritis, who may get little relief from routine medications.
- As drug tolerance develops, the person may become less responsive to analgesics, requiring a higher medication dosage to relieve chronic discomfort.
- Additional drugs may be added to the primary analgesic for greater pain relief.
- The person with chronic pain easily builds up a tolerance to analgesics—a cause-and-effect reaction—so analgesics may provide little relief in long-term chronic pain, leading to pseudoaddiction.

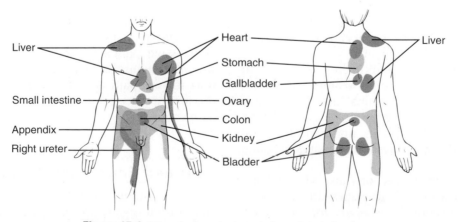

Figure 15-1 Sites of referred pain, anterior and posterior views.

Analgesics are, by definition, medications used for pain relief. Analgesics include opioid and opiate substances (controlled by the Drug Enforcement Administration) and nonopioid medications, which may be prescription or over-the-counter (OTC) drugs. Many of nonopioid and nonopioid-opioid preparations also work as antipyretics and antiinflammatory agents for a desirable therapeutic effect.

Patient Education for Compliance

1. Pain level is what the patient perceives it to be. Pain is evaluated by the patient on levels from 1 to 10.
2. The patient, family, and significant others (with the patient's permission) should be oriented to the benefits of adequate pain management. The patient's perception of pain and past use of pain medication are important factors to be considered with pain control.
3. Addiction and drug dependence (see Chapter 31) are not a problem when pain medication is used for a short period of time and should not be considerations in treating terminal pain. Addiction and drug dependence become a problem with long-term chronic pain.
4. The goal of using analgesics is to achieve sufficient pain control to ensure patient comfort, especially in terminal illnesses.
5. Patients should be taught that various pain medications are available to manage different levels of pain—from OTC to prescription opioids and opiates. Pain relief management is individual and must be evaluated by the patient and physician together for an appropriate regimen.
6. The patient should be taught that for best pain management, medications should be taken before pain becomes severe. Waiting until mild to moderate pain becomes excessive to severe will keep the patient from receiving the full analgesic effect. Also, apprehension of further pain can heighten perception of pain's intensity.

Important Facts about Pain

- Pain is based on the patient's psychologic, physiologic, and cultural background and is one of the most common symptoms that cause patients to seek medical attention.
- Reaction to chronic or acute pain depends on the person's pain perception, threshold, and tolerance; thus pain relief must be individualized.
- Analgesics may also work as antipyretics or antiinflammatory agents, or both.
- The objective of analgesia is to produce pain relief that is more effective if used before the onset of severe pain. Pain is more easily controlled while it is mild to moderate.
- Analgesics may be given by mouth, by injection, by suppository, or transdermally, depending on how fast relief is needed, the intensity of the pain, the ability of patient to self-administer medication, and the availability of the medication form.

TYPES OF ANALGESICS

Opioid and opiate medications are strong analgesics capable of reducing pain of any origin. Nonopioids may require a prescription or may be bought OTC. Because of ease and popularity of self-medication, OTC medications are often used today to relieve mild to moderate pain and fever. Nonopioids may also be used in coanalgesia or as adjuvant therapy. Coanalgesics such as *codeine* and *acetaminophen* are most often used for chronic pain but may be used for acute pain that requires opioid use. Adjuvant medications, such as *diazepam,* given with opioids are not true analgesics but are used with analgesics to potentiate pain relief and reduce pseudoaddiction.

🔹 CLINICAL TIP

Pseudoaddiction occurs when inadequate analgesic therapy to reduce primary pain takes place, leading to mistrust between patient and medical care giver.

Opioid and Opiate Analgesics

Narcotic analgesics are derivatives of opium or synthetic chemicals that produce pharmaceutic effects similar to those of opium. If purified opium is naturally found in the medication, such as codeine and *morphine,* the drug is called an *opiate.* Opioids are synthetic manufactured narcotics such as *meperidine* (Demerol) and *fentanyl* (Duragesic) (Table 15-1).

Did You Know?

Morphine, used for severe pain, is considered the standard for narcotic analgesia. This means that the analgesic amount achieved with a particular drug is compared with amount of analgesia achieved with the equivalent of morphine.

Morphine was first isolated from dried seeds of the opium poppy in 1815. It was named for the Greek god of dreams, Morpheus, who was the son of the Greek god of sleep, Hypnos. Morphine was used in the Civil War, leaving many veterans addicted after the war. *Heroin* was introduced in 1898 as a nonaddicting substitute for morphine. In 1939 meperidine was introduced with the same assumption. Both meperidine and heroin were later found to be addicting.

Because sedation is one of the side effects of narcotic analgesia, anxiety that accompanies pain is also reduced. Most people stop taking the medication when pain

TABLE 15-1 SELECT ANALGESICS REQUIRING A PRESCRIPTION THAT ARE COMMONLY USED IN AMBULATORY CARE

GENERIC NAME	TRADE NAME	USUAL ADULT DOSE, ROUTE, AND FREQUENCY	INDICATIONS FOR USE	MAJOR SIDE EFFECTS	DRUG INTERACTIONS
CONTROLLED SUBSTANCES				Respiratory depression, constipation, urinary retention, confusion, euphoria, sedation, dizziness, lightheadedness, orthostatic hypotension, respiratory arrest*	Alcohol, muscle relaxants, antipsychotics
morphine sulfate (II)[†‡]	MSIR, Astramorph, Duramorph	5-15 mg SC, IM 10-30 mg PO q3-4hr, SC, IM	Moderate to severe pain		
codeine (II)[†‡]	Same	15-60 mg PO q4h, SC, IM	Moderate to severe pain		MAOIs
meperidine (II)[†‡]	Demerol	50-150 mg PO q4h, SC, IM	Moderate to severe pain	Circulatory collapse*	MAOIs
fentanyl (II)[†]	Duragesic; Actiq	12-100 mcg transdermal; 50-100 mcg IM, IV; 200-800 mcg buccal	Severe chronic pain including cancer		Many intravenous incompatibilities
oxycodone (II)[†]	OxyContin	10-40 mg PO q4h	Moderate to severe pain		
methadone (II)[†]	Dolophine	2.5-10 mg PO q8-12h, SC, IM	Severe pain; opioid withdrawal		
pentazocine[§]	Talwin Nx, Talwin	50 mg PO q3-4h 30 mg SC, IM q3-4h	Moderate pain	Hypertension	
NONSCHEDULED DRUGS					
tramadol	Ultram	50-100 mg PO q4-6h	Moderate chronic pain	Dizziness, hallucinations, GI bleeding	MAOIs, neuroleptics, carbamazepine
pregabalin	Lyrica	150 mg daily in divided doses	Peripheral neuropathy, postherpetic neuralgia	Dizziness, somnolence	Oxycodone, lorazepam

GI, gastrointestinal; *IV*, intravenously; *IM*, intramuscularly; *MAOIs*, monoamine oxidase inhibitors; *PO*, orally; *SC*, subcutaneously.

*Life-threatening adverse reaction.

[†]Opioid medications interact with central nervous system medications and depressants such as psychotropics, alcohol, sedatives, hypnotics, muscle relaxants, antihistamines, antiemetics, antiarrhythmics, and antihypertensives.

[‡]Idiosyncratic reactions include agitation, restlessness, itching, and nausea.

[§]Not scheduled at present but is being evaluated by the Food and Drug Administration.

stops, preferring not to have sedation and confusion. Tolerance to these medications and potential for dependence keep opiate and opioid medications from being routinely used for chronic pain, except in terminally ill patients or those with pain unresponsive to other relief methods. Most narcotics are Schedule II drugs because of their danger of addiction and dependence (see Chapter 1 for a list of schedules). Drugs containing small amounts of a narcotic in combination with another medication—such as some of the antitussives that contain a narcotic, usually codeine, to control the cough reflex—may be placed on Schedules III, IV, and V. Because of their limited abuse potential, other medications can be found on Schedule V, depending on state statutes.

Uses of Opioids and Opiates

Opiates and opioids, used to treat acute pain of moderate to severe intensity, alter the perception of pain by mimicking endorphins to block neurotransmission of painful impulses and increase the pain threshold.

The World Health Organization (WHO) has described a three-step analgesic ladder in pharmacologic treatment of pain, using adjuvant analgesics in conjunction with opioids and opiates with each type of pain.

- *Mild pain*—Use acetaminophen, ***aspirin***, or another **nonsteroidal antiinflammatory drugs (NSAIDs)** around the clock.
- *Moderate pain*—If pain persists or increases, add a mild opioid such as codeine or ***hydrocodone***.
- *Severe pain*—If pain persists or if it is moderate to severe at outset, give a strong opioid or opiate such as morphine, fentanyl, or meperidine. A nonopioid medication may also be continued to assist with pain control or discontinued.

Analgesics are prescribed based on age, severity of pain, cultural norms, and patient's pain tolerance and pain threshold. Some patients need more than a standard dose, and others need less with analgesic dosages being adjusted to these idiosyncrasies. Metabolism of the narcotic—faster in older children and adolescents and slower in the elderly—will determine how often medication is administered. The analgesic must provide relief without causing unacceptable side effects. The **ceiling effect**, seen with opiates not pure opioids, results in side effects of increased occurrence and intensity if the dose is increased without providing increased relief.

CLINICAL TIP

The patient must be taught to take ordered medications consistently to maintain serum levels sufficiently high to produce relief without having breaks in pain control. This may mean having the patient take medication on a regular basis for a few days or until acute pain subsides.

Important Facts about Opioids and Opiates

- Opioids and opiates are derivatives of opium or opium-like chemicals that produce similar results to elevate pain thresholds and alter pain perception.
- Opiates and opioids have antitussive effects and may cause respiratory depression, especially in the elderly.
- Opioids and opiates are used for acute pain of moderate to severe intensity and in terminal illnesses.
- Addiction and psychologic dependence may occur with use of strong analgesics for chronic pain. These analgesics are effective and safe for short-term usage.
- Around-the-clock administration of opioids and opiates is used for severe, acute pain and chronic pain of terminal illnesses.

Opioid and Opiate Analgesic Precautions

- Use of opioid and opiate medications may lead to confusion and respiratory depression.
- If the person has liver and kidney impairment, meperidine, and ***pentazocine*** (Talwin) should be used with caution because of slowed excretion time.
- Constipation is often a side effect.
- The cough reflex is suppressed, and respiratory centers are especially sensitive to narcotics.
- Meperidine and morphine are physically incompatible drugs when administered in the same syringe and should not be used together because of dangerous potentiation.
- Men with benign prostatic hypertrophy should be educated about urinary retention that occurs with opioids and opiates.

Fentanyl (Duragesic), a transdermal patch applied every 72 hours, provides continuous opioid administration for chronic persistent pain in adults (Box 15-3).

BOX 15-3 USE OF TRANSDERMAL FENTANYL

- Skin should be cleansed with water before application of a patch. Do *not* use soap, oil, lotion, alcohol, or other products because absorption of the medication is altered.
- The patch should be applied as supplied to a nonhairy body surface, preferably on the upper body.
- Do not use heat sources (e.g., heating pads) because they increase absorption rate and toxic effects.
- Because of slow onset of action, short-term analgesics may be needed for pain until the transdermal patch takes effect.
- Fever increases the rate of absorption by about one third.
- Patches should be kept away from children and pets. To discard a patch, fold it together on the adhesive side and flush it down the toilet.

- Three pharmacologic uses—antiinflammatory, analgesic, and antipyretic—are found with nonopioid analgesics.
- Aspirin has all three qualities, which is why it is so widely used.
- Acetaminophen has analgesic and antipyretic actions but little antiinflammatory effect, except in high doses.
- Ibuprofen has antipyretic and antiinflammatory effects with less analgesia.
- Nonopioid analgesics do not alter consciousness or mental function to the same degree as opioids and opiates.
- They relieve inflammation and associated mild to moderately intense pain, dull aches, and vague pains that occur at times throughout the body.
- Most reduce fever.

Patient Education for Compliance

1. Cultural, psychologic, and physiologic aspects of pain are interwoven in a person's pain perception and response to analgesics.
2. Analgesics should be taken before pain becomes severe, to ensure needed relief. Previous doses should still be in effect to maintain optimum relief.
3. Opioid and opiate analgesics are for short-term treatment of moderate to severe pain.
4. The patient should be warned about sudden position changes because orthostatic hypotension occurs with use of analgesics.
5. Fiber in diets and fluids should be increased to relieve constipation that occurs as a side effect.
6. Pain medications should be taken with food to minimize gastrointestinal distress.
7. Patients should avoid driving, operating machinery, or performing other hazardous activities after taking pain medications, because of possible sedation.
8. Alcohol and other central nervous system (CNS) depressants should not be taken with opioids because of the enhanced analgesic effect and further suppression of the CNS and respiration.
9. Important for men with benign prostatic hypertrophy, urinary retention is possible.

Nonopioid Analgesics

Nonopioid analgesics, usually the first step in pain control, with mild to moderate pain differ from narcotic analgesics in several ways (Box 15-4). Most of the nonopioid analgesics, such as aspirin, *ibuprofen,* and acetaminophen, are available as OTC drugs and are not as expensive or addictive as narcotics (Table 15-2). Some of

these drugs, when combined with pain medications such as opioids or opiates, require a prescription.
- Although not chemically or structurally related to morphine, some nonopioid analgesics do produce CNS effects.
- Most nonopioid analgesics act on the peripheral nervous system rather than the CNS. Acetaminophen is centrally active with little to no peripheral action.
- Nonopioid analgesics alone are not effective for acute, severe, sharp, or visceral pain.
- Nonopioid analgesics usually do not produce physical dependency or tolerance, although gastrointestinal (GI) bleeding as an adverse reaction is possible.
- A ceiling effect does occur; in these cases adverse reactions increase in proportion to increased amount of drug being taken.
- Under the Controlled Substances Act of 1970, some of these prescription medications are listed as controlled substances because of potency.

Salicylate Analgesics

Salicylates, including aspirin (acetylsalicylic acid), are the oldest, most frequently used nonopioid analgesics. Aspirin has fewer side effects than most nonopioid analgesics when taken over a prolonged period of time. Salicylates may be combined with caffeine to potentiate their action (e.g., Anacin, Excedrin). Others are combined with antacids or are enteric coated to reduce possible GI problems (e.g., Bufferin, Ecotrin).

Aspirin has four distinct therapeutic actions:
1. It is an analgesic, relieving pain by inhibiting synthesis of prostaglandin from damaged tissue.
2. It is an antiinflammatory, decreasing inflammation by reducing synthesis of prostaglandin.
3. It is an antipyretic, reducing fever by causing vasodilation and sweating, causing heat loss from skin. It also resets the temperature control in the hypothalamus to normal.
4. It is an anticoagulant, prolonging clotting time by preventing clot formation by aggregation of platelets. Some laypeople may think of this as "thinning the blood," but clot prevention is the cause of decreased chance of heart attacks.

Non-salicylates for Pain

Another common OTC nonopioid analgesic is acetaminophen, a non-salicylate analgesic and antipyretic, that acts within the CNS to increase the pain threshold by inhibiting prostaglandin synthesis. Acetaminophen is used to treat mild pain and has been found to be effective as an antiinflammatory when administered in high doses for osteoarthritis. Advantages of acetaminophen over aspirin include the following:

TABLE 15-2 OVER-THE-COUNTER NONOPIOID ANALGESICS*

GENERIC NAME	TRADE NAME (EXAMPLES)	USUAL ADULT DOSE, ROUTE, AND FREQUENCY	INDICATIONS FOR USE	MAJOR SIDE EFFECTS	DRUG INTERACTIONS
SALICYLATES				Bleeding, including GI bleeding	
aspirin[†‡§] (also available TR, ER)	Bayer Bufferin,[‡¶] Alka-Seltzer	81-325 mg suppository, 325-650 mg PO q4h, age dependent	Antiplatelet for MI, fever in children, mild to moderate pain; analgesic, antipyretic, antiinflammatory		NSAIDs, anticoagulants, some anticonvulsants, antidiabetic agents
NONSALICYLATES				Nausea	
acetaminophen	Tylenol	325-650 mg PO q4-6h, 80-650 mg suppository	Mild to moderate pain, analgesic, antipyretic	Renal failure, liver toxicity	Alcohol (causes liver damage)
NSAIDS				GI distress, gastric ulcer, GI bleeding	
ibuprofen	OTC: Motrin, Advil R: Motrin	200-400 mg PO q4-6h 600 800 mg PO qd	Mild pain analgesic, antipyretic, antiinflammatory		aspirin, Coumadin
naproxen	OTC: Aleve, Midol R: Naprosyn, Anaprox	250 mg PO bid 250-500 mg PO bid 275-550 mg PO bid	Mild to moderate pain, analgesic, antiinflammatory		Coumadin, aspirin

ER, Extended release; *GI*, gastrointestinal; *MI*, myocardial infarction; *NSAIDs*, nonsteroidal antiinflammatory drugs; *OTC*, over the counter; *PO*, orally; *TR*, time release.
*Major side effects are relatively rare.
[†]Aspirin should not be administered to children with viral diseases, especially chickenpox.
[‡]Bulk-forming laxatives will reduce the absorption of aspirin and reduce the analgesic effect.
[§]Aspirin and Pepto-Bismol (bismuth subsalicylate) both contain salicylates and should not be used together.
[¶]Contains buffering agents, which reduce gastric distress.

1. All age groups, from infants to the elderly, may use acetaminophen with relative safety.
2. Acetaminophen rarely causes GI upset and bleeding problems, which can occur with aspirin.
3. Acetaminophen may be used in children because it has not been associated with Reye syndrome.
4. Acetaminophen can be taken with anticoagulant medications.
5. Acetaminophen can be used by people who are allergic to aspirin and aspirin-like drugs.

The main disadvantage of acetaminophen is liver damage when used for a prolonged period of time or with intake of alcohol. If medication is used at less than 4 g/day for most patients and 2 g or less for elderly and alcoholic patients, the medication is relatively safe.

Did You Know?

Extra-strength OTC drugs such as Extra-Strength Tylenol and Anacin usually contain 500 mg of analgesic per tablet, whereas regular-strength formulations contain 325 mg per tablet.

Nonsteroidal Antiinflammatory Drugs

NSAIDs are used for mild to moderate pain when opioids are not indicated. Most NSAIDs are used for inflammatory conditions such as arthritis (see Chapter 23) and for dysmenorrhea and dental pain. NSAIDs are available in OTC formulations in lower dosages and by prescription in stronger doses, such as ibuprofen 200 mg found OTC and ibuprofen 600 mg or 800 mg as prescription medications. NSAIDs should not be taken with other OTC analgesics (aspirin, acetaminophen, or other NSAIDs). The acceptable time limit for taking NSAIDs is 10 days for pain, 3 days for fever, or as prescribed by a health care provider. These medications should not be used in the last 3 months of pregnancy because they could have an adverse effect on the fetus and may cause complications during delivery. Alcohol with many of these medications may result in drug interactions (see Table 15-2).

Combination Nonopioid Medications

Medications may be combinations of several drugs to enhance medicinal qualities of each. More common OTC combinations include acetaminophen with salicylates, buffers, or caffeine such as Goody's Powder or Excedrin.

- Antacids, such as found with Bufferin and Alka-Seltzer, decrease gastric irritation, although some researchers believe the amount of antacid in these medications is too little to be effective.
- Effervescent antacids found in such medications as Alka-Seltzer speed medication dissolution, resulting in a more rapid analgesic absorption.
- Adding caffeine is thought to produce better pain relief than an analgesic given alone because it slows aspirin excretion and keeps blood levels elevated for longer periods of time.

CLINICAL TIP

Effervescent drugs often contain large amounts of sodium and should be avoided by patients with cardiac or renal problems.

Patient Education for Compliance

1. If someone is allergic to one nonopioid analgesic, care should be taken before taking another nonopioid analgesic.
2. Patients with liver and kidney disease, as well as pregnant or breast-feeding mothers, should avoid analgesics and should take only the dosage suggested by their health care provider.
3. If symptoms worsen, if new symptoms occur, or if pain increases when taking nonopioids, the health care provider should be contacted.
4. If stomach distress occurs, the medication should be taken with meals.
5. Aspirin and aspirin-like medications should be stopped at least 5 days before elective surgery. These drugs slow blood clotting by preventing aggregation of platelets, and continued use could lead to bleeding complications.
6. Aspirin should not be placed on gums or mucous membranes or on teeth because it may irritate or burn tissues.

Patient Education for Compliance—cont'd

7. If aspirin has a strong vinegar odor, it should not be used, as the odor is a sign of medication deterioration.
8. The health care provider should be notified if pain persists more than 5 days, if fever lasts more than 3 days, or if redness or swelling develops.
9. These drugs may cause drowsiness and will reduce the coordination needed to drive, operate machinery, or perform manual tasks.
10. Patients should not exceed the recommended daily dose of an OTC medication.
11. Acetaminophen may cause a false-positive decrease in blood glucose levels.
12. Use of acetaminophen with intake of alcohol increases the risk of liver damage.
13. Aspirin and ibuprofen should not be taken during the same time period because two medications slow the action of each other and increase side effects such as GI bleeding and the decreased antiplatelet effect of aspirin. However, if low doses of aspirin are prescribed to decrease platelet aggregation, the aspirin-ibuprofen combination may be used if aspirin is taken 2 hours before ibuprofen.

Important Facts about Nonopioid Analgesics

- Nonopioid analgesics may be prescription or OTC items. Opioid and nonopioid analgesics may be coanalgesics for more effective pain relief and to decrease inflammation.
- Use of OTC analgesics may lead to polypharmacy, especially in the elderly, because these medications are readily available and widely used for mild to moderate pain.
- OTC medications with analgesic, antipyretic, and antiinflammatory effects include salicylates, acetaminophen, and nonsteroidal antiinflammatory drugs (NSAIDs).
- Salicylates are also used to prolong clotting times.
- NSAIDs are used for treatment of musculoskeletal diseases.
- Nonopioids, especially OTC medications, have a therapeutic ceiling effect: when the maximum effect is achieved, an increasing dose does not increase the effect.

Combining Analgesics for Greater Effectiveness

Narcotic and nonnarcotic medications are often given in combination because the nonnarcotic agent provides a foundation for analgesic relief, allowing narcotics to be more effective; combination medications will reduce pain from stimulation of nerve endings or pain intensified by the patient's anxiety. When used together, combination medications provide greater relief of moderate to severe pain than if used separately. Combinations with acetaminophen should not be given with additional acetaminophen; the same is true of aspirin with other salicylate drugs (Table 15-3).

Did You Know?

Medications with the word *compound* in their name usually contain aspirin. Drugs ending in *-cet,* such as Percocet, contain acetaminophen; drugs ending in *-dan,* such as Percodan, contain aspirin.

TABLE 15-3 SELECTED COMBINATION MEDICATIONS FOR ANALGESIA

GENERIC NAME (SCHEDULE)	TRADE NAME (EXAMPLES)	USUAL ADULT DOSE, ROUTE, AND FREQUENCY	INDICATIONS FOR USE	DRUG INTERACTIONS
COMBINATIONS OF NARCOTICS AND NONNARCOTICS				
aspirin with codeine	Empirin with codeine	1 or 2 tabs PO q4-6h	Moderate to severe pain	Alcohol, CNS depressants, anticoagulants
15 mg (IV)	#2			
30 mg (IV)	#3			
60 mg (III)	#4			
acetaminophen–codeine 30 mg–butalbital (III)	Fioricet with Codeine	1 or 2 tabs PO q4h	Moderate to severe pain	Alcohol, CNS depressants
aspirin-butalbital–codeine 30 mg (III)	Fiorinal with Codeine	1 or 2 tabs PO q4h	Moderate to severe pain	Alcohol, CNS depressants, anticoagulants
acetaminophen-hydrocodone (III)	Lortab, Vicodin, Lorcet	1 tab PO q4-6h 1 cap PO q4-6h	Moderate to severe pain	Alcohol, CNS depressants
acetaminophen-oxycodone (II)	Percocet, Tylox	1 or 2 tabs PO q6h	Moderate to severe pain	Alcohol, CNS depressants
aspirin-oxycodone (II)	Percodan	1 or 2 tabs PO q6h	Moderate to severe pain	Alcohol, anticoagulants
ibuprofen-hydrocodone (III)	Vicoprofen	1 or 2 tabs PO q4-6h		
NONNARCOTIC COMBINATIONS				
aspirin-caffeine	OTC Anacin	1 or 2 tabs PO q6h	Mild pain	Coumadin
aspirin–sodium bicarbonate	OTC Alka-Seltzer	1 or 2 effervescent tabs in water PO q4h	Mild pain	Coumadin
acetaminophen-aspirin-caffeine	Excedrin, Goody's Powders	1 or 2 tabs PO q6h 1 pkg in water PO q6h		
acetaminophen-butalbital-caffeine* (III)	Fioricet	1 or 2 tabs PO q4h	Moderate to severe pain	CNS depressants, alcohol
aspirin-butalbital-caffeine (III)	Fiorinal	1 or 2 tabs PO q4h	Moderate to severe pain	Coumadin, CNS depressants, alcohol
acetaminophen-tramadol	Ultracet	1 or 2 tabs PO q4-6h	Moderate to severe pain	

Major Side Effects of Combination Medications:
Sedation, dizziness, constipation, lightheadedness, orthostatic hypotension as found with separate drugs in other tables. Major side effects would be the same as those found with each active ingredient.

CNS, central nervous system; *OTC,* over the counter; *PO,* orally.
Note: Medications containing aspirin should not be used in persons taking anticoagulants such as warfarin.
*Not scheduled in some states but scheduled in others.

TABLE 15-4 SELECTED ADJUVANT MEDICATIONS

DRUG CATEGORY/DRUG	USUAL ADULT DOSE, ROUTE, AND FREQUENCY	DESIRED EFFECT	MAJOR SIDE EFFECTS	TYPE OF PAIN
TRICYCLIC ANTIDEPRESSANT				
amitriptyline (NTN)	10-25 mg PO hs	To elevate mood, enhance opioids, direct analgesic effect	Sedation, dizziness, confusion, nausea and vomiting, constipation, urinary retention	Neuropathic pain described as dull, aching, or throbbing, as found in headaches, herpes, arthritis, back pain
doxepin (NTN)	25-50 mg PO hs			
imipramine (Tofranil)	25-50 mg PO qd			
nortriptyline (Pamelor)	50-100 mg PO daily in divided doses			
ANTICONVULSANTS				
carbamazepine (Tegretol)	200 mg PO bid	To suppress spontaneous nerve stimuli	Same as above	Neuropathic pain described as sharp, shooting, or burning, as found in neuralgia, cancer, and herpes
phenytoin (Dilantin)	100-200 mg PO qd			
lorazepam (Ativan)	0.5-1 mg PO daily in divided doses			
topiramate (Topamax)	25-50 mg PO qd			
gabapentin (Neurontin)	900-1800 mg PO qd			
CORTICOSTEROIDS				
dexamethasone (Decadron)	0.75-2 mg PO qd	To elevate mood, strong antiinflammatory action, to stimulate appetite	Nausea and vomiting, weight gain, fluid retention	Pain of cerebral or spinal cord edema or peripheral nerve pain
prednisone (NTN)	10 mg PO daily in divided doses			
ANTIHISTAMINES				
hydroxyzine (Vistaril)	10-25 mg PO qd	To relieve anxiety, insomnia, nausea, and itching	Constipation	Pain with nausea, and anxiety

NTN, no trade name; *PO,* orally.

ADJUVANT MEDICATIONS FOR ANALGESIA

A decrease in the amount of pain medication with an increase in pain control is the object of adjuvant therapy. Adjuvant analgesics enhance analgesic efficiency of opioid and opiate medications, treat symptoms that might exacerbate pain, and provide analgesia for specific types of pain. Adjuvant analgesics may also be used to reduce side effects common to analgesics, such as nausea, while also acting as synergists to analgesics (Table 15-4).

Route of administration of analgesics must be considered because of related side effects. Side effects may be rapid if the analgesic is given by injection or slow when given by mouth. Knowing the side effects and disadvantages of analgesics and adjuvant medications is a necessary lego-ethical consideration when administering medications together (Table 15-5).

Important Facts about Adjuvant Analgesics

- Drugs may be given with analgesics to prevent nausea, vomiting, constipation, and other side effects.
- OTC and prescription medications may be used as adjuvant drugs to prolong effects of prescription medications.
- When two analgesics are given together, the action is coanalgesia. When analgesics and medications to enhance the analgesic are given together, adjuvant medication administration occurs. Prescription and OTC medications for coanalgesia and adjuvant medications may be prescribed with the stronger analgesics to provide pain relief at a higher level.

CHILDREN AND ANALGESICS

Children and adults experience pain, but young children cannot express themselves to describe the degree of pain or site of pain. Comfort measures to control pain and

TABLE 15-5 ADVANTAGES AND DISADVANTAGES OF SELECTED ADMINISTRATION ROUTES FOR ANALGESICS

MEDICATION TYPE	ADVANTAGES	DISADVANTAGES
NONPRESCRIPTION		
Oral analgesics (acetaminophen, aspirin, NSAIDs)	Used for many types of mild to moderate pain reduces fever Easily obtained, some OTC Used as adjuvant-additive medications with opioids Easily administered by patient or family Nonaddictive, nonlegend medications Relatively inexpensive	Ceiling effect for analgesia Gastric and renal side effects May affect bleeding time Increased effects in elderly and children Children: no aspirin for viral diseases
Rectal analgesics (acetaminophen)	Same as above Can be used with nausea and vomiting	Same as above May cause rectal irritation
PRESCRIPTION		
Oral (NSAIDs, [Schedules III, IV] opioids)	For generalized and localized pain Ceiling effect only from possible side effects or long-term use Sedation and anxiety relief useful for moderate to severe pain Multiple drug choices Easily administered by patient or family Inexpensive to expensive	Side effects limit analgesic effects Regulated by strict prescription regulations Less effective in patients with alcohol or drug dependence Stigma or fear of use Gastric bleeding
Transdermal opioids (fentanyl)	Long duration of action (24-72 hr) Used in outpatient settings for patients who cannot tolerate morphine or related medications Used for chronic severe pain Easy use Continuous release without invasive techniques Easily administered by patient or family	Side effects not easily reversed because of time of action Slow onset of relief May require additional medications for breakthrough pain Skin irritation Expensive
Rectal opioids	Relatively easy to use as an alternative to oral administration Can be administered by family Moderately expensive Faster onset of action than oral Can be used with nausea and vomiting	Rectal suppositories not easily accepted by patients Rectal irritation Slower than injectable medications May be expelled before complete absorption owing to stimulation of the rectal muscles

NSAIDs, nonsteroidal antiinflammatory drugs; *OTC*, over the counter.

fever should be used with children so they do not suffer unnecessarily. In pediatrics a low level of analgesia appropriate for the child's age should be administered, and parenteral administration should be avoided if possible.

Poisoning may result from inappropriate use of analgesics by children, especially because some of these medications are easily obtained without a prescription. Aspirin use in children, including teenagers, with acute viral infections has been associated with possible development of Reye syndrome, so aspirin therapy should be avoided, especially with viral diseases.

Table 15-6 lists safe doses for OTC analgesics in children.

Did You Know?

Pharmaceutical companies are aware of the danger of children taking baby aspirin as candy, so OTC bottles of baby aspirin contain only 36 tablets—less than a lethal dose if an entire bottle is taken. Federal law requires all aspirin to be in lock-top bottles for children's safety.

TABLE 15-6 TYPICAL SAFE DOSE OF OTC ANALGESICS IN CHILDREN*

OTC DRUG	INFANT	2-3 YR OLD	4-5 YR OLD	6-12 YR OLD	12 YR OLD AND OLDER
aspirin (chewable tablets, 81 mg)	By physician's order only	162 mg or 2 tabs	243 mg or 3 tabs	325 mg or 4 tabs (equal to 1 adult aspirin)	650 mg or 2 adult aspirin tabs
acetaminophen 80 mg/2.5 mL liquid (infant strength)	0-3 mo: 40 mg 4-11 mo: 80 mg 1-2 yr: 120 mg	160 mg	240 mg	6-8 yr: 320 mg 9-10 yr: 400 mg 12 yr: 480 mg	325-500 mg
160 mg/5 mL elixir 160 mg/5 mL liquid 120-mg suppositories 80-mg chewable tablets (children's strength) 160-mg chewable tablets (junior strength) 80- or 160-mg sprinkle	May also be based on body weight at 10-15 mg/kg/dose				

ibuprofen
    40 mg/mL oral drops
    100 mg/5 mL suspension
    50-mg chewable tablets
    100-mg chewable tablets
    200-mg tablets
		Based on body weight of 5-10 mg/kg, depending on amount of fever or pain, or physician's suggestion; not to exceed 40 mg/kg/24 hr			

*These doses were determined for children of normal weight for age.

Patient Education for Compliance

Chewable analgesics should not be called "candy," because children are attracted to sweet-flavored colored tablets. The result might be toxic to a child who chews more tablets than recommended.

THE ELDERLY AND ANALGESICS

The geriatric patient may have undesirable effects because of age, coexisting medical conditions, and polypharmacy. Altered pharmacokinetics and pharmacodynamics in the elderly can result in a greater risk of adverse effects and in drug interactions. Also, the elderly frequently take multiple medications to relieve multiple symptoms of pain, which also leads to interactions and adverse reactions. Although nonopioid analgesics, including NSAIDs and acetaminophen, are appropriate for pain management in the elderly, pentazocine (Talwin) is considered inappropriate because of prolonged excretion time. However, heightened awareness of possible OTC analgesic abuse and a thorough assessment of the pain by the health care professional are important steps in safe patient care.

Elderly patients are more prone to gastric irritation and for greater risk for GI bleeding, as well as renal toxicity and constipation. Taking analgesics with food will decrease this possibility. In addition, these patients experience higher peak levels and longer duration of action with opioid medications. Sedation, depression of the respiratory system, and urinary retention may occur in elderly individuals who are given opioids. Confusion, ototoxicity, nausea, tinnitus, and orthostatic hypotension are common side effects and need careful evaluation because of prolonged half-life of pain medications in older adults whose body functions have slowed.

Patient Education for Compliance

Polypharmacy in the elderly increases the likelihood of side effects and adverse reactions. Care should be taken to ensure safety about polypharmacy because OTC medications for pain are so readily available leading to use of multiple pain medications.

SUMMARY

Pain, a major worldwide health consideration, is often disabling. For pain to be treated, the intensity and type of pain must be evaluated so proper therapy can be prescribed. Cultural, psychologic, and physiologic considerations play important roles in how a patient perceives pain and responds to medication. Analgesics vary from OTC analgesics such as aspirin, acetaminophen, and NSAIDS, which are also antipyretic and anti-inflammatory agents, to opioids and opiates, which are tightly regulated because of the potential for addiction or dependency. In cases of moderate to severe pain, coanalgesia and adjuvant medications may be used for increased therapeutic effects.

Some analgesics such as aspirin and pentazocine are administered orally, whereas other medications such as morphine and often meperidine are given by injection for faster absorption. The severity of pain and ease of administration are important factors to consider in selecting drugs and routes of administration. Polypharmacy in the elderly necessitates careful analysis of pain and its relief including any adjuvant or alternative therapies that are available and being used.

Societal attitudes often contribute to unnecessary undertreatment of pain. Fear of addiction or dependency with opiates and opioids is a consideration when scheduled drugs are used. An opioid is typically used for moderate to severe pain over a short period of time. For chronically ill people, these medications may lead to dependency. For the terminally ill, the risk of dependence is no reason to withhold medications.

OTC analgesics are easily obtained and may be abused if taken over long periods of time. A common misnomer is that OTC medications are completely safe, with no chance of overdose or reaction. Analgesics are perhaps the most frequently administered and most abused medications. Pain should be relieved and evaluated on a personal basis to be sure analgesics are being used properly.

CRITICAL THINKING EXERCISES

Scenario

Mrs. Jones, age 76, takes an aspirin as anticoagulant therapy. When the rheumatologist sees her, she is given a prescription for ibuprofen 800 mg tid for arthritis.

1. Will taking these two medications together affect the absorption rate of either drug? Explain your answer.
2. What side effects and adverse reactions should Mrs. Jones watch for with aspirin?
3. What are some of the age-related polypharmacy problems associated with chronic pain control?

DRUG CALCULATIONS

1. Dose ordered: Tylenol 650 mg PO stat and q4-6h prn pain
   Available medication:

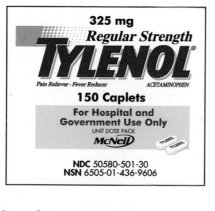

Interpret the order: _____

_____

Dose to be given: _____

_____

2. Demerol 75 mg stat and then 50 mg q4-6h prn pain
   Available medication:

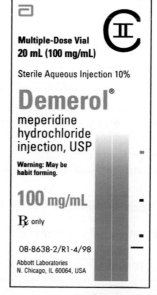

Question 2 continued on next page

Show the start dose to be given on the syringe.

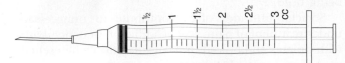

Interpret the order: _____

_____

Volume dose to be given stat: _____

Volume dose to be given prn: _____

REVIEW QUESTIONS

1. What families of drugs are Schedule II medications? What is the difference between an opioid and an opiate? _____

_____

_____

2. What is an analgesic? What is an antipyretic medication? What is an antiinflammatory agent? Give examples of each. What are three types of medications that have all of these characteristics? _____

_____

_____

_____

_____

3. When are coanalgesics used? Name two drugs that are used as coanalgesics. _____

_____

_____

4. Why are salicylates not administered to children with viral diseases, especially chickenpox and influenza? _____

_____

_____

5. Why are opioids, opiates, and other Schedule II analgesics used for short-term acute pain rather than long-term chronic pain except in the terminally ill patient? _____

_____

_____

6. Name salicylates, acetaminophens, and NSAIDs commonly used as analgesics, antipyretics, or antiinflammatory agents. _____

_____

_____

_____

_____

7. Why are adjuvant medications given with analgesics? _____

_____

_____

8. Describe the routes of administration of the various analgesics, giving the advantages and disadvantages of each. _____

_____

CHAPTER 16

Immunizations and the Immune System

OBJECTIVES

After studying this chapter, you should be capable of doing the following:

- Defining various types of agents used in active and passive immunity and their appropriate routes of administration.
- Describing public health guidelines for immunizations and the indications and contraindications for administering each agent.
- Discussing agents that provide passive immunity.
- Describing use of immunoglobulins following an Rh-O–incompatible mother and child birth.

- Describing why immunosuppressants are necessary after transplantation of organs and for autoimmune and allergic conditions.
- Discussing medical needs for immunostimulants.
- Providing patient education for compliance with medications used as immunizations and in the immune system.

Michelle is an allied health professional in a pediatric setting. Dr. Jones, using the accepted schedule, has ordered DTP, MMR, and IPV vaccines for an 18-month-old child to provide immunity.

Are all immunizations that are appropriate for a child this age being administered?
What information does Michelle need to document in the chart both before Dr. Jones decides in favor of giving the immunizations and after the immunizations have been administered?
What law requires this documentation?

KEY TERMS

Acquired
  immunity
Active immunity
Antibody
Antibody titer
Antigen
Antigen-antibody
  response
Antiserum
Antitoxin
Artificial active
  immunity

Artificial passive
  immunity
Attenuated
Avirulent
Carcinogenic
Endemic
Endogenous
Genetic immunity
  (inborn or natural
  immunity)
Immunity
Immunization

Immunodeficiency
Immunoglobulins or
  immune globulins
Immunostimulant
Immunosuppressant
Inactivated vaccines
Live or live attenuated
  vaccines
Macrophage
Mutagenic
Natural active
  immunity

Natural immunity
Natural passive
  immunity
Passive immunity
Serum
Teratogenic
Toxoid
Vaccination
Vaccine
Virulence

EASY WORKING KNOWLEDGE OF MEDICATIONS USED IN IMMUNOLOGY

DRUG CLASS	PRESCRIPTION	OTC	PREGNANCY CATEGORY	MAJOR INDICATIONS
Active immunizing agents (e.g., toxoids, vaccines)	Yes; administered by physician's order or by state guidelines	No	Most category C. rubella, measles (rubeola), mumps, varicella vaccines should not be given to pregnant women or those who might become pregnant within 1 month of vaccine administration	Active immunization against specific diseases
Passive immunizing agents (e.g., immune globulins, antitoxins)	Yes; administered by physician's order	No	Used with pregnant women who have been exposed to certain viral diseases such as measles or those needing short term immunity to specific diseases	Used in immunosuppressive conditions to achieve passive immunity over a short period of time to reduce or prevent disease processes
Immunosuppressants	Yes	No	C, D, X	Organ transplantation; immunosuppression
Immunostimulants	Yes	No	C, D	Stimulation of immune response

EASY WORKING KNOWLEDGE OF INDICATIONS AND SIDE EFFECTS

Common Indications for Immunizations
Initial immunizations against diseases in children
Booster immunizations against diseases as indicated by age and disease process—potential and actual
Passive immunization for those who cannot take active immunizations
Passive immunization in illnesses where active immunization is not available or applicable

Common Indication for Immunosuppressants
Organ transplantation

Common Indications for Immunostimulants
Cancer
Acquired immunodeficiency syndrome (AIDS)
Autoimmune diseases

Common Side Effects of Immunizations
Tenderness at the injection site
Fever
Erythema and induration at the injection site
Arthralgia, myalgia

Common Side Effects of Immunosuppressants and Immunostimulants
Nausea, vomiting, diarrhea
Insomnia
Fever
Arthralgia
Increased susceptibility to infections

The immune system is based on cells, factors, and responses all working together to either destroy microorganisms by cell-mediated mechanisms or be the mechanism that uses antibodies to neutralize or destroy invading microorganisms. Production of antibodies is significant for immunity after immunizations. Antibodies, gamma globulins found in plasma, are the body's defense system against disease invaders. Immunity may be either inborn or acquired and is selective—a person immune to one disease may not be immune to another. Generic immunity (inborn and natural immunity) is found because of genetic factors and is species specific. A substance must be delivered into the body to produce acquired immunity. It may be obtained by natural or artificial sources, such as immunizations or immune serums, and may produce active or passive immunity (Figure 16-1 and Table 16-1).

The development of vaccines has enabled remarkable advances in disease prevention via acquired immunity. Work on new vaccines offers hope for treating new diseases as they emerge. Vaccines for shingles and human papillomavirus (HPV) are some of the latest introductions, with a vaccine to prevent human immunodeficiency virus (HIV) and possibly forms of cancer on the horizon. Widespread use of immunizations has had a great impact on health of people in the United States by reducing the incidence of many severe infections by 99%. Two diseases have been dramatically decreased through vaccinations: polio, which has been virtually eliminated from the Western Hemisphere, and smallpox, which has been successfully eliminated from most of the world. Through increased parental education and community participation, the goal of immunizing all susceptible populations and the elimination

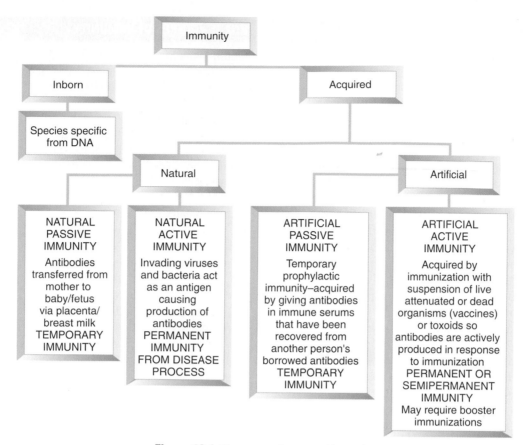

Figure 16-1 The types and extents of immunity.

TABLE 16-1 COMPARISON OF ACTIVE AND PASSIVE IMMUNITY		
CATEGORY	**ACTIVE IMMUNITY**	**PASSIVE IMMUNITY**
Purpose	Disease prevention	Disease prevention and therapeutics
Source	Individually produced from various sources—self-produced immunity	Other immune humans or animals—immunity from another source
Effectiveness	High	Low to moderate over periods of time; high for immediate protection
Methods of immunity	1. Contraction of the disease 2. Immunization with toxoid or vaccine	1. From mother to fetus or baby 2. Administration of antibody by injection
Response time	5-21 days	Immediate
Duration	Long term, up to a lifetime	Short term, days to a few months
Ease of reactivation	Booster dose	New administration; anaphylaxis possible, can be dangerous

of many immunizable diseases would become more of a reality.

ROLE OF LYMPHOCYTES IN IMMUNITY

Lymphocytes, cells produced to fight infections, reside in lymphoid tissue, such as the spleen, tonsils, lymph nodes, or thymus or in the reticuloendothelial system and in circulating blood. Once the body has produced a specific **antibody** in response to an antigen, the antibodies circulate throughout the body and attach to a specific **antigen,** labeling these for destruction.

T cells are responsible for cell-mediated immunity by directly attacking the invading antigen found with viruses, cancer cells, foreign tissue cells, fungi, and protozoa. For example, T cells are involved whether organ or tissue transplantation is accepted or rejected. **Macrophages** work with T cells to recognize "self" from "nonself" and to boost the immune system. T cells release substances that stimulate other lymphocytes or macrophages to destroy antigens and suppress the immune response; thus the second exposure to the antigen will elicit a more powerful response from the T cell than the first exposure.

B cells, or B lymphocytes, are responsible for antibody-mediated immunity (humoral immunity) and are dormant in lymphoid tissue until a foreign antigen appears. Exposure to specific antigens stimulates the B cells to multiply rapidly and produce immunity by producing antibodies that circulate in body fluids. Unlike T cells, B cells do not neutralize the antigen; rather, these cells take up residence in lymphoid tissue and continue to produce small amounts of antibodies after the infectious state has been conquered. Select B and T cells become memory cells that will remember the pathogen encountered and will mount a strong response if the pathogen is detected again.

Specific antibodies are formed in response to specific antigens. The shape of the antibody that circulates in the bloodstream matches the shape of the antigen, and they bind together, destroying or inactivating the antigen. This is called the antigen-antibody response and is present in some way from birth until death. This immunity protects the person from foreign substances that invade the body, or self, while not overreacting and damaging the body itself under normal circumstances.

INBORN VERSUS ACQUIRED IMMUNITY

Inborn or generic immunity, found with inherited factors making a human immune to diseases found in animals, may also be called species specific, natural, or inherited immunity. A person who seems resistant to certain diseases is also considered to have inborn immunity. Individual immunity may result from a genetic makeup that prevents the person from responding to antigens, resulting in immunity to certain diseases or conditions (Box 16-1).

Acquired immunity develops during a lifetime as the person encounters various agents that may be disease causing or as the person is immunized with agents that stimulate a similar immune response as would occur during exposure to the disease itself. The formation of antibodies to the antigens by the body produces an immune response (see Box 16-1). Acquired by the host over a length of time, antibody response will become more potent with each exposure to the antigen (Figure 16-2).

Natural Passive Immunity

When antibodies come from sources other than the individual's own body, the immunity is called passive immunity. Natural passive immunity, transfer of

---

BOX 16-1 TYPES OF IMMUNITY

Inborn Immunity
Inborn immunity results from the genetic makeup of an individual, an ethnic group, or a species.

Acquired Immunity
Acquired immunity results from the introduction into the body of substances (e.g., antigens) that prompt the immune system to produce antibodies or substances that already contain antibodies (e.g., mother's milk, immune serum from another person).

Natural Immunity
No vaccines or toxoids are involved; the process is largely endogenous.
- Natural active immunity—Acquired by exposure to invading pathogens (viruses, bacteria) that act as antigens and activate the immune system to produce antibodies (e.g., an unvaccinated person is exposed to a seasonal influenza virus, gets sick, produces antibodies to the virus, and is immune when exposed again to the same viral strain); usually permanent immunity.
- Natural passive immunity—Immunity acquired by the fetus or infant on transfer of maternal antibodies through the placenta or breast milk, resulting in temporary immunity.

Artificial Immunity
Acquired by exogenous immunization.
- Artificial active immunity—Acquired by immunization with vaccines or toxoids; antibodies are actively produced in response to presence of a foreign antigen to provide semipermanent to permanent immunity.
- Artificial passive immunity—Acquired by immunization with serum from another person or animal source that contains antibodies for immediate but temporary immunity.

---

antibodies from mother to baby through the placenta or breast milk, especially in colostrum, is the only example of natural passive immunity. Because antibodies are transferred from an outside source, they do not last as long as antibodies produced as a response to specific antigens by the infant, but the transfer does provide protection for an infant until his or her own immune system is fully functional, at approximately 6 months to 1 year of age (see Figure 16-1).

Natural Active Immunity

Natural active immunity is permanent immunity gained by having a disease. Antigens force the body to make antibodies to counteract or fight the disease; these

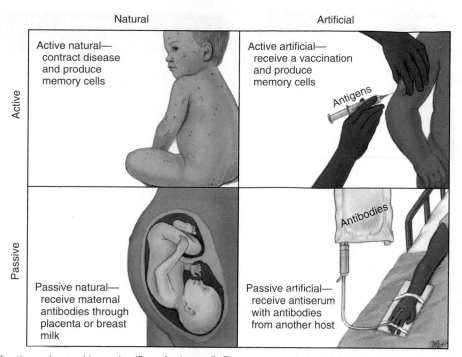

Figure 16-2 Types of active and natural immunity. (From Applegate E: *The anatomy and physiology learning system,* ed 4, St Louis, 2011, Saunders.)

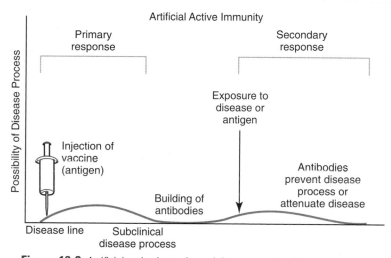

Figure 16-3 Artificial active immunity and the response to disease processes.

remain in the body after the disease has subsided (Figure 16-3). Natural active immunity may last for years or even for a lifetime. The host is engaged in the formation of antibodies in response to a disease or toxic process. Even if the infection is subclinical or mild, the host's cells are stimulated to form antibodies for **active immunity**. If sufficient antibodies are produced, the person will not contract the disease in most cases during further exposure unless initial exposure to the disease was too mild to provide immunity.

Artificial Active Immunity

Most immunity found within the wellness concept of medical practice is **artificial active immunity**—a purposefully initiated immunity for protection of the susceptible person from a specific disease. With artificial active immunity, an antigen is introduced into the body by artificial means to stimulate production of antibodies when the person has not had the disease process and immunity is desired. Rather than introducing the virulent agent that might be pathogenic, **virulence** in the immune producing agent is reduced, or **attenuated,** for administration, to allow the body to produce antibodies without causing the person to have a serious illness. The process of **immunization** may also be called **vaccination** because the agent used is usually a vaccine for bacterial and viral pathogens.

Artificial Passive Immunity

A person with no immunity who has been exposed to a virulent organism is at danger for contracting the disease. To prevent the disease process, the person needs borrowed or "ready-made" antibodies found in immune **serum** to counteract the microorganisms and to give short-term immunity rapidly. The process of providing a person with antibodies from another source is **artificial passive immunity.** With use of immune serum globulins (or **antiserum**) found in the blood from another source, the immunity is immediate and effective but short-lived (Figure 16-4).

The sera prepared for immune purposes in emergencies are often derived from human or animal sources, such as horses, and are used when there is no time for the body to develop its own antibodies or when the disease process would cause imminent danger, as with exposure to rubella in nonimmune pregnant woman.

Use of animal antibodies may produce a sensitivity reaction called *serum sickness.* The patient should be skin tested for hypersensitivity before administration; however, this sensitivity reaction is not likely to occur if human gamma globulins are used.

Some immune sera contain antibodies known as *antitoxins* (Box 16-2).

TYPES OF ACTIVE AND PASSIVE IMMUNIZING AGENTS

Vaccines and toxoids are available to provide artificial active immunity. Blood derivatives, such as plasma, and antitoxins provide artificial passive immunity.

Vaccines

Vaccines contain a suspension of whole or fractionated microorganisms that, on administration, causes the recipient's immune system to produce antibodies for the antigen or microbe found in the vaccine. Two major types of vaccines, inactivated and live attenuated, exist:

BOX 16-2 SOURCES OF IMMUNE GLOBULINS OR SERA

1. Diphtheria antitoxin, for diphtheria, is obtained from immunized horses.
2. Tetanus immune globulin, used in prevention of tetanus or lockjaw, is from human sources.
3. Immune globulins from human plasma are used for hepatitis A, measles, polio, and chickenpox.
4. Human hepatitis B immune globulins are used to supply immunity to infants born to mothers who have hepatitis B.
5. Rabies antiserum may be obtained from humans to treat victims of bites from rabid animals.
6. Botulism antitoxin, obtained from horses, must be used soon after exposure to be effective.
7. Anti-snakebite serum is an antivenom specific to combat the effects of bites from poisonous snakes such as rattlesnakes.

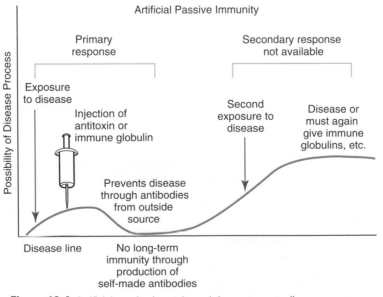

Artificial Passive Immunity

Primary response — Secondary response not available

Possibility of Disease Process

Exposure to disease

Injection of antitoxin or immune globulin

Prevents disease through antibodies from outside source

Second exposure to disease

Disease or must again give immune globulins, etc.

Disease line

No long-term immunity through production of self-made antibodies

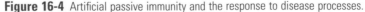

Figure 16-4 Artificial passive immunity and the response to disease processes.

- **Inactivated vaccines** are made of whole killed or inactivated microbes or some of their components. Examples include injected influenza, pertussis, and rabies vaccines.
- **Live vaccines** or **live attenuated vaccines** are composed of live microbes that have been weakened or rendered **avirulent;** examples are vaccines for polio (OPV); rotavirus; and measles, mumps, and rubella combined (MMR). Immunocompromised individuals may be unable to fight the live or attenuated vaccine, and pregnant women may have a risk for fetal teratogenicity. Therefore these patients should not receive these vaccines.

Toxoids

Toxoids are bacterial toxins that have been changed to a nontoxic state. The toxicity of the bacterial toxin has been weakened to the point that it does not cause the disease, but the toxin is still capable of stimulating the body to form antibodies. An example is tetanus toxoid (TT).

Immune Globulins

Serum or plasma derivatives, or specific **immunoglobulins** or **immune globulins,** contain large concentrations of antibodies to a specific antigen or disease. These preparations are made from blood products and provide immediate short-term passive immunity. Immune globulins are used in acute exposure to diseases such as hepatitis B and rabies.

Antitoxins

Antitoxins are antibodies produced in response to specific toxins and when administered have the ability to neutralize these specific toxins (e.g., diphtheria, tetanus) for a person at high risk for the disease or condition. Antitoxins are also used for short-term prophylaxis in a person without active immunity who has been exposed to a specific toxin.

WHO SHOULD BE IMMUNIZED?

In today's health care environment, immunizations for wellness are routine patient care. The period of required immunization is from birth through school entry, with continuation through the school years, but currently immunizations are recommended to continue through adulthood to prevent outbreaks of disease in adults. The required immunizations are suggested by the Centers for Disease Control and Prevention (CDC), with the various state immunization requirements based on age groups. On entry into school, the child must meet the criteria set by the state and by local schools. Adults should continue

to receive certain immunizations such as diphtheria-tetanus toxoid every 10 years and influenza vaccine yearly to maintain immunity.

Certain populations have been found to be at high risk for contracting immunizable diseases:

- Adolescents, because of the declining need for immunizations to meet requirements for school attendance
- New parents who have allowed their immunity to wane and who are now exposed to childhood diseases or who may carry an illness potentially detrimental to the newborn
- Debilitated persons, whether from physical disabilities or from age-related problems, who are now more susceptible to illness
- Migrant workers and new immigrants who are inadequately immunized or may not have been immunized at all
- Health care workers who are not properly immunized and are exposed to diseases

In patients who have been exposed to a disease, an **antibody titer** may be performed to determine immunity. Persons intending to travel to areas where a disease is **endemic** should obtain the required and recommended immunizations before traveling. The local health department, in cooperation with the CDC, can provide a list of needed immunizations for travel.

Patient Education for Compliance

The need to be current with immunizations as a means of disease prevention is obvious. Vaccinations do carry some risks, but the more serious risk is contracting a disease for which a vaccine is available. An example of the future hazards from disease processes that appear in adults is chickenpox leading to shingles later in life or mumps being associated with development of diabetes mellitus. Concerns about vaccines causing attention-deficit/hyperactivity disorder, autism, diabetes, and sudden infant death syndrome have caused parents to question immunizing children. However, data from clinical trials do not support neurologic or developmental harm. Vaccines have reduced and even eliminated many diseases that killed or severely disabled persons several generations ago. Parents should be educated regarding the benefits of vaccination.

Important Facts about Immunizations

- Immunizations are vital to the maintenance of public health.
- Vaccines promote production of antibodies against bacteria and viruses; toxoids promote the building of antibodies against bacterial toxins, not bacteria themselves.
- Inactivated vaccines are made of whole killed microbes or their components. Live vaccines are made from attenuated or weakened live microbes, rendering these avirulent in most persons.

INDICATIONS FOR IMMUNIZATIONS

- Vaccines may be safely administered, after authorization by a health care provider, to a person with a mild acute illness with or without fever unless chest congestion is present. *Care should be taken that immunizations are not needlessly postponed because of mild to moderate symptoms.*
- Mild to moderate local reactions from previous immunizations, such as soreness, erythema, or swelling, are not contraindications to further immunization.
- Taking antimicrobials, recovering from disease processes, and having recently been exposed to an infectious disease do not preclude the administration of the vaccines.
- A fever, even a high fever, is no longer considered a reason for not giving an immunization, nor are diarrhea, vomiting, and otitis.

CLINICAL TIP

If a patient has sustained a wound, especially a puncture wound, information concerning the level of immunity to tetanus should be obtained including when the last immunization against tetanus was given. If the patient does not remember or the record is unavailable, the health care provider will usually administer a booster of tetanus toxoid.

CONTRAINDICATIONS TO IMMUNIZATIONS

Live vaccines should not be given to the following individuals:
- Patients receiving steroids, radiation therapy, or antineoplastics
- Patients who are immunosuppressed or have a current moderate to severe infection that suppresses the immune system
- Patients who have received immune serum within the past 3 months; the immune serum may prevent adequate production of antibodies.

Care must also be taken to ensure that those who are immunized cannot harm susceptible persons in their home or work environment. Live vaccines take up to 30 days to be shed from the body, so the immunosuppressed person must be protected during this time. An example is the immunized child who is living in a home with a chronically ill grandparent or in a home where someone is undergoing chemotherapy.

Vaccines should not be administered to persons who are allergic to the substance or any component used in manufacturing the vaccine, because of the danger of anaphylaxis. Some vaccines have egg as a component, others are made with preservatives such as mercury, and some vaccines contain antibiotics such as neomycin or polymyxin B that were used to attenuate the microorganisms.

Rubella and varicella vaccines are contraindicated in pregnancy because of a rare but possible risk of teratogenicity to the developing fetus caused by viral exposure.

A closer evaluation of the person who gives a history of seizures or high-pitched screams over a prolonged time after the administration of vaccines should occur before the administration of the immunization.

If a question exists concerning whether or not to administer the vaccine, the physician will make a decision by weighing the potential for benefit against the potential for risks and will provide sufficient information for parents to make informed decisions about immunizations. (See Evolve site for the specific published contraindications and precautions for immunizations for pediatric patients and common vaccine contraindications for adults.)

ADVERSE REACTIONS TO IMMUNIZATIONS

The importance of immunizations as protection from infectious diseases cannot be stressed enough, but immunizations also have associated risks that can be controlled by such measures as *acetaminophen* in appropriate doses before and after immunizations and sponge baths. The side effects are usually mild and transient, with such symptoms as a slight fever, minor rashes, or soreness at the injection site. Joint pain and malaise may be found with live and inactivated vaccines. Though these effects of immunization are common and uncomfortable, the need for vaccines to prevent disease may tip the balance in favor of giving the immunization.

Some people have unusual and severe reactions that are monitored by the Food and Drug Administration (FDA) and CDC. With any serious problem encountered with a vaccine, data must be sent to the Vaccine Adverse Event Reporting System (VAERS) to permit detection of uncommon, severe, previously unseen, or rare reactions. Some of these rare reactions have included Guillain-Barré syndrome with influenza vaccines, encephalitis with measles vaccine, and peripheral neuropathy with rubella vaccine.

Anaphylactic reactions are a possibility with immunizations, as they are with any medication (Box 16-3).

The advantages of immunity far outweigh the dangers of vaccines in most instances. Health care professionals should encourage parents to immunize their children. Adults should also be reminded of the need for proper

BOX 16-3 TYPICAL SIDE EFFECTS AND ADVERSE REACTIONS FROM SELECTED VACCINES OR TOXOIDS

Vaccine or Toxoid	Serious Side Effects
Measles, mumps, rubella	Anaphylaxis, thrombocytopenia, dangers of teratogenicity in pregnancy, encephalitis
Diphtheria, tetanus, pertussis	Encephalopathy, convulsions, shocklike states
Hepatitis B	Anaphylaxis
Varicella	Anaphylaxis
Influenza	Guillain-Barré syndrome

immunization on a regular basis to protect public and personal health.

Did You Know?

In early 2006 and 2010, outbreaks of mumps and pertussis were both documented, although both diseases had been virtually eradicated in the United States. The pathogens were originally thought to have been brought to the country by world travelers who had visited countries where immunizations are not enforced and were passed to persons whose antibody levels were not sufficient to prevent the diseases, especially in adults who had not been sufficiently immunized.

DOCUMENTATION OF IMMUNIZATIONS

The National Childhood Vaccine Injury Act of 1986 provided for the compilation of Vaccine Information Statements (VISs) by the CDC for certain immunizations. Documents are available from the CDC's website (www.cdc.gov/vaccines/pubs/vis/default.htm), or a set may be ordered by calling the CDC Immunization Hotline at 800-232-2522. Further statute requirements include the following:

- A parent or legal guardian of a child, or the adult being vaccinated, must be provided with a copy of the VIS and have time to read the materials showing the risks and benefits of a vaccine before the administration. The medical office may add an identifier on the VIS, but the CDC must approve any other change.
- A permanent record of each mandated vaccination must be given to a patient.
- VIS documents must be provided for DTaP, DTP, Td, MMR, varicella, polio, Hib, or hepatitis B vaccines.
- VIS documents are not required but are recommended for influenza, pneumococcal, and hepatitis A vaccines.

- The medical record must show documentation of the VIS publication date because revisions occur from time to time. The revision date appears under the CDC logo.
- From a legal standpoint, the immunization should always be recorded in the patient's medical record to show that the medication has been given. The following data must be included in documentation:
  - Date of vaccination
  - Route and site of vaccination
  - Vaccine type, manufacturer, lot number, and expiration date
  - Name, address, and title of person administering the vaccine
  - Delivery of VIS to the appropriate person and the date of VIS publication
  - Signing of permission to give medication by parent or guardian before administration

These records ensure the person, especially a child, receives the appropriate immunization and the records reduce chance of errors such as duplicative vaccinations. Reporting adverse reactions to the CDC by vaccine, lot number, manufacturer, and so on is important for tracking possible links to the reactions.

AGENTS FOR ARTIFICIAL ACTIVE IMMUNITY

Artificial active immunity produces a level of immunity that requires frequent immunizations after the initial rounds. Live attenuated virus vaccine produces a mild, subclinical form of the disease to produce antibodies for immunity. Agents containing inactivated bacteria are shorter acting and require multiple doses to produce a proper immune response; revaccination doses (boosters) may be required for continued protection.

Vaccines for Diphtheria, Tetanus, and Pertussis (DTaP, Tdap, Td)

- **DTaP** (diphtheria, tetanus, and acellular pertussis) vaccine is for patients younger than 7 years of age. DTaP contains acellular pertussis, a form less likely to cause adverse reactions.
- **Tdap** (tetanus, diphtheria, and acellular pertussis), containing a lower dose of the pertussis component, is used as booster dose after the initial immunization series for adolescents when adverse reactions are less likely to occur. Adults should receive Tdap as a booster dose instead of one of the booster doses of Td to maintain pertussis immunity.
- The tetanus-diphtheria vaccine **(Td)** should be administered every 10 years throughout the adult years (Table 16-2).

TABLE 16-2 SELECT AGENTS THAT PROVIDE ACTIVE IMMUNITY

IMMUNIZING AGENT	TRADE NAME	DOSE, ROUTE, AND FREQUENCY	INDICATIONS FOR PROTECTION	SIDE EFFECTS
DTaP (inactivated bacterial components)	Daptacel, Infanrix, and Tripedia	0.5 mL IM q4-8 wk × 4 doses beginning at 2 mo, with boosters at 15-18 mo; 4-6 yr; 11-12 yr	Diphtheria, tetanus, pertussis, ages >2 mo to <7 yr	Swelling, local reactions, fever, irritability, crying, drowsiness, anorexia
DTaP-IPV/Hib	Pentacel	0.5 mL IM × 4 doses at 2, 4, 6, and 15-18 mo	Protections for listed diseases for children aged 6 wk through 4 yr	Same as for DTP
DTaP-IPV	Kinrix	0.5 mL IM	Single dose booster for DTaP for ages 4-6 yr	Same as for DTP
Diphtheria and Tetanus toxoids (Tc; adult)	Decavac	0.5 mL IM q10yr (adult). >7 yr: 0.5 mL IM x 3 doses pediatric (initial, then 4-8 wk, then 6-12 mo after 2nd, then q10yr)	Diphtheria, tetanus in children >7 yr old through adulthood; may be used with children who have contraindications to pertussis vaccine	Local reactions, headaches, myalgia, hypotension, joint pain, stuffiness
Diphtheria and Tetanus toxoids (DT; pediatric)	NTN	0.5 mL IM at 2, 4, 10-16 mo; booster at 6-12 mo after 3rd dose	Tetanus and diphtheria	
Tetanus, reduced diphtheria, acellular pertussis (adult Tdap)	Adacel	0.5 mL IM × 1 dose for persons aged 11-64 yr	Tetanus, diphtheria, and pertussis in adults	Same as Td
Tetanus toxoid (TT)	NTN	0.5 mL SC 1-12 yr 1 dose after 12 mo of age; 12 yr to adults: 0.5 mL SC followed by a second dose in 4-8 wk, then as needed	Possible tetanus due to injury and for prophylaxis	Local reactions, fever, chills, malaise, myalgia
MMR	M-M-R II	1 dose SC after 12-15 mo, with booster at 4-6 yr; 1-2 doses >17 yr	Rubeola, mumps, rubella	Fever, rash, jaw pain, headache, myalgia, sore throat
Rubella vaccine	Meruvax II	1 dose SC	Rubella	Same as MMR except jaw pain and sore throat
Mumps vaccine	Mumpsvax	0.5 mL SC	Mumps	Same as MMR
Polio vaccine Inactivated IPV (Salk)	IPOL	0.5 mL IM × 2 doses at 4- to 8-wk intervals beginning at 2 mo with booster at 6-18 mo, then 1 booster at 4-6 yr	Polio (in children or adults)	Tenderness at injection site, fever, erythema

EL, Elisa units; *GI*, gastrointestinal; *IM*, intramuscularly; *IPV*, inactivated poliomyelitis vaccine; *MMR*, measles, mumps, rubella; *NTN*, no trade name; *PO*, orally; *SC*, subcutaneously; *URI*, upper respiratory infection.

Vaccine	Brand (Doses)	Dose/Schedule	Indication	Side Effects
Haemophilus influenza B (Hib) vaccine	ActHIB (4 doses)	0.5 mL IM at 2, 4, and 6 mo with booster at 12-15 mo	Diseases caused by *Haemophilus influenzae* B such as sepsis, osteomyelitis, septic arthritis, bacterial meningitis, pneumonia	Redness at injection site, fever, vomiting, diarrhea
	PedvaxHIB (3 doses)	0.5 mL IM at 2 and 4 mo; booster at 12-18 mo		Same as for DTwP and Hib
Hepatitis B vaccine	Recombivax HB, Engerix-B	Birth, 1-2 mo, 6-18 mo IM (see package inserts and CDC schedule for doses, as these vary with brand and age)	Given to children and adults for hepatitis B protection	Redness at injection site, headache, nausea, myalgia, jaw pain, fever
Hepatitis A vaccine	Havrix	1440 EL units for adults >18 yr old; 720 EL units for 12-18 yr old—2 doses 6 mo apart	Hepatitis A	Local side effects, fever, malaise, anorexia, headache, nausea,
	VAQTA	50 units in adults; 25 units in children		
Hepatitis A and B vaccine	Twinrix	1 mL IM × 3 doses, with the second dose scheduled 1 mo after the first, and the third dose 6 mo after the first dose for ages <18 yr	Hepatitis A and B	Pain, redness and swelling at injection site, headache, lethargy, loss of appetite, fever, and GI symptoms
Varicella vaccine	Varivax	0.5 mL SC >12-15 mo, with second dose at 4-6 yr Adults: 0.5 mL SC, with second dose in 4-8 wk	Varicella	Local reaction at injection site, rash, fever
Influenza vaccine	NTN	6 mo-35 mo, 0.25 mL × 2 doses 2 mo apart >3 yr, 0.5 mL yearly	Annual vaccination for influenza, especially indicated for those susceptible to URIs	Local redness, fever, myalgia, malaise
Influenza vaccine A and B, live	Fluvirin, Fluzone	Adults: 0.5 mL IM single dose IM as single dose		Runny nose, nasal congestion, cough, sore throat, low-grade fever, myalgia, chills, headache, lethargy
	Fluvirin	0.5 mL intranasal	For use with healthy persons aged 2-49 yr	
Pneumococcal 23-valent vaccine (PPV)	Pneumovax 23	Certain children 2-6 yr and adults 0.5 mL SC, IM as single dose	Pneumococcal pneumonia and bacteremia, adults and children >2 yr	Local reaction, fever, arthralgia, myalgia, rash
Pneumococcal 7-valent conjugate vaccine (PCV)	Prevnar	0.5 mL IM based on initial immunization age; 4 doses for infants at 2, 4, 6, and 12-15 mo; 3 doses for 7-11 mo; 2 doses for 12-23 mo; 1 dose for 24 mo-9 yr	Invasive pneumococcal infections in infants and toddlers	Local reaction, irritability, restless sleep, drowsiness, decreased appetite
BCG (bacille Calmette-Guérin) vaccine	Generic, TICE	0.2-0.3 mL percutaneously by small puncture wounds	Tuberculosis if person is at high risk	Swollen lymph nodes

Continued

TABLE 16-2 SELECT AGENTS THAT PROVIDE ACTIVE IMMUNITY—cont'd

IMMUNIZING AGENT	TRADE NAME	DOSE, ROUTE, AND FREQUENCY	INDICATIONS FOR PROTECTION	SIDE EFFECTS
Rotavirus vaccine	RotaTeq	3 (2 mL) doses PO at 2, 4, 6 mo	Prevents rotavirus	Diarrhea, vomiting, fever, runny nose, sore throat, wheezing or coughing, and ear infection
	Rotarix	2 (1 mL) doses PO at 6 wk and 4 wk later	Immunity to rotavirus	Crying, fussing, cough, runny nose, fever, loss of appetite, vomiting
Meningococcal vaccine—MCV4	Menactra	0.5 mL IM for 11-55 yr	Meningitis	Fever, rash
Human papillomavirus (HPV) recombinant vaccine	Gardasil (HPV4)	0.5 mL IM for each dose in females; first dose followed by second dose 1 mo later, and third dose 6 mo after first dose	Women aged 11-26 yr for HPV, a cause of cervical cancer	Pain, itching, swelling, and redness at injection site; fever, nausea, dizziness
	Cervarix (HPV2)	0.5 mL IM for each dose in males or females; first dose followed by second dose 2 mo later, and third dose 6 mo after first dose	Women same as above; males 9-18 yr	
Herpes zoster vaccine	Zostavax	0.65 mL SC to adults >60 yr, single dose	Herpes zoster (shingles)	Facial reddening, rash, fever
Rabies vaccine	Imovax	Preexposure: 1 mL IM × 4 doses; Postexposure: 1 mL IM × 5 doses	Rabies	Local reaction, headache, nausea, abdominal pain, muscle aches
SUPER SHOTS				
Diphtheria and tetanus toxoids, (DTaP), Hepatitis B and IPV vaccines	Pediarix	0.5 mL IM at 2, 4, and 6 mo	Diphtheria, tetanus, pertussis, hepatitis B, poliomyelitis	Same as with the individual vaccines listed earlier
MMR and varicella vaccines	ProQuad	0.5 mL SC at 12 mo and 12 yr	Rubeola, rubella, mumps, and chickenpox	Same as with the individual vaccines listed earlier

Tetanus Toxoid (TT)

Tetanus toxoid should be given to:
- The person with less than three doses of a vaccine containing TT at any time
- The person with a wound who has met the proper schedule of three or more vaccine doses but who has not had a booster in more than 10 years
- The person, including children, with a severe or dirty wound who has not had a tetanus immunization in 5 years (see Table 16-2)

Vaccines for Measles (Rubeola), Mumps, and Rubella (MMR)

The *MMR vaccine*, a live virus vaccine, immunizes against the three diseases. The vaccine is given at ages 12 to 15 months and 4 to 6 years, with doses being at least 4 weeks apart, and to persons who have not had the diseases or whose antibody titer shows insufficient numbers of antibodies for immunity. Pregnant and breast-feeding women and persons who are immunosuppressed because of HIV or tuberculosis (TB) should not be given this vaccine.
- Women who might become pregnant within 1 month should not receive this immunization.
- MMR must be reconstituted using a fluid supplied with the vaccine or fluid with no antibacterial or bacteriostatic additives.
- Rubella vaccine (Meruvax II), rubella and mumps vaccine (Biavax), and mumps vaccine (Mumpsvax) are available for those persons requiring immunity for a single disease (see Table 16-2).

Did You Know?

Some states now require a rubella antibody titer for all women of childbearing age to show their immune state before issuing a marriage license; however, the person may decline immunity testing.

Poliomyelitis Vaccines (IPV, OPV)

Two polio vaccines are available for immunization against poliomyelitis: *IPV* (inactivated poliovirus vaccine [Salk vaccine]) and *OPV* (oral poliovirus vaccine [Sabin vaccine], which is no longer available in the United States). The use of IPV is now recommended because of the chance of acquiring polio as a disease from OPV. However, in other countries where polio is still a threat, OPV is still used. Polio vaccine is generally not given to adults older than the age of 18 years unless they have not been vaccinated, are traveling to an endemic area, or are in a high-risk health care occupation (see Table 16-2).

Vaccine for Haemophilus Influenzae Type B

Haemophilus influenzae type B (Hib) vaccine is used to provide protection against the virus that is a common cause of meningitis in young children. The child who is allergic to Hib vaccine or its components or is younger than 6 weeks of age should not be given the vaccine (see Table 16-2).

Vaccines for Hepatitis A and B

Hepatitis B vaccine (Recombivax HB, Engerix-B) is an inactive noninfectious viral antigen vaccine. The vaccine is required in many states for childcare facilities and school attendance and is recommended for health care workers, patients on hemodialysis or who receive blood products, persons at high risk for sexually transmitted diseases, drug users, and persons in contact with hepatitis B. Hepatitis B vaccine is now given to infants, beginning with the first dose either at birth or at 1 month of age, then at 2 and 4 months, with the fourth injection at 6 to 18 months of age.

Hepatitis A vaccine (Havrix), also an inactive viral antigen, is provided to persons who are traveling to endemic areas for hepatitis A and to all children 1 year of age, with a second dose in 6 months. Persons with chronic liver disease, those with employment situations, such as health care workers, or lifestyles that put the individual at risk may be given the vaccine prophylactically. Length of protection is unknown but is believed to be up to 10 years.

A combination of *Hepatitis B and A vaccine* (Twinrix) is available (see Table 16-2).

Vaccine for Chickenpox

Varicella vaccine (Varivax), an attenuated viral vaccine, is recommended at age 12 months of age and is required in most states for admission to school. Adults with no evidence of immunity should receive two doses of the vaccine 4 weeks apart. The length of immunity against chickenpox using this live attenuated varicella virus has not been confirmed, but studies indicate that immunity lasts at least six years, with the need for a booster not established. All adults with no evidence of immunity to varicella should receive two doses of varicella vaccine 4 weeks apart.

Varivax should not be given to persons with hypersensitivity to components of the vaccine, with active untreated TB, with febrile infections, with neoplasms of the bone marrow or lymphatic system, or in an immunosuppressed state. This vaccine should not be given to pregnant women or those who may be pregnant within 3 months of vaccination (see Table 16-2).

Vaccines for Influenza

Influenza vaccines, including injectable and intranasal types, produce immunity to only those strains of influenza viruses expected to cause disease in the United States in a given year. Some strains of influenza have vaccines developed on a yearly basis based on the viral strains that will possibly be prevalent—for example, the H1N1 (swine flu) vaccine in 2009 to 2010. These immunizations are recommended yearly for all persons older than 6 months of age. Those who have a special need for immunization are persons older than age 65 years; those with chronic medical conditions; those in long-term care facilities; people with chronic pulmonary or cardiovascular conditions or with chronic metabolic, renal, immunosuppressive, or hematopoietic blood diseases; children 6 months to 18 years of age on aspirin therapy (reducing the chance of influenza virus causing Reye syndrome); and health care workers or members of households with persons at high risk. People with an allergy to eggs or neomycin should not receive any influenza vaccine unless desensitized. A person with a moderate to severe illness should delay taking this vaccine.

For children younger than 2 years of age and nonpregnant persons aged 5 to 49 years without severe medical conditions, an acceptable alternative to parenteral immunization is *FluMist*, a live attenuated influenza vaccine (LAIV) that is administered intranasally (see Table 16-2).

Vaccine for Pneumonia

Two types of pneumococcal vaccine are available—one for children and the other for adults. *Pneumococcal conjugated vaccine (PCV)* is recommended for all children aged 2 to 23 months, with alternative schedules for some children aged 24 to 59 months, for *Streptococcus pneumoniae*. A final dose should be given at 12 years of age. The vaccine also gives protection against meningitis and offers some protection against otitis media.

All adults older than age 65 years should receive one dose of *pneumococcal polysaccharide vaccine (PPV)*. Persons with chronic disorders and adults aged 19 to 64 years should receive PPV. Persons over age 65 should be revaccinated if the initial vaccination was more than 5 years previously and if the person was younger than 65 when the initial vaccine was administered. This

vaccine should be delayed in people with fever (see Table 16-2).

Vaccine for Tuberculosis

Bacille Calmette-Guérin (BCG) vaccine is used to immunize against TB. The vaccine is commonly used only for persons at high risk for exposure to TB, such as those traveling to areas with high incidence of TB, persons with family members with active TB, or health care workers who are routinely exposed to the disease. The administration of BCG vaccine is percutaneous, by rubbing 0.2 to 0.3 mL of the vaccine on the skin and then making small punctures in that area. The area should be kept dry for 24 hours without a dressing. The person receiving the medication should be aware that any subsequent tuberculin skin tests should show positive results and a radiograph will be necessary for further testing for TB (see Table 16-2).

Vaccine for Rotavirus

The vaccine for rotavirus, a common cause of diarrhea in children younger than 3 years of age, contains five strains of rotaviruses. *Rotavirus vaccine (RotaTeq)*, given orally in three doses at 2, 4, and 6 months of age, may be administered with other vaccines for infants. Rotarix is given to infants in two doses at 6 weeks and 24 weeks (see Table 16-2).

Vaccine for Meningitis

Meningococcal vaccine is available in two forms—one that contains *inactivated bacteria (MPSV4)* and one containing bacterial components conjugated to *diphtheria toxoid protein (MCV4)*; however, this vaccine does not contain live bacteria. The meningococcal conjugate vaccine protects against four different strains of the causative bacteria for meningitis, *Neisseria meningitides*. The MCV4 vaccine is to be administered to 11- to 55-year-olds, but especially to college students living in dormitories or other persons at risk because of travel or working conditions. MPSV4 is an acceptable alternative for children and adolescents. Usually one dose of vaccine is adequate, but a second dose 5 years later may be indicated in persons at high risk for contracting the disease. Some colleges now require that all freshmen be immunized before admission to prevent outbreaks of the disease. The vaccine may be administered to anyone who has been exposed during an outbreak, including pregnant women (see Table 16-2).

Vaccine for Human Papillomavirus

HPV vaccines (*Gardasil* and *Cervarix*) have been developed to prevent cervical cancer, precancerous genital lesions, and genital warts caused by HPV. The vaccines are 70% effective for cervical cancer and 90% effective for genital warts. The CDC recommends routine HPV vaccination for females from 11 to 26 years of age using either vaccine, to be given in three doses. For males aged 9 to 26 years, Gardasil is the recommended vaccine. The length of immunity is unknown at present but is at least 5 years (see Table 16-2).

Vaccine for Shingles

The *zoster vaccine (Zostavax)* provides protection against shingles and the associated chronic pain. In October 2006 the CDC recommended that zoster vaccine be administered to all people age 60 and older including those who have previously had shingles. Only one dose is necessary at present. The vaccine is not a substitute for herpes zoster vaccine for chickenpox in children (see Table 16-2).

"Super Shots"

Researchers have developed and continue to test what are being called "super shots"—combinations of vaccines that give a child protection for more diseases with fewer injections. Children can now receive up to 16 immunizations in the first 2 years of life; the new combination immunizations reduce this number. By combining vaccines, it is hoped that the likelihood of completion of the immunization schedule will be increased, and pain for children and parents will be reduced (see Table 16-2).

One of the most important developments is a super shot for *diphtheria, tetanus, pertussis, hepatitis B, and polio vaccine (Pediarix)*. Another approved super shot is the combination of MMR vaccine with varicella vaccine *(ProQuad)*. *Pentacel* (a combination of DTaP, Hib, and IPV) is also approved for multiple immunizations in one injection.

VACCINES FOR SPECIFIC POPULATIONS

Vaccine for Rabies

Rabies vaccine is given prophylactically to those persons whose occupation or travel puts them at high risk for potential contact with rabid animals. This vaccine is an exception to the rule of immunization because the vaccine is given in most cases after potential exposure to the disease organism following an animal bite. Additional doses may be required after exposure is confirmed. Rabies is slow to develop, and the affected persons may be vaccinated after transmission of the organism and still have sufficient time to build antibodies against the invading organisms, providing active immunity. After

receiving a dose of rabies immune globulin for short-term immunity, the affected person is then given the killed virus vaccine.

PATIENT SAFETY WITH AGENTS FOR ACTIVE IMMUNIZATION

With all immunizations, the patient should remain in the office for 15 to 30 minutes after administration to observe for adverse reactions such as shortness of breath, wheezing, or a drop in blood pressure. If the patient does not remain, documentation of the leaving as well as the time of immunization provides legal protection if needed. Because adverse reactions are often not reported until the next appointment, the patient or parent should be told to immediately report reactions such as high fever (temperature >104° F to 105° F), collapse, persistent cough (in excess of 3 hours), and seizures.

Do not combine separate vaccines into the same syringe for administration unless the health professional approves and the package inserts state FDA approval of compatibility. Each vaccine should be given as a single medication to prevent adverse reactions and possible interactions among the active immunization components. Table 16-3 gives the recommended schedule of the most common immunizations for children and adults, and Box 16-4 gives a quick reference of the proper route of administration for selected vaccines.

SAFETY WITH VACCINES

The CDC, as a means of providing continued safety for vaccines, has supplied information to the immunization provider for storage and maintenance of vaccines for patient safety. Box 16-5 provides some safety tips related to vaccines. Others may be found at the CDC website (www.cdc.gov/od/science/iso/about_iso.htm).

Important Facts about Agents for Artificial Active Immunity

- Immunizations provide antibody-antigen reactions to produce antibodies for long-term immunity, whereas immune globulins and antitoxins provide antibodies for short-term immunity.
- Active immunity provides long-term disease protection, with the person producing antibodies to the disease process, whereas passive immunity provides short-term disease prevention, with immunity provided with antibodies from other sources.
- Immunizations are administration of vaccines or toxoids. These produce artificial active immunity, with antibodies

Continued

TABLE 16-3 RECOMMENDED IMMUNIZATION SCHEDULE

Recommended Immunization Schedule for Persons Aged 0 Through 6 Years—United States • 2010

For those who fall behind or start late, see the catch-up schedule

Vaccine ▼ Age ▶	Birth	1 month	2 months	4 months	6 months	12 months	15 months	18 months	19–23 months	2–3 years	4–6 years
Hepatitis B[1]	HepB	HepB				HepB					
Rotavirus[2]			RV	RV	RV[2]						
Diphtheria, Tetanus, Pertussis[3]			DTaP	DTaP	DTaP	see footnote[3]	DTaP				DTaP
Haemophilus influenzae type b[4]			Hib	Hib	Hib[4]	Hib					
Pneumococcal[5]			PCV	PCV	PCV	PCV					PPSV
Inactivated Poliovirus[6]			IPV	IPV		IPV					IPV
Influenza[7]						Influenza (Yearly)					
Measles, Mumps, Rubella[8]						MMR		see footnote[8]			MMR
Varicella[9]						Varicella		see footnote[9]			Varicella
Hepatitis A[10]						HepA (2 doses)				HepA Series	
Meningococcal[11]										MCV	

Range of recommended ages for all children except certain high-risk groups

Range of recommended ages for certain high-risk groups

This schedule includes recommendations in effect as of December 15, 2009. Any dose not administered at the recommended age should be administered at a subsequent visit, when indicated and feasible. The use of a combination vaccine generally is preferred over separate injections of its equivalent component vaccines. Considerations should include provider assessment, patient preference, and the potential for adverse events. Providers should consult the relevant Advisory Committee on Immunization Practices statement for detailed recommendations: **http://www.cdc.gov/vaccines/pubs/acip-list.htm**. Clinically significant adverse events that follow immunization should be reported to the Vaccine Adverse Event Reporting System (VAERS) at **http://www.vaers.hhs.gov** or by telephone, **800-822-7967**.

1. **Hepatitis B vaccine (HepB).** (Minimum age: birth)
   At birth:
   • Administer monovalent HepB to all newborns before hospital discharge.
   • If mother is hepatitis B surface antigen (HBsAg)-positive, administer HepB and 0.5 mL of hepatitis B immune globulin (HBIG) within 12 hours of birth.
   • If mother's HBsAg status is unknown, administer HepB within 12 hours of birth. Determine mother's HBsAg status as soon as possible and, if HBsAg-positive, administer HBIG (no later than age 1 week).
   After the birth dose:
   • The HepB series should be completed with either monovalent HepB or a combination vaccine containing HepB. The second dose should be administered at age 1 or 2 months. Monovalent HepB vaccine should be used for doses administered before age 6 weeks. The final dose should be administered no earlier than age 24 weeks.
   • Infants born to HBsAg-positive mothers should be tested for HBsAg and antibody to HBsAg 1 to 2 months after completion of at least 3 doses of the HepB series, at age 9 through 18 months (generally at the next well-child visit).
   • Administration of 4 doses of HepB to infants is permissible when a combination vaccine containing HepB is administered after the birth dose. The fourth dose should be administered no earlier than age 24 weeks.

2. **Rotavirus vaccine (RV).** (Minimum age: 6 weeks)
   • Administer the first dose at age 6 through 14 weeks (maximum age: 14 weeks 6 days). Vaccination should not be initiated for infants aged 15 weeks 0 days or older.
   • The maximum age for the final dose in the series is 8 months 0 days
   • If Rotarix is administered at ages 2 and 4 months, a dose at 6 months is not indicated.

3. **Diphtheria and tetanus toxoids and acellular pertussis vaccine (DTaP).** (Minimum age: 6 weeks)
   • The fourth dose may be administered as early as age 12 months, provided at least 6 months have elapsed since the third dose.
   • Administer the final dose in the series at age 4 through 6 years.

4. ***Haemophilus influenzae* type b conjugate vaccine (Hib).** (Minimum age: 6 weeks)
   • If PRP-OMP (PedvaxHIB or Comvax [HepB-Hib]) is administered at ages 2 and 4 months, a dose at age 6 months is not indicated.
   • TriHiBit (DTaP/Hib) and Hiberix (PRP-T) should not be used for doses at ages 2, 4, or 6 months for the primary series but can be used as the final dose in children aged 12 months through 4 years.

5. **Pneumococcal vaccine.** (Minimum age: 6 weeks for pneumococcal conjugate vaccine [PCV]; 2 years for pneumococcal polysaccharide vaccine [PPSV])
   • PCV is recommended for all children aged younger than 5 years. Administer 1 dose of PCV to all healthy children aged 24 through 59 months who are not completely vaccinated for their age.
   • Administer PPSV 2 or more months after last dose of PCV to children aged 2 years or older with certain underlying medical conditions, including a cochlear implant. See *MMWR* 1997;46(No. RR-8).

6. **Inactivated poliovirus vaccine (IPV)** (Minimum age: 6 weeks)
   • The final dose in the series should be administered on or after the fourth birthday and at least 6 months following the previous dose.
   • If 4 doses are administered prior to age 4 years a fifth dose should be administered at age 4 through 6 years. See *MMWR* 2009;58(30):829–30.

7. **Influenza vaccine (seasonal).** (Minimum age: 6 months for trivalent inactivated influenza vaccine [TIV]; 2 years for live, attenuated influenza vaccine [LAIV])
   • Administer annually to children aged 6 months through 18 years.
   • For healthy children aged 2 through 6 years (i.e., those who do not have underlying medical conditions that predispose them to influenza complications), either LAIV or TIV may be used, except LAIV should not be given to children aged 2 through 4 years who have had wheezing in the past 12 months.
   • Children receiving TIV should receive 0.25 mL if aged 6 through 35 months or 0.5 mL if aged 3 years or older.
   • Administer 2 doses (separated by at least 4 weeks) to children aged younger than 9 years who are receiving influenza vaccine for the first time or who were vaccinated for the first time during the previous influenza season but only received 1 dose.
   • For recommendations for use of influenza A (H1N1) 2009 monovalent vaccine see *MMWR* 2009;58(No. RR-10).

8. **Measles, mumps, and rubella vaccine (MMR).** (Minimum age: 12 months)
   • Administer the second dose routinely at age 4 through 6 years. However, the second dose may be administered before age 4, provided at least 28 days have elapsed since the first dose.

9. **Varicella vaccine.** (Minimum age: 12 months)
   • Administer the second dose routinely at age 4 through 6 years. However, the second dose may be administered before age 4, provided at least 3 months have elapsed since the first dose.
   • For children aged 12 months through 12 years the minimum interval between doses is 3 months. However, if the second dose was administered at least 28 days after the first dose, it can be accepted as valid.

10. **Hepatitis A vaccine (HepA).** (Minimum age: 12 months)
   • Administer to all children aged 1 year (i.e., aged 12 through 23 months). Administer 2 doses at least 6 months apart.
   • Children not fully vaccinated by age 2 years can be vaccinated at subsequent visits
   • HepA also is recommended for older children who live in areas where vaccination programs target older children, who are at increased risk for infection, or for whom immunity against hepatitis A is desired.

11. **Meningococcal vaccine.** (Minimum age: 2 years for meningococcal conjugate vaccine [MCV4] and for meningococcal polysaccharide vaccine [MPSV4])
   • Administer MCV4 to children aged 2 through 10 years with persistent complement component deficiency, anatomic or functional asplenia, and certain other conditions placing them at high risk.
   • Administer MCV4 to children previously vaccinated with MCV4 or MPSV4 after 3 years if first dose administered at age 2 through 6 years. See *MMWR* 2009;58:1042–3.

The Recommended Immunization Schedules for Persons Aged 0 through 18 Years are approved by the Advisory Committee on Immunization Practices (**http://www.cdc.gov/vaccines/recs/acip**), the American Academy of Pediatrics (**http://www.aap.org**), and the American Academy of Family Physicians (**http://www.aafp.org**).

Department of Health and Human Services • Centers for Disease Control and Prevention

CS207330-A

From the Centers for Disease Control and Prevention, Atlanta.

BOX 16-4 PROPER ADMINISTRATION ROUTES FOR IMMUNIZATIONS

Subcutaneous	Intramuscular	Intranasal	Oral
MMR	DTaP, DT, Td	Hepatitis A	RotaTeq
IPV	Hepatitis B	FluMist	
Pneumococcal polysaccharide	Hib	H1N1 (swine flu)	
Varicella	IPV		
Meningococcal polysaccharide	Meningococcal conjugate		
Pneumococcal conjugate	Tetanus toxoid		
Hepatitis A			

Important Facts about Agents for Artificial Active Immunity—cont'd

developing over a period of time to provide immunity for years.
- Vaccines contain a suspension of whole or fractionated microorganisms. Toxoids are bacterial toxins that have been changed to a nontoxic state.
- Vaccines are safe, although mild reactions are fairly common. Serious adverse effects rarely occur.
- Live vaccines should not be given to immunocompromised patients. For persons who have recently received gamma globulins, immunity may not occur.
- Yearly the Centers for Disease Control and Prevention (CDC) issues statements of recommended vaccines, which should be checked on a regular basis to ensure proper vaccination of patients.
- For diseases with specific vaccines, the routine for administration of these should be obtained from the CDC to ensure safety for travel to susceptible areas, exposure to disease, or specific circumstances that indicate use of these vaccines.

Did You Know?

The vaccines of the future include those for cytomegalovirus, human immunodeficiency virus (HIV), herpes simplex virus, *Staphylococcus aureus*, group B streptococci, and malaria.

AGENTS FOR ARTIFICIAL PASSIVE IMMUNITY

Passive immunity occurs when antibodies are injected into the body for an immediate, rapid but short-lived type of immunity, lasting for only a few weeks or months.

BOX 16-5 SAFE STORAGE OF VACCINES

- Inspect vaccines on delivery and monitor refrigerator and freezer temperatures to ensure maintenance of the proper temperature during delivery.
- Vaccines are fragile and must be kept at recommended temperatures at all times. It is better to not vaccinate than to administer a dose of vaccine that has been mishandled.
- Rotate vaccine stock so that the oldest vaccines are used first, being sure of the expiration date.
- If reconstitution of medication is required, be sure to use specified diluent.
- Administer vaccines within the prescribed time period after reconstitution.
- Wait to draw vaccines into syringes until immediately before administration.
- Anyone who received compromised vaccine will have to be revaccinated, making parents or caregivers unhappy because the recipient must receive repeat doses of vaccines.
- If errors in vaccine storage and administration occur, take corrective action immediately to prevent recurrence, and notify public health authorities.

CLINICAL TIP

To lessen pain of vaccines with children, one technique is to have children blow on a feather to blow away the pain. Blowing lessens perceived pain. Another technique is to swab the forearm with alcohol and have the child blow on the spot. The person cannot perceive the difference in the cold of blowing and the pain from the immunization at the same time.

Antitoxins

Antitoxins are immune agents produced in response to an antigen and capable of neutralizing toxins. Before administration the patient should be skin tested to protect from anaphylaxis caused by allergies. Antitoxins from human and animal sources are used for prophylactic and therapeutic purposes for specific toxins.

Immune Globulins

Immune globulins are antibodies found in serum that are used in the prevention of diseases such as hepatitis B, tetanus, and rabies. Active immunizing agents should not be administered at the same time as immune globulins, because the immune globulins may stop the actions of the immunizing agents to produce antibodies.

Immune Globulins for Specific Conditions

Rho(D) immune human globulin (RhoGAM) is an antibody preparation given after delivery to desensitize Rh-negative mothers who delivers an Rh-positive baby (Figure 16-5). The sensitization of the mother occurs when any of the blood cells from the infant enter the bloodstream of the mother, usually at birth, causing antibody formation in the mother. If that mother has a subsequent Rh-positive infant, the produced antibodies may cause erythroblastosis fetalis in the second infant. RhoGAM must be administered within 72 hours after delivery to diminish antibody formation by the mother.

Respiratory Syncytial Virus Immune Globulin

Respiratory syncytial virus (RSV) immune globulin for lower respiratory diseases caused by RSV is produced using DNA technology. Immunization with *polyvalent RSV-10 (Respigam)* and *palivizumab* (a monoclonal antibody) are often used with premature babies to prevent respiratory problems. Patients, including those who develop an RSV infection, should continue to receive monthly doses throughout the RSV season. Other selected agents for artificial passive immunity are found in Table 16-4.

EDUCATION CONCERNING IMMUNIZATIONS

In today's world, many childhood diseases that were fatal several generations ago are now almost eradicated in the United States because of immunizations. Parents must understand the need for immunizing children. State and federal laws require immunizations for school, although some parents may refuse to immunize their child because of cultural or religious beliefs. For the child to obtain maximum effect of immunizations, spacing of immunizations should be at the CDC-suggested time intervals. Although time intervals longer than those recommended may be acceptable in some cases, shorter intervals for obtaining immunizations required by law are unacceptable. The child who is not properly immunized during the first year and a half of life and whose parents then wait until school age in most cases will not be allowed to attend school until immunizations have been administered. Administering multiple vaccines over a short period of time puts the child at greater risk for adverse reactions.

Adults have a higher incidence of noncompliance than children. The allied health professional should assist the adult patient in keeping current with vaccines such as diphtheria-tetanus (Td) vaccine. The at-risk patient should be encouraged to have influenza immunizations yearly, and the pneumococcal vaccine as recommended. As vaccines are available for artificial active immunity, such as HPV and shingles vaccines, adults and

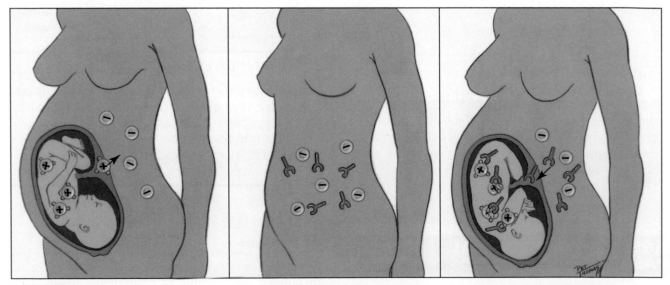

First pregnancy Rh− mother exposed to Rh+ agglutinogens.

After exposure, Rh− mother produces anti-Rh agglutinins.

Second pregnancy with Rh+ fetus. Anti-Rh agglutinins cause agglutination of fetal red blood cells.

Figure 16-5 RhoGAM is necessary to prevent hemolytic disease in an infant whose Rh-mother has been exposed to an Rh-positive fetus. (From Applegate E: *The anatomy and physiology learning system*, ed 4, St Louis, 2011, Saunders.)

TABLE 16-4 SELECT AGENTS FOR ARTIFICIALLY ACQUIRED PASSIVE IMMUNITY

IMMUNIZING AGENT	TRADE NAME	DOSE, ROUTE, AND FREQUNECY	INDICATIONS	SIDE EFFECTS
ANTITOXINS				
Diphtheria antitoxin (from horses, so must skin test for allergies)	NTN	Prophylactic: 10,000 units IM Therapeutic: 20,000-120,000 units IM or IV	Prevention or treatment of diphtheria	Redness at injection site
SERUMS AND IMMUNE GLOBULINS				
Botulism immune globulin	BabyBIG	See package insert	Prevention and treatment of botulism	Given IV with the resultant side effects and dangers
Rabies immune globulin	Imogam, HyperRab	20 units/kg IM ($\frac{1}{2}$ of dose may be used to infiltrate the wound)	Exposure to rabies	Fever, soreness at injection site
Tetanus immune (human) globulin	HyperTET	Prophylactic: 250-500 units IM (children based on weight) Therapeutic: 500-3000 units IM	Passive immunization to tetanus	Tenderness and muscle stiffness
Hepatitis B immune globulin	HBIG, HyperHep B, Nabi-HB, HepaGam B	0.06 mL/kg IM within 7 days of exposure for most situations	Postexposure prophylaxis to hepatitis B	Local reaction, fever, urticaria
Immune human serum globulin	IV: Carimune NF, Felbogamma, Gammunex, Octagam, Privigen, Gammagard IM: GamaSTA SD	100-200 mg/kg IV q mo 200-400 mg/kg IV q mo 0.02-1.3 mL/kg IM (1.3-2 mL/kg for adults) depending on reason for use	Passive immunity for rubeola, hepatitis A, varicella, and so on; use IV for immunodeficiency syndrome	Local reaction, fever, urticaria
RSV monoclonal antibody (palivizumab)	Synagis	Based on body weight IM during RSV season	RSV in premature infants and susceptible children	Local reaction, rash, diarrhea, cough, otitis
Respiratory syncytial immune globulin	RespiGam	750 mg/kg IV	Reduce lower respiratory tract infections from RSV in children <24 mo old at high risk	Fever, diarrhea, vomiting, wheezing
Rho(D) immune globulin	RhoGam	300 mg IM at 26-28 wks, within 72 hr or after 72 hr have passed if Rh status is unknown	Desensitization to RhoD in Rh negative mothers	Lethargy, myalgia, irritation at injection site

IM, intramuscularly; *IV,* intravenously; *NTN,* no trade name; *RSV,* respiratory syncytial virus; *SC,* subcutaneously.

children should be encouraged to avail themselves of this protection.

Immunizations save indirectly in medical and societal costs. Parents must do their part to make sure their children are immunized with current vaccines and new immunizations as these become available. Although 95% of all school children have been vaccinated, parents and children of migrant workers, new immigrants, and others who may not be aware of the need for and benefits of immunization must be educated. *The risk of acquiring the disease is much greater than the risk associated with vaccines.* When large numbers of a population are not immunized, chances of exposure to infectious diseases are increased.

Persons traveling to foreign countries should contact their health care provider or local health department well in advance of the departure date for needed (either required or suggested) immunizations. These immunizations must be given in advance to produce adequate immunity before traveling (Table 16-5).

Important Facts about Education For Immunizations

- The CDC sets requirements to meet public health needs.
- Educating parents about the need for immunizations for children is an important role for the allied health professional. Continued immune states in adult patients should be checked and proper immunizations given as indicated.
- If a question of whether to administer an immunization or not exists, the potential for benefit must be weighed against the potential for risks.
- Documentation of immunizations is specific, and the National Childhood Vaccine Act of 1986 provides the guidelines for charting.

IMMUNOSUPPRESSANTS

With the advent of transplantation of body organs such as the liver, heart, and kidney, a new drug category was necessary to decrease or prevent normal antigen-antibody

---

TABLE 16-5 IMMUNIZATIONS FOR TRAVEL TO FOREIGN COUNTRIES OR FOR SPECIFIC SITUATIONS

IMMUNIZING AGENT	TRADE NAME	DOSE, ROUTE, AND FREQUENCY	INDICATIONS FOR PROTECTION	SIDE EFFECTS
Cholera vaccine	NTN	0.5 mL SC or IM 2 doses 1 wk to 1 mo apart	Cholera for travelers in areas of high risk	Local reaction, fever, malaise, headache
Plague vaccine	NTN	First dose: 1 mL IM; second dose: 0.2 mL IM 2-3 mo after first dose and again at 6 mo, followed by 0.1 to 0.2 mL boosters q6 mo while in the endemic region	Plague for those at risk for exposure	Malaise, headache, local erythema
Rabies vaccine	Imovax	See package insert;1 mL IM × 4 doses pre-exposure, second dose 7 days after first, third dose 3-4 wk after first; 4 doses post-exposure	Rabies: preexposure and postexposure for those at risk; and	Local reactions, nausea, headache, myalgia, abdominal pain
	RabAvert	3 doses: 1 mL IM pre-exposure, 7 days, 14 days, 21-28 days; 5 doses post-exposure	Prophylaxis (preexposure)	
Typhoid Parenteral	NTN Typhim VI	0.5 mL SC with booster in 4 wk or more 0.5 mL IM x 1 dose Children <10 yr 0.25 mL, booster 0.5 mL SC or 0.1 mL ID q3 yr 0.5 mL IM and q 2 yr if needed owing to travel to endemic areas	Travelers who will be in countries where typhoid is endemic	Local reactions, malaise, myalgia, fever
Oral	Vivotif Berna Vaccine	1 cap 1 hr ac × 4 doses (at least 1 week before potential exposure) with booster in 5 years		GI symptoms, rash
Yellow fever vaccine	YF-VAX	0.5 mL SC	Travelers who will be in countries where yellow fever is endemic	Headaches, myalgia, rash, GI symptoms

AC, before meals; *GI,* gastrointestinal; *ID,* intradermally; *IM,* intramuscularly; *NTN,* no trade name; *SC,* subcutaneously.

response of the body. This new group of drugs, known as **immunosuppressants,** is used mainly in transplantation but has other uses such as in autoimmune diseases and severe allergic reactions. When a foreign substance or organ is transplanted into the body, the body's immune response processes transplanted matter as a foreign substance. Without these agents, tissue destruction and rejection of the transplanted organs would certainly occur. The main adverse effects of using immunosuppressive medications are that these agents lower the body's ability to fight diseases, leaving the patient more susceptible to infections, infectious diseases, and the possibility of malignancies, and the inherent side effects of each medication.

Corticosteroids have the ability to suppress immune responses and are used to produce potent antiinflammatory and antiallergic effects by causing lymphocytes in blood to be redistributed in the bone marrow, lowering the number of lymphocytes in the blood. Corticosteroids are most frequently used in conjunction with other immunosuppressive agents (see Chapter 20).

Other immunosuppressive agents are used, including the following:

- **Azathioprine** (Imuran), a derivative of the antineoplastic mercaptopurine, suppresses formation of new B and T cells by suppressing DNA and RNA synthesis. Azathioprine is **mutagenic, teratogenic,** and **carcinogenic.**
- **Cyclosporine** (Sandimmune), a metabolite produced by a fungus, is a potent immunosuppressive agent but is not cytotoxic. It suppresses T-cell function, thus depressing the immune response. When this medication is discontinued, normal T-cell function resumes. Administered along with corticosteroids, cyclosporine is used to prevent organ rejection after transplantation.
- **Mycophenolate mofetil** (CellCept) and **mycophenolic acid** (Myfortic) inhibit the activity of T cells and B cells to reduce the effectiveness of the immune system. The primary use of both of these drugs is prevention of rejection in renal transplantation, but mycophenolate may also be used with liver and heart transplantation (Table 16-6).

Patient Education for Compliance

1. A person taking immunosuppressant drugs is susceptible to infectious disease because these agents lower the body's immune response.
2. No immunizations with live virus vaccines should be administered to people taking immunosuppressants.
3. Report unusual bleeding or bruising, as well as sore throat and mouth sores, to health care provider when taking immunosuppressants.
4. Women of childbearing age should not take these medications; pregnancy must be avoided.

Patient Education for Compliance—cont'd

5. Avoid grapefruit juice and grapefruit when taking cyclosporine.
6. Cyclosporine should be taken consistently at the same time(s) each day with meals.
7. Maintain good dental hygiene.

IMMUNOSTIMULANTS

Drugs used to increase or stimulate the immune system response to treat cancer and HIV infection are called **immunostimulants.** The first agents, which became available in the 1980s with the advent of DNA technology, are used to stimulate the immune system when deficiencies exist and are a rapidly increasing group of medications. The acquired **immunodeficiency** may be caused by medications such as chemotherapy or it may be acquired through viral infections such as HIV. Immunostimulants are expected to provide control of pain and discomfort found with many illnesses. **Interferon alfa** and **interleukin-2** (Proleukin) are two of the earliest medications to stimulate the production of B cells and killer T cells. By increasing the number of killer T cells, it is thought that these drugs provide the needed T cells to attack and destroy infections or cancers in the affected person. Many of these drugs are more commonly used and approved for use as antineoplastics (see Chapter 18) or in the treatment of hepatitis C infection (see Table 16-6 for a sample of these agents).

Important Facts about Immunosuppressants and Immunostimulants

- Immunosuppressants are used to prevent organ rejection after transplants and to treat autoimmune diseases such as rheumatoid arthritis.
- Immunosuppressants increase the risk of infections and lymphomas.
- Cyclosporine is one of the most effective immunosuppressants.
- Corticosteroids are often given as adjunct medications with other immunosuppressants.
- Azathioprine and other cytotoxic drugs suppress immune responses by B and T cells. Many antineoplastic agents produce immunosuppression as a side effect.
- Research regarding immunostimulants is increasing because of their potential use in the treatment of human immunodeficiency virus (HIV) infection and other acquired immunodeficiencies.

TABLE 16-6 SELECTED AGENTS OF IMMUNOTHERAPY

DRUG (GENERIC)	TRADE NAME	USUAL ADULT DOSE, ROUTE, AND FREQUENCY	MAJOR SIDE EFFECTS	INDICATIONS FOR USE	DRUG INTERACTIONS
IMMUNOSUPPRESSANTS					
azathioprine	Imuran, Azasan	3-5 mg/kg/day PO initially; 1-3 mg/kg/day as maintenance dose	Nausea, vomiting, decrease in blood cells, depression of bone marrow	Kidney transplantation	allopurinol, live virus vaccines, other immunosuppressants
cyclosporine	Sandimmune, Neoral, Gengraf	10-14 mg/kg/day PO, IV for 1-2 wk; then taper to maintenance dose of 5-10 mg/kg/day	Renal damage	Heart, kidney, or liver transplant	Same as azathioprine, plus cimetidine, danazol, diltiazem, ACE inhibitors, K-sparing diuretics, erythromycin, K supplements, ketoconazole
mycophenolate mofetil	CellCept	2-3 g/day PO, IV in 2 divided doses (to be given with corticosteroids and cyclosporine)	Renal damage, insomnia, dysrhythmias, arthralgia	Kidney, heart, liver transplantation	acyclovir, ganciclovir, antacids, probenecid, cholestyramine, other immunosuppressants, live virus vaccines
mycophenolic acid	Myfortic	720 mg PO bid	Renal damage, insomnia, dysrhythmias, arthralgia	Kidney transplant	Same as above
sirolimus	Rapamune	6 mg PO stat, then 2 mg/day PO		Kidney transplant	None given
tacrolimus	Prograf	See package insert		Heart, liver, and kidney transplant	Antifungals, aminoglycosides, calcium channel blockers, cimetidine, erythromycin
IMMUNOSTIMULANTS					
interferon alfa	Roferon-A	Varies among patients; IM, IV, SC	Fever, flulike symptoms, nausea, diarrhea	AIDS-related conditions, Kaposi's sarcoma, other malignancies	aminophylline, zidovudine

ACE, Angiotensin-converting enzyme; *AIDS,* acquired immunodeficiency syndrome; *IM,* intramuscularly; *IV,* intravenously; *PO,* orally; *SC,* subcutaneously.

SUMMARY

Vaccines were one of the greatest achievements in the medical field in the twentieth century. Immunizations have altered the way Americans look at quality of life, from childhood through adolescence into aging. Vicious diseases, such as smallpox, have been virtually erased, and polio is expected to be eradicated early in this century.

Immunizations may provide artificial active immunity, in which the body builds its own antibodies to foreign antigens. This immunity is usually long acting, sometimes lasting a lifetime. Artificial active immunity begins at birth and continues throughout life. Parents must be taught the dangers of not immunizing children and the importance of laws requiring that certain vaccines be administered before a child attends school.

Artificial passive immunity, or short-term immunity, is introduced through antitoxins from human or animal sources or as immune globulins in serum. Passive immunity is effective immediately, as the serum or antitoxin contains antibodies needed to fight the specific disease.

Immunizations are indicated for lifelong medical care—from infants obtaining hepatitis B vaccine to chronically ill older adults who receive influenza and pneumonia vaccines. To achieve the full potential of vaccines, adults must recognize that vaccines mobilize the body's natural defenses, and they should seek vaccinations for themselves and their children. Health care workers are susceptible to many disease processes and should avail themselves of specific immunizations for protection against pathogens found in medical settings. The vaccine delivery must be extended to adolescents and adults to ensure that they are protected from such diseases as tetanus, influenza, hepatitis B, and pneumococcal disease.

Immunosuppressants are used to prevent tissue rejection by the antibody-antigen reaction when foreign tissue is introduced into the body, such as with organ transplants. HIV, cancers, and other autoimmune diseases respond to immunostimulants, or agents that increase the activity of the immune system. The introduction of new immunostimulants is one of the most rapidly growing medical fields. Immunotherapy is a relatively new area of medicine coming into the forefront by imitating the action of the immune system for the treatment of HIV and with organ transplants.

CRITICAL THINKING EXERCISES

Scenario

Previc Wadhwa, who has an Rh-negative blood type, has just given birth to Jason, who is Rh-positive.

1. What medication is indicated for Mrs. Wadhwa to prevent erythroblastosis fetalis if she should become pregnant again?
2. What is the time limit for giving this medication after childbirth?
3. Would Mrs. Wadhwa need the medication if Jason had been an Rh-negative infant? Why or why not?
4. What would you tell Mrs. Wadhwa if she asked about the dangers of RhoGAM immunization?
5. How would you answer if she asked about the source of the medication?

DRUG CALCULATIONS

1. Drug ordered: CellCept 500 mg
   Available medication:

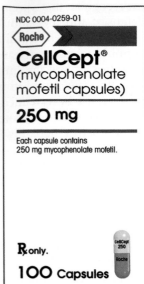

   Dose to be administered: _____

2. Drug ordered: Imuran 4 mg/kg/day PO for a person who weighs 165 lb
   Available medication: azathioprine 50 mg/tab
   Dose to be administered: _____

REVIEW QUESTIONS

1. What is naturally acquired passive immunity? Naturally acquired active immunity? Artificially acquired passive immunity? Artificially acquired active immunity? _____

   _____

   _____

   _____

2. Which of the types of immunity listed in question 1 uses vaccines and toxoids? Which uses antitoxins and immune globulins? Which immunity lasts longer? Why? _____

   _____

   _____

   _____

3. Discuss instances in which immunizations would be contraindicated. Do contraindications always prevent the administration of an immunization? How are the circumstances evaluated? _____

   _____

   _____

   _____

4. List the data required to be included in documentation of immunizations, mandated by the National Childhood Vaccine Act of 1986. _____

   _____

   _____

5. Adults have a higher incidence of nonconformance with immunizations. What can the allied health professional do to lower the incidence of nonimmunization? _____

_____

_____

6. What is the main indication for using immunosuppressants? _____

_____

_____

7. What is the main activity of an immunostimulant? _____

_____

_____

CHAPTER 17

Antimicrobials, Antifungals, and Antivirals

OBJECTIVES

After studying this chapter, you should be capable of doing the following:

- Explaining the difference between pathogenic and nonpathogenic bacteria.
- Describing various forms of bacteria that are pathogenic in the body.
- Describing factors that are important in choosing an antibiotic or antimicrobial agent.
- Explaining the difference between *bacteriostatic* and *bactericidal* agents.
- Explaining how bacteria can acquire resistance to specific antibiotics.

- Knowing why antibiotics, antimicrobials, antivirals, and antifungals may be used prophylactically and when prophylactic use is inappropriate.
- Explaining why some infections are best treated with a multidrug regimen.
- Identifying and classifying by family antibiotics, antimicrobials, antivirals, and antifungals commonly used today.
- Providing patient education for compliance with medications used as antimicrobials, antifungals, and antivirals.

Richard is seen in Dr. Merry's office with an infected lesion on his leg. Dr. Merry examines Richard and gives him a prescription for a topical antibiotic to be applied to the lesion three times a day. Richard is concerned because Dr. Merry did not give him an antibiotic to take orally.

What is your response?

In the past, Richard has taken multiple antibiotics for illnesses. How might this affect the effectiveness of antibiotics he takes in the future?

Why is a topical antibiotic more likely to be used for localized infections? When is a systemic antibiotic more likely to be indicated?

KEY TERMS

Aerobic bacteria
Anaerobic bacteria
Antibacterial drugs
Antibiotic
Antimicrobial
Antiseptic
Bacteria (singular, *bacterium***)**
Bactericidal
Bacteriostatic
Broad-spectrum antibiotic

Disinfectant or germicidal agent
Empiric
Endemic
Facultative bacteria
Fungicidal
Fungistatic
Fungus (plural, *fungi***)**
Germicide
Germistatic agent
Helminths

Host
Microbe
Microbiology
Morphology
Narrow-spectrum antibiotic
Normal flora
Opportunistic infection
Parasite
Pathogen

Photosensitivity
Protozoa (singular, *protozoan***)**
Sanitization
Semisynthetic
Spore
Sterilization
Superinfection
Synthetic
Vector
Virus

EASY WORKING KNOWLEDGE OF INDICATIONS AND SIDE EFFECTS

Common Indications for Antimicrobials, Antifungals, and Antivirals

Infections caused by bacteria, fungi, or viruses
Prevention (prophylaxis) of infection or contamination in select procedures
Disinfectants, germicidals, and antiseptics used in medical settings for asepsis and cleaning

Common Side Effects of Antimicrobials, Antifungals, and Antivirals

Anorexia and changes in taste sensation
Nausea, vomiting, and diarrhea
Photosensitivity
Dizziness, headache, insomnia (fluoroquinolones)
Skin rashes and eruptions

EASY WORKING KNOWLEDGE OF ANTIMICROBIALS, ANTIFUNGALS, AND ANTIVIRALS

DRUG CLASS	PRESCRIPTION	OTC	PREGNANCY CATEGORY	MAJOR INDICATIONS
Antibiotics (penicillins, cephalosporins, macrolides, tetracyclines, aminoglycosides, chloramphenicol, fluoroquinolone antibacterials)	Yes	Some topical ointments and creams	B and C for most antibiotics; D for aminoglycosides and tetracycline	Bacterial infections
Sulfonamides	Yes	No	B and C; D near term of pregnancy	Bacterial infections, especially urinary tract infections
Antitubercular drugs	Yes	No	B, C	Tuberculosis
Antifungal drugs	Yes	Yes (topical)	B, C (nystatin is preferred)	Fungal infections
Antiviral drugs	Yes	No	B, C, X	Viral infections, including human immunodeficiency virus (HIV)
Antimalarial drugs	Yes	No	B, C	Malaria
Antiseptics, disinfectants, and germicides	Yes, including pHisoHex in some states	Yes	N/A	Cleaning and sanitizing animate and inanimate objects to remove microbes

With discovery of sulfonamides in the 1930s and availability of penicillin in the 1940s, a new era in infection treatment began. Since then, many drugs have been produced to either kill or inhibit the growth of bacteria, fungi, and viruses. These drugs have cured diseases such as tuberculosis and some types of pneumonia that until the 1950s were permanently debilitating to fatal. The average human life span in developed countries lengthened greatly, and fewer years of life were lost to devastating infectious disease.

In the 1940s, during World War II, the U.S. government secretly researched penicillin to treat infections among the service members. With the advent of antimicrobials, patients could be given relatively nontoxic medications to control infections until the immune system could fight the infection. Today, these medicines come from plants, animals, or chemical synthesis.

Most people have infections at some point in life and will be treated for the pathogen with medications. Because pathogens are multitudinous and common, affect all body systems, and spare no one, health care professionals in all fields can expect to spend time administering, documenting, and providing patient education about antimicrobials.

WHAT IS AN ANTIBIOTIC?

The term antibiotic (anti, against, plus Greek bios, life; hence, "against life") began with a description of a group of diverse chemicals, some of which were produced to inhibit the growth of or kill other microorganisms when given in low concentrations. Major antibiotic families were discovered before 1955 by screening thousands of cultures from a variety of sources. For example, cephalosporins were derived from the mold of genus *Cephalosporium*, found in the ocean near sewage outflow; streptomycin was derived from *Streptomyces*, a bacterial genus found in the throat of a contaminated chicken; and lincomycin, produced by a variant of *Streptomyces lincolnensis*, came from the soil in Lincoln, Nebraska.

Through use of artificial means, chemists have produced drugs resulting in the creation of families of antibiotics. Each antibiotic in a family is similar to the original chemical, with properties making it useful for treating infections. Antibiotics that contain an original chemical molecule from a microorganism but are further altered are called semisynthetics—for example, penicillin V. Those made completely in a laboratory are called synthetics, such as cephalosporins.

Antibiotics are further classified according to susceptible bacteria against which they are effective, or their *antibacterial spectrum*. Some drugs, called broad-spectrum antibiotics, have a wide range of effectiveness against both gram-positive and gram-negative bacteria. With broad-spectrum antibiotics it is possible to eliminate pathogens without initially performing laboratory tests to identify the exact pathogen involved, so treatment is not delayed. Other antibiotics are effective against a few or specific bacteria and are called narrow-spectrum antibiotics.

CLASSIFICATION OF MICROORGANISMS

Microbiology is the study of microscopic organisms, or microbes, such as fungi, molds, bacteria, and protozoa. Many microorganisms live freely in soil and water, where they are relatively harmless. When these microorganisms leave the free environment and enter a susceptible host, they may become pathogens. Normal flora with beneficial relationships for our bodies are the many microorganisms normally living on our skin or in our bodies. Examples are certain strains of *Escherichia coli* that exist in the gastrointestinal (GI) tract to assist with digestion of food.

Bacteria are a large group of one-celled organisms without a nucleus; bacteria are found everywhere.

Viruses, minute infectious cell particles, are so small that they are visible only through an electron microscope. They are actually small amounts of genetic material wrapped in a protein coat. They can replicate only within living cells and so are parasites on their hosts for nutrition, metabolism, and reproduction. Some can mutate quickly in their hosts, making it difficult to develop effective antiviral treatment. Although viruses are not truly living microorganisms, they are often included when discussing microbiology and antimicrobials.

Did You Know?

Some researchers consider viruses to be parasitic particles; others consider them to have once been primitive organisms that lost all characteristics outside of the host.

Growing as a single cell (such as yeast) or in colonies (such as mushrooms or molds), certain fungi are pathogenic and may cause serious disease in susceptible persons. Protozoa are unicellular animals that may colonize and become pathogenic in susceptible persons.

Parasites do not live freely and require interaction with other organisms, being dependent on their hosts. Fungi and viruses are parasitic, as are other members of the animal kingdom such as lice and helminths. Of importance in the medical field is the high dependency of parasites on host cells for livelihood and ability to reproduce.

IDENTIFICATION OF MICROORGANISMS

For the best effective treatment of an infection, the causative microorganism should be identified, along with drug susceptibility to the medication known. This requires the identification of the microbe by its morphology.

Shape

- *Cocci* are round or spheric bacteria and are further subdivided by the way they combine in groups: *diplococci*, cocci in pairs; *streptococci*, cocci in chains; *staphylococci*, clusters of cocci looking much like bunches of grapes
- *Bacilli* are rod shaped.
- *Spirilla* are spiral shaped.

Gram Staining

Gram staining, a test for narrowing bacterial classification, entails applying crystal violet and iodine, followed by an agent that decolorizes the stain.
- Gram-positive bacteria stain purple.
- Gram-negative bacteria do not keep the stain.

Need for Oxygen

- Aerobic bacteria require oxygen to live.
- Anaerobic bacteria require an oxygen-free environment. Anaerobic organisms, which thrive in the oxygen-free interior of the body, tend to produce virulent infection and may be difficult to eradicate.
- Facultative bacteria can survive in either environment.

ANTIMICROBIALS VERSUS ANTIBIOTICS

Antimicrobials and antibiotics, both having the capability to kill or suppress growth of microorganisms, are distinguished by their origins. The term antimicrobial is broader, including antibiotics, antifungals, antiparasitics, and drugs such as mercury. Antimicrobials reach target cells either through localized activity of the drug at the site of application (e.g., topical, otic, or ophthalmic preparations) or through systemic distribution of the drug. Drugs absorbed systemically can upset the balance of normal body flora, eradicating some and allowing overgrowth of other organisms, resulting in an imbalance that causes a second, new infection at a different site and with a different causative organism—necessitating treatment of the new infection.

Antibiotics are enhanced natural substances or synthetically formed substances originally obtained from organic sources; each antibiotic—a term used to describe those drugs that treat bacterial infections—bears a chemical resemblance to the original chemical substance. The goal of therapy with antibiotics is to destroy or suppress growth of the infecting organism for sufficient time to allow normal host defenses to control the infection, providing a resultant cure. Antibiotics alone cannot always produce a cure. These drugs may be used in conjunction with surgical procedures such as incision and drainage, débridement of wounds, and excision of infected tissue.

BACTERICIDAL VERSUS BACTERIOSTATIC

Antibiotics may function as bacteriostatic agents or as bactericidal agents. By inhibiting the growth of bacteria, bacteriostatic agents inhibit growth of the microorganism without causing death, allowing the body's defense mechanisms extra time to control and eradicate the infection. Bactericidal agents cause either death or destruction of the bacterial cell. The antimicrobial action, whether bacteriostatic or bactericidal, is not firm with some antibiotics because dosage of the drug, drug concentration at infection site, and virulence of the microorganism all contribute to whether the cell is destroyed outright or simply inhibited in its growth. Thus for some medications the same agent may be either bacteriostatic or bactericidal against the given microorganism. See the families of agents discussed later in this chapter for the effective action of each against microorganisms.

FACTORS IN THE CHOICE OF ANTIBIOTICS

When treating infections the goal is to achieve the maximal antimicrobial effect while causing minimal patient harm. Antimicrobial therapy tries to "match the bug and the drug" while considering the patient's physical condition. The appropriate antibiotic choice for each individual is based on the causative organism, its drug

sensitivity, the drug's ability to penetrate the infection's site, and the host factors present. The best antimicrobial therapy occurs when the infecting organism has been identified and is sensitive to the drug selected for the infection's causative organisms. However, in some cases a broad-spectrum medication may be prescribed before the results of testing are obtained; drug therapy may then be narrowed once the results and sensitivities are known.

Drug Sensitivity

The likely microbial that is effective against the microorganism should be considered when the medication is being selected. If a tentative identification of the infective organism is difficult to make, a broad-spectrum antibiotic can be prescribed, or several antibiotics may be prescribed to be taken concurrently. It is widely thought that use of more than one antibiotic for empiric treatment may delay the rapid increase in bacterial resistance to antimicrobial drugs.

A certain medication may be preferred for reasons such as greater efficacy, lower toxicity, or greater sensitivity of the microorganisms to the medication or for such personal factors as cost. Alternative agents may be required if the patient is allergic to the drug of choice or because of toxic effects.

💊 CLINICAL TIP

If therapy must be started before culture and sensitivity results are available, specimens for culture should be obtained before therapy begins. If the laboratory sample is obtained after the patient has started antimicrobial therapy, infecting agents may be suppressed and their identification impeded.

MEDICATION ALERT

The goal of antibiotic therapy is not to kill all the infecting organisms; rather, the goal is to suppress the growth of the microorganisms to allow the host's immune system to subdue the infection and resolve the patient's signs and symptoms of disease.

Patient Factors

Patient factors may influence the choice of drug, route of administration, or dosage. In the immunosuppressed individual, the immune system is important because the compromised state and drugs alone may suppress diseases. Pacemakers, prosthetic joints, and other foreign objects may cause attacks on healthy cells at the site of implantation, requiring the use of antibiotics to prevent an infection that might necessitate removal of the prosthesis. Neonates and the elderly are particularly susceptible to drug toxicity because of accumulation and toxic drug levels in the blood. Pregnancy and lactation pose specific problems in antibiotic treatment because some drugs can cross the placenta or are excreted in breast milk.

Severe allergic reactions are more common with antibiotics, especially **penicillin,** than with any other drug classification. The general rule is that a person who has had an allergic reaction to penicillin should not receive it again. Symptoms of hypersensitivity to antibiotics range from a mild rash, fever, and urticaria with pruritus to generalized erythema or even anaphylaxis.

Did You Know?

A person can become sensitized to a drug even through indirect exposure such as eating foods from animals given antimicrobials. Sensitization may also be caused by a previous use of topical antibiotics. Microbe resistance caused by exposure to antimicrobials in the environment, food, and water supplies is now considered a major public health problem that is being studied by the Centers for Disease Control and Prevention (CDC).

ANTIBIOTIC RESISTANCE

In recent years many discoveries about the growing resistance of many microorganisms to antimicrobials have been made. Resistance often occurs by mutation of the microbe, or changing of the genetic structure, so that currently available medications are no longer effective. Several bacteria—*Staphylococcus aureus*, *E. coli*, and *Mycobacterium tuberculosis*—are now serious clinical problems because of drug resistance.

As a rule, microorganisms resistant to a certain drug will tend to be resistant to other chemically-related antimicrobials, a phenomenon known as *cross-resistance. The person does not become resistant to the antimicrobial; the microbe becomes resistant to the drug.* Thus any person who is infected by the drug-resistant microbe is now affected because the medication will not be as effective. The microorganism may be disease causing, and the more resistant microbe will grow in the environment because of the drug ineffectiveness.

The primary reason for development of drug-resistant bacteria is inappropriate use of antibiotics. The more an antibiotic is used, the faster virulent-resistant microorganisms emerge. Inept prescribing and inappropriate use of medications may also increase the resistance of normal flora, turning them into possible pathogens. Environmental factors such as overcrowding and poor sanitation may play a role in microorganisms developing resistance because of the repeated infections and/or repeated use of antimicrobials to fight infections.

SUPERINFECTION AND ANTIBIOTIC USE

A *superinfection* is a secondary infection appearing during the course of treatment for a primary infection, such as a yeast infection that arises during the course of treatment with penicillin for bacterial pneumonia. Superinfection most often occurs when the antimicrobial inhibits or alters the balance of normal flora within the body.

Broad-spectrum antibiotics tend to kill off more normal flora than targeted drugs, and they also promote drug resistance of multiple organisms. Drugs that change the body's immune responses, such as corticosteroids and immunosuppressive drugs, may also permit the emergence of superinfections.

PROPHYLACTIC USE OF ANTIBIOTICS

From 30% to 50% of antibiotics prescribed in the United States are used for prophylactic reasons rather than to treat a current infection. Much of prophylactic use is not necessary, but in some situations it is appropriate and effective. An example of appropriate prophylaxis is the use of **ciprofloxacin** for those persons who have been exposed to anthrax through bioterrorism.

The risks of toxic effects, superinfections, and other adverse reactions of using antimicrobials should be weighed against the advantages before drugs are used prophylactically. People with congenital or valvular heart disease, those with some prostheses, and those who have had rheumatic fever may need prophylactic antibiotics before surgery or dental procedures to decrease normal flora, reducing the chance of endocarditis. Neutropenia (low neutrophil counts) increases the risk of infections and may be another indication for prophylactic use. Finally, antimicrobial agents are given prophylactically in single large doses to effectively treat persons who have been exposed to sexually transmitted diseases but have not yet shown signs of infection.

MISUSE OF ANTIBIOTICS

Antibiotics are among the most commonly prescribed medications and some of the most incorrectly used medications. Patients who are given clear explanations of why an antibiotic is prescribed are more likely to complete the full course of therapy and will not seek unneeded medications.

TABLE 17-1 COMMON PENICILLINS

GENERIC NAME/ TRADE NAME	USUAL ADULT DOSE, ROUTE, AND FREQUENCY OF ADMINISTRATION	INDICATIONS FOR USE	DRUG INTERACTIONS
NARROW SPECTRUM			
First Generation			
penicillin G* (Pfizerpen)	600,000-4,000,000 units IM, IV q4-6h	*Types of bacteria:* Gram-positive and gram-negative bacteria, gram-positive aerobic cocci, gram-positive aerobic and anaerobic bacilli, spirochetes *Types of infection:* Upper respiratory tract infections, pneumonia, dental prophylaxis, urinary tract infections	Probenecid increases and prolongs penicillin levels in the blood
penicillin V* (NTN)	250-500 mg PO q6h		Decreased effectiveness of tetracyclines
Antistaphylococcal (Penicillinase Resistant)			
nafcillin (NTN)	2-12 g IM, IV	*Type of bacteria:* Staphylococci *Type of infection:* Staphylococcal infections	Probenecid increases and prolongs penicillin levels in the blood
oxacillin (NTN)	2-12 g IM, IV		
dicloxacillin (NTN)	125-500 mg PO q6hr		
BROAD SPECTRUM (AMINOPENICILLINS)			
Second Generation			
ampicillin* (Omnipen and generic)	500 mg-2 g PO qid, IM, IV	*Types of bacteria:* Gram-positive and gram-negative bacteria, gram-positive aerobic cocci, gram-positive aerobic and anaerobic bacilli, spirochetes *Types of infection:* Respiratory tract infections, urinary tract infections, otitis media	No significant interaction
amoxicillin* (NTN for immediate release)	250-500 mg PO tid		
EXTENDED SPECTRUM (ANTIPSEUDOMONAL PENICILLINS)			
Third Generation			
piperacillin (NTN)	1.5-4 g IM, IV q4-6h	*Type of bacteria:* Pseudomonas *Type of infection:* Pseudomonas infections	No significant interaction
EXTENDED SPECTRUM PENICILLINS WITH β-LACTAMASE INHIBITORS			
Fourth Generation			
amoxicillin-clavulanate (Augmentin)	250-750 mg PO q8h	*Types of bacteria:* Gram-positive cocci, non-*Pseudomonal* gram-negative and anaerobic species	See amoxicillin
(Augmentin ES-600) (susp)†	600 mg PO 2 divided doses for 10 days		
(Augmentin XR)	2000 mg PO q12h		
ampicillin-sulbactam (Unasyn)	1.5-3 gm IV q6h		See ampicillin
piperacillin-tazobactam (Zosyn)	3.375 g IV q6h	*Types of bacteria:* Non—methicillin resistant staphylococci, *Pseudomonas,* and other gram-negative and anaerobic species	
ticarcillin-clavulanate (Timentin)	3.1 g IV q4-6h	Same as for Zosyn	

Major Side Effects of Penicillins: Nausea and vomiting, diarrhea, sore mouth, hives, itching, anaphylaxis

IM, intramuscularly; *IV,* intravenously; *NTN,* no trade name; *PO,* orally.
*The effectiveness of oral contraceptives may be reduced with these penicillins.
†Pediatric medication.

Patients contribute to the problem of misuse of antibiotics by failing to take the entire prescribed course of an antibiotic because the person feels better; the abbreviated course of treatment kills off only the more susceptible microorganisms, allowing more resistant ones—those that need to be eradicated—to grow with less competition. Antibiotics are usually given for 5 to 14 days, with the most commonly ordered duration being 10 days. Longer treatment courses may be prescribed for serious bacterial infections or when appropriately using antifungals or antiviral drugs for certain susceptible illnesses. The danger of taking antimicrobial medications too briefly is the potential development of drug-resistant microorganisms and relapse of the disease. "Saving" unused medications until another illness occurs is another misuse of antibiotics; this practice allows remaining microbes to grow, and the patient will feel that the medicine "didn't work." Even though a patient may no longer be experiencing the symptoms, the medication may not have had time to kill the more virulent microorganisms.

For most viral infections, when antibiotic therapy is inappropriately begun, the patient is exposed to all of the drug risks without receiving benefits because viruses are not microorganisms susceptible to treatment with antibacterials. However, antibiotics *can* be appropriately used, either preventatively or therapeutically, to treat secondary infections that may occur with viral disease.

For most antibiotics to be most effective, they should be taken at evenly spaced intervals to maintain a therapeutic blood level throughout a 24-hour period. For example, if the order reads "three times a day," the medicine should usually be taken every 8 hours. Not taking medications because of sleep or other activities causes erratic dosing and fluctuations in blood levels, making the antibiotic less effective.

Taking medications prescribed for another person without obtaining appropriate medical care is misuse, abuse, or both.

Fever is a symptom of more diseases than just a bacterial infection; therefore giving antibiotics just because someone has a fever is inappropriate. The one situation in which fever alone is an indication for antibiotics is in the immunosuppressed patient (Box 17-1).

BOX 17-1 IMPLICATIONS IN ANTIBIOTIC THERAPY

1. Selected antibiotic should be known to be effective against common organisms isolated from infection site.
2. Minimum number of drugs necessary to treat infection should be used.
3. Drug of first choice should be used unless it is contraindicated. In children and elderly, caution is needed. For all patients, dosage should take into account weight or body surface area, organ function, and concurrent diseases.
4. Unless benefit outweighs risk, a drug should not be used when previous allergic or adverse reactions to that drug have occurred.
5. Antibiotic therapy should be continued as long as infection is present but should not exceed usual treatment time for suspected infective organisms.

Important Facts about Antibiotics

- Antibiotics should be carefully chosen on the basis of the determined or suspected sensitivity of infecting organisms.
- Antibiotics may be given prophylactically for surgery or on exposure to unusual diseases such as anthrax or malaria.
- Narrow-spectrum antibiotics are effective against few microorganisms, whereas broad-spectrum antibiotics are used against a wide range of microbes.
- The emergence of drug-resistant microorganisms is a major concern; therefore antibiotics should be prescribed only when indicated by a disease process.
- *Bactericidal* drugs kill microorganisms. *Bacteriostatic* drugs suppress bacterial growth until the person's immune system can effectively bring the body into homeostasis.

ANTIBACTERIAL DRUGS

Antimicrobial therapy became a pharmacologic entity when Alexander Fleming discovered that when mold fell on a Petri dish containing *Staphylococcus,* growth of the bacteria was inhibited by the mold. Some penicillins today are still made from the same molds found to be effective by Fleming. Several categories of antibacterial drugs are effective against bacterial infections. This section discusses each family and the use of individual drugs.

Penicillins

Penicillin, the first true antibiotic, has been derived from a number of strains of common molds found on bread and fruit. Natural and semisynthetic penicillins and their related antibiotics remain the most effective and least toxic of antimicrobials. These substances act by inhibiting bacterial cell-wall synthesis, an action that makes

Patient Education for Compliance

1. Misuse of antibiotics is common and should be discouraged. Fever is only a symptom and is not an indication to begin antibiotic therapy.
2. Antibiotics are ineffective for the treatment of viral infections unless secondary bacterial infections are present.

most penicillins *bactericidal,* although in low doses they may be *bacteriostatic.* Adverse reactions are generally allergic reactions that tend to occur more frequently and severely than with other medications.

Penicillins are categorized by their antimicrobial spectrum into four major groups: (1) narrow-spectrum penicillins, (2) narrow-spectrum antistaphylococcal penicillins, (3) broad-spectrum penicillins (aminopenicillins), and (4) extended-spectrum penicillins.

Did You Know?

Most generic names for penicillins end in *-cillin,* and many older trade names have *pen* in their names. As an example, **penicillin G** (generic name) is known as Pfizerpen by trade name.

Narrow-Spectrum Penicillins

Penicillin G was the first penicillin developed and is still the drug of choice for treating many infections. The narrow-spectrum penicillins are considered first-generation penicillins; in general, they are effective against (1) many gram-positive organisms such as streptococci and staphylococci; (2) gram-negative bacteria such as *Neisseria* and *E. coli;* (3) spirochetes; and (4) some anaerobic bacteria. Diseases susceptible to penicillin are infections such as pneumonia, throat and ear infections, gonorrhea, and syphilis (Table 17-1).

Narrow-Spectrum Antistaphylococcal (Penicillin-Resistant) Penicillins

The antistaphylococcal penicillins (e.g., **oxacillin, nafcillin**) have a narrow spectrum of action for infections and are specific for penicillin-resistant staphylococci strains (see Table 17-1).

Broad-Spectrum Penicillins (Aminopenicillins)

By altering naturally occurring semisynthetic broad-spectrum penicillins, second-generation penicillins are effective against a broader spectrum of microorganisms (including some gram-negative bacteria). However, these medications are not effective for *S. aureus* infections. Many are available in oral preparations (e.g., **ampicillin** and **amoxicillin**) (see Table 17-1).

Extended-Spectrum Penicillins

Third-generation penicillins (e.g., **ticarcillin**), also known as *extended-spectrum penicillins,* have a wider antimicrobial action than second-generation penicillins. These medications are used for more serious urinary tract and respiratory tract infections and for infections caused by gram-negative bacteria such as *Pseudomonas* and *Proteus* species (see Table 17-1).

Fourth-generation penicillins (e.g., **piperacillin**), extended-spectrum antimicrobials with antipseudomonal activity, are used for the most serious infections

that are difficult to treat. These penicillins are given parenterally, often in combination therapy with other antimicrobials (see Table 17-1).

✎ CLINICAL TIP

A person allergic to any penicillin should be considered allergic to all penicillins. If a question arises about the possibility of allergic penicillin reactions, the person should be considered allergic.

PATIENT ALERT

- Patients should be asked about allergies each time they are seen in health care settings with questions concerning any possible allergic reactions to any medication, such as rashes, hives, and itching.
- Patients with penicillin allergies should wear or carry identification to prevent inadvertent administration of penicillin.

Patient Education for Compliance

1. Penicillins are best taken on an empty stomach with a full glass of water 1 hour before meals or 2 hours after meals.
2. All penicillin-class oral suspensions require refrigeration after reconstitution.
3. As a precaution, women taking ampicillin, amoxicillin, or penicillins G and V and who are also taking estrogen-containing contraceptives should use a different form of contraception while taking these antibiotics. Reports have indicated a decreased effectiveness of birth control pills when penicillin derivatives are used concurrently.

Important Facts about Penicillins

- Penicillins weaken cell walls, causing lysis and cell death, making them bactericidal.
- Gram-negative bacteria are resistant to many penicillins.
- Penicillins cause a high incidence of allergic reactions relative to other antibiotics.
- A patient allergic to one penicillin should be considered allergic to all penicillins. Even mild reactions should be considered an allergic reaction.
- The principal differences among the penicillins are their spectrum of antibacterial action, their stability in stomach acids, and their duration of action.
- Narrow-spectrum penicillins G and V are naturally occurring substances. Penicillin G is administered by injection because it is not stable in gastric acids. However, penicillin V can be administered orally.

Cephalosporins

Like penicillins, cephalosporins were originally derived from a mold and are structurally related to penicillins. Cephalosporins weaken the bacterial cell wall, resulting in lysis and death of the bacterial cell; thus they are bactericidal. Cephalosporins are active against a broad spectrum of pathogens. Because of the chemical relationship of cephalosporins to penicillin, patients who are allergic to penicillin should be given cephalosporins with caution because of the slight chance of cross allergy.

Did You Know?

Most cephalosporins have the prefix *ceph-* or *cef-* in their name. An example is **cefadroxil** (generic name), which is Duricef (trade name).

Classified in four generations, cephalosporins are most often used as substitutes for penicillins with drug-resistant bacteria and in treatment of certain gram-negative infections.

- First-generation cephalosporins (e.g., **cephalexin**) are primarily active against gram-positive bacteria.
- Second-generation drugs (e.g., **cefaclor**) have increased effectiveness against gram-negative microorganisms.
- Third and fourth generations are more active against gram-negative microbes, with the third generation (e.g., **cefdinir**) not as effective against gram-positive cocci. Fourth-generation drugs (e.g., **cefepime**) are more resistant to the inactivating intestinal enzymes that cause other cephalosporins to be ineffective.

The expense of first- and second-generation cephalosporins rarely makes these medications the drug of choice for treating most infections (Box 17-2 and Table 17-2).

BOX 17-2 SUMMARY OF PENICILLIN VERSUS CEPHALOSPORIN GENERATIONS

Penicillin generations are based on general potency and ability to treat increasingly broader microbial spectrum.

Cephalosporin generations are based on effectiveness against the gram-negative or gram-positive microbes, not on the breadth of the drug effectiveness spectrum.

Each generation of penicillins represents an increase in potency, whereas cephalosporins generations work on different microbial spectrums.

Patient Education for Compliance

1. Cephalosporins should be taken with food if gastric upset occurs.
2. Depending on package labels, many cephalosporin suspensions should be refrigerated once reconstituted, but a few may be stored at room temperature.
3. A few cephalosporins cannot be combined with alcohol. Individuals who are taking these medications should not consume alcohol during treatment.
4. Select cephalosporins tend to intensify bleeding tendencies. Individuals who take oral anticoagulants may be more at risk for this side effect.
5. Patients with diabetes mellitus who check their urine should be aware that cephalosporins tend to raise blood glucose levels and may interfere with certain urine testing methods.
6. Report any excessive diarrhea and easy bruising.

Important Facts about Cephalosporins

- Cephalosporins weaken the cell wall, causing death to bacteria so these drugs are bacteriacidal.
- Cephalosporins are closely related to penicillins in their chemical structure.
- Cephalosporins are grouped into four generations. As drugs progress through the generations, there occurs increased activity against gram-negative bacteria.
- The most common adverse reactions to cephalosporins are diarrhea and allergic reactions. Persons allergic to penicillin should be watched carefully when administered cephalosporins because up to 3% to 5% of people allergic to penicillin will also prove to be allergic to cephalosporins.

Carbapenems

Four carbapenems (**imipenem, meropenem, ertapenem, and doripenem**) have low toxicity rates while having broad antimicrobial spectra but are not active against methicillin-resistant *S. aureus* (MRSA). Parenteral administration is necessary for all of these drugs at present. Most drugs are well tolerated, with GI symptoms, rashes, and headaches being possible adverse effects. People allergic to cephalosporins may also be allergic to these drugs (Table 17-3).

Macrolides

The macrolide antibiotics, called *macro* because of the large size of the chemical compounds, are broad-spectrum antimicrobials that act by inhibiting protein synthesis in bacteria. These drugs are primarily bacteriostatic but may be bactericidal in large doses. Macrolides have a unique role in treating Legionnaires disease and

TABLE 17-2 SELECT CEPHALOSPORINS

GENERIC NAME/ TRADE NAME	USUAL ADULT DOSE, ROUTE, AND FREQUENCY OF ADMINISTRATION	INDICATIONS FOR USE	DRUG INTERACTIONS
FIRST GENERATION			
cefadroxil (Duracif)	0.5-1 gm PO q12h	*Types of bacteria:* Streptococci and some staphylococci	Aminoglycoside, polymyxin B, vancomycin
cefazolin (Ancef)	500 mg-1 g PO q8h	*Types of infection:* Staphylococcal and streptococcal infections, some urinary tract infections, bone and joint diseases, upper respiratory tract infection	Probenecid increases the activity of some cephalosporins
cephalexin (Keflex, Panixine)	250-500 mg PO q6-12h		Some cephalosporins cause Antabuse-like reactions
			Decrease the effectiveness of oral contraceptives
SECOND GENERATION			
cefaclor (NTN)	250-500 mg PO q8h	Same as for first generation, plus *Haemophilus influenzae* and *Neisseria gonorrhoeae*	cefadroxil plus aspirin, anticoagulants, NSAIDs (because medication may promote bleeding)
cefotetan (Cefotan)	1-2 g IM, IV q12-24h		
cefoxitin (NTN)	1-2 g IM, IV q6-8h		
cefuroxime (Zinacef)	750-1.5 g/kg IM, IV q6-8h		
Ceftin	250-500 mg PO q12h		
cefprozil (Cefzil)	250-500 mg PO q12-24h		
THIRD GENERATION			
cefdinir (Omnicef)	300 mg PO q12h	*Types of bacteria:* Less effective against streptococci and pneumococci; more effective against gram-negative and anaerobic bacteria; generally used with serious infections	No significant interactions
cefixime (Suprax)	400 mg PO/d divided q12-24h		
ceftibuten (Cedax)	400 mg PO qd		
cefotaxime (Claforan)	1-2 g IM, IV q8h		
ceftazidime (Fortaz, Tazicef)	1-2 g IM, IV q8-12h	*Pseudomonas*	
ceftriaxone (Rocephin)	1-2 g IM, IV q24h	Drug of choice for meningitis	
cefpodoxime (NTN)	100-500 mg PO q12h		
cefditoren (Spectracef)	200-400 mg PO q12h		
FOURTH GENERATION			
cefepime (Maxipime)	0.5-2 g IM, IV q8-12h	*Types of infection:* Similar to third generation— gram-negative coverage	Aspirin, other NSAIDs, anticoagulants, alcohol

Major Side Effects of Cephalosporins: Headache, dizziness, weakness, fever, diarrhea, anorexia, nephrotoxicity, rash, dyspnea, blood dyscrasias

IM, intramuscularly; *IV,* intravenously; *NSAIDs,* nonsteroidal antiinflammatory drugs; *NTN,* no trade name; *PO,* orally.

TABLE 17-3 SELECTED CARBAPENEMS

GENERIC NAME/ TRADE NAME	USUAL ADULT DOSE, ROUTE, AND FREQUENCY OF ADMINISTRATION	INDICATIONS FOR USE	DRUG INTERACTIONS
imipenem-cilastatin/Primaxin	250-500 mg IM, IV q6h	Serious gram-positive and gram-negative infections	Antagonistic with other antibiotics
meropenem/Merrem	1 g IV q8h		
ertapenem/Invanz	1 g IM, IV qd		probenecid
doripenem/Doribax	500 mg IV q8h		

Major Side Effects of Carbapenems: Headaches, diarrhea, nausea

IM, intramuscularly; *IV,* intravenously.

Chlamydia infections and in treating and preventing atypical pneumonias, especially with human immuno-deficiency virus (HIV) patients. Macrolides are often used as an alternative to penicillin in penicillin-allergic patients.

Erythromycin was the first macrolide and is a treatment of choice for several infections. The newer macrolides, including **azithromycin** and **clarithromycin,** may cause GI symptoms, as well as headaches and dizziness. A significant change in the QT interval with large doses may result in sudden cardiac death. Persons taking antidysrhythmics, calcium channel blockers, azole antifungals, and HIV protease inhibitors should avoid erythromycin (Table 17-4).

CLINICAL TIP

Erythromycin is most effective if taken on an empty stomach, but it may be given with food if gastrointestinal upset occurs.

Did You Know?

The names of macrolide drugs typically end in -*mycin.* The same suffix is also used in naming some aminoglycosides (e.g., erythromycin, a macrolide, and neomycin, a member of the aminoglycoside family). Thus the drug suffix cannot always be used as identification of the drug family.

Important Facts about Macrolides

- Erythromycin is the prototype of macrolides and is bacteriostatic in its mechanism of action.
- Erythromycin, often used for patients with penicillin allergies, is effective against the basic spectrum of microbes.

Tetracyclines

The tetracyclines (e.g., ***tetracycline, doxycycline***), medications that are bacteriostatic and bactericidal, were the first group of broad-spectrum antibiotics. They are used to treat organisms including those causing acne, Rocky Mountain spotted fever, Lyme disease, urinary tract infections (UTIs), bronchitis, and periodontal disease. Some bacteria have become resistant to tetracyclines (Table 17-5).

PATIENT ALERT

- Unused tetracycline products should be thrown away after their expiration date; decomposing tetracycline can be harmful if ingested.
- The patient should avoid the sun because of danger of rapid sunburning; therefore care should be used in prescribing tetracycline for teenagers with acne because teens like to sunbathe. The use of sunscreens is necessary with these medications.
- These medications also cannot be used in children younger than 8 years old or in pregnant women because of the permanent discoloration of developing teeth.
- Superinfections of the bowels occur with all antibiotics, but especially with tetracyclines, so significant diarrhea should be reported, as should vaginal and rectal itching or a black, furry appearance of the tongue. These are signs of fungal superinfections.

Did You Know?

The suffix -*cycline* is found with the tetracyclines such as doxycycline and **minocycline.**

TABLE 17-4 SELECTED MACROLIDES

GENERIC NAME/ TRADE NAME	USUAL ADULT DOSE, ROUTE, AND FREQUENCY OF ADMINISTRATION	INDICATIONS FOR USE	DRUG INTERACTIONS
ERYTHROMYCINS*			
erythromycin (Erythrocin) erythromycin succinate (EES, EryPed)	250-500 mg PO, IV qid, 400 mg PO q6h	*Types of bacteria:* Gram-positive and some gram-negative microorganisms *Types of infection:* Respiratory illnesses, gastrointestinal tract, skin, and soft tissue; drugs of choice for Legionnaires disease	carbamazepine, cyclosporine, statins, ergot alkaloids, rifabutin theophylline, and warfarin anticoagulants

Major Side Effects of Erythromycins: Abdominal cramping, diarrhea, oral or vaginal candidiasis, hearing loss, headache, dizziness

ERYTHROMYCIN DERIVATIVES			
azithromycin (Zithromax)	250-600 mg PO qd	*Types of bacteria:* Especially gram-negative organisms and anaerobic organisms	Aluminum magnesium antacids, theophylline, Coumadin, carbamazepine
clarithromycin (Biaxin)	250-500 mg PO q12h	*Types of infection: Haemophilus influenzae,* Legionnaires disease, *Chlamydia,* Lyme disease	
(Biaxin XL)	1000 mg PO qd		
dirithromycin (Dynabac†)	500 mg PO	Soft tissue infections with *Streptococcus pneumoniae* and *Staphylococcus aureus;* Legionnaires disease	

Major Side Effects of Erythromycin Derivatives: Same as for erythromycins, plus change in taste sensation

KETOLIDES			
telithromycin (Ketek)	800 mg PO qd	Bronchitis, sinusitis, pneumonia	Same as for erythromycins, plus phenobarbital, phenytoin

Major Side Effects of Ketolides: Nausea, vomiting, diarrhea

EES, erythromycin ethylsuccinate; *IV,* intravenously; *NTN,* no trade name; *PO,* orally.
*Also available in topical and ophthalmic preparations.
†Increased absorption with food.

TABLE 17-5 SELECT TETRACYCLINES

GENERIC NAME/ TRADE NAME	USUAL ADULT DOSE, ROUTE, AND FREQUENCY OF ADMINISTRATION	INDICATIONS FOR USE	DRUG INTERACTIONS
SHORT ACTING			
tetracycline (NTN)	250-500 mg PO qid	*Types of bacteria:* Rickettsiae, *Mycoplasma pneumoniae* *Types of infection:* Cholera, *Chlamydia,* Lyme disease, acne	Pregnancy category D Decreases effectiveness of contraceptives, antacids, calcium supplements, iron supplements, magnesium laxatives, milk products
LONG ACTING			
doxycycline (Vibramycin, Doryx, Adoxa, Periostat)	100-200 mg PO bid	Same as short-acting agents, plus gastrointestinal diseases	
	As directed topically	Periodontal disease	
minocycline (Minocin)	200 mg PO then 100 mg q12h	Same as short-acting agents, plus acne	

Major Side Effects of Tetracyclines: Photosensitivity, permanent stains in developing teeth in fetus and in children <8 yr of age

IM, intramuscularly; *IV,* intravenously; *NTN,* no trade name; *PO,* orally.

Patient Education for Compliance

1. Tetracyclines should not be taken with milk products, iron supplements, or antacids. Many antacid and mineral supplements interfere with absorption of tetracyclines. Do not administer any medications, including multivitamins, with the minerals aluminum, calcium, magnesium, iron, or zinc within 4 hours of injesting oral tetracyclines.

2. Tetracycline should be taken on an empty stomach, but medications in this class can cause gastrointestinal distress, which can be reduced by taking the medication with meals if necessary. Doxycycline and **minocycline** may be given with dairy products as necessary, but milk products should be avoided with other tetracyclines.

Aminoglycosides

Aminoglycosides (e.g., **gentamien**) are a group of potent bactericidal agents that inhibit protein synthesis; they are usually reserved for serious or life-threatening infections. Generally the main spectrum sensitive to these drugs consists of gram-positive bacilli, but gram-positive microbes may also be affected. Aminoglycosides may be used with cephalosporins or **vancomycin** for synergistic effects and with penicillin with certain conditions such as neonatal sepsis. Topical, ophthalmic, and otic use of aminoglycosides is relatively safe, with few side effects. Patients receiving systemically administered aminoglycosides must be carefully monitored to avoid renal toxicity and ototoxicity (Table 17-6).

PATIENT ALERT

Patients receiving parenteral aminoglycosides should be watched closely for tinnitus, vertigo, weakness, and changes in respiration, as well as for scant urinary output and proteinuria.

Important Facts about Aminoglycosides

- Aminoglycosides—narrow-spectrum antibiotics that are bactericidal—are used against gram-negative bacilli.
- Aminoglycosides are nephrotoxic and can be ototoxic.
- The topical use of aminoglycosides is relatively safe, but some adverse reactions are possible.

Quinolones

Fluoroquinolones (e.g., **ciprofloxacin**), broad-spectrum antimicrobials and bactericidals, act by inhibiting enzymes needed for the bacteria's DNA. Easily absorbed on oral administration, these antimicrobials are used to treat bone and joint infections, UTIs, prostatitis, gonorrhea, pneumonia, and other diseases. Antacids decrease

TABLE 17-6 AMINOGLYCOSIDES

GENERIC NAME/ TRADE NAME	USUAL ADULT DOSE, ROUTE, AND FREQUENCY OF ADMINISTRATION	INDICATIONS FOR USE	DRUG INTERACTIONS
amikacin (Amikin)	10-15 mg/kg/day divided q8-12h IV, IM, PO	*Types of bacteria:* Serious gram-negative and some gram-positive organisms	Extended-spectrum penicillins inactivate aminoglycosides if mixed, increase action of some muscle relaxants; use with caution with other nephrotoxic medications
gentamicin (NTN)	3-5 mg/kg/day divided q8h IV, IM topical	*Types of infection:* Those caused by above bacteria, plus tuberculosis (Kantrex)	
(Gentak)	ophthalmalogic		
kanamycin (NTN)	15 mg/kg/day qd IM, IV		
neomycin* (NTN)	1 g PO prior to GI surgery	Topical for skin and ocular infections	
Neobiotic	Topical Nebulizer		
tobramycin (NTN)	3-5 mg/kg/day tid IM, IV	*Pseudomonas aeruginosa,* plus other gram-negative infections	
(Tobrex)	Ophthalmic		
(TOBI)	Nebulizer		

Major Side Effects of Aminoglycosides: Ototoxicity, blood dyscrasias, nephrotoxicity, nausea, vomiting, and anorexia

GI, gastrointestinal; *IM,* intramuscularly; *IV,* intravenously; *NTN,* no trade name; *PO,* orally.
*Also available in ophthalmic and topical preparations.

the absorption of these drugs and should not be given for 2 hours after the administration of the antibiotic (Table 17-7).

Important Facts about Fluoroquinolones

- Fluoroquinolones are broad-spectrum antimicrobials and bactericidals.
- The oral absorption of fluoroquinolones may be reduced by ingestion of dairy products, antacids, calcium, magnesium or iron supplements, or laxatives.

Other Antibiotics

Chloramphenicol

Chloramphenicol, a broad-spectrum antibacterial and antirickettsial agent, is bacteriostatic to a wide variety of gram-positive and gram-negative organisms, but it may be bactericidal in large doses. Bone marrow toxicity is a major drawback to its use. Chloramphenicol is used to treat forms of meningitis, paratyphoid and typhoid fever, typhus, Rocky Mountain spotted fever, and bacterial sepsis in life-threatening situations when other treatment options have not been effective. It should not be used in newborns unless no acceptable alternative is available because of the potential risk of "gray baby syndrome," a life-threatening adverse effect. It is not recommended for use in pregnant or breast-feeding women (Table 17-8).

Lincomycin and Derivatives

Lincomycin derivatives are primarily bacteriostatic but may be bactericidal in high doses. **Clindamycin** (Cleocin) is a semisynthetic derivative of lincomycin used for bone and joint diseases, gynecologic diseases, skin and soft tissue infections, and septicemia. It may be administered either systemically or topically. Oral doses should be administered with a full glass of water. Diarrhea and GI side effects are common with oral therapy. Lincocin, a natural antibiotic, is used to treat serious streptococcal, pneumococcal, and staphylococcal infections (see Table 17-8).

Oxazolidinones

Linezolid (Zyvox) is the first member of the oxazolidinones, a new class of drugs that are important for use with multidrug-resistant gram-positive pathogens,

TABLE 17-7 FLUOROQUINOLONES (QUINOLONE ANTIMICROBIALS)

GENERIC NAME/ TRADE NAME	USUAL ADULT DOSE, ROUTE, AND FREQUENCY OF ADMINISTRATION	INDICATIONS FOR USE	DRUG INTERACTIONS
ciprofloxacin (Cipro)	500-750 mg PO q12h 400 mg IV q12h	*Type of bacteria:* Gram-positive and gram-negative microorganisms; drug of choice for anthrax infection or prophylaxis for anthrax infection	Increases effect of anticoagulants, caffeine; causes photosensitivity; should not be used in children and infants
(Cipro XR Proquin XR)	500 mg PO bid	*Type of infection:* Wide variety	
levofloxacin (Levaquin)	250-500 mg PO, IV qd	Bronchitis, urinary tract infections, upper respiratory infections, skin infections, pneumonia	
norfloxacin (Noroxin)	400 mg PO q12h	Urinary tract infections and sexually transmitted diseases	
ofloxacin (Floxin*)	200-400 mg PO q12h	Upper respiratory infections, urinary tract infections, gonorrhea, prostate infections	
gemifloxacin (Factive)	320 mg PO qd	Same as for Cipro	
moxifloxacin (Avelox)	400 mg PO, IV qd	Gram-positive upper respiratory infections	

Major Side Effects of Fluoroquinolones: Dizziness, drowsiness, restlessness, insomnia, rashes, GI symptoms; ligament and cartilage damage, hypersensitivity; additionally ototoxicity with norfloxacin

GI, gastrointestinal; *IV,* intravenously; *PO,* orally.
*Also available as ophthalmic and otic preparations.

TABLE 17-8 MISCELLANEOUS ANTIBIOTICS

GENERIC NAME/ TRADE NAME	USUAL ADULT DOSE, ROUTE, AND FREQUENCY OF ADMINISTRATION	INDICATIONS FOR USE	DRUG INTERACTIONS
chloramphenicol (NTN)	50-75 mg/kg/day IV q6h	*Types of bacteria:* Gram-negative aerobic organisms *Types of infection:* Meningitis, Rocky Mountain spotted fever, paratyphoid fever, typhoid fever, bacterial sepsis, typhus fever when not responsive to other medications	Decreased antidiabetic agents and increased blood glucose levels, increased barbiturates, phenytoin, warfarin Decreased by erythromycin lincomycin, and clindamycin
metronidazole (Flagyl)	500 mg-1 g PO tid 500 mg IV tid	*Types of infection:* Trichomoniasis, giardiasis, amebiasis	Alcohol-containing medications, disulfiram; increases effectiveness of anticoagulants
rifaximin (Xifaxan)	200 mg PO tid	*Escherichia coli,* diarrhea	Basically none

Major Side Effects:

chloramphenicol—Blood dyscrasias, nausea, diarrhea, dizziness, depression; *metronidazole*—Dizziness, headache, GI disturbances, CNS toxicity, candidiasis

OTHER AGENTS

clindamycin (Cleocin)	100-300 mg PO, IM, IV q6h	*Types of infection:* Streptococcal, pneumococcal, and staphylococcal	erythromycin and chloramphenicol, antidiarrheals
vancomycin (Vancocin)	125-500 mg PO q6h 1 g IV q12h	*Types of infection:* Severe septicemia, meningitis, pseudomembranous colitis	aspirin, furosemide, aminoglycosides, and other antibiotics, because increases likelihood of ototoxicity and nephrotoxicity
linezolid (Zyvox)	600 mg PO, IV q12h	Broad-spectrum antiinfective	MAOIs, SSRIs, INH
quinupristin-dalfopristin (Synercid)	7.5 mg/kg IV q8h	MRSA (safe for persons allergic to PCN and cephalosporins)	Decreased metabolism of many drugs
tigecycline (Tygacil)	100 mg IV initially, then 50 mg IV q12h	Broad-spectrum microbes	Similar to tetracyclines
aztreonam (Azactam)	1-2 g IM, IV q6-12h	Antiinfective, UTIs	Allergies to PCN, cephalosporins

Major Side Effects:

linezolid, quinupristin-dalfopristin, tigecycline, and aztreonam—Diarrhea, superinfections, headache, pruritus, nausea, vomiting

TOPICAL ANTIBIOTICS

bacitracin and polymyxin B (Neosporin)	Apply locally several times a day topically	Dermatologic infections	No significant interactions
retapamulin* (Altabax, mupirocin*, Bactroban)			

CNS, central nervous system; *GI*, gastrointestinal; *IM*, intramuscularly; *INH*, isoniazid; *IV*, intravenously; *MAOIs*, monoamine oxidase inhibitors; *MRSA*, methicillin-resistant *Staphylococcus aureus*; *PCN*, penicillin; *PO*, orally; *SSRIs,* selective serotonin reuptake inhibitors; *UTI,* urinary tract infection.
*See Chapter 22.

including MRSA. Usually well tolerated, it may cause GI symptoms and headaches (see Table 17-8).

Ketolides

Telithromycin (Ketek) is in a new class of antibiotics, ketolides, that is closely related to the macrolides. Although telithromycin is an effective drug, it is associated with a high risk of liver damage. This medication should be used only when absolutely necessary (see Table 17-8).

Vancomycin

A bactericidal, ***vancomycin*** is usually the drug of last resort and should be reserved for severe infections with drug-resistant *Staphylococcus* and *Clostridium*. Vancomycin given intravenously requires careful therapeutic monitoring because of the potential risks for nephrotoxicity and ototoxicity to help limit the chance that these adverse reactions will occur. Vancomycin is not well absorbed orally but does have some oral indications (see Table 17-8).

Metronidazole

Metronidazole (Flagyl), a short-acting bactericidal agent that is toxic to cells, is used to treat infections caused by anaerobic bacteria, protozoa, and diarrhea associated with *Clostridium difficile*. The patient may experience a metallic taste and diarrhea. Alcohol should be avoided when taking metronidazole because of a disulfiram-like adverse reaction (see Table 17-8).

Tigecycline

Tigecycline (Tygacil), a tetracycline derivative, was developed to overcome tetracycline drug resistance. The agent is active against a broad spectrum of bacteria. Adverse effects are similar to those of tetracycline (see Table 17-8).

Topical Over-the-Counter Antibiotics

Many antibiotics are found in over-the-counter (OTC) preparations for topical use. A commonly recognized brand is Neosporin, a combination of ***polymyxin B, neomycin,*** and ***bacitracin.*** These OTC antibiotics are first-aid remedies for use either prophylactically or therapeutically for minor wounds and abrasions; the individual components are available in other forms for other uses.

- Bacitracin is used topically for bacterial infections such as staphylococcal and group A streptococcal infections.
- Neomycin is a member of the aminoglycoside family of antibiotics.
- Polymyxin B, a bactericidal agent with a broad spectrum of action against aerobic gram-negative bacilli and used as a sterile topical treatment of eye

(by prescription), ear, and skin infections, is not systemically absorbed, so systemic effects, such as neurotoxicity and nephrotoxicity, do not occur.

Important Facts about Miscellaneous Antibiotics and Topical OTC Preparations

- Vancomycin, with the potential to be nephrotoxic and ototoxic, is reserved for treating serious infections, such as drug-resistant gram-positive organisms.
- Chloramphenicol causes serious blood dyscrasias and should be used only when clearly indicated.
- Metronidazole is useful with protozoa and anaerobic bacteria.
- Topical antibiotic preparations, usually containing combinations of neomycin, bacitracin, and polymyxin B, are not absorbed systemically when applied topically.

SULFONAMIDES (SULFA DRUGS)

Sulfonamides, or sulfa drugs, are not antibiotics (the drugs did not originate in a microorganism) but are *antibacterials* used to combat infection by slowing bacterial growth while the body builds its own defenses. Most of the sulfonamides are synthetically produced and are primarily bacteriostatic, but some are bactericidal. These agents are used in areas where fluids can flush away the wastes of infection (such as the eyes, urinary tract, and sinuses) and for pneumonia and soft tissue infections.

Sulfonamides were discovered in the 1930s as a byproduct of the dye industry. They were initially effective against gram-positive and gram-negative microorganisms. However long-term use of these drugs has led to increased bacterial resistance.

Sulfonamides are subdivided into two groups on the basis of their duration of action—short-acting and intermediate-acting agents. Because sulfonamides are rapidly excreted, high doses given at short intervals are necessary to maintain effective blood levels. The major indication for the sulfonamides is UTIs, but these medications are also used for toxoplasmosis, malaria, *Haemophilus influenzae* infection, and topically for burns. Sulfa derivatives (e.g., ***sulfasalazine***) have been used in colitis of the lower GI tract for their antiinflammatory action. In the urinary tract, effectiveness is increased because the drug is actively secreted in urinary tubules.

Sulfonamides in Combinations

Sulfonamides are combined with each other or with other medications such as ***trimethoprim*** (TMP) to increase the antimicrobial action and the spectrum of action. **Sulfamethoxazole** with TMP (SMZ-TMP), the most commonly encountered, is used for UTIs, otitis media, bronchitis, shigellosis, and *Pneumocystis jiroveci*, such as for prophylaxis and treatment of *Pneumocystis* pneumonia (PCP) in patients with acquired immunodeficiency syndrome (AIDS). The combination drugs are generally well tolerated, with rare toxic effects. The drug forms of tablets, suspensions, and intravenous solutions consist of one part TMP to five parts SMZ.

Topical Sulfonamide Preparations

Topical preparations of sulfonamides are available in several forms. Ophthalmic preparations such as **sulfacetamide** (Sulamyd) are used for conjunctivitis and corneal ulcers. Skin lotions are occasionally used for seborrheic dermatitis, acne vulgaris, and skin infections. Other topical preparations such as powders and ointments are used to treat burns. These topical preparations do have some systemic absorption (Table 17-9).

PATIENT ALERT

While taking sulfonamides, the patient must take large quantities of fluids to prevent drug crystallization in the kidneys, a minimal danger when urine is kept dilute.

TABLE 17-9 SELECT SULFONAMIDES

GENERIC NAME/ TRADE NAME	USUAL ADULT DOSE, ROUTE, AND FREQUENCY OF ADMINISTRATION	INDICATIONS FOR USE	DRUG INTERACTIONS
LONG-ACTING AGENT			
sulfasalazine (Azulfidine)	3-4 g PO q8h	*Types of diseases:* Ulcerative colitis, Crohn disease, juvenile rheumatoid arthritis	Increases the action of anticoagulants and oral hypoglycemics; decreases the effectiveness of oral contraceptives
COMBINATION SULFONAMIDES			
trimethoprim (TMP)-SMZ (Bactrim, Septra)	80 mg TMP/400 mg SMZ PO qd, IV	*Types of infection:* Urinary tract infections, otitis media, vaginal	
double-strength TMP-SMZ (Bactrim DS, Septra DS)	160 mg TMP/800 mg SMZ PO q12h		
erythromycin-sulfisoxazole (Pediazole)	400 mg PO q6h 1200 mg PO q6h	Otitis media	

Major Side Effects of Systemic Sulfonamides: GI disturbances, kidney damage, drug-induced fever, diarrhea, headache, rashes, pruritus when taken PO or by parenteral routes

TOPICAL PREPARATIONS			
sulfacetamide ophthalmic ointment, solution (Sulamyd)	As directed, usually 1 drop in eye with solution	*Type of infection:* Ophthalmologic infection	
silver sulfadiazine (Silvadene Cream)	Apply topically to affected area	Burns and skin infections	

GI, gastrointestinal; *IV*, intravenously; *PO*, orally.

Patient Education for Compliance

1. Oral sulfonamides should be taken with a full glass of water on an empty stomach. The person should drink 8 to 10 glasses of water a day to prevent crystallization of sulfa in the kidneys.
2. Sulfonamides may cause photosensitivity reactions, so protective clothing should be worn and sunscreen used when in the sun.

Important Facts about Sulfonamides

- Sulfonamides are used primarily to treat urinary tract infections and are used in combination for other antiinfective therapy with other infections such as malaria and toxoplasmosis.
- Combinations of trimethoprim-sulfamethoxazole inhibit bacteria in sequential steps, making these drugs more powerful than when used alone.
- *Escherichia coli*, the most common cause of uncomplicated urinary tract infections, is susceptible to sulfonamides.

DRUGS TO TREAT TUBERCULOSIS

With the emergence of multidrug-resistant mycobacteria associated with AIDS, tuberculosis has again become a global public health problem. *M. tuberculosis,* the cause of tuberculosis, is most often found in the lungs, but it may infect other body areas where the bacillus can grow in a high oxygen level. The bacilli may be dormant in the body for years and reemerge when the immune system has a lowered ability to fight disease. Multidrug resistance has been a recent development, and resistance to *isoniazid* (INH) and *rifampin,* the two mainstays of tuberculosis therapy, has caused particular concern.

In general, antitubercular drugs can be divided into two groups: (1) medications that are fairly effective and not too toxic and (2) drugs that are more toxic and should be used only as necessary.

As preventive medicine for tuberculosis, a single drug is usually recommended—most frequently INH, with rifampin being the second choice. For the treatment of tuberculosis, two or more drugs should be used; initial treatment regimens combine four agents until susceptibility results are known. Drug therapy may even include three or more medications given for prolonged periods of time. The combination of medications not only decreases the risk of resistance but also reduces the chance of a disease relapse.

Some drugs, such as INH and rifampin, are most effective against rapidly dividing bacilli, whereas others such as **pyrazinamide** (PZA) are active against intracellular activity. The four recommended drugs in combinations are INH, rifampin, PZA, and either ***ethambutol*** or ***streptomycin;*** these agents will provide the best treatment over prolonged periods of time, often a year or more.

- PZA, a bactericidal most often used for active tuberculosis, may also be used in combination with rifampin or ***rifabutin*** as a prophylactic medication for INH-resistant infections.
- Ethambutol should always be given in combination with other medications.
- ***Vitamin B₆ (pyridoxine)*** may be added to the therapy to prevent neuropathies (Table 17-10).

PATIENT ALERT

- Because tubercular drugs are hepatotoxic, ingestion of alcohol should be avoided. Jaundice, pale stools, or other signs of liver disease should be reported.
- Rifampin will discolor urine, sweat, and saliva to a red-orange color and may permanently stain soft contact lenses.

Patient Education for Compliance

1. With medications for tuberculosis, the reason for prolonged multidrug therapy must be explained to the patient. The length of therapy may make compliance a significant problem.
2. Isoniazid (INH) and rifampin should be taken on an empty stomach unless gastrointestinal upset occurs, in which case they may be taken with meals.
3. Any changes in vision while taking ethambutol should be reported because of the possibility of ocular toxicity.

Important Facts about Drugs to Treat Tuberculosis

- The principal cause of drug-resistant strains of tuberculosis is inadequate drug therapy.
- The prolonged use of multiple medications contributes to lapses in medication therapy.
- To prevent drug resistance, tuberculosis should always be treated with at least two drugs.
- The usual four-drug regimen to treat tuberculosis includes isoniazid, rifampin, pyrazinamide, and either ethambutol or streptomycin. These drugs can be used in all areas of tuberculosis treatment including drug-resistant tuberculosis.
- Isoniazid is the only drug that has been proved effective in preventing tuberculosis.

TABLE 17-10	SELECT ANTITUBERCULOSIS DRUGS		
GENERIC NAME/ TRADE NAME	**USUAL ADULT DOSE, ROUTE, AND FREQUENCY OF ADMINISTRATION**	**INDICATIONS FOR USE**	**DRUG INTERACTIONS**
FIRST-LINE DRUGS			
isoniazid (INH) (NTN)	5-10 mg/kg PO (usually 300 mg) qd	Preventive therapy for contacts of persons with tuberculosis and as treatment for those whose skin test results have recently converted from negative to positive	Increased absorption with alcohol intake Decreased Dilantin metabolism Increased hepatotoxicity when combined with drugs that cause hepatotoxic effects
rifampin (Rifadin)	600 mg PO, IV qd	Prophylactic treatment for tuberculosis	Increased absorption with alcohol intake Decreased Dilantin metabolism Increased hepatotoxicity when combined with drugs that cause hepatotoxic effects Increased metabolism of antidiabetic medications
pyrazinamide (PZA)	15-30 mg/kg PO qd	Therapy for active tuberculosis	
ethambutol (Myambutol)	15-25 mg/kg PO, usually 1000 mg qd		
streptomycin (an aminoglycoside) (NTN)	0.5-1 g IM (for short-term therapy) qd	Also for tularemia and plague	
rifampin-INH (Rifamate)	600/300 mg PO qd 600/300 mg PO qd	Preventive therapy for tuberculosis and treatment of active tuberculosis	

Major Side Effects of First-Line Drugs:

Hepatotoxicity, neurotoxicity, ocular toxicity with ethambutol; arthritis, gout, arthritis-like reactions with pyrazinamide

SECOND-LINE DRUGS			
kanamycin (see Table 17-6)		Therapy for active tuberculosis	
p-aminosalicylic acid (PAS) (NTN)	3-4 g PO tid		

IM, intramuscularly; *NTN*, no trade name; *PO*, orally.

DRUGS TO TREAT FUNGAL INFECTIONS

Fungi, including yeasts and molds, are spore-forming, plantlike, colorless microorganisms. More complex than viruses or bacteria, fungi are found in soil, air, and contaminated food. Thriving on dead plants and on animals to produce many irritating symptoms, they also cover the entire body, eating dead tissue from the skin, hair, and nails. Bacteria and the immune system keep fungi under control, but multiplication is possible, causing pathogenicity in susceptible persons. Fungal cell membranes have little resemblance to bacterial cells; therefore antibiotics are ineffective. Long-term antibiotic therapy or radiation therapy can create an environment conducive to rapid fungal growth by altering the balance of normal flora or suppressing the immune system.

Antifungal drugs, both systemic and topical, can be fungicidal or fungistatic based on their concentration in the body tissues. Therapy is usually prolonged, taking several weeks because mycoses resist treatment, and toxic effects from treatment may occur before a cure is achieved. These drugs are fairly specific for the disease processes (Table 17-11).

Topical Antifungals

Dermatologic mycotic infections, with symptoms such as intense itching, discolored scaling of the skin, loss of hair and skin pigmentation, and blistered or broken skin between the toes, are typically more annoying than serious. Two of the most common fungal infections are ringworm infections (tinea corporis or tinea capitis) and athlete's foot (tinea pedis). **Undecylenic acid** as a topical agent for superficial mycoses is active against tinea infections. The major indication is tinea pedis. Another fairly common fungal condition is infection caused by *Candida albicans,* such as thrush in the mouth and candidiasis in the vagina. Undecylenic acid, used to treat tinea infections, is not effective against candidiasis. Many topical and vaginal agents are available as OTC medications (see Chapter 22 for more on topical antifungals).

Systemic Antifungals

Systemic fungal or mycotic infections are divided into two categories: (1) opportunistic infections (e.g., candidiasis, aspergillosis, cryptococcosis, mucormycosis) and (2) nonopportunistic uncommon infections (e.g.,

TABLE 17-11 SELECT ANTIFUNGAL DRUGS

GENERIC NAME/ TRADE NAME	USUAL ADULT DOSE, ROUTE, AND FREQUENCY OF ADMINISTRATION	INDICATIONS FOR USE	DRUG INTERACTIONS
SYSTEMIC DRUGS			
amphotericin B (Fungizone)	0.25-1.5 mg/kg IV qd topical	Aspergillosis, candidiasis, coccidioidomycosis, blastomycosis	Increased potential for digitalis toxicity
micafungin sodium (Mycamine)	50-150 mg IV qd	Candidiasis	prednisone, tacrolimus, sirolimus
caspofungin (Cancidas)	50-70 mg IV qd	Candidiasis, aspergillosis	
flucytosine (Ancobon)	50-150 mg/kg/day q6h	*Candida,* cryptococci	quinidine, cytosine
Major Side Effects of Systemic Drugs:			
Headache, anemia; GI disturbances; blurred vision, confusion, hallucinations; bone marrow suppression			
AZOLE ANTIFUNGALS			
fluconazole (Diflucan)	100-200 mg PO, IV qd	Candidiasis, cryptococcal infections, histoplasmosis; similar to amphotericin B	Increased liver toxicity with alcohol, increased effects of oral hypoglycemics, and phenytoin
ketoconazole (NTN)	200-400 mg PO qd	Same as for amphotericin B	See drug literature
itraconazole (Sporanox)	200-400 mg PO qd	Same	pimozide, quinidine. dofetilide
posaconazole (Noxafil)	100-200 mg PO tid	Prophylaxis for *Aspergillus* and *Candida* infections in immunosuppressed individuals	cyclosporine, tacrolimus, sirolimus, cimetidine, and others
OTHER ANTIFUNGALS			
griseofulvin (Grifulvin-V)	500 mg PO qd	Tinea infections Tinea pedis, onychomycosis	Decreased anticoagulant therapy such as Coumadin and oral contraceptives
nystatin (Mycostatin, Nilstat)	400,000-600,000 mg PO qid, 500,000-1,000,000 mg PO qid as lozenge, suspension, tablets	*Monilia,* candidiasis	No significant interactions
terbinafine (Lamisil)	250 mg PO qd topical	Onychomycosis; tinea infections	Alcohol

GI, gastrointestinal; *IV,* intravenously; *NTN,* no trade name; *PO,* orally.

histoplasmosis and blastomycosis). ***Amphotericin B*** is active against a broad spectrum of fungi and is the drug of choice for most systemic mycoses. Other medications frequently used for systemic fungal infections include the azole group (see Table 17-11).

Drugs for dermatologic fungal conditions are discussed in Chapter 22.

PATIENT ALERT

- Cotton socks should be worn during treatment for foot fungal infections. All shoes should be worn with socks.
- For treating fungal infections of the genitals or tinea of the groin, men and women should preferably wear breathable cotton undergarments.

Patient Education for Compliance

The feet, groin, and underarm areas are moister than other skin areas, thus requiring the use of powders for topical treatment of fungal infections, rather than creams or lotions, because powders tend to absorb moisture.

Important Facts about Antifungals

- Antifungals may be either fungicidal or fungistatic and are found as prescription and OTC preparations.
- Antifungals are designed to be used for 4 weeks unless they are being used on nails where a longer period of time is needed. However, the agent and organism may require a time variance.
- Vulvovaginal candidiasis may be treated with a single oral dose of fluconazole.

DRUGS TO TREAT VIRAL INFECTIONS

Viruses are strands of genetic material wrapped in a protein coating that prevents the virus from sustaining itself independently. Viruses are parasitic on host cells where the virus reproduces and range from viruses that cause the common cold to those that cause devastating illnesses such as HIV and AIDS. Therefore difficulty lies in the inability to suppress viral replication without doing significant harm to the host.

Viruses attach to the outer membrane of the cell and enter the cell nucleus, where DNA or RNA is covered with a protein capsule. HIV virus, a retrovirus, attaches to the RNA and replicates on DNA, causing new viruses to be placed in circulation.

By the time signs and symptoms of a viral infection appear, viral replication is complete and the disease course has been determined. To be effective for all viral diseases, antivirals would need to be given prophylactically, which is not practical, safe, or effective in most instances. An exception is the use of antivirals prophylactically in certain settings with influenza outbreaks. Most antiviral drugs work by preventing the virus from entering the host's cell or by interrupting replication.

Classification of Antiviral Drugs

The antiviral drugs are classified according to their use for either HIV infection or for non-HIV infection. Drugs for HIV infection are called *antiretroviral drugs*, whereas drugs for non-HIV infections are active against a narrow spectrum of viruses.

Non-HIV Antiviral Medications

The non-HIV antiviral medications have limited ability to treat infections because the viruses depend on host cells for replication. The herpes group includes herpes simplex virus (HSV) infections of the genitalia, mouth and face, and other sites and varicella zoster virus (VZV), the causative virus for varicella (chickenpox) and herpes zoster (shingles). The effective drug of choice for these conditions is ***acyclovir*** (Zovirax), which is available in topical, oral, and IV forms (see Table 17-12 for other drugs used for herpes infections).

Cytomegalovirus (CMV) and Epstein-Barr virus (infectious mononucleosis) are also members of the herpes viral group. Transmission of CMV occurs through body fluids, blood transfusion, and organ transplants. By age 40, harboring of the virus is common and is of little concern in healthy persons; however, immunocompromised people are at high risk for the disease. Five drugs, oral and intravenous, are used for treatment. Ophthalmic preparations for these diseases are discussed in Chapter 21.

Influenza, a serious viral respiratory condition, is caused by influenza A and B viruses. Highly contagious, it can be minimized by vaccination (Chapter 16) and with medications for the prevention and treatment of the disease (Chapter 25).

Viral hepatitis is the most common liver disease. See Chapter 24 for related drugs.

HIV Antivirals

Although no cure for HIV infection has been found, advances in drug treatment have been dramatic, and presently the ability to delay progression of HIV infection to AIDS occurs with appropriate use of antiretroviral drugs. Advances in pharmaceutical preparations are also increasing quality of life for those affected; the trend is

TABLE 17-12 SELECT ANTIVIRAL DRUGS

GENERIC NAME/ TRADE NAME	USUAL ADULT DOSE, ROUTE, AND FREQUENCY OF ADMINISTRATION	INDICATIONS FOR USE	DRUG INTERACTIONS
NON-HIV ANTIVIRALS			
cidofovir (Vistide)	5 mg/kg IV weekly to every other wk	Cytomegalovirus (CMV), CMV retinitis	No significant interactions
ganciclovir (Cytovene)	5 mg/kg IV daily to bid 1000 mg PO tid	CMV	zidovudine (AZT)
valganciclovir (Valcyte)	450-900 mg PO daily-bid	CMV	
acyclovir (Zovirax)	200 mg PO qid	Herpesvirus types 1 and 2 and zoster	No significant interactions
famciclovir (Famvir)	125 mg PO daily-tid 500 mg PO daily-tid	Genital herpes Herpes zoster	No significant interactions
penciclovir (Denavir)	Apply topically at site	Herpes simplex	No significant interactions
valacyclovir (Valtrex)	500 mg PO bid	Genital herpes, herpes zoster	No significant interactions
foscarnet (Foscavir)	40 mg/kg IV q8-12h	Herpes viruses, CMV, Epstein-Barr virus, varicella-zoster	No significant interactions

Major Side Effects of Non-HIV Antivirals:
GI distress, dizziness, tinnitus, unpleasant taste; may be toxic, causing nephrotoxicity, hepatic dysfunction, blood dyscrasias

HIV ANTIVIRALS

Nucleoside Reverse Transcriptase Inhibitors (NRTIs)

abacavir (Ziagen)	300 mg PO bid	HIV	Alcohol, St John's wort
didanosine, ddl (Videx)	200 mg PO bid	Advanced HIV	Care with anti-TB drugs, alcohol, furosemide, estrogens, tetracyclines, nitrofurantoin, diuretics
emtricitabine (Emtriva)	200 mg PO bid	HIV	No significant interactions
lamivudine (Epivir)	150 mg PO bid	HIV	St. John's wort
nelfinavir (Viracept)	750 mg PO tid	HIV	prednisone, rifampin, oral contraceptives, ketoconazole, St. John's wort
stavudine (Zerit)	40 mg PO bid	HIV	zidovudine
tenofovir (Viread)	300 mg PO qd	HIV	No significant interactions
zalcitabine (Hivid)	0.75 mg PO tid	HIV	probenecid, cimetidine, Maalox, metoclopramide, didanosine
zidovudine (Retrovir)	600 mg/day PO in divided doses 1 mg/kg IV 5-6 times/day	HIV with impaired immunity	ganciclovir

Nonnucleoside Reverse Transcriptase Inhibitors (NNTIs)

delavirdine (Rescriptor*)	400 mg PO tid	Advanced HIV	Multiple, see drug literature
nevirapine (Viramune*)	200 mg PO bid	HIV	Same as nelfinavir Numerous life-threatening interactions (see literature)
efavirenz (Sustiva)	600 mg PO qd	HIV	Benzodiazepines, ergot products
etravirine (Intelence)	200 mg PO bid	HIV	May interact with other HIV medications

CNS, central nervous system; *GI,* gastrointestinal; *HIV,* human immunodeficiency virus; *IV,* intravenously; *PO,* orally; *TB,* tuberculosis.
*Used in combination with other antivirals.

Continued

TABLE 17-12 SELECT ANTIVIRAL DRUGS—cont'd

GENERIC NAME/ TRADE NAME	USUAL ADULT DOSE, ROUTE, AND FREQUENCY OF ADMINISTRATION	INDICATIONS FOR USE	DRUG INTERACTIONS
Protease Inhibitors (PI)			
indinavir (Crixivan)	800 mg PO q8h	HIV infection	cisapride, midazolam, triazolam, rifampin, Rescriptor, ketoconazole
ritonavir (Norvir)	600 mg PO bid	HIV	Antianxiety agents, cisapride, meperidine, piroxicam, propoxyphene
saquinavir (Invirase)	1000 mg PO bid	HIV	Anti-TB, Dilantin, nonsedating antihistamines
fosamprenavir (Lexiva)	700-1400 mg PO bid	HIV	See drug information
atazanavir (Rayataz)	300-400 mg PO qd	HIV	See drug information
darunavir (given with efavirenz) (Prezista)	600 mg PO bid	HIV	See drug information
Other HIV Antivirals			
raltegravir (Isentress)	400 mg PO bid	HIV	TB medications
maraviroc (Selzentry)	150-600 mg PO	HIV	St John's wort, TB medications, anticonvulsant medications

Major Side Effects of HIV Antivirals:
Nephrotoxicity, nausea, vomiting, anorexia, renal failure, diarrhea, headache, blood dyscrasias, fat redistribution, pancreatitis, blood glucose alterations

for once-daily dosing with fewer tablets and no food restrictions.

Medications for HIV, which have been rapidly approved by the Food and Drug Administration (FDA), require a triple-drug regimen, often known as a "cocktail." These drugs act to reduce HIV levels in plasma, thereby slowing loss of immune function, preserving health, and prolonging life. For this reason, combination medicinal products have been FDA approved for decreasing the need for administration of multiple doses of different medications at the same time.

The benefits of the antiretrovirals for HIV are complex, cost is high, and toxicity is great. HIV antivirals exhibit multiple drug interactions and cause noticeable side effects. Treatment does not eliminate the HIV virus, but drugs reduce viral levels, sometimes to the point of being undetectable.

Nucleoside or nucleotide reverse transcriptase inhibitors (NRTIs), by preventing healthy T cells in the body from becoming infected with HIV, are the prime focus for once-a-day therapies and are the backbone for most current regimens. NRTIs are chemical relatives of the nucleosides in DNA; they suppress viral DNA, preventing conversion of RNA to DNA in infected T cells. These drugs must undergo intracellular conversion to be effective. Nonnucleoside reverse transcriptase inhibitors (NNRTIs) bind to the active center of reverse transcriptase and are effective as administered. Rashes, headaches, and GI symptoms occur with these compounds.

Protease inhibitors (PIs) are the most effective HIV-drugs available. Although these agents are well tolerated, GI symptoms do occur. Other significant side effects include hyperglycemia, fat maldistribution, increased bleeding tendencies, hyperlipidemia, and decreased bone mineral density. These drugs should not be used alone. Drug informational materials should be read when these medications are prescribed, because of multiple side effects that are found with individual drugs.

The only absolute contraindication to the use of an HIV antiviral drug is hypersensitivity to the medication or concurrent conditions or drug therapy that prevents the drug use. Because HIV is treated with combinations of antivirals, many drugs are now found in set combinations for patient convenience, but the possibility of nephrotoxicity is very real (see Table 17-12).

PATIENT ALERT

To be effective, antivirals for AIDS and HIV-related diseases must be administered continuously for life. Stopping treatment causes a danger of producing drug-resistant HIV.

Patient Education for Compliance

1. Drugs, especially acyclovir and valacyclovir, decrease symptoms of genital herpes simplex infection, but they do not produce a cure. If lesions are present, the disease is communicable.
2. Persons with HIV should adhere closely to prescribed dosage schedules.

Important Facts about Antiviral Medications

- Viruses live on host cells, so it is difficult to suppress viral reproduction without the host's body cells also being harmed.
- Acyclovir and valacyclovir are drugs of choice for herpes simplex and varicella-zoster viral infections.
- Resistance to antiviral drugs is a major concern. To reduce the emergence of resistant strains, drugs for HIV should be given in combination.
- New drugs given to HIV patients should be agents that the patient has not previously taken and are not cross-resistant with already taken drugs.

DRUGS TO TREAT MALARIA

Malaria, a parasitic disease transmitted by a mosquito that acts as a vector, is characterized by high fever with recurrent chills, severe sweating, and jaundice brought about by involving the liver.

Antimalarial drugs, with **chloroquine** being the drug of choice except with drug sensitivity issues, are administered for prophylaxis and to prevent disease development after exposure. Prophylaxis should begin 1 to 2 weeks before travel to an area where malaria is endemic and should continue for 6 weeks after the individual leaves the area. Drugs used during an acute attack of malaria selectively stop the multiplication of microorganisms and arrest the disease.

Choice of antimalarial medications is based on the strain of malaria-causing protozoa involved and the stage in organism's life cycle. Travelers to areas where malaria is endemic should contact the CDC for current prophylaxis requirements (Table 17-13).

CHEMICAL AGENTS USED AS ANTISEPTICS AND GERMICIDES AND DISINFECTANTS

Microorganisms are everywhere, migrating on skin, hair, furniture, and even in the air currents. Even in an optimal environment, microorganisms can produce infection. Antiseptics and disinfectants are used to reduce microbial growth, wound contamination, and ultimately the risk of wound infection. See Figure 17-1 for the chain of infection. The terms antiseptic and disinfectant or germicidal agent are not interchangeable, although both types of agents are used to control and prevent infection.

TABLE 17-13 SELECT ANTIMALARIALS

GENERIC NAME/ TRADE NAME	USUAL ADULT DOSE, ROUTE, AND FREQUENCY OF ADMINISTRATION	INDICATIONS FOR USE	DRUG INTERACTIONS
chloroquine/Aralen	300-700 mg/wk PO 2 wk before exposure and for up to 8 wk after leaving endemic area	Acute malaria and prophylaxis	No significant interactions
hydroxychloroquine/Plaquenil	400 mg/wk PO 2 wk before and 4 wk after leaving	Acute attacks and prophylaxis	No significant interactions
mefloquine/Lariam	5 tabs PO once (treatment), 250 mg/wk PO prophylactic	Same as for Plaquenil	quinine, beta blockers, calcium channel blockers
pyrimethamine/Daraprim	25 mg PO once a wk up to 10 wk	Prophylaxis	No significant interactions
pyrimethamine with sulfadoxine/Fansidar	50 mg PO qd	Acute attack for chloroquine-resistant disease	No significant interactions
doxycycline* (tetracycline)/ Vibramycin	100 mg/day PO for 1-2 days before travel, continuously throughout travel, and 4 wk after travel	Prophylaxis	See interactions for tetracyclines in Table 17-5

Major Side Effects of Antimalarials: Nausea, diarrhea, headaches, blurred vision, vertigo, rashes

PO, orally.
*See Antibiotics.

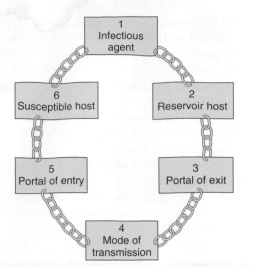

Figure 17-1 Chain of infection. (From Young AP, Proctor DB: *Kinn's the medical assistant,* ed 11, St Louis, 2011, Elsevier.)

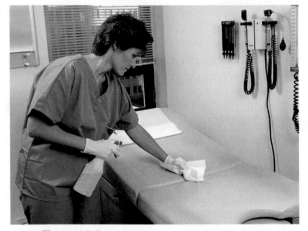

Figure 17-2 Disinfectants used to sanitize rooms.

Antiseptics versus Disinfectants and Germicides

Antiseptics are agents applied to living tissue to clean wounds or to prepare skin for procedures, surgery, or injections. The objective of antiseptic therapy is to decrease the number of bacteria and eliminate disease or to serve as prophylaxis with activities such as hand washing. Antiseptics and disinfectants should not be taken orally because of their toxicity when ingested or absorbed through the skin.

Too harsh for living tissue, disinfectants are applied to inanimate objects to reduce bacterial growth (Figure 17-2). Disinfectants may not kill all types of microorganisms, especially mold spores, viruses, and fungi. Germicides, which kill microorganisms, may be used on either living or nonliving objects. Germicides may be further subdivided into bactericides, fungicides, virucides, and amebicides. Germistatic agents may be used

for **sanitization** but do not kill microbes for sterilization.

In clinical use, effectiveness of antiseptics and disinfectants is extremely variable, depending on the product, how it is applied, and the situation in which it is used. Antiseptic and disinfectant solutions vary in their antimicrobial potency, their spectrum of activity, and the time they take to act, as well as their duration of action with exposure to chemicals. For example, *70% ethanol* reduces bacteria on skin by 50% in 36 seconds, whereas *benzalkonium chloride 1:1000* requires 7 minutes of exposure for the same effect.

Some chemicals are broad spectrum or nonselective in their action, such as *formaldehyde, glutaraldehyde,* and *iodine. Hexachlorophene* and benzalkonium chloride are primarily effective against both gram-positive and gram-negative bacteria. *Alcohol* is bactericidal to vegetative forms of both gram-positive and gram-negative bacteria.

✒ CLINICAL TIP

After cleansing an instrument, allied health professionals should be sure the instrument is dry before placing it in a disinfectant to prevent diluting the disinfecting solution and decreasing its effectiveness.

Antiseptics

Iodine Preparations
Iodine preparations (iodophors) are rapid-acting, potent germicides that are superior for effectively removing microorganisms such as bacteria, viruses, and protozoa from skin. *Tincture of iodine* is especially effective, but it causes residual skin staining and also local stinging because of its alcohol base. Iodine preparations such as *povidone-iodine* (Betadine) are used to disinfect skin before surgery. Allergic reactions to iodine are common and should be carefully evaluated because the resultant stain may mask redness and swelling.

Alcohol
Alcohol preparations can be used as antiseptics either alone or in combination with other topical agents to prepare skin for surgery or injection. Ethyl alcohol is effective in concentrations of less than 70%; *isopropyl alcohol* is bactericidal in concentrations of 50% to 90%, with 70% being the desired concentration. Alcohol is added to other antiseptics to increase the antiseptic effect, but this additive may cause skin irritation. The swabs or prep wipes for giving injections contain isopropyl alcohol for its bactericidal effects. The area should be air-dried for ultimate cleaning.

Hexachlorophene

Hexachlorophene, used as a surgical scrub or skin cleanser, is effective against gram-positive microorganisms, the usual bacteria found on skin. With repeated use, hexachlorophene accumulates on skin to maintain antibacterial activity.

Hydrogen Peroxide

Hydrogen peroxide is an excellent disinfectant and sterilizing agent but is useless as an antiseptic because it does not penetrate skin and breaks down rapidly into oxygen and water. Its effervescence may facilitate mechanical cleaning of debris from a wound, but this contact terminates germicidal action. Use may be detrimental by causing new tissue to slough.

Silver Preparations

Silver preparations are antiseptics. **Silver nitrate** is used as an ophthalmic antiseptic in eyes of newborns to prevent gonococcal infections. **Silver sulfadiazine** (Silvadene) is used topically for burns because of its ability to better penetrate wounds.

Disinfectants

Disinfectants are used for cleaning and storage of surgical instruments, disinfection of operating rooms, and sterilization of objects that cannot be exposed to high temperatures. Formaldehyde and glutaraldehyde are irritating to skin and should be used only on inanimate objects. Other common disinfectants that are also antiseptics are **sodium hypochlorite** (bleach) and alcohol (Table 17-14).

Weakened sodium hypochlorite (10% dilution) may be used as an antiseptic to disinfect countertops, floors, and other surfaces as a virucide. Weaker solutions are available (**Dakin solution**), with a maximum concentration of 0.5% at full strength, to irrigate wounds.

Boric acid is a mild nontoxic bacteriostatic and fungicidal most commonly used as a surgical eyewash or irrigant. This compound is also found in medications for first-aid treatments (see Table 17-14).

✐ CLINICAL TIP

Any dilute hypochlorite solution used for disinfecting surfaces should be made in the office daily because it remains fully potent for only 24 to 36 hours. Dilution should be 1:10 for the solution to be effective for disinfecting surfaces. Care must be taken to dilute sodium hypochlorite solution to prevent discoloration of surfaces or clothing. Some facilities purchase a prediluted product because of convenience and solution stability.

Important Facts about Antiseptics and Disinfectants

- *Antiseptics* are used on living tissue, and *disinfectants* are used on inanimate objects. *Germicides* may be used on either animate or inanimate objects.
- *Bactericidals* kill microorganisms, whereas antiseptics and *bacteriostatics* only inhibit the growth of microbes.
- If sodium hypochlorite is used as a disinfectant, the solution should be diluted to prevent discoloration of surfaces to which it is applied.
- Antiseptics prevent development of local infections. For an established infection, systemic antiinfectants are preferred for treatment.

SUMMARY

With the advent of penicillin and sulfonamides, a new era in health care was launched. Since the time penicillin was first used in the early 1940s, antimicrobials have been used in medical offices on a daily basis. As bacteria, fungi, and viruses become resistant to one type of antimicrobial agent, new agents must be developed to replace the agents that are no longer effective. The FDA approves new antimicrobials many times a year, with special rapidity for agents used to treat debilitating diseases such as HIV infection.

Patient education in the use of antimicrobials, a major responsibility of the allied health professional, should include not saving medications but to complete the full prescription. If the drug is not taken for the prescribed time, drug-resistant bacteria become victors in the battle against disease (two of the major strains of drug-resistant bacteria are those that cause tuberculosis and those that cause staphylococcal infections). When drugs are taken correctly, virulent bacteria are killed or controlled until the body's own defense system suppresses any remaining microorganisms. Without the body's defense system, antibiotic therapy would rarely be successful. *People do not become drug resistant; the microorganism becomes drug resistant, and microbes will continue to multiply in a drug-resistant state.*

The key to treating infection is to match the medication to the microorganism. Some antimicrobials are effective against a broad spectrum of organisms; others have narrow spectra. The best match can be obtained by performing culture and sensitivity testing. Effectiveness of the antibiotic depends on its ability to concentrate at the infection site as well as other factors. Superinfections can become a problem with antibiotic therapy, especially when treatment is over a prolonged period of time.

Antibiotics are available in several categories such as penicillins, cephalosporins, macrolides, tetracyclines,

TABLE 17-14 ANTISEPTICS AND DISINFECTANTS/GERMICIDALS*

GENERIC NAME	TRADE NAME OR COMMON NAME	PRIMARY ANTIMICROBIAL USE	ANTISEPTIC	DISINFECTANT
ALCOHOLS				
ethanol	Ethyl alcohol	Vegetative bacteria	X	
isopropyl (70%)	Rubbing alcohol		X	
ALDEHYDES				
formaldehyde (10%-37%)		Bacterial spores, viruses, fungi		X
glutaraldehyde (2%)	Cidex			X
IODINE PREPARATIONS				
povidone-iodine (0.5%-10%)	Betadine, Iodine	Vegetative microorganisms and spores	X	X
iodine solution (2%)			X	
tincture of iodine (2%)		Bacteria, spores, fungi, viruses	X	
CHLORINE COMPOUNDS				
sodium hypochlorite 10%—disinfectant 0.15%-0.5%—antiseptic	Clorox	Bacteria, spores, fungi, viruses	X	X
oxychlorosene	Clorpactin	Useful with local infections that are drug resistant	X	
PHENOL COMPOUND				
hexachlorophene	Dial soap, pHisoHex ℞	Vegetative gram-positive bacteria	X	
OTHERS				
chlorhexidine 1%	Exidine cleanser, Hibiclens	Spores, bacteria, fungi, viruses	X	
boric acid		Bacteria, fungi	X	
gentian violet		Yeast infections	X	
hydrogen peroxide (1.5%)		Vegetative microorganisms		X
benzalkonium chloride (0.02%-0.5%)	Zephiran	Vegetative gram-positive bacteria	X	X
silver nitrate (0.1%-0.5%)		Vegetative bacteria and fungi	X	
silver sulfadiazine (1%)[†]	Silvadene	Vegetative bacteria and fungi	X	

*Antiseptics and germicidals and disinfectants may cause such side effects as skin irritation, rashes, and skin dryness.
[†]Requires a prescription.

aminoglycosides, and some miscellaneous groups. Antibiotics are found for systemic use by prescription and in many OTC preparations for topical use. OTC preparations are first-aid medications used therapeutically or prophylactically with lacerations, abrasions, insect bites, and so on.

Sulfonamides are not antibiotics but are antibacterials used to treat an infection while the body responds with its own defense mechanisms.

Tuberculosis has traditionally been treated with rifampin and INH, but as the causative organism is becoming resistant to these drugs, new drugs are being introduced. Medications for tuberculosis must be given in combination to prevent development of drug-resistant bacteria, to effectively eradicate organisms, and to achieve synergistic effects.

Topical or systemic medications for fungal infections require long-term use. Fungal infections are difficult to cure because fungi live on dead body skin or within body tissues. Long-term antibiotic therapy or radiation therapy allows naturally occurring fungi on skin to grow without natural controls, leading to superinfections.

Because viruses do not respond to antibiotics, these should not be administered in viral infections unless a secondary bacterial infection is present. The problem with developing antiviral medications is that often the virus is virulent within the body before signs and symptoms of the disease are evident, and many viruses rapidly mutate and change as they replicate.

Drugs for malaria may be given prophylactically before travel to regions where malaria is endemic and therapeutically for the treatment of active malaria.

Antiseptics, disinfectants, and germicidals are mainstays of the physician's office. Antiseptics are used on living tissue, disinfectants on inanimate objects, and germicides on both. The agent should be chosen to match medical use. Disinfectants include sodium hypochlorite, used to decontaminate surfaces where body fluids may be found. Sodium hypochlorite is an excellent virucide, but care must be taken to avoid discoloration of surfaces where it is used.

Care must be taken in treating individuals who might have had allergic reactions to antibiotics in the past. Medications should not be prescribed when they are not indicated because of the danger of drug-resistant microorganisms developing.

CRITICAL THINKING EXERCISES

Scenario

Janie comes to the office complaining of a sore throat, hoarseness, cough, and runny nose. Dr. Merry has examined Janie and told her that she has a virus. Janie tells you as she leaves that she just does not understand why Dr. Merry did not give her an antibiotic. Janie's health history is nonsignificant except for symptoms of the present respiratory tract infection.

1. What reason do you give Janie to explain why Dr. Merry did not prescribe an antibiotic?
2. What do you tell Janie about the misuse of antibiotics?
3. Is a prophylactic prescription for an antibiotic indicated in this case?

DRUG CALCULATIONS

1. Order: ampicillin 125 mg IM stat
   Available medication:

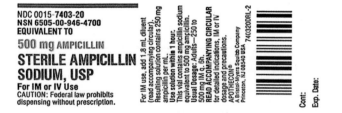

What volume of diluent should be added to the vial? _____

_____

What volume of medication should be administered for the order? _____

_____

How long is the solution stable after reconstitution?

_____

Show on the syringe the amount of Cefadyl that should be administered.

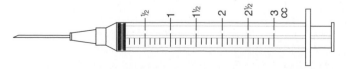

2. Order: clindamycin oral solution 150 mg q8h
   Available medication:

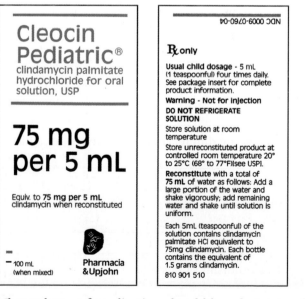

What volume of medication should be administered with each dose? _____

How can this medication be administered using a household measurement when a dose spoon is not available? _____

Show on the cup the amount of medication that
should be given to the child.

```
2 TBS ————— 30 mL
         ————— 25 mL
         ————— 20 mL
1 TBS ————— 15 mL
2 TSP ————— 10 mL
1 TSP ————— 5 mL
```

REVIEW QUESTIONS

1. Why are antibiotics effective against bacteria but not viruses? _____

   _____

   _____

2. What is acquired antibiotic resistance? How does a bacterium become drug resistant? _____

   _____

   _____

3. What spectra are used to classify penicillins? Name a commonly used medication in each spectrum. _____

   _____

   _____

   _____

   _____

4. What is meant by *generation* when discussing penicillin? _____

   _____

   _____

5. What is the main indication for the use of sulfonamides? Are these drugs bacteriostatic or bactericidal? What does
   the patient need to be told concerning fluid intake? _____

   _____

   _____

   _____

   _____

6. What is the difference in use between an antiseptic and a disinfectant? _____

   _____

   _____

7. What are the uses of antiseptics in the medical office? _____

   _____

   _____

8. How do disinfectants work? _____

   _____

   _____

CHAPTER 18

Antineoplastic Agents

After studying this chapter, you should be capable of doing the following:

- Defining use of antineoplastic medications.
- Explaining the difference between curative and palliative uses of chemotherapeutic agents.
- Classifying tumors by tissues in which they originate.
- Describing the role of the allied health professional in chemotherapy.
- Describing how to safely handle and administer antineoplastics.
- Identifying and classifying various chemotherapeutic medications.
- Providing patient education for compliance with medication used as antineoplastic agents.

Jack has esophageal cancer and is undergoing chemotherapy. After chemotherapy treatments, Jack has nausea and anorexia. His tongue is red, swollen, and sore.

Is this an expected effect of antineoplastics? Why or why not?
What suggestions do you have to help with his dietary intake?
Can Jack expect alopecia from all types of chemotherapy? Why or why not?
How would you explain to Jack what stage II carcinoma indicates?

KEY TERMS

Adenocarcinoma	Biotherapy	In situ	Neoplasm
Alkylating agent	Cancer	Malignant	Nystagmus
Alopecia	Carcinogenic	Metastasis	Palliative
Anaplastic	Cell cycle phase	Mitotic alkaloids	Plant alkaloids
Antimetabolite	Chemotherapy	Mitotic inhibitors	Proliferation
Antineoplastic agent	Cytotoxic agent	Morbidity	Radioisotope
Antitumor antibiotics	Diffusion	Morphology	Stomatitis
Ascites	Extravasation	Mortality	Teratogenic
Ataxia	Hormone	Mutagenic	Tumor
Benign	immunosuppressant		

EASY WORKING KNOWLEDGE OF ANTINEOPLASTICS

DRUG CLASS	PRESCRIPTION	OTC	PREGNANCY CATEGORY	MAJOR INDICATIONS
Alkylating agents	Yes	No	C, D, X (especially in first trimester)	Carcinomas, sarcomas, lymphomas, leukemias, and polycythemia vera
Antimetabolites	Yes	No	D	Carcinomas, trophoblastic tumors, osteogenic sarcomas
Antitumor antibiotics	Yes	No	C, D	Carcinomas, sarcomas, lymphomas, leukemias
Mitotic inhibitors (plant alkaloids)	Yes	No	D	Carcinomas, leukemias, Hodgkin disease, Ewing sarcoma
Hormone therapy	Yes	No	C, D, X	Prostate cancer, breast cancer, endometrial cancer, adrenal cancer
Immunosuppressants	Yes	No	C, D	Kaposi sarcoma, leukemias
Radioisotopes	Yes	No	C, D	Thyroid cancer, polycythemia vera, metastatic cancer

EASY WORKING KNOWLEDGE OF INDICATIONS AND SIDE EFFECTS

Seven Warning Signs of Cancer for Adults
Change in bowel or bladder habits
A sore that will not heal
Unusual bleeding or discharge
Thickening or a lump in the breast or elsewhere
Indigestion or difficulty swallowing
Obvious change in a wart or mole
Nagging cough or hoarseness

Common Signs of Childhood Cancer
Continued unexplained weight loss
Headaches, often with early morning vomiting
Increased swelling or persistent pain in bones, joints, back, or legs
Lump or mass, especially in the abdomen, neck, chest, pelvis, or armpits
Development of excessive bruising, bleeding, or rash

Constant infections
A whitish color behind the pupil
Nausea that persists or vomiting without nausea
Constant tiredness or noticeable paleness
Eye or vision changes that occur suddenly and persist
Recurrent and persistent fevers of unknown origin

Common Side Effects of Antineoplastic Medications
Stomatitis
Nausea and vomiting
Diarrhea
Alopecia
Local tissue injury
Suppression of blood elements

A neoplasm (*neo-*, new, plus Greek *-plasma*, formation), also known as a **tumor,** is a new or unusual growth of tissue in plants or animals. If the tumor has uncontrolled growth and spread of abnormal cells, it is known as **cancer.** Neoplasms, named for site of origin, may be **benign** or **malignant** (Figure 18-1). Named using originating tissue, benign neoplasms are named by the site plus the suffix *-oma.* (Note: Some malignant tumors also end with *-oma.*) Malignant neoplasms are characterized by the names ending in *sarcoma* (Table 18-1).

Drug treatment of tumors and malignancies, or **chemotherapy,** is increasingly important as an adjunct to surgery and radiation therapy. Chemotherapy is performed using **antineoplastic agents** that do not directly kill cancer cells; rather, they interfere with cell reproduction and growth, causing death to cells. Because cancer cells are prone to rapid **proliferation,** they are more vulnerable to chemotherapy than healthy, noncancerous cells. Nevertheless, many healthy cells die in the course of chemotherapy, and the individual undergoing such therapy can expect significant side effects from these toxic drugs. With **morbidity** and **mortality** from cancer continuing to pose a major health problem in the United States, research for more effective treatment is an ongoing quest and new drugs are introduced to the field often.

WHAT IS CANCER?

Cancer is not a single disease. With uncontrolled division of abnormal cells and with cancer cells reproducing faster than normal cells, more than 100 different types of cancer have been identified. Cancer, a mass of cells with no useful function, can cause dysfunction and structural alterations in surrounding tissues. As the tumor increases in size, normal cells lack the necessary nutrition or blood supply and thus decrease in number. This alteration causes loss of normal body functions, especially in the late stages of the disease.

The original site of a tumor is called the *primary site.* As the tumor undergoes metastasis to new locations in the body, each new site is referred to as a *secondary site.* First, cells may metastasize directly to neighboring tissue, causing ulceration or hemorrhagic masses with local infiltration and distortion of the structures.

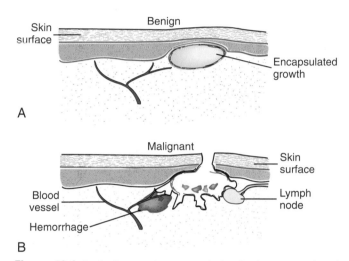

Figure 18-1 A, Benign neoplasms remain localized, are smooth and freely movable, compress local tissue, and do not break the skin. **B,** Malignant neoplasms metastasize to new and distant tissues through the lymph system and blood vessels, causing hemorrhage. They also have an irregular shape, invade local tissue, and often ulcerate through the skin.

Second, detached cells may move along lymphatic vessels or to regional lymph nodes as an embolism. Thus lymphatic tissue is the usual site for invasion and spread of abnormal cells. Cells may also form an embolus that moves through blood vessels to organs throughout the body. Finally, cells may invade a body cavity by diffusion.

Metastatic tumors mimic the primary tumor, permitting disease diagnosis by cell morphology. Cancers tend to metastasize to specific secondary sites at some distance from the primary site by traveling through the circulatory or lymphatic systems. The secondary tumors tend to resemble cells at the primary site and are so named, such as *lymphomas* for tumors originally found in the lymphatic system (see Table 18-1).

Classifying Tumors

Tumors are classified by stage (invasion) and grade (degree of metastasis). These are used for overall treatment plan for a neoplasm. The grade and stage are used to describe the abnormal cells and the extent of the spread of the disease. The tumor grade is a system used to classify cancer cells in terms of how abnormal they look under a microscope, giving some idea of how fast the tumor will grow and how fast it will spread. Grade 0 is normal tissue. Grade 1 tumor is the most differentiated, looking more like the parent tissue, and is the least malignant. Grade 2 is moderately well differentiated with some structural change from normal tissue. Grade 3 is poorly differentiated and has extensive change from normal tissue. Grade 4 has no resemblance to the tissue of origin and is anaplastic.

The stages of tumors show the extent of the spread of the cancer. Stage 0 is cancer in situ or without invasion

TABLE 18-1 EXAMPLES OF BENIGN AND MALIGNANT NEOPLASMS BY TISSUE OF ORIGIN		
TISSUE OF ORIGIN	**BENIGN**	**MALIGNANT**
Connective, nerve, and muscle tissue	Site + *-oma* (lipoma, a benign neoplasm of adipose tissue)	*Sarcoma* (liposarcoma = malignant neoplasm of adipose tissue)
Epithelial tissue	Adenoma, a benign neoplasm of glands	*Carcinoma* (adenocarcinoma = malignant neoplasm of glands)
	Nevus, a neoplasm of pigmented cells	*Melanoma* (malignant neoplasm of pigmented cells)
Blood-forming tissue including lymphoid tissue, plasma cells, and bone marrow	Lymphangioma, a benign neoplasm of lymph vessels	*Lymphoma* (lymphangiosarcoma = malignant neoplasm of lymph vessels; leukemias)
Nerve tissue ganglion cells	Ganglioneuroma, a benign neoplasm of nerve ganglion cells	*Blastoma* (neuroblastoma = malignant neoplasm of ganglion cells)

Note: Headings "Benign" and "Malignant" are not all-inclusive but are examples of naming of tumors. Entities in *italics* are malignant neoplasms.

of surrounding tissue. Stage 1 is a tumor limited to its site of origin. Stage 2 is cancer with only local spread. Stage 3 has extensive local to regional spread. Stage 4 has widespread metastasis throughout the body.

ANTINEOPLASTIC AGENTS

Antineoplastic agents, also called *chemotherapeutic agents,* kill tumor cells directly while interrupting cell replication of normal and abnormal cells to shrink tumors and to provide palliation and/or cure (Figure 18-2). When antineoplastic agents are chosen and administered for treatment of a malignant tumor, its type, size, site, grade, and stage are considered. Chemotherapy may be the primary treatment or may be used in combination with surgical removal and radiation. If the tumor is extensive, chemotherapy may first be used to reduce its size, followed by the surgical procedure and then further use of chemotherapeutics. In other cases the tumor may be excised, then chemotherapy and radiation may be used. The second course of chemotherapy is aimed at destroying cancer cells not destroyed by the immune system.

Cancers with fast growth factors and short cell replications are the most vulnerable to chemotherapeutic agents. Each antineoplastic agent has a specific point of effective action in cell replication (Figure 18-3). **Antimetabolites** interfere with DNA synthesis, whereas plant alkaloids, or mitotic inhibitors, interfere with cell reproduction in the metaphase. Some drugs, such as the

alkylating agents, antibiotics, and hormones, are active in several stages of the cell cycle and are not specific to a single phase. In combination therapy the goal is to destroy cancer cells at various stages of the cell replication process.

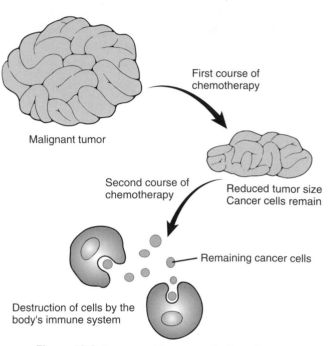

Figure 18-2 A cancer cell's response to chemotherapy.

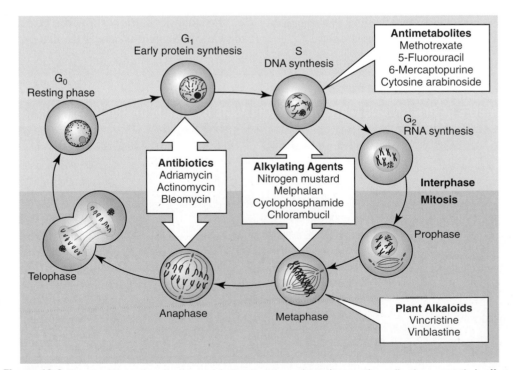

Figure 18-3 Phases of the cell replication cycle, showing where chemotherapeutic medications exert their effects.

BOX 18-1 DISORDERS AND SYMPTOMS OF ORGAN TOXICITY FROM ANTINEOPLASTICS

Cardiotoxic Effects
Congestive heart failure
Changes in ST waves
Angina while receiving medication
Shortness of breath
Ventricular fibrillation; death

Nephrotoxic Effects
Weight gain
Change in vital signs
Fluid overload
Swelling
Decreased urine output
Changes in urine color or components

Neurotoxic Effects
Change in cognitive abilities
Nystagmus
Ataxia
Dizziness, difficulty changing positions (cerebellar dysfunction)
Tingling of face, fingers, toes

Hepatotoxic Effects
Jaundice
Nausea and vomiting
Ascites
Clay-colored stools
Dark urine
Bleeding disorders, pruritus

Antineoplastic agents are most frequently given in combinations for **palliative** effect. **Cytotoxic agents** are used for long-term treatment in the hope of either curing the disease or placing it in remission. Because the metabolic rate of a malignant tumor cell is more rapid than that of a normal cell, malignant cells are more sensitive to products that interfere with cell growth.

Side Effects of Antineoplastics

The most serious cell destruction from antineoplastics occurs in the bone marrow, epithelium of the gastrointestinal (GI) tract, nervous system, hair follicles, and reproductive cells. Each chemotherapeutic agent differs in the likelihood to cause these adverse effects. Bone marrow suppression may lead to infection, bleeding, and anemia. The digestive tract epithelium is especially sensitive to cytotoxic drugs, leading to **stomatitis** and diarrhea because loss of epithelial cells prevents fluids from being absorbed in the intestines. **Alopecia** results from injury to the hair follicles and typically begins 7 to 10 days after the start of treatments that cause these effects. Some hormonal treatments may cause symptoms similar to menopause, creating hot flashes. In the reproductive system, certain teratogenic agents cause effects on the growing fetus and on the germinal epithelium of the testes. Women undergoing chemotherapy should be advised not to become pregnant because of the danger of fetal malformations. Male patients should be told that anticancer drugs might cause irreversible sterility. Nervous system effects can include numbness and tingling in the extremities, headaches, dizziness, confusion, or, in rare cases, seizures. Nausea and vomiting from chemotherapy are usually more severe than nausea and vomiting from most medications. Premedication with a combination of antiemetics, such as *prochlorperazine,*

trimethobenzamide, dexamethasone, metoclopramide, lorazepam, and serotonin agonist drugs may reduce symptoms. Weight loss and resultant malnutrition may occur because of the many GI symptoms including anorexia.

Certain chemotherapeutic agents have dose-limiting adverse reactions that occur when the maximum permissible dose has been given to the individual patient (Box 18-1).

PATIENT ALERT

- If hair loss is expected and the patient desires to wear a hairpiece, this should be selected before treatment is begun so that hair color and style will look as normal as possible. Hair begins to regrow in 1 to 2 months after therapy. When hair grows, it may not have the same texture or thickness as before chemotherapy.
- Patients undergoing chemotherapy should avoid highly seasoned foods and foods with strong odors. Eating small, frequent meals of complex carbohydrates and drinking liquids 30 to 60 minutes before meals will help manage nausea. Eating tart foods either cold or at room temperature enhances food intake.
- Any of the following should be reported to the physician: rashes; loss of taste; tingling in face, fingers, and toes; dizziness, headache, confusion, slurred speech, convulsions; and unusual bleeding, bruising, fever, sore throat, mouth sores.
- Because of immune system compromise, patients should avoid contact with communicable diseases and should have limited contact with persons who may have a subclinical illness, such as children who have fever or signs of possible disease.

Important Facts about Antineoplastic Agents

- Antineoplastic agents are used most often for malignant growths, although they may be used for other chronic diseases such as rheumatoid arthritis.
- Cancer treatment may entail surgery, radiation therapy, and chemotherapy, singly or in any combination. Surgery and radiation therapy are the treatments of choice for solid tumors, whereas antineoplastic agents are the treatment of choice for cancers that are found in several sites throughout the body.
- Most antineoplastic drugs work best on tumors formed by cells rapidly multiplying rather than on slow-growing tumors.
- Anticancer drugs are more effective when used as combination therapy rather than single-drug therapy because the cancer cells are less likely to mutate and become drug resistant.
- Toxic effects on normal cells are a major obstacle to successful chemotherapy.
- Antineoplastics must have one of three possible benefits to be used: cure, palliation, or prolongation of life.

Patient Education for Compliance

1. Because anxiety is an expected response, cancer patients should be made aware of the need for emotional support for themselves and their families.
2. Good nutrition is essential during chemotherapy. The patient should follow instructions to meet specific nutritional needs.
3. Lesions in the mouth and bleeding gums are common with chemotherapy. Good oral hygiene is essential.
4. Cool, sweetened beverages are best tolerated.
5. Fever, sore throat, infections, and suppression of blood counts are common side effects of chemotherapy.

FACTORS TO CONSIDER WITH CHEMOTHERAPY

Not all patients or types of cancer are candidates for chemotherapy. The decision to begin medical treatment is made on an individual basis after informing the patient of possible risks and benefits of therapy and after informed consent has been obtained. Patients should not be put at great risk for little to gain. What is unacceptable to one patient might be eagerly pursued by another, depending on a variety of life factors.

CLASSES OF ANTINEOPLASTIC AGENTS

Alkylating or Alkylating-Like Agents

Some of the earliest agents used to treat neoplasms were alkylating agents that poison cancer cells. These agents are based on chemical warfare from World War I when use of **nitrogen mustard** was introduced. Alkylating agents were observed to inhibit cell growth, and so were investigated to inhibit the growth of malignant cells. Because cell reproduction has irreversible binding to DNA, eventually the cell dies from inability to maintain cell metabolism. This group of chemotherapeutics also includes nitrosoureas and platinum compounds and alkylating agents (see Figure 18-3).

Alkylating medications are highly toxic compounds used to treat metastatic ovarian, testicular, and bladder cancer and for palliative treatment of undesirable symptoms of other cancers, such as brain tumors (Table 18-2).

Antimetabolites

Antimetabolites are effective against cells by interfering during the synthesis phase of metabolism, blocking the chemical reactions necessary for normal cell growth and reproduction. Certain antimetabolites such as **mercaptopurine** (Purinethol) are also used in immunosuppressive therapy (such as for organ transplantation), as antiviral medications, and in treatment of gout (see Tables 18-2 and 18-3).

Mitotic Inhibitors (Plant Alkaloids)

The primary **mitotic inhibitors** are derived from periwinkle and May apple plants. Thus these medications as a group are known as **plant alkaloids** or **mitotic alkaloids.** They prevent the chromosomes from dividing and migrating to the end of the cells, stopping further cell replication or mitosis. If **extravasation** occurs with these medications, tissue injury is expected. Alopecia is not as common as with other cytotoxic drugs (sees Tables 18-2 and 18-3).

Did You Know?

Vinca, the periwinkle plant, is an evergreen ground cover. It takes more than 6 tons of the leaves to produce 1 ounce of vinca compound.

Hormones and Hormone Antagonists

Hormones and hormone antagonists, the least toxic of anticancer medications, act on specific hormone

Text continued on p. 319

TABLE 18-2 SELECT ANTINEOPLASTIC AGENTS*

GENERIC NAME/ TRADE NAME	USUAL ADULT DOSE, ROUTE, AND FREQUENCY	MAJOR SIDE EFFECTS	INDICATIONS FOR USE	DRUG INTERACTIONS
ALKYLATING AND ALKYLATING-LIKE DRUGS				
		Nausea, vomiting, bone marrow suppression, diarrhea, dermatitis, hepatic or renal toxicity, alopecia, myalgia, fever, malaise		
nitrogen mustard or mechlorethamine (Mustargen)	0.4 mg/kg IV		Lymphosarcoma, Hodgkin disease	No immunizations, alcohol
cyclophosphamide (Cytoxan)	50-100 mg/m² /day PO; 400-1800 mg/m² 40-50 mg/kg IV		Broad spectrum of neoplasms	Antigout medications
chlorambucil (Leukeran)	0.1-0.2 mg/kg/day PO		Leukemias, malignancies of the lymphatic system	Antigout medications and live virus vaccines
melphalan (Alkeran)	6 mg daily PO		Multiple myeloma, carcinoma of breast and ovary, lymphocytic leukemia, lymphomas, mycotic fungus, polycythemia vera	Antigout medications
Platinum Compounds and Alkylating Agents				
				Aspirin, NSAIDs, alcohol, aminoglycosides, loop diuretics
oxaliplatin (Eloxatin)	85 mg/m² BSA IV		CA of colon	
cisplatin (Platinol)	IV; varies with neoplasm type		Metastatic testicular and ovarian cancers, bladder cancer	Antigout medications
NITROSOUREAS				
carmustine (BiCNU) Gliadel wafer	75-100 mg/m² BSA IV 62.6 mg/wafer for brain implant	Severe nausea and vomiting with liver and kidney toxicity, bone marrow suppression	CA of CNS	Anticoagulants, other antineoplastics, cimetidine, digoxin, phenytoin
lomustine (CCNU)	100-130 mg/m² BSA PO	Hepatotoxicity, renal failure, pulmonary fibrosis, anemia	Hodgkin disease and CNS CA	Same as for carmustine
streptozocin (Zanosar)	500 mg/m² BSA IV	Severe nausea and vomiting, changes in glucose levels, diarrhea, chills and fever	Pancreatic CA	Same as for carmustine

BSA, body surface area; *CA*, cancer *CNS*, central nervous system; *GI*, gastrointestinal; *IM*, intramuscularly; *IV*, intravenously; *NSAIDs*, nonsteroidal anti-inflammatory drugs; *PCN*, penicillin *PO*, orally; *SC*, subcutaneously.

*Medications used as antineoplastics have highly individualized doses based on the BSA of the patient and the neoplasm being treated. The doses in this table are provided as typical doses only.

Because of the many drug interactions, when administering all chemotherapeutic agents, the accompanying literature should always be read and compared with medications being taken by the person receiving treatment.

A table with more agents can be found on Evolve.

Continued

TABLE 18-2 SELECT ANTINEOPLASTIC AGENTS—cont'd

GENERIC NAME/ TRADE NAME	USUAL ADULT DOSE, ROUTE, AND FREQUENCY	MAJOR SIDE EFFECTS	INDICATIONS FOR USE	DRUG INTERACTIONS
ANTIMETABOLITES				
		Severe bone marrow suppression, mouth and stomach ulcers, anorexia, diarrhea, nausea, vomiting, chills and fever, alopecia		
methotrexate (folic acid analogue), amethopterin (Mexate, Rheumatrex, MTX, Trexall)	3.3 mg/m^2 PO daily, IM, IV		Acute lymphocytic leukemia, breast cancer, lymphoma, psoriasis, uterine choriocarcinomas, lymphosarcomas	Alcohol, NSAIDs, probenecid, salicylates, live virus vaccine, digoxin, PCN
mercaptopurine (purine analogue) (Purinethol, 6-MP)	2.5 mg/kg PO qd		Acute lymphocytic leukemias; Hodgkin disease; tumors of the lymphatic system; carcinomas of the reproductive tract, liver, pancreas, GI tract, and breast; actinic keratosis	Antigout medications
fluorouracil (pyrimidine analogue) (Adrucil, Efudex)	varies with administration IV, topical		Acute myelocytic leukemias Basal cell carcinomas, actinic keratoses	Other antineoplastics
MITOTIC INHIBITORS (PLANT ALKALOIDS)				
		Stomatitis		
vincristine (Oncovin)	0.5-1.5 mg/m^2 IV	Peripheral neurotoxic effects	Acute leukemia	Antigout medications, live virus vaccines, doxorubicin
vinblastine (Velban, Velsar)	3-11 mg/m^2 BSA IV	Bone marrow suppression, nausea and vomiting	Hodgkin disease, lymphosarcomas, choriocarcinoma	Antigout medications, live virus vaccines
paclitaxel (Taxol)	135-250 mg/m^2 BSA IV	Tachycardia, peripheral neuropathy, blood dyscrasias, tissue necrosis	Ovarian cancer, breast cancer, Kaposi sarcoma	Same as for vinblastine
HORMONE THERAPY *Estrogens*				
		Feminization in males, blood clots		
estramustine (Emcyt)	14 mg/kg PO qd		Prostate cancer	Dairy products
diethylstilbestrol (DES) (Stilphostrol)	500 mg IV qd initially, increase to 1 g qd for next 5 days		Prostate cancer and breast cancer	

TABLE 18-2 SELECT ANTINEOPLASTIC AGENTS—cont'd

GENERIC NAME/ TRADE NAME	USUAL ADULT DOSE, ROUTE, AND FREQUENCY	MAJOR SIDE EFFECTS	INDICATIONS FOR USE	DRUG INTERACTIONS
Androgen		Masculinization of females	Breast cancer in premenopausal women	Oral anticoagulants
fluoxymesterone (Halotestin)	10-40 mg PO daily in divided doses		Metastatic breast cancer	Hypoglycemics, cephalosporins, anticoagulants
Antiestrogens		Hot flashes and weight gain in females		
tamoxifen (Nolvadex)	20-40 mg PO bid		Treatment and prevention of breast cancer	Estrogens
anastrozole (Arimidex)	1 mg PO qd		Breast cancer	None
exemestane (Aromasin)	25 mg PO qd		Breast and prostate cancer	
Antiandrogens		Impotence in males		
goserelin (Zoladex)	1 implant q28d		Metastatic prostatc cancer	None
Progestins				
megestrol (Megace)	40 mg PO qid		Endometrial and breast cancer	None
leuprolide gonadotropin-releasing hormone (Lupron)	1 mg SC; 2.5 mg IM 7.5 mg IM mo; 22.5 mg IM q3mo; 30 mg q4mo	GI bleeding, myocardial infarction, edema, hot flashes, impotence	Prostate cancer, endometriosis	None
ANTITUMOR ANTIBIOTICS		Nausea, vomiting, anorexia, alopecia, dermalitis, hepatotoxicity, cardiotoxicity, nephrotoxicity, blood dyscrasias		
dactinomycin (Actinomycin D, Cosmegen)	500 mcg IV × 5 days		Testicular cancer, Wilms tumor, lymphoma	Antigout medications, live virus vaccines
doxorubicin (traditional) (Adriamycin)	60-75 mg/m^2 BSA IV		Solid tumors, CA of lungs, stomach, breast sarcomas and brain tumors	Antigout medications, live virus vaccines
doxorubicin (liposomal) (Doxil)	20-50, mg/m^2 BSA		Ovarian cancer, Kaposi sarcoma	
mitomycin (Mutamycin)	20 mg/m^2 BSA IV		Adenocarcinomas, squamous cell carcinomas, malignant melanomas	None
daunorubicin (Cerubidine)	30-60 mg/m^2 BSA IV		Leukemias	Antigout medications, live virus vaccines

Continued

TABLE 18-2 SELECT ANTINEOPLASTIC AGENTS—cont'd

GENERIC NAME/ TRADE NAME	USUAL ADULT DOSE, ROUTE, AND FREQUENCY	MAJOR SIDE EFFECTS	INDICATIONS FOR USE	DRUG INTERACTIONS
IMMUNOSUPPRESSANTS AND BIOLOGIC RESPONSE MODIFIERS				
		Hematuria, gum hyperplasia, tremors, headaches, nausea, vomiting, hematologic dangers		
interferon alfa-2a (Roferon)	Various, IM, IV, SC		Chronic hepatitis C, malignant melanomas, Kaposi sarcoma, leukemias	Glucocorticoids, thiazide diuretics, alcohol
interferon alfa-2b (Intron)	2,000,000 IU/m^2 BSA, IM, IV		Leukemia, Kaposi sarcoma	
RETINOIC ACID DERIVATIVE				
tretinoin (Vesanoid)	45 mg/m^2 PO daily in 2 divided doses		Kaposi sarcoma	
TARGET DRUGS				
cetuximab (Erbitux)	250-400 mg/m^2 BSA IV	See literature	Colorectal cancer, head and neck cancer	See drug literature
imatinib (Gleevec)	400-600 mg PO qd	CNS symptoms, Heart failure, hepatotoxicity, vomiting, dyspepsia	Myeloid leukemias, gastrointestinal stromal tumors	See drug literature
nilotinib (Tasigna)	400 mg PO bid	See drug literature	Myeloid leukemias	See drug literature
dasatinib (Sprycel)	70-100 mg PO qd	See drug literature	Myleoid leukemias	See drug literature
rituximab (Rituxan)	375 mg/m^2 BSA IV	See drug literature	Non-Hodgkin lymphoma (also used for rheumatoid arthritis)	See drug literature
MISCELLANEOUS ANTINEOPLASTICS				
asparaginase (Elspar)	200 units/kg IM, IV	Hepatotoxicity, pancreatitis, thrombocytopenia, anemia	Acute lymphocytic leukemias	Steroids, vincristine, antigout medications, methotrexate, live virus vaccines
erlotinib (Tarceva)	150 mg PO qd	GI symptoms, rash, eye pain, fatigue, mouth ulcers	Lung cancer	None
trastuzumab (Herceptin)	2-4 mg/kg IV	Pain, fever, chills, headaches, back pain, infection, GI symptoms, cough, dyspnea	Breast, lung, ovarian, pancreatic cancers	Cyclophosphamide, epirubicin

receptors or target lesions, making their action on malignant cells highly selective.

Adrenocorticosteroids—hormones (or steroids) naturally found in the adrenal cortex—produce remission in certain malignancies by retarding proliferation of lymphocytes, such as in treating acute lymphocytic leukemia. Often these hormones are used in conjunction with radiation therapy to decrease radiation edema. (See Chapter 20 for hormones.)

Sex hormones are used for palliation and for some cures in carcinomas of the reproductive tract. Estrogens may be administered to relieve symptoms of prostate cancer and to treat breast cancer in postmenopausal women. Androgens, male hormones, are used in premenopausal women with breast cancers.

Antiestrogens, such as **tamoxifen** (Nolvadex), and antiandrogens are used to inhibit hormone production in advanced stages of hormonally responsive cancer. Tamoxifen, used for breast cancer, may increase the risk of endometrial cancer, but the benefits greatly outweigh the known risks (see Table 18-2 and Figure 18-3).

Antitumor Antibiotics

Antitumor antibiotics, used only to treat cancer, bind to DNA, inhibiting DNA and RNA synthesis. These medications are not used to treat infections. Antitumor antibiotics are poorly absorbed through the GI tract and therefore are given parenterally, usually intravenously (see Table 18-2).

Immunosuppressants

Immunosuppressants may be produced naturally by white blood cells or synthetically using recombinant DNA techniques. **Interferon** exerts a variety of effects on tumor cells, with an antiproliferative action that stops rapid cell production and increases the efficacy of antineoplastic drugs. Some immunosuppressants can even render cancer cells nonmalignant. The exact action of these drugs is unknown, but cancer research is exploring the potential for immunotherapy to bring about cures (see Table 18-2).

Radioisotopes

Radioactive isotopes, or **radioisotopes,** are used to treat many types of cancer. The isotopes may be inserted locally as pellets, administered as radiation therapy, or administered systemically as capsules or solutions. The patient and family *must* be made aware that these treatments cause exposure to ionizing radiation so that necessary precautions can be taken (see Table 18-2).

NEWER DRUGS AND DRUG DELIVERY SYSTEMS

Many new drugs are being studied to treat acquired immunodeficiency syndrome (AIDS)–associated cancers and to improve the treatment and survival of cancer patients. New medications that have been approved address different cell-type malignancies occurring in specific body organs. The use of liposomes as a delivery system for lipid-soluble drugs, such as **liposomal doxorubicin** and **Herceptin,** is Food and Drug Administration (FDA)–approved. By attaching to liposomes, drugs become "smart bombs" targeting tumor cells but not normal cells. Drugs to treat or slow the progression of breast cancer are another area of intense research interest. The cancer gene *HER-2/neu* produces a protein that alters genes.

A new group of drugs, signal transduction inhibitors, target specific molecules that drive tumor growth, in the hope that the targeted cell is affected while leaving normal cells untouched. Many of these drugs are very expensive for treatment. Unfortunately, the responses to these drugs have been less than impressive, with more severe adverse effects than simply their high cost.

Important Facts about Specific Antineoplastic Agents

- Many anticancer drugs are effective only in specific cell cycle phases. These medications must be in place when cells enter the phase in which the medication works. Hormones and hormone antagonists are not specific to any phase in the cell cycle.
- Alkylating agents injure cells by binding to DNA and inhibiting DNA and RNA synthesis.
- Antimetabolites are similar to natural metabolites and are able to disrupt metabolic processes by damaging the DNA template by acting on the folic acid needed for cell metabolism.
- Antitumor antibiotics are used to treat malignancies, not infections. Many antitumor antibiotics are cardiotoxic.
- Hormonal anticancer drugs act on target cells through specific hormone receptors and are highly selective in their action.

Continued

Important Facts about Specific Antineoplastic Agents—cont'd

- Glucocorticoids, a subset of hormonal adrenocorticosteroids, are toxic to malignancies of lymphoid organs.
- Tamoxifen is an antiestrogen used in the adjuvant treatment of breast cancer after surgery and/or radiation. It is also used prophylactically in certain women at high risk for breast cancer.
- Prostate cancers are treated with gonadotropin-releasing hormone agonists and androgen suppressants, which reduce the stimulation of prostate cells.
- New drugs for treating tumors target specific cell types, with the intention of affecting malignant cells while not harming "normal" cells.

HANDLING AND ADMINISTERING ANTINEOPLASTIC AGENTS

In 2004 USP 797, a regulation developed by the *United States Pharmacopoeia*, was initiated to provide safety in preparing sterile drugs. The FDA has the responsibility of enforcing the standards of this edict in facilities where sterile products are prepared or where drug manipulations are performed during compounding of sterile products. Products that are covered may be biologics, diagnostics, drugs, and cytotoxics. The monitoring of the facility's environment is also included to enhance patient safety and decrease the chance for cross-contamination of sterile preparations.

The drugs to treat cancer are **mutagenic, teratogenic,** and **carcinogenic** when absorbed through skin, lungs, or GI tract. Because of these characteristics, direct contact of the drug with skin, eyes, and mucous membranes can cause local injury to the patient or health care professional preparing or administering the medication. Personnel must observe recommendations and regulations to prevent chronic exposure to cytotoxic drugs. Box 18-2 outlines precautions found in written policies and procedures.

Most antineoplastics cause tissue damage if given subcutaneously or intramuscularly. For medications given by these routes, the medication should be drawn and the needle should be changed to the smallest possible gauge to prevent damage to normal tissue as drugs are administered. The most reliable and most commonly used route of administration for very toxic antineoplastics is the intravenous route.

One goal when administering antineoplastics is to prevent unwanted exposure of the allied health professional to drugs that disrupt natural biologic processes. The exact protocol for administering antineoplastic

BOX 18-2 PRECAUTIONS IN HANDLING ANTINEOPLASTIC AGENTS

- Follow Occupational Safety and Health Administration (OSHA) and *United States Pharmacopeia* 797 guidelines.
- Follow written guidelines for handling antineoplastic drugs.
- Protect and secure packages of hazardous drugs.
- Educate all people who are handling hazardous drugs—patient, family, and other health care workers—in procedures needed for safely handling hazardous drugs. Be sure drugs do not escape from containers while being prepared and administered.
- Maintain a register of the staff members who administer these drugs.
- Use a biologic safety cabinet with a laminar air flow hood for preparation.
- Medications should be prepared in a closed room with excellent ventilation and with equipment for irrigating skin and eyes in case of spills. An OSHA spill kit should be available.
- Dispose of biohazard wastes properly.
- Use personal protective equipment including long-sleeved clothing, a plastic apron, gloves, safety glasses, and a face mask when working with chemotherapeutic agents.
- Reconstituted medications must not be sprayed into the atmosphere. Diluents must be allowed to slowly run down the sides of containers to prevent back spray. Air in the syringe must be expelled into sterile cotton or gauze to prevent spray. Powders must be reconstituted so no excess pressure in the vial would allow medication to spray through the needle hole. Syringes, intravenous sets, and needles should have locked fittings, and all fittings should be secured.
- All materials used in preparing and administering chemotherapy should be disposed of in leakproof, puncture-resistant containers marked "BIOHAZARD."
- Because of the teratogenicity of antineoplastics, health care workers who are pregnant, breast-feeding, or trying to conceive a child should not handle cytotoxic medications or provide direct care for patients who are receiving cytotoxic medications. These precautions should also be used with patients receiving radioisotopes, to prevent unnecessary exposure to radiation.

medications will vary with each medical setting and drug administered, but as a general guideline, strict aseptic technique should be used, following all safety measures, and one must stay within their scope of practice. The complexity of chemotherapeutics and hazards associated with their administration require administration under direct supervision of a specialist. Although allied health professionals would infrequently, if ever, be asked to administer antineoplastics, these drugs may be found in their practice setting. Understanding the toxic nature of these drugs, practicing personal safety measures, and following precautions for handling these medications must be appreciated. Giving support to the patient and family is an important duty of the health professional.

Because antineoplastic agents are toxic, hematologic testing and blood chemistry studies may be done to monitor hematologic, renal, and hepatic function. Testing is begun before the first treatment and is repeated throughout the course of chemotherapy and during follow-up. Dosage may be based on either body weight or body surface area and may be altered during treatment based on any toxicities that the patient is exhibiting and their severity. For many chemotherapeutic agents, use of a nomogram is the best means of dosage calculation because body surface area—weight and height—is considered for safe administration. Too much medication will cause toxicity, whereas too little will not be effective.

SUMMARY

Rapid changes are occurring in the area of antineoplastics because of the rapid approval of investigational medications used to prolong patients' lives. New categories of medications have been shown to be effective and are being used to alter DNA and RNA to prevent abnormal cell mitosis.

Antineoplastic medications are classified according to their effect on specific phases in a cell's replication cycle or based on their ability to target certain cellular functions. According to their potential mechanism of action, the main medication categories include but are not limited to antimetabolites, alkylating agents, mitotic inhibitors, antitumor antibiotics, hormones, immunosuppressants, and radioactive agents. Most malignancies are treated by some combination of surgery, chemotherapy, and radiation therapy.

Many antineoplastic agents are nonselective in their actions, affecting both normal cells and cancerous cells. Cells that replicate quickly are more susceptible to the chemotherapeutic agents than cells with a slower growth rate. Most side effects of antineoplastic therapy occur in bone marrow, the GI tract, and hair follicles because these organ systems are dominated by cells that grow and reproduce quickly. Patients should be educated about these side effects because patients who know what to expect in advance will be more compliant with treatment.

CRITICAL THINKING EXERCISES

Scenario

Jane has been diagnosed with carcinoma of the breast. She has undergone a mastectomy and is now scheduled to undergo chemotherapy that will cause alopecia. She tells you she is afraid of hair loss, nausea, and vomiting. Her friends have told her these are the worst problems associated with chemotherapy.

1. How do you help Jane prepare for alopecia?
2. How do you help her prepare for nausea and vomiting?
3. What do you tell Jane about her dietary needs while she is receiving chemotherapy?
4. What should Jane be taught about contact with people with infectious diseases?

DRUG CALCULATIONS

1. Order: doxorubicin hydrochloride 20 mg/m^2 for a person who is 5'4" tall and weighs 125 lb
   Dose to be given: _____

2. Order: vincristine 1.2 mg/m^2 for a person who is 73" tall and weighs 185 lb
   Dose to be given: _____

REVIEW QUESTIONS

1. Define antineoplastic medications and their general mode of action. _____
   _____
   _____

2. What is an immunosuppressant? Why are these agents beneficial in treating malignancies but harmful to the
   patient? _____
   _____
   _____

3. Describe the more common side effects that patients receiving chemotherapy might expect. _____
   _____
   _____

4. List the precautions necessary when preparing and administering cytotoxic medications. _____
   _____
   _____
   _____
   _____
   _____

5. Why should patients expecting alopecia buy hairpieces before beginning chemotherapy? _____
   _____
   _____

6. How can the patient undergoing chemotherapy have some relief from nausea and vomiting without taking
   medications? _____
   _____
   _____

CHAPTER 19

Nutritional Supplements and Alternative Medicines

Carol has a long history of severe arthritis in her knees. She has a limited income and cannot afford to buy prescription medications for her arthritis. She drinks milk to which vitamin D has been added.

Why is milk with vitamin D important to Carol?

If Carol is allergic to milk, what OTC preparations other than calcium tablets may be used to provide calcium?

If Carol has a history of epigastric burning, what OTC preparation could she use to enhance her calcium intake and also help her epigastric discomfort?

What are the implications of using glucosamine?

EASY WORKING KNOWLEDGE OF NUTRITIONAL SUPPLEMENTS AND ALTERNATIVE MEDICINES

DRUG CLASS	PRESCRIPTION	OTC	PREGNANCY CATEGORY	MAJOR INDICATIONS
Vitamins	Yes	Yes	A, C, X (retinol A)	Supplement to food sources of vitamins
Minerals	Yes	Yes	None	Supplement to food sources of minerals
ALTERNATIVE MEDICINES				
Home remedies	No	Yes	None	Folk medicine (to treat disease by folklore)
Herbals and plants	No	Yes (regulated by U.S. Department of Agriculture [USDA])	None, regulated by USDA under the Dietary Supplements Health Education Act (DSHEA)	Alternative medicine (to treat disease by herbals)

EASY WORKING KNOWLEDGE OF INDICATIONS AND SIDE EFFECTS

Common Signs and Symptoms of Nutritional Imbalance
Nonspecific complaints
Abnormal bone formation
Abnormal heartbeat (palpitations)
Neurologic damage
Inability to build and repair tissue
Change in energy levels
Intellectual impairment
Muscle wasting
Obesity, emaciation
Loss of hair
Delayed wound healing

Common Side Effects of Vitamins, Minerals, and Herbs
Irritability
Anorexia
Headaches, flushing
Indigestion, nausea, diarrhea, constipation
Abdominal cramping and pain
Discolored stools
Insomnia
Hypotension

Vitamins and minerals, called **micronutrients,** are essential compounds normally obtained from plant and animal products and fluids we ingest for body functions such as growth, maintenance, and reproduction. Microorganisms require few raw materials from their environment, but as life forms become more sophisticated with highly specialized cells and organs, the ability to synthesize necessary nutrients is lost. Thus the human body is more dependent on exogenous sources for nourishment, especially for vitamins.

The OTC market for nutritional and dietary supplements is one of the largest in the pharmaceutical field, with more than half of U.S. citizens taking vitamins, minerals, and herbal preparations without a prescription. A working knowledge of vitamins and minerals, their sources, symptoms of vitamin deficiencies, and possible toxic effects from overdose is necessary for patient safety.

VITAMINS

Vitamins are required for metabolism of fats, carbohydrates, and proteins. Although vitamins are not themselves a source of energy, they are essential for energy production and for regulation of metabolic processes.

These compounds, or **nutrients,** regulate body functions and are necessary in trace amounts for growth and health. The needed amount varies somewhat over the life cycle. A vitamin deficiency or **hypovitaminosis** produces certain symptoms, just as excessive supplementation produces toxic effects. Exactly how vitamins work and indications for their use are not completely understood, but we do know that a vitamin deficiency may result in compromise of homeostasis. Some vitamins occur in a usable dietary form; others are inactive in their natural form but are converted to active chemical compounds within the body. Bacteria in the gastrointestinal (GI) tract help activate vitamin K, vitamin D is synthesized on exposure to sunlight, and vitamin B is manufactured in small amounts in the GI tract. Vitamins are important as the enzyme system breaks down food sources during the metabolic process.

Insufficient intake of vitamins may be caused by an inadequate diet as a result of cultural, religious, or personal preferences, fad dieting, alcoholism, poverty, lack of food availability, or ignorance. Signs of vitamin deficiency are primarily abnormal tiredness, aches, pains, and general malaise. In the United States, the severe **avitaminosis** that produces diseases such as beriberi, **pellagra**, rickets, or scurvy is rarely seen. An adequate diet of proper foods, prepared in ways to retain vitamins, is the best way to prevent hypovitaminosis.

Some experts believe that the average American diet contains adequate vitamins and that vitamin supplements are not necessary to meet the U.S. Recommended Dietary Intakes (RDIs) set by the Food and Nutrition Board of the National Academy of Sciences. The RDIs should not be considered the minimum daily requirement for persons at risk for deficiencies because RDIs apply to people in good health. Ill individuals, the elderly, growing children and teenagers, pregnant and nursing women, and people who smoke may need supplements to compensate for dietary deficiencies. Although the practice of taking vitamins is widespread, in most cases vitamin supplementation is not necessary and excessive consumption can be harmful and lead to **hypervitaminosis.**

Classification of Vitamins

Vitamins are divided into two major groups: fat-soluble and water-soluble vitamins. Fat-soluble vitamins—A, D, E, and K—are stored in the liver and fatty tissues. A deficiency of these vitamins would occur only after a long period of deprivation, either from lack of food intake or from a disease preventing absorption. Excessive intake, particularly of vitamin A, may lead to toxic effects because of prolonged storage time of fat-soluble vitamins.

Water-soluble vitamins, B complex vitamins—B_1 (thiamine), B_2 (riboflavin), B_3 (niacin), B_5 (pantothenic acid), B_6 (pyridoxine), B_9 (folic acid), and B_{12} (cyanocobalamin)—and vitamin C, are not stored in large amounts, and even a brief period of deprivation can lead to deficiency. Toxic effects of water-soluble vitamins are rare because excess amounts are excreted from the body.

Did You Know?

Successive letters of the alphabet were assigned as new vitamins were isolated, with some letters being assigned out of order. Because vitamin K is necessary for blood clotting, it was named for the German word *Koagulation*. Later it became evident that vitamin B was not a single vitamin but actually a group of vitamins. Subscript numbers were then added. Missing numbers had been assigned to fractions of the group that were later found to be identical to an already named vitamin. In fact, all water-soluble vitamins but C are actually groups of related substances to which subscript numbers are assigned (e.g., B_1, B_2, B_3).

The many vitamin preparations on the market today, both as prescription products and as OTC products, vary from a single vitamin to multivitamin capsules and

TABLE 19-1 FOOD AND DRUG ADMINISTRATION (FDA) PREGNANCY CATEGORIES FOR VITAMINS

PREGNANCY CLASSIFICATION	VITAMIN
A	B_1 (thiamine), B_6 (pyridoxine), B_9 (folic acid), B_{12} (cyanocobalamin as nasal spray or PO), E, B_2 (riboflavin)
C	D, B_{12} (cyanocobalamin as injectable), C (ascorbic acid), B_3 (niacin), K
X	A

Note: These categories are for vitamins administered it the Recommended Daily Allowances (RDA). With increased amounts, the pregnancy category may change to a higher level.

tablets. The most popular OTC multivitamin preparations contain all of the vitamins needed to meet daily requirement without regard to dietary vitamin content. Extra-strength or high-potency vitamins are rarely necessary for the average person.

The U.S. Food and Drug Administration (FDA) pregnancy risk classification for the major vitamins is found in Table 19-1.

Patient Education for Compliance

1. Vitamins taken in addition to dietary sources are called *vitamin supplements.* Specific vitamin supplements may be useful at designated times in the life cycle. However, healthy, nonsmoking, nonpregnant adults who eat a well-rounded diet generally should not need vitamin supplements.
2. Foods with synthetic vitamins added during processing are labeled "fortified" or "enriched."
3. Vitamins that are purchased over the counter generally have lower vitamin content, especially of fat-soluble vitamins and folic acid, than prescription medications.

Fat-Soluble Vitamins

Because storage time of the fat-soluble vitamins—A, D, E, and K—medications containing these vitamins should be used only when a medical condition has been found for which a particular vitamin is needed. Fat-soluble vitamins are of clinical importance because persons who have diseases that interfere with absorption of fats will eventually develop fat-soluble vitamin deficiencies (Table 19-2).

Water-Soluble Vitamins

The water-soluble vitamins—the B complex and C vitamins—are not stored in fatty tissue. The B vitamins, varying in structure and function, are grouped together

Text continued on p. 330

TABLE 19-2 MICRONUTRIENTS—VITAMINS

DRUG NAME, DOSAGE, ROUTE	FUNCTION IN BODY	INDICATIONS FOR USE	FOOD SOURCES	HYPOVITAMINOSIS	HYPERVITAMINOSIS	DRUG INTERACTIONS	OTHER INFORMATION
FAT-SOLUBLE VITAMINS							
A retinol (Aquasol A)*—4000-5000 international units PO, IM	Visual adaptation, especially night vision; structural and functional integrity of skin and mucous membranes; development of teeth and bones	Malabsorption syndrome caused by GI diseases; acne, wrinkles	Fish oils, butter, yellow fruits and vegetables, milk, cheese, liver	Night blindness, skin lesions, dryness of conjunctiva, softening of cornea in children	Acute confusion, irritation, diarrhea, dizziness, skin peeling and cracking; vomiting alopecia; headache	orlistat	Pregnancy category X
D calciferol (Calderol)—25 mcg-1.5 mg PO; ergocalciferol (Calciferol, Drisdol)—10,000-80,000 mcg PO, IM; calcitriol (Rocatrol)—0.25 mcg PO A and D Ointment—topical	Absorption of calcium, phosphorus in GI tract; calcification of bones	Maintenance of proper bone health; metabolic bone disorders, hypocalcemia with dialysis, hypoparathyroidism, topically for diaper rash and chafed skin	Fortified cereals, dairy products, candy, liver, eggs, fish	Rickets, **osteomalacia**, osteoporosis, bone and muscle pain, weakness, **tetany**	*Early*—diarrhea, headache, high thirst and urination, N/V *Late*—bone and muscle pain, high B/P, pruritus, lethargy, mood swings, pancreatitis, CVD, renal calculi	orlistat, isotretinoin, antacids, thiazide diuretics, aminoglycosides, Ca preparations	Must have 10 minutes of sunlight per day for proper synthesis and active conversion
E alpha tocopherol (Aquasol E)—individualized PO; (Vita E Cream)—topical	Antioxidant; protects RBCs from hemolysis; role not clearly understood	Menopause when not taking estrogen; diaper rash	Wheat germ oil, vegetable oils, leafy vegetables	Slows reflexes, lowers muscle mass, coordination; anemia; chapped skin	*Acute*—visual disturbances, headache, nausea, abdominal pain, weakness *Chronic*—higher bleeding tendencies, impaired sexual function; altered thyroid metabolism	orlistat, oral anticoagulants, iron, antilipemics, mineral oil	Temporary relief for minor burns, chapped skin

BP, blood pressure; *CAD*, coronary artery disease; *CVD*, cardiovascular disease; *GI*, gastrointestinal; *IM*, intramuscularly; *INH*, isoniazid; *IV*, intravenously; *N&V*, nausea and vomiting; *PO*, orally; *RBC*, red blood cell; *SC*, subcutaneously.

*Name in parentheses is the trade name; dosage and route of administration follow trade names.

	Function	Use	Source	Deficiency	Toxicity	Interactions	Comments
K phytonadione (Mephyton)—25 mg PO; (AquaMEPHYTON)—0.5-1 mg IM in newborn	Synthesis of blood clotting factor; producing prothrombin in liver	Hypoprothrombinemia; prevent excessive bleeding in newborn; warfarin toxicity	Green vegetables, cabbage, cauliflower, fish liver oils, eggs, milk, meat	Bleeding and hemorrhage	Flushing, dyspnea, chest pain, taste alterations, brain damage, **hematuria**	orlistat, antilipemics, oil preparations, antiseizure medications, coumarin anticoagulants, antiinfectives	Malabsorption syndrome in intestines leads to deficiency; antibiotic therapy may eliminate bacteria needed for synthesis

WATER-SOLUBLE VITAMINS

	Function	Use	Source	Deficiency	Toxicity	Interactions	Comments
B₁ thiamine (Betalin, Biamine)—10-20 mg PO, IM	Normal function of nervous system	Prevent beriberi, malabsorption and metabolic disorders, alcoholism	Pork products	Peripheral neuritis; loss of muscle tone and strength; **paresthesia**; depression; memory loss; dyspnea; anorexia	Very low toxicity; excess excreted	alcohol	
B₂ riboflavin—5-30 mg PO	Promotes metabolism of carbohydrates, fats, and proteins; synthesis of DNA	Riboflavin deficiency	Milk and milk products, meats, grains	Sore throat, swollen tongue, anemia, pitching changes in cornea in children, dermatitis of face and burning	None	alcohol, probenecid	May turn urine orange
B₃ niacin, nicotinic acid (Nicobid)—100 mg PO, IM; (Niaspan)—500-2000 mg/day PO 5× daily	Metabolism of food, builds tissue proteins	Prevent pellagra, hyperlipoproteinemia, lowers cholesterol	Meats, legumes, enriched grains, peanuts	Skin eruptions, sore mouth, diarrhea, headache, dizziness, insomnia, dementia, memory loss	Flushing, pruritus, dizziness, dysrhythmias, muscle pain, N&V, diarrhea, dry skin	statin medications, probenecid	More like a drug than a vitamin and should be used with medical supervision

Continued

TABLE 19-2 MICRONUTRIENTS—VITAMINS—cont'd

DRUG NAME, DOSAGE, ROUTE	FUNCTION IN BODY	INDICATIONS FOR USE	FOOD SOURCES	HYPOVITAMINOSIS	HYPERVITAMINOSIS	DRUG INTERACTIONS	OTHER INFORMATION
B₆ pyridoxine—dose varies	Metabolism of amino acids, formation of blood, maintenance of nervous system	pyridoxine deficiency, INH neurotoxicity	Chicken, fish, eggs, whole grains	Seborrheic-like lesions of skin, sore mouth, peripheral neuritis, seizures	Very little toxicity except with chronic overuse	INH, levodopa, alcohol, some antiinfectives, oral contraceptives, immunosuppressants	
B₉ folic acid (Folvite)—use; PO, IM, SC, IV, varies with age, gender	Synthesis of DNA and RNA	Megaloblastic and macrocytic anemia	Green leafy vegetables, milk, eggs, yeast	Glossitis, diarrhea	Redness of skin, fever, rashes, pruritus	sulfonamides, alcohol, methotrexate, steroids, estrogen, oral contraceptives	March of Dimes suggests that all women of childbearing age take folic acid supplements of at least 400 mg/day to prevent neural tube defects in developing fetus; requirements usually increase in actual pregnancy, and most pregnancy supplements contain 1 mg/day

B12 cyanocobalamin (NTN)—dose varies, IM, SC; (Nascobal Nasal Spray) topical	Promotes normal cell function, especially in nervous system; blood formation; metabolism of carbohydrates, fats, proteins, folates; synthesis of DNA and RNA	Pernicious anemia, B12 deficiency	Fresh shrimp, oysters, milk, eggs, cheese	Nervous system damage, poor coordination, memory loss, confusion, dementia, abnormal blood cell formation	No toxic effects	chloramphenicol, alcohol	Many people take B12 injections to provide feeling of well-being, lifelong treatment may be necessary for malabsorption diseases, cannot be administered by IV
C ascorbic acid (Cecon)—70-500 mg PO, IM, SC, IV	Building and maintaining tissue for wound healing, resistance to infections, enhanced iron absorption	Prevent scurvy, vitamin C deficiency with burns	Citrus fruits, tomatoes, melons, cabbage, strawberries, broccoli	Gingivitis, scurvy, anemia, bruising, delayed wound healing	Kidney stones, dizziness, N&V, diarrhea	salicylates, primidone, iron	Prophylactically given for the common cold; adjunct therapy for cancer, may protect against cataracts
B5 pantothenic acid—found in multiple vitamins in various amounts	Component of coenzyme A used in metabolism of carbohydrates and fatty acids		Virtually all foods	No deficiency reported	No reports of toxicity	None known	No need for supplementation because readily found in most foods
B7 biotin—found in multivitamins; dosage varies	Metabolism of carbohydrates and fats		In many foods	Experimentally, dermatitis, hair loss, conjunctivitis, muscle pain, paresthesias	No toxicity noted	None noted	Intrinsically synthesized by intestinal bacteria

TABLE 19-3 LIFESTYLE CHOICES AND VITAMIN SUPPLEMENTS

LIFESTYLE CHOICE	VITAMIN SUPPLEMENT NEEDED
Restricted diet	B_{12}
Extensive exercise	B_2
Oral contraceptives	B_3, B_6, B_9, B_{12}, C
Smoking	C
Alcohol	B_1, B_9, B complex
Caffeine	B complex, C
Excessive stress	B complex

Patient Education for Compliance

1. For best absorption and limited gastrointestinal (GI) distress, vitamins should not be taken on an empty stomach.
2. Vitamin B_{12} is not readily absorbed through the GI tract and should be given by injection or intranasally for better absorption.
3. Some vitamins may change the color of urine and stools.
4. Experts suggest that those who take excessive amounts of a micronutrient should not stop taking it completely but should cut back about half of the current dosage so the body can adjust before stopping medication completely.

because they were first isolated from the same sources, yeast and liver. Because these vitamins are rapidly used or excreted through urine, a daily dietary supply is necessary to prevent deficiency. Under normal circumstances, hypervitaminosis does not occur. The most common condition causing a deficiency in water-soluble vitamins in adults is alcoholism because of the associated anorexia, decreased food intake, and damage to the digestive and metabolic systems. Fasting, metabolic diseases, and anorexia nervosa may also lead to a deficiency, as may excessive cooking and boiling of foods. As a rule, any condition that predisposes a person to a water-soluble vitamin deficiency will reduce levels of multiple B vitamins at the same time (see Table 19-2).

Some lifestyle choices are important in supplementation and vitamin absorption (Table 19-3).

Use of Vitamin Supplements in the Elderly

The need for dietary supplements increases as people age because geriatric people cannot absorb and store nutrients as easily as at a younger age. In elderly individuals who do not eat adequate foods containing sufficient nutrients, vitamins might be indicated. The goal of therapy is to boost energy and strength, provide nutrition for weight gain as appropriate, aid in recovery from illnesses, and provide extra minerals to maintain health. Many formulations of vitamins and supplements are available in liquid and solid forms for persons older than 50 years of age. Multivitamins designed for use with younger adults may not contain adequate supplements for geriatric patients. Drug companies have formulated many products to meet specific needs such as cardiovascular health, prostate health, and protection against osteoporosis in postmenopausal women. Vitamin and mineral supplements may even contain the wording "for age 50+" to indicate products for use by older adults.

Important Facts about Vitamins

- Vitamins are compounds required in minute amounts for growth and maintenance of health. Vitamins are needed for energy transformation and food metabolism.
- For most people, proper diet alone will supply the necessary vitamins.
- Vitamins are divided into two groups: fat-soluble vitamins (A, D, E, and K) and water-soluble vitamins (B complex and C).
- Fat-soluble vitamins are stored in the body and do not require daily replenishment. Water-soluble vitamins not immediately used by the body are excreted in urine and need to be replenished daily.

MINERALS

Minerals, inorganic solid substances such as those occurring as part of the earth's crust, are important parts of body composition and are necessary in small amounts for normal body function. Humans obtain minerals by eating plants grown in mineral-rich soil or from secondary sources of food products obtained from animals. Like vitamins, minerals have no energy value but are necessary to regulate body processes and serve as structural components of cells while accounting for approximately 4% of body weight.

As minerals dissolve in body fluids, they exist as **acids, alkalines (or bases),** and **salts.** The dissolved minerals are called **electrolytes** because they have the ability to form charged particles called **ions** that are needed for metabolism. Water is the **solvent,** and electrolytes are the **solutes.** The normal salt concentration found in body fluids is 0.9% concentration of sodium chloride, or **isotonic.** Changes in this concentration as a consequence of either raising or lowering the percentage of the salt in the solution will disrupt body homeostasis.

Most minerals in foods occur as salts, which are soluble in water. Mineral supplements may be necessary during periods of rapid growth and in some clinical situations—for example, iron for patients with anemia. People taking potassium-depleting diuretics may need potassium supplementation.

Minerals are subdivided into two classes, major minerals and trace minerals, based on body needs and not on chemical importance. The major electrolytes in the body are sodium, chloride, potassium, calcium, phosphorus, and magnesium. The most important trace minerals for homeostasis are iron, zinc, fluorine, iodine, and copper (Table 19-4).

Use of Mineral Supplements

Mineral supplements should be used with care because excessive supplemental amounts can be hazardous. A healthy person who eats a balanced diet should obtain sufficient minerals to counteract normal losses through perspiration, saliva, urine, and feces. Mineral supplements should be taken only on health care provider advice.

Important Facts about Minerals

- Minerals are essential for normal body function.
- Minerals called *electrolytes* are essential for homeostasis.

Patient Education for Compliance

1. The patient should pay attention to any special labels on medicine bottles to check exact contents of vitamins and minerals. Multivitamin-mineral combinations can cause toxicity of some components.
2. Minerals not necessary should not be taken because of the danger of changing electrolyte balances.
3. Liquid iron preparations should be taken with a dropper or straw after dilution to prevent staining of teeth and mucous membranes. The mouth should be rinsed after each administration.
4. Iron should be taken on an empty stomach, but it may be taken with food if GI upset occurs.
5. Iron supplements may cause constipation.
6. Antacids and iron should not be taken at the same time.
7. Calcium carbonate (e.g., Tums) is a good replacement for calcium in postmenopausal women who have GI upset from taking other calcium supplements.
8. Oral fluoride drops should not be taken with milk or dairy products. Fluoride dental rinses should be used at bedtime after brushing teeth to ensure nothing is eaten after use.

ALTERNATIVE MEDICATIONS

Over the past 20 to 30 years, use of alternative medicine is an approach to illness that has rapidly increased in the United States. One of the most rapidly growing types of alternative therapy is the treatment of osteoarthritis using such drugs as glucosamine or chondroitin, which are nutritional supplements. Some research supports the fact that glucosamine aids in the repair and formation of cartilage. Chondroitin is a protein that allows for elasticity of the cartilage.

The terms **complementary medicine** and **alternative medicine** describe a group of diverse medical and health care system practices and products that are generally considered part of conventional medicine. Complementary therapies include diet, exercise, counseling, biofeedback, massage therapy, relaxation techniques, and hypnosis, which generally are not invasive. Home remedies and folk remedies (Table 19-5) are still popular in many cultures and may coexist with modern pharmacologic therapy.

CULTURAL DIFFERENCES IN USING ALTERNATIVE MEDICINE

The first alternative medicines were home remedies. Many **folk medicine** treatments or **home remedies** are used on a daily basis, with each culture having its primary folk medicine providers. In the United States, most cultural groups use some form of complementary or alternative therapies, using both medicinal treatments and social or psychic adjustments.

Among Native Americans, medicine men and women used plants and herbs blessed for medicinal use. Illness was prevented through prayer, charms, and the use of objects with power to protect the owner. Some of these forms of healing and health maintenance continue today.

Certain African and Latin American cultures have attributed disease to disharmony in relationships between humans and supernatural forces. Discord may occur between the person and ancestral spirits, evil spirits, or living relatives. Treatments are provided by trained, culturally accepted healers, who may be elderly women healers ("grannies"), shamans, or root doctors. Herbs, roots, and oils are used for healing. Talismans are worn to ward off evil spirits. Religious rituals such as the laying on of hands are used to treat disease.

Latin American populations, including immigrants to the United States, practice a fusion medicine. Illness is viewed as having a natural cause, as an act of God, as punishment, or as result of witchcraft or a curse. The

Text continued on p. 336

TABLE 19-4 MICRONUTRIENTS—MINERALS

DRUG NAME, DOSAGE, ROUTE	FUNCTION IN BODY	INDICATIONS FOR USE	FOOD SOURCES	MINERAL DEFICIENCY	EXCESSIVE MINERALS	DRUG INTERACTIONS	OTHER INFORMATION
MAJOR MINERALS							
Calcium (Ca) Ca citrate (Citrical)—varies, PO; Ca carbonate (Os-Cal, Titralac, Tums, Vivactiv)—varies, PO, chewable; Ca gluconate (NTN)—varies, PO, IV	Bone formation; contraction and relaxation of muscles; blood clotting; nervous system transmission to and from brain; secretion of insulin; need vitamin D metabolism	Nutritional supplement; hypocalcemic tetany; replacement therapy in menopause; antacid; phosphate-lowering agent for renal failure	Milk, sardines, cheese, salmon, green leafy vegetables, whole grains	Bone deformities, rickets, osteomalacia; osteoporosis	Confusion, headaches, N&V, coma	dairy products, digoxin, thyroid hormones, tetracycline, fluoroquinolone antibiotics	May be deposited in joints and soft tissues, causing pain, limitation of motion; postmenopausal women need Ca supplements at 1500 mg/day
Phosphorus (P+) potassium phosphate (Neutra-Phos, K-Phosphate)—varies, PO, IV; sodium phosphate (Na phosphate)—varies, IV	Bone and tooth formation; energy production; maintenance of intact cell membranes; storage of fats; metabolism of nutrients	Nutritional supplement; urinary acidifiers	Fish, beef, pork, cheese, milk, legumes, carbonated beverages, processed meat, foods prepared with phosphoric acid	Confusion, anemia, weakness, bone brittleness	Low Ca blood levels, kidney stones	antacids, sevelamer, Ca products, ACE inhibitors, K supplements, K-sparing diuretics	Phosphorus supplements, K, Ca, Na cause GI upsets and bone and joint pain

ACE, angiotensin-converting enzyme; *CNS*, central nervous system; *CVD*, cardiovascular disease; *GI*, gastrointestinal; *KI*, potassium iodine; *N&V*, nausea and vomiting; *NSAIDs*, nonsteroidal antiinflammatory drugs; *PO*, orally.

*Name in parentheses is the trade name; dosage and route of administration follow trade names.

	Action	Use	Food Sources	Signs of Deficiency	Signs of Toxicity	Drug Interactions	Nursing Considerations
Magnesium (Mg+) magnesium chloride (Slow-Mg), PO; magnesium citrate (Citroma)—varies, PO; magnesium hydroxide (MOM)—varies, PO; magnesium oxide (Epsom salts)—varies, PO, soaks; magnesium sulfate—varies, PO, IM, IV	Synthesis of proteins; stimulates muscle contractions and nerve transmissions; activates enzymes; aids in bone formation	All but magnesium sulfate—used with Ca, aluminum, simethicone for antacids, laxatives, and dietary supplements; magnesium sulfate—seizures	Green leafy vegetables, whole grains, legumes	Spasms, convulsions, tetany, diarrhea	Spasms, convulsions, tetany, CNS depression, coma, hypotension	cefditoren, tetracyclines, fluoroquinolones	Magnesium and calcium interdependent
Sodium (Na+) sodium chloride (Salinex, Ocean Nasal Mist, normal saline, NaCl for injection)—SC, IM, IV ophthalmic, nasal solution, injectable	Necessary for extracellular fluid; body fluid balance; acid-base balance; regulates nerve transmission; irritates cell membrane irritability	Flushing, hydration, fluid and electrolyte balance, acid-base balance	Table salt, milk, meat, processed foods, carrots, celery	Nausea, headache, mental confusion, hypotension, weakness, anxiety, muscle spasms	Edema, hypertension, CVD disturbances		Table salt is the primary source; intake by diet, excretion by kidneys
Potassium (K+) potassium acetate—40-100 mEq PO; potassium citrate and potassium bicarbonate (K-Lyte)—varies, PO, IV; potassium chloride (K-Lor, K-Dur, Klor-Con, Slow-K, Micro-K)—40-100 mg PO, IV; potassium gluconate (NTN)—40-100 mg PO	Intracellular fluid; maintenance of cell structure; regulates muscle function, including cardiac muscle; protein synthesis; carbohydrate metabolism	Vitamin K deficiency; acid-base balance	Oranges, bananas, prunes, red meats, vegetables, milk and milk products, yams, coffee, salt substitutes	Tissue breakdown, acid-base imbalance, loss of muscle tone, weakness, paralysis, cardiac arrhythmias	Lethargy, confusion, diarrhea, N&V, decreased urinary output, muscle weakness	digitalis, NSAIDs, diuretics, salt substitutes	Salt substitutes cause K increases, main cause of digitoxin toxicity

Continued

TABLE 19-4 MICRONUTRIENTS—MINERALS—cont'd

DRUG NAME, DOSAGE, ROUTE	FUNCTION IN BODY	INDICATIONS FOR USE	FOOD SOURCES	MINERAL DEFICIENCY	EXCESSIVE MINERALS	DRUG INTERACTIONS	OTHER INFORMATION
Chloride (Cl⁻)							
In combination with other electrolytes	Extracellular fluid; buffer; enzyme activator; component of gastric hydrochloric acid	Balance of tissue fluids	Table salt, milk, meat, processed foods	Rare except in those taking medications that cause NaCl loss over long term	Nonexistent	None	
TRACE MINERALS							
Iron (Fe⁺)							
ferrous sulfate (Feosol, Slow FE)—325 mg PO; ferrous gluconate (Fergon)—325-600 mg PO; ferrous fumarate (Feostat)—200 mg PO; iron dextran (Imferon, INFeD)—IM; iron sucrose (Venofer)—100 mg/dialysis treatment IV	Essential component in hemoglobin; antibody formation	Iron deficiency anemia, pregnancy, dialysis	Lean red meat, whole grains, egg yolks, legumes, raisins, prunes, apricots	Anemia	Iron poisoning	antacids, cefdinir, tetracyclines, fluoroquinolones, mycophenolate, thyroid hormones, proton-pump inhibitors	Men generally do not need supplement; ferrous sulfate is drug of choice; iron causes constipation; injectable iron should be given via Z-track; iron dextran—shock, seizures; coffee and tea interfere with absorption
Zinc (Zn⁺)							
Zinc acetate (Galzin)—25 mg PO; prenatal vitamins—varies, PO; zinc oxide—topical	Component of RNA and DNA; skin irritation	Wilson disease, sexual development, wound healing, normal taste and smell, prevention of common cold	Meat, oysters, eggs, milk, whole grains	Skin lesions	Poor muscle coordination, vomiting, diarrhea, renal failure	fluoroquinolones, tetracyclines	Excess zinc inhibits copper

	Action	Use	Source	Deficiency	Adverse Effects	Interactions	Comments
Fluorine (Fl⁻) fluoride, fluorine (Fluoritab Luride)—varies, PO; (Poly-Vi-Flor) drops, PO	Dental and bone formation and integrity	Dietary supplement, osteoporosis, dental caries	Fluorinated water, toothpaste and rinses, tea, seafood	Dental caries	Mottled tooth stains	Aluminum hydroxide, milk, dairy products	Fluoride supplements for children living where water supply not fluorinated; experimentally for treating osteoporosis
Iodine (I⁺) In combination with other medications	Thyroid gland synthesis, basal metabolic rate	Goiter, cretinism	Iodized table salt, seafood	Physical deformity, dwarfism, mental retardation in children, coma, hypothermia, respiratory depression in adults	Acne-like lesions	thyroid hormones; if using KI, be alert to interactions with K-containing medications or those that help retain K (e.g., ACE inhibitors)	
Copper (Cu⁺) In multiple vitamins and prenatal vitamins in various strengths, PO	Component of cell enzyme, energy production, hemoglobin synthesis	Wilson disease with zinc intake with liver and nerve damage	Organ meats, seafood, nuts, seeds, legumes, grains	Found with total parenteral nutrition (TPN)	Rare	As with other minerals in other combination drugs	

TABLE 19-5 EXAMPLES OF HOME AND FOLK REMEDIES

REMEDY AND METHOD OF USE	USED FOR
Hot chicken soup—oral	Fever, cold, flu
Lemon in water—oral	Cold and congestion
Potato juice—oral	Arthritis
Orange juice and gelatin—oral	Arthritis
Onions	
topical to feet	Fever
oral	Cold
inhaled	Congestion
topical hot packs	Earache
topical, raw, on neck or soles	Headache
oral	Stomach or intestinal distress
oral	Blood clotting disorders
oral	Heart disease
Vinegar	
gargled	Sore throat
topical	Sunburned skin
topical	Pruritus, contact dermatitis
oral	Chronic fatigue syndrome
Dandelion tea—oral	Urinary tract infections
Gelatin—oral	Diarrhea
Garlic	
topical or oral	Antiseptic
oral	Antibiotic, coronary heart disease, decrease blood cholesterol, hypertension, antitumor agent

healers are *curanderos* (native healers), *yerberos* (herbalists), *espiritualistas* (spiritualists), or *brujos* (those who use witchcraft or magic). Hot and cold foods such as herbal teas are used to treat some conditions. Massage may be used, and religious medals may be worn. Some Hispanic Americans wear an *azabache*, a black stone, to ward off the evil eye that causes disease.

In Eastern (Asian) medicine, the objective is to keep the body in balance between opposing forces of yin (cold) and yang (hot) for maintenance of good health, with illness occurring when the body is out of balance. The Chinese physician prescribes a variety of therapies, including herbs, acupuncture, diet changes, exercise, meditation, or services of spiritual healers. Herbs may be applied externally or taken orally to correct physical disorders. The goal of Eastern medicine is health promotion and stabilization.

In Western medicine, in which the scientific-medical paradigm of illness and treatment predominates, physicians identify illness as a physical, chemical, or physiologic disturbance in the body. Focus is on interventions, often invasive in some manner, to correct disturbances. Aggressive treatment of symptoms and their causes has been the norm; however, alternative therapies such as massage, acupuncture, yoga, and dietary changes are increasingly accepted.

SAFETY AND REGULATION OF HERBAL SUPPLEMENTS

Herbal supplements (see Table 19-6 for commonly used herbs) are minimally regulated by the FDA and U.S. Department of Agriculture. The FDA regulates these as dietary supplements with labeling for content but not for medicinal uses, doses, and dangers. In 1994 Congress passed the Dietary Supplement Health and Education Act, defining supplements such as vitamins, minerals, amino acids, and herbs. Minimal quality control exists, and false claims are numerous. The maker of a supplement must only prove that it is a "food substance" and label it as a dietary supplement, so these products are not subject to the stringent rules and testing before marketing that are required for pharmaceuticals. The FDA must prove that a supplement is unsafe before it can be legally removed from the market. Because many patients do not have complete knowledge about interactions of pharmaceutical products and herbal products, health professionals should interview the patient about all medications and supplements being taken, whether prescription or OTC. Patients should be encouraged to discuss herbal preparations used without reproach and understand the physician is interested in discussing supplement use to prevent drug-supplement interactions.

Different parts of an herb—blossoms, seeds, stems, and roots—may be used for medicinal purposes. Some leading uses of supplement products are listed in Box 19-1. Consumers should be aware that "natural" does not necessarily mean "safe." Some herbal supplements can be harmful because of the herb itself, amount consumed, part of plant used, or contaminants that have entered during growing or processing stages. Herbals may have interactions with prescribed medications and OTC items, causing toxic or allergic responses. Of true concern is the possibility that the patient is being treated with herbal supplements and foregoing a medical diagnosis and treatment until the disease has become too advanced to treat effectively.

TABLE 19-6 SELECT HERBS USED BY CONSUMERS*

HERB NAME	FUNCTION IN BODY	INDICATIONS FOR USE
Echinacea (caution during pregnancy and lactation)	May have antibiotic action	*Internal:* Colds, influenza, URIs, ear infections, septicemia, bladder infections *External:* Cuts, boils, abscesses, wounds, hives, eczema, insect bites, herpes
Garlic	Strengthens cardiovascular system, decreases cholesterol, decreases BP	*Internal:* Digestive disorders, diarrhea, liver and gallbladder problems, URIs, influenza, rheumatoid arthritis, bladder infection *External:* Hookworm, roundworm, ringworm, athlete's foot, swelling, minor skin infections
Ginkgo (not during pregnancy or lactation)	Vasodilatation, improves blood circulation, decreases blood clots, decreases retinal damage from macular degeneration	*Internal:* Vertigo, Alzheimer disease, tinnitus, phlebitis, leg ulcers, peripheral vascular disease, cerebral atherosclerosis, headaches, depression, strokes, heart attacks, lack of concentration
Golden seal (not during pregnancy or in young children)	Dries secretions, reduces inflammation, mild antimicrobial, aids in digestion	*Internal:* Diarrhea, irritable bowel syndrome, colitis, ulcers, gastritis, gingivitis, vaginal yeast infections, otitis
Saw palmetto	Reduces size of prostate gland; dries secretions; aids with digestion, sleep, and coughs	*Internal:* Benign prostatic hypertrophy, nasal congestion, asthma, bronchitis, URIs, sinusitis, sedative, diuretic, expectorant, bladder infections *External:* Antiseptic
Aloe	Decreases pain of burns and skin irritations, antihistamine, laxative	*Internal:* Digestive disorders, gastric ulcer, laxative *External:* Burns, wound infections, insect bites, skin irritations, chickenpox, acne, poison ivy
Panax ginseng (may cause asthma attacks, increased BP, heart palpitations, postmenopausal bleeding)	Calms stomach, stimulates vital organs	*Internal:* Depression, fatigue, stress, URIs, influenza, inflammation, respiratory tract disorders
Astragalus	Strengthens body, speeds metabolism, promotes tissue regeneration, increases energy	*Internal:* General weakness or fatigue, loss of appetite, diarrhea, blood abnormalities, URIs, AIDS, cancer, chronic fatigue
Cayenne	Stimulates heart, increases circulation, improves digestion, boosts energy	*Internal:* Poor circulation, indigestion, physical or mental exhaustion, lowered energy *External:* Pain, arthritis, strains, sore muscles and joints; increases blood flow, stops external bleeding
Siberian ginseng (may cause asthma, increased BP, heart palpitations, postmenopausal bleeding)	Increases immune system; increases resistance to disease, stress, and fatigue	*Internal:* Depression, fatigue, stress, URIs, influenza, respiratory problems, damaged immune system
Bilberry (cannot be used for long period of time)	To treat eye problems such as glaucoma and cataracts, decreases plaque in arteries; diarrhea; decreases blood sugar	*Internal:* Eye strain, cataracts, glaucoma, night blindness, nearsightedness, diarrhea, constipation, stomach cramps *External:* Spider veins, varicose veins, hemorrhoids, burns, skin disorders
Dong quai	Gynecologic complaints	*Internal:* Menstrual irregularity, stabbing pain, poor circulation, carbuncles, palpitations, blurred vision, lightheadedness
St John's wort (headaches, increased BP, photosensitivity, multiple drug interactions)	Germicidal, antiinflammatory, antidepressant	*Internal:* Depression *External:* Wounds, scar tissue

Continued

TABLE 19-6 SELECT HERBS USED BY CONSUMERS—cont'd

HERB NAME	FUNCTION IN BODY	INDICATIONS FOR USE
Valerian	Mild tranquilizer, improves sleep	*Internal:* Insomnia, anxiety, nervousness, anxiety-induced palpitations, headaches, intestinal pain, menstrual cramps
Feverfew (may alter clotting times)	Blocks inflammatory substances in blood	*Internal:* Migraine headaches
Ginger	Motion sickness, digestion, dizziness, burns, may prevent heart disease and strokes by decreasing BP and internal clotting	*Internal:* Vomiting, abdominal cramping, cough, menstrual irregularities, motion sickness, morning sickness, colds, flu, arthritis; increases BP and cholesterol
Kava kava*	Antidepressant, diuresis, antiseptic and antiinflammatory agent for urinary tract	*Internal:* Urinary tract disorders, prostate inflammation, gout, rheumatism, insomnia, depression, muscle spasms
Ephedra (similar to ephedrine)	Bronchial decongestant, CNS stimulant, increases heart rate, increases BP	*Internal:* Fever, coughing, wheezing, nasal or chest congestion, indigestion, asthma, obesity
Alfalfa	Nutritional supplement, body cleanser	*Internal:* Inflammation of bladder, diuresis, indigestion, constipation, halitosis
Kelp	Goiter remedy, thyroid disorders (iodine-rich)	*Internal:* Hypothyroidism, goiter
Parsley	Expectorant, diuretic, laxative	*Internal:* Indigestion, congestion, asthma, irregular menstrual periods, PMS; increases BP; congestive heart failure
Rose hips	Nasal and chest congestion	*Internal:* Colds and flu
Tea tree oil	Skin disorders	*External:* Cuts, abrasions, insect bites, acne, fungal infections, flea shampoo for pets
Melatonin	Tranquilizer, sedative	Sleep

AIDS, acquired immunodeficiency syndrome; *BP,* blood pressure; *CNS,* central nervous system; *PMS,* premenstrual syndrome; *URI,* upper respiratory infection.

*FDA has indicated that kava kava should not be used because of liver toxicity.

BOX 19-1 COMMON REASONS FOR USE OF DIETARY SUPPLEMENTS

Disorder	Herb or Substance Commonly Used
Upper respiratory infection	*Echinacea,* elderberry, *Astragalus*
Burns	Calendula, tea tree, aloe, lavender oil
Headaches	Feverfew, black cohosh, willow bark
Allergies	Freeze-dried nettle leaf, *Coleus,* grape seed
Rashes	Calendula, tea tree, flaxseed oil
Insomnia and stress	Valerian, passion flower, kava, melatonin
Premenstrual syndrome	Vitex, black cohosh, dong quai
Depression	St John's wort, SAM-e
Diarrhea	Blueberry leaf, bilberry
Symptoms associated with menopause	Black cohosh, soy isoflavones, Vitax, evening primrose oil
Nausea	Peppermint, ginger
Urinary tract irritability	Cranberry
Cholesterol and lipid control	Flax seed oil
Prostate health	Saw palmetto
Memory enhancement	Ginseng

Note: This box is not an endorsement of the uses stated.

TABLE 19-7 EXAMPLES OF HERBS WITH A POTENTIAL FOR TOXIC EFFECTS

HERB	TOXIC EFFECT
Echinacea	Immunosuppression with long-term use
Garlic	Reacts with anticoagulants; hypoglycemic effects, so may affect antidiabetic treatments
Ginkgo	Reacts with anticoagulants
Goldenseal, *Cunica* flowers, wolfsbane *(Aconitum)*, mountain tobacco	Affects heart and vascular system; *Cunica* induces toxic gastroenteritis, nervous system disturbances, muscle weakness, and death
Wormwood, absinthe, mugwort, madwort *(Alyssum)*	Narcotic poison (oil of wormwood); damage nervous system, cause mental impairment
Belladonna, deadly nightshade *(Solanum)*	Alkaloids of atropine and hyoscyamine—anticholinergic symptoms ranging from blurred vision, mydriasis, dry mouth, and inability to urinate to unusual behavior and hallucinations
Buckeye, horse chestnut *(Aesculus hippocastanum)*	Coumadin glycoside—interfere with blood clotting
Hemlock *(Conium)*, spotted parsley, St Bennett's herb, spotted cowbane, fool's parsley	Toxic alkaloid *conium* and other related alkaloids
Lobelia, Indian tobacco, wild tobacco, asthma weed, emetic weed	Excessive use—severe vomiting, pain, sweating, paralysis, decreased body temperature, coma, and death
Ephedra (ma huang)	Contains ephedrine, pseudoephedrine, sympathomimetic—likely to mimic actions of epinephrine, increases blood pressure, increases heart rate; used to make methamphetamine
Periwinkle, vinca	Alkaloids—cytotoxic, causing liver, kidney, and neurologic damage; base for antineoplastic agents
Black cohosh, chaparral, comfrey, kava kava	Hepatotoxicity
Foxglove, squill, licorice, lily of the valley	Potential cardiac effects, such as arrhythmia

It is difficult to evaluate the safety of herbs because herbal supplements may contain a mixture of plants and other materials. When potent herbs are compared with equally potent medications, side effects of herbs are comparable or more severe. To date no study has shown herbs to be more effective than chemicals purified from them, and safety of these products cannot be proven because chemicals have not been tested for purity. Prescription medications from herbs produce essentially the same actions as quantities of herbs themselves and have a higher safety factor because of the quality standards required for medications. Supplements should always be used with caution.

Some serious problems such as toxic effects on the liver and heart, fetal malformations, and production of abnormal cells leading to cancer have been reported with indiscriminate supplement use. The actual rate of adverse reactions to these supplements cannot be determined because they are not reportable by law. Products with potential to cause toxic effects and interactions with certain drugs are listed in Table 19-7.

Patient Education for Compliance

1. Special care should be taken with herbals by patients with allergies, those sensitive to medications, those taking medicines for chronic illnesses, and those older than 65 years of age or younger than 12 years of age.
2. The lowest possible dose should be taken to protect against adverse reactions. Herbal supplements are best absorbed on an empty stomach, but they should be discontinued if nausea consistently develops within 2 hours after ingestion.
3. Pregnant or lactating women are advised not to take dietary supplements without a physician's advice.
4. Supplements should be purchased from a reputable source rather than home grown because toxic contaminants such as pesticides and heavy metals may be found in some herbal products. Reputable sources also are more likely to have some method of quality control during the production of the product.
5. Patients should be careful about taking prescription medications and herbal supplements together.
6. Before taking dietary supplements, the consumer should acquire as much information as possible about the products.

SUMMARY

Vitamins and minerals are essential compounds needed to keep the body in homeostasis. If adequate diets are consumed, most people will not need vitamin and mineral supplements. The FDA considers vitamin supplements to be medications and therefore regulates their production and use. Young children and elderly people, pregnant or lactating women, and patients undergoing chemotherapy and dialysis generally need to take vitamin and mineral supplements. Absorption disorders and immune system deficiencies may also necessitate daily intake of additional vitamins. Some diseases, such as scurvy and beriberi, are the result of insufficient vitamins or minerals; other diseases such as osteoporosis and anemias may be improved by supplementation.

Vitamins are divided into two groups. The fat-soluble vitamins—A, D, E, and K—are absorbed and stored by the body, therefore not requiring replacement on a daily basis. Vitamin B complex and vitamin C, water-soluble vitamins, are not stored, and the excess is excreted in the urine; a well-balanced diet provides a continuing supply of these vitamins.

Minerals, like vitamins, usually occur adequately in foods and are absorbed from supplements depending on body needs. Some OTC supplements are formulated as vitamin and mineral combinations.

Complementary and alternative medicine practices are not universally professionally accepted treatment by traditional Western medical care. Folk medicines and home remedies, based on herbs, have been used throughout history, with some cultures having deeper roots in these traditions than others.

Herbal supplements contain many biologically active ingredients to be used primarily for the treatment of mild or chronic illnesses. Many pharmaceuticals originating from plants contain these same ingredients but in a highly purified form. The danger with herbal supplements is that they are not subject to strict supervision by the FDA. As well, many of their interactions with prescription medicines are unknown or just coming to light. Documentation of all herbal supplements being used by a patient is essential for patient safety as well as being required by law.

CRITICAL THINKING EXERCISES

Scenario

Kim, a young adult, is in good health and eats a well-balanced diet. She has heard that taking vitamins may make her feel better, and she is considering taking multivitamins that contain water-soluble and fat-soluble components.

1. What do you tell her about excessive water- and fat-soluble vitamins? Should she need vitamins?
2. What can Kim expect to gain by using these vitamins?
3. What risks will she be taking?
4. Kim says that when she was pregnant she had to take vitamins. Why were vitamins important then and not necessary now?
5. What vitamin does the March of Dimes suggest Kim take?

DRUG CALCULATIONS

1. Order: potassium chloride 80 mEq
   Available medication:

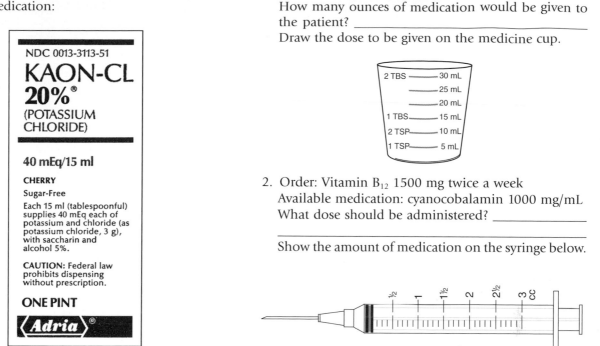

Dose to be given: 30 mL
How many ounces of medication would be given to the patient? _____
Draw the dose to be given on the medicine cup.

2. Order: Vitamin B_{12} 1500 mg twice a week
   Available medication: cyanocobalamin 1000 mg/mL
   What dose should be administered? _____

   _____

   Show the amount of medication on the syringe below.

REVIEW QUESTIONS

1. Name three groups of people who might need vitamin supplements. _____

   _____

2. What are vitamins? Minerals? Electrolytes? _____

   _____

   _____

   _____

   _____

3. Which vitamins are water soluble? Fat soluble? _____

   _____

   _____

4. Why is toxicity with fat-soluble vitamins a possibility? Why is toxicity not as likely with water-soluble vitamins?

   _____

   _____

   _____

   _____

   _____

5. What vitamin is necessary for calcium to be effective? What are two sources of this vitamin? _____

   _____

   _____

SECTION

V

Medications Related to Body Systems

CHAPTER 20

Endocrine System Disorders

OBJECTIVES

After studying this chapter, you should be capable of doing the following:

- Describing hormones and their functions.
- Explaining how hormones secreted by anterior and posterior pituitary glands affect diseases and their treatment.
- Describing the role of the thyroid gland and its replacements and antagonistic medications.
- Discussing forms of steroids and corticosteroids and their role in treating disorders.

- Describing the role of antidiabetic agents and adjunctive agents in treating diabetes mellitus (DM).
- Describing role of glucose and glycogen in maintaining homeostasis.
- Providing patient education for compliance with medications used to treat diseases and conditions of the endocrine system.

Dianne, age 45, has recently been diagnosed as having T2DM. She had no idea she had any medical problems until she went to her physician and her blood glucose test result was elevated above 300 and the HgA_{1c} above 15.

What symptoms do you think may have been present that she might not have realized were important?
What role will exercise and diet play in control of glucose levels with this type of diabetes? What is the role of weight loss with T2DM?
Can Dianne expect to take insulin for this type of illness? Why or why not?
If not insulin, what classes of medications might be used?
Can oral antidiabetic medications be used during pregnancy for gestational diabetes? Why or why not?

KEY TERMS

Action onset	Goiter	Lipodystrophy	Replacement therapy
Action peak	Growth hormone	Mineralocorticoid	Repository action
Bolus	Hormone	Negative feedback	Steroid
Corticosteroids	Hyperglycemia	Osteoporosis	Target organ
Endogenous	Hypoglycemia	Polydipsia	Tropic hormone
Exogenous	Hypothalamus	Polyphagia	
Glucocorticoid	Islets of Langerhans	Polyuria	

EASY WORKING KNOWLEDGE OF DRUGS USED IN THE ENDOCRINE SYSTEM

DRUG CLASS	PRESCRIPTION	OTC	PREGNANCY CATEGORY	MAJOR INDICATIONS
Anterior pituitary hormones	Yes	No	B, C	Growth stimulants, thyroid-stimulating hormone, adrenocorticotropin, gonadotropin
Posterior pituitary hormones	Yes	No	C	Antidiuretic hormone, oxytocin
THYROID HORMONES				
Triiodothyronine (T_3), Thyroxine (T_4)	Yes	No	A, C	Hypothyroidism
Calcitonin	Yes	No	C	Osteoporosis
Thyroid-inhibiting preparations	Yes	No	D, X (I-131)	Thyroid malignancies, hyperthyroidism
STEROIDS/CORTICOSTEROIDS				
Glucocorticoids	Yes	Yes—topical	C	Chronic inflammations, allergies, exacerbation of chronic lung disease
Mineralocorticoids	Yes	No	C	Antiinflammatory, Addison disease
Corticosteroid-inhibiting agents	Yes	No	C, D	Cushing disease, malignancies of adrenal glands
ANTIDIABETIC AGENTS				
Insulin	Yes	Yes (Regular and NPH)	B, C	T1DM, T2DM in some cases
Oral and other injectable antidiabetic agents	Yes	No	B, C, (should not be used in pregnancy)	T2DM
HYPERGLYCEMICS				
Glucagon	Yes	No	B	Hypoglycemia

T1DM, Type 1 diabetes mellitus; *T2DM*, type 2 diabetes mellitus.

EASY WORKING KNOWLEDGE OF INDICATIONS AND SIDE EFFECTS

Common Symptoms of Endocrine Diseases
Mental deviations
Exceptional changes in energy levels
Growth abnormalities
Skin, hair, and nail changes
Weakness and atrophy of muscles
Emotional disturbances or psychologic disorders
Edema
Changes in blood pressure and heart irregularities
Sexual irregularities
Changes in urinary output

Common Side Effects of Medications for Endocrine Diseases
Corticosteroids: Short-term—increased appetite and swelling; long-term—cushingoid syndrome, decreased density of minerals in bones
Thyroid preparations: palpitations, tremors, nervousness, tachycardia, increased blood pressure, headache, exophthalmos, weight loss, and irritability
Antidiabetic agents: hypoglycemia, nausea, heartburn, diarrhea, headache, weight gain

The endocrine system is a network of internal glands without ducts that secrete **hormones** directly into the bloodstream to be carried by blood or the lymphatic system to tissues or other glands throughout the body for vital functions (Figure 20-1). Hormones stimulate various tissues to increase their activity. Hormone action is slower in onset and of longer duration when stimulated by the nervous system. Some hormones are effective only in certain types of tissues or organs, called **target organs**, with specific receptors for the specific hormone. As the hormone attaches to this receptor site, it acts as a key to release the hormone to produce its effect. Hormone specificity and cellular receptor sites together form a complex regulatory system to ensure homeostasis. Only specific receptor material binds the hormone so it

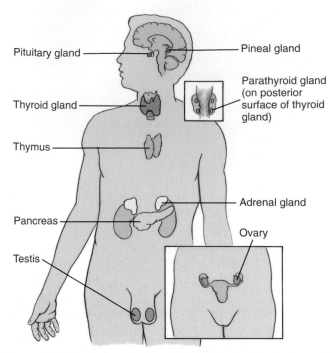

Figure 20-1 The major endocrine glands of the body. (From Applegate E: *The anatomy and physiology learning system,* ed 4, Philadelphia, 2011, WB Saunders.)

may begin activity when recognized by cell or site. Therefore hormones have no effect on tissues not having specific receptors for the specific hormone (Figure 20-2).

The **hypothalamus,** located in the brain, regulates hormone secretions, much as a thermostat regulates temperature in a heating-cooling system. Influenced by the body itself and by environmental factors, the hypothalamus causes production of releasing hormones that are received in the pituitary gland to maintain homeostasis. With the hypothalamus responding to the body's internal environment to control hormone release by **negative feedback,** a physiologic response inhibits further secretions of hormone. Similarly, increased hormone secretions may cause cessation of external stimuli, ending the secretion response internally. This response is a positive-negative response much like turning a light off and on in response to light and darkness (Figure 20-3).

WHAT ARE HORMONES?

Hormones are substances from steroids (lipids) or are nonsteroidal (derived from amino acids). Some hormones regulate the activity of other hormones and have a specific physiologic effect on metabolism, including substances causing the anterior and posterior pituitary glands to release tropic or stimulating hormones. These integrated relationships are between different glands of the endocrine system (Figure 20-4).

Hormones are necessary for regulation of vital processes such as secretion of gastric enzymes and fluids and

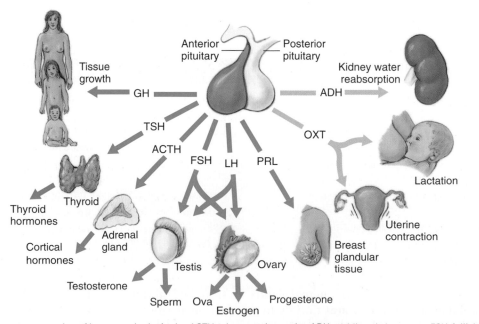

Figure 20-2 Hormone-receptor action of hormones in the body. *ACTH,* adrenocorticotropin; *ADH,* antidiuretic hormone; *FSH,* follicle-stimulating hormone; *GH,* growth hormone; *LH,* luteinizing hormone; *OXT,* oxytocin; *PRL,* prolactin; *TSH,* thyroid-stimulating hormone. (From Applegate E: *The anatomy and physiology learning system,* ed 4, Philadelphia, 2011, Saunders.)

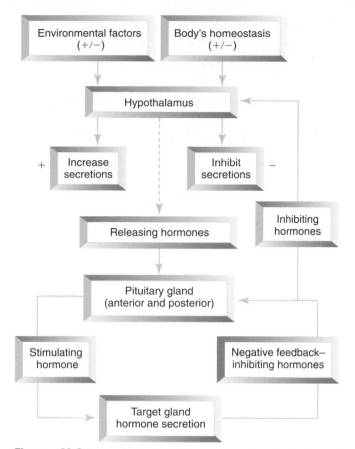

Figure 20-3 The relationship between negative feedback and homeostasis.

motor activities of the digestive tract; production of energy; composition and volume of extracellular fluid; adaptation of the body to external environment; growth and development; and reproduction and lactation.

Steroid hormones, secreted by adrenal and sex glands and manufactured from cholesterol by endocrine cells, are lipid soluble to be transported in plasma. These chemicals act as messengers to regulate the body's inner environment in conjunction with the nervous system.

Nonsteroid hormones, synthesized from amino acids, are characterized by the following:
- Protein hormones such as insulin and glucagons, parathyroid hormones (PTHs), calcitonin, **growth hormones** (GHs), and *adrenocorticotropin hormone (ACTH)*
- Glycoproteins, including follicle-stimulating hormone (FSH), luteinizing hormone (LH), thyroid-stimulating hormone (TSH), and chorionic gonadotropin
- Peptides such as antidiuretic hormone (ADH), oxytocin, and releasing hormones
- Amino acid derivatives that include epinephrine, norepinephrine, melatonin, thyroxine, and triiodothyronine

The endocrine system has extensive flexibility in length of action, as the hormone leaves the bloodstream to access target organs. Most hormones have short half-lives of 10 to 20 minutes, exerting their effect immediately and reflecting their rapid use or excretion. The effects of other hormones may persist for hours, resulting in prolonged organ stimulation.

Hormones not used completely must be inactivated by enzymes in blood, intracellular spaces, liver, kidneys, or target organs or are excreted for the body to stay in homeostasis. Excretion is primarily in urine but may be found in bile.

Two major therapeutic uses of hormones exist. In case of a deficiency, the needed hormone is administered as **replacement therapy.** Second, large doses of hormones may be given therapeutically, such as **corticosteroids** for inflammation or arthritis. Hormones may also be used for endocrine diagnostic testing, such as ACTH for adrenal insufficiency testing. When used either therapeutically or diagnostically, as in the situations cited, the hormone becomes a pharmacologic agent.

PITUITARY GLAND HORMONES

The pituitary gland, located below the hypothalamus and about the size of a pea, is called "the master gland," as it regulates the endocrine system. Pituitary hormones regulate hormone secretions from other endocrine glands. The anterior pituitary lobe secretes **tropic hormones,** named for the affected gland, such as thyrotropin, which affects the thyroid. Responding to neurohormones or hypothalamic-releasing factors, these hormones cause other endocrine glands to secrete their specific hormones.

Anterior Pituitary Gland

The anterior pituitary gland with the hypothalamus communicates by releasing regulating factors delivered through blood vessels. The anterior pituitary gland secretes six major hormones controlled by the hypothalamus, with three being used therapeutically (see Figure 20-4).
1. GH—stimulates almost all tissues and organs for growth
2. Adrenocorticotropic hormone (ACTH), or adrenocorticotropin—acts on the adrenal cortex to promote synthesis and release of its hormones
3. Thyrotropin (TSH)—acts on the thyroid gland to promote synthesis and release of hormones
4. Prolactin—stimulates milk production and secretion in women
5. FSH—promotes follicular ovarian growth and testicular spermatogenesis
6. LH—promotes ovulation and the development of corpus luteum in the female and acts on testes to

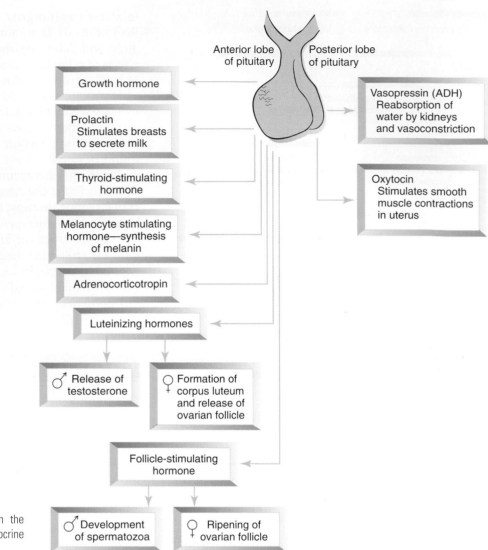

Figure 20-4 The relationship between the pituitary gland and other glands of the endocrine system.

promote androgen production in the male (These last three hormones are discussed in Chapter 28 in the sections on the reproductive system.)

Somatotropin, or GH, is produced by the anterior pituitary gland to help in regulation of growth. Absence of this hormone during childhood is the reason for dwarfism in most cases. Main replacement of GH is with children who have growth failure because of lack of production of **endogenous** somatotropin. Some people develop antibodies with prolonged treatment, but these rarely decrease the effectiveness of treatment (which may increase growth by as much as 6 inches). Somatotropin replacement is expensive (approximately $2000 per year). The efficacy of GH replacement therapy declines as the person grows older, with its therapy becoming ineffective by age 20 to 24 years. **Octreotide** (Sandostatin), a GH inhibitor, is used therapeutically to lower blood GH levels with acromegaly or gigantism

(Table 20-1). Excessive production of GH in adults causes *acromegaly,* whereas *gigantism* occurs if excessive stimulation occurs before epiphyseal lines in children are closed.

Adrenocorticotropic hormone (or adrenocorticotropin), used primarily for diagnostic testing, is rarely used therapeutically because its effects are highly variable. It cannot be given orally, and undesired side effects may be produced because it stimulates production of other hormones (see Table 20-1).

Thyroid-stimulating hormone (TSH, thyrotropin) stimulates thyroid gland function by increasing the uptake of iodine, increasing thyroid hormone synthesis and release, and promoting thyroid growth (Figure 20-5). It is used diagnostically to differentiate primary hypothyroidism from secondary hypothyroidism, and it may also be used to test for anterior pituitary gland deficiencies (see Table 20-1).

TABLE 20-1 SELECT DRUGS USED AS AGENTS OF THE PITUITARY GLAND

GENERIC NAME/ TRADE NAME	USUAL ADULT DOSE AND ROUTE	INDICATIONS FOR USE	MAJOR SIDE EFFECTS	DRUG INTERACTIONS
ANTERIOR PITUITARY GLAND				
Growth Hormone				
somatotropin (recombinant DNA) (Humatrope, Genotropin, Omnitrope)	Varies by product	Prader-Willi syndrome Patients with growth failure	Weakness, transient edema	insulin
Growth Hormone Inhibitor				
octreotide (Sandostatin)	Initially 50 mcg SC, IV	Inhibits rapid or excessive growth (acromegaly)	Sinus bradycardia, diarrhea, headache, cardiac dysrhythmias, changes in blood glucose levels	antidiabetic medications, glucagon
Adrenocortical Hormones				
corticotropin (Acthar) ACTH	Varies with patient, and Dx IM, SC, IV Varies with patient, and Dx IM, IV	Diagnostic testing	Insomnia, acne, abdominal distress, delayed wound healing, increased susceptibility to infection hypertension, mood changes, edema, weight gain	amphotericin, insulin, oral hypoglycemics, digoxin, diuretics, potassium supplements, live virus vaccines
Thyroid-Stimulating Hormone				
thyrotropin alfa (Thyrogen)	0.9 mg IM	Diagnostic testing and treatment of thyroid cancer	Headache, nausea	No major interactions
POSTERIOR PITUITARY GLAND				
Antidiuretic Hormone (ADH)				
vasopressin (Pitressin)	Varies, SC, IM, IV	Diabetes insipidus, acute massive hemorrhage, abdominal distention	Abdominal pain and distress, nausea and vomiting, headache, chest pain, confusion, arrhythmias	carbamazepine, lithium, chlorpropamide, clofibrate, norepinephrine
desmopressin (DDAVP)	Varies, PO, nasal spray, IV	Diabetes insipidus, primary nocturnal enuresis, control bleeding in hemophilia	abdominal pain, headache, change in BP	Same as for vasopressin

ACTH, Adrenocorticotropic hormone; *BP,* blood pressure; *CHF,* congestive heart failure; *Dx,* diagnosis; *IM,* intramuscularly; *IV,* intravenously; *PO,* orally; *SC,* subcutaneously.

Posterior Pituitary Gland

The posterior pituitary gland, with only neuronal stimulation and no direct contact through blood vessels, produces two hormones: **oxytocin** (active on the reproductive system) and ADH (**vasopressin**; active on the urinary system). Oxytocin (see Chapter 28) and ADH (see Chapter 27) are synthesized in the neurosecretory cells of the hypothalamus. ADH promotes renal conservation of water, whereas oxytocin functions during labor and

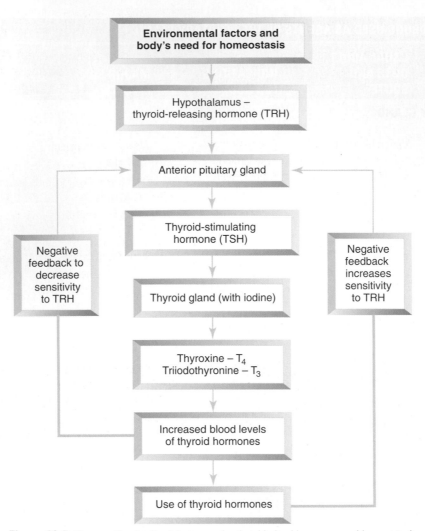

Figure 20-5 The negative feedback between the thyroid gland hormones and homeostasis.

delivery and therefore is not discussed in depth in this book. Hypofunction of the posterior pituitary gland results in diabetes insipidus, causing profuse voiding of large amounts of dilute urine, leading to dehydration (see Table 20-1).

Important Facts about Pituitary Hormones

- Release of hormones from the anterior pituitary gland is influenced by the hypothalamus and is inhibited by negative feedback.
- Growth hormone (GH) replacement therapy is indicated only for children deficient in GH, not for children who are simply short.
- Elevated blood glucose levels occur in children taking GH.

Patient Education for Compliance

1. When using somatotropin (growth hormone [GH]) therapy, regularly scheduled medical visits are important so that height and weight can be measured.
2. When receiving adrenocorticotropin hormone (ACTH), notify the physician of any signs of infection. Do not stop ACTH injections abruptly; this drug must be tapered off.
3. Patients taking antidiuretic hormone (ADH) should monitor fluid intake and output, as well as weight, as indications of dehydration. Report shortness of breath, chest pain, or headaches with ADH therapy.

THYROID GLAND HORMONES

The thyroid gland, located in the anterior neck, secretes TSH on stimulation by the anterior pituitary gland, to control secretion of T_3, T_4, and calcitonin (see Figure 20-5). T_3 and T_4 stimulate protein synthesis, increase blood sugar levels, decrease serum cholesterol levels, increase metabolism for production of heat and energy, and enable normal mental development and normal growth. Diets deficient in iodine lead to **goiter**, as T_3 and T_4 require iodine for production and the thyroid increases in size in an effort to secrete the needed iodine.

Hyposecretion may be caused by glandular destruction from radiation therapy, lack of iodine, surgical thyroid removal, or pituitary dysfunction. Oral thyroid replacements may be extracted from endocrine glands of animals or be synthetically prepared. Two hormones, T_3 and T_4, or a combination of the two, may be used, with the dose gradually adjusted for lifelong therapy according to an individual's needs. Thyroid hormones are approved for supplemental or replacement needs of hypothyroidism and are not indicated or approved for treatment of obesity, although they do affect metabolism. Doses that would be necessary for weight reduction could produce life-threatening cardiovascular effects.

Thyroid hormones are usually initiated in small doses and are individualized until adequate response is reached. Physiologic effects of overdose are symptoms of psychotic behavior, diarrhea, increased blood pressure and heart rate, and angina. Long-term overuse of thyroxine has been associated with **osteoporosis** in postmenopausal women. Thyroxine is contraindicated in patients who have had a myocardial infarction and may exacerbate diabetes mellitus (DM), leading to an increased need for antidiabetic medications. With estrogen therapy the amount of thyroid hormone needed may increase because estrogens tie up circulating hormones, thereby decreasing the amount available at target tissues.

Thyroid replacement medications do not readily cross the placenta, so their needed use in pregnancy does not affect fetal development (Table 20-2).

✏ CLINICAL TIP

Patients with diabetes taking thyroid replacements and antidiabetic medications should be watched closely. Discontinuing thyroid medication when taking hypoglycemics may lead to severe hypoglycemic reactions because thyroid medications tend to increase blood sugar levels and the need for increased hypoglycemics for control of glucose levels.

Patient Education for Compliance

1. Lifelong thyroid replacement therapy should not be discontinued without consulting a physician.
2. When counseling patients who are beginning thyroid replacement therapy, inform them that it should be taken in the morning (on an empty stomach) to avoid insomnia from increased metabolism.
3. Palpitations, nervousness, and headaches may be signs of toxicity of thyroid medication.
4. Iodized salt is an excellent source of the iodine needed for proper thyroid function.

ANTITHYROID MEDICATIONS

Hypersecretion of thyroid hormones may be the result of tumors or autoimmune diseases such as Graves disease. Excessive secretion and circulation of T_3 and T_4 result in increased cell metabolism, weakness, anxiety, and heat production. Treatment for hyperthyroidism is use of antithyroid medications, irradiation of the thyroid gland, or surgical thyroid tissue removal.

Antithyroid medications, such as **iodine** or iodide ions, radioactive iodine, and thionamide derivatives, interfere with synthesis of thyroid hormones by saturating the thyroid gland and decreasing the vascularity of the thyroid gland to decrease secretions. These agents will cross the placenta to stop fetal thyroid development and can cross into breast milk to affect the infant. **Radioactive iodine, iodine 131 (^{131}I),** may be used to destroy tissue of thyroid gland (see Table 20-2).

Patient Education for Compliance

1. **Propylthiouracil** should be taken at regular intervals around the clock.
2. Iodine solutions should be diluted in fruit juices or beverages to make them palatable.
3. Brassy taste, burning sensation in the mouth, and soreness of gums and teeth are signs of excessive iodine and should be reported to the physician immediately.

Important Facts about Thyroid Medications

- The thyroid gland produces two active hormones—triiodothyronine (T_3) and thyroxine (T_4)—to stimulate energy production, stimulate the heart, and promote growth and development.
- Thyroid replacement therapy is for treatment of hypothyroidism, not for treatment of obesity or for weight loss.
- Antithyroid medications benefit patients with hyperthyroidism by suppressing the secretion of T_3 and T_4.

Calcitonin

Calcitonin is secreted by the thyroid gland, but blood calcium levels are regulated by PTH and an adequate absorption of vitamin D. These hormones work together to ensure an adequate supply of calcium for neuromuscular and endocrine function. **Calcitonin salmon** and calcium have the same effects as human calcitonin and is safer for treatment of osteoporosis in postmenopausal women. Calcium and vitamin D intake must be adequate for calcitonin salmon to be effective (see Table 20-2).

TABLE 20-2 SELECT DRUGS USED AS AGENTS OF THE THYROID AND PARATHYROID GLANDS

GENERIC NAME/ TRADE NAME	USUAL ADULT DOSE AND ROUTE	INDICATIONS FOR USE	MAJOR SIDE EFFECTS	DRUG INTERACTIONS
SYNTHETIC THYROID REPLACEMENT				
levothyroxine (T_4) (Levothroid, Synthroid, Unithroid, Levoxyl)	0.1-0.2 mg PO qd	Hypothyroidism	Weight loss, tremors, nervousness, headaches, sweating, exophthalmos, insomnia	cholestyramine, anticoagulants
liothyronine (T_3) (Cytomel, Triostat)	0.25-1 mg PO qd	Same as for levothyroxine		same as levothryoxine
liotrix (T_3, T_4) (Thyrolar)	60-120 mg PO qd			same as liothyronine
NATURAL THYROID REPLACEMENT				
desiccated thyroid (T_3, T_4) (Armour Thyroid, Nature-throid, Westhroid)	60-120 mg PO qd	Hypothyroidism	Same as for synthetic thyroid replacement	Same as for synthetic thyroid
ANTITHYROID PREPARATIONS				
thionamide derivatives, propylthiouracil (Propyl-Thyracil)	300-400 mg PO qd initially; 100-150 mg PO maintenance	Hyperthyroidism	Rashes, nausea and vomiting, myalgia, stomach pain, fever, increased bleeding tendencies	anticoagulants, iodine 131 (^{131}I)
methimazole (Tapazole)	15-60 mg PO tid initially; 5-15 mg PO tid maintenance	Same as for propylthiouracil		Same as for propylthiouracil
^{131}I, RAI (Iodotope)	4-10 millicuries PO qd, IV			Same as for propylthiouracil, except ^{131}I
CALCITONIN				
calcitonin salmon (Fortical)	100 units IM, SC	Paget disease, elevated Ca levels, osteoporosis	Local irritation, GI upset	Lithium
(Miacalcin)	1 spray in alternating nostrils			
PARATHYROID GLAND MEDICATION				
teriparatide (Forteo)	20 mcg SC	Osteoporosis, for those at high risk for fractures	Dizziness, headache, depression, hypertension, symptomatic orthostatic hypotension, arthralgia, nausea and vomiting, diarrhea	digoxin

GI, Gastrointestinal; *IM,* intramuscularly; *IV,* intravenously; *PO,* orally; *RAI,* radioactive iodine; *SC,* subcutaneously.

Patient Education for Compliance

Teach patients how to activate a nasal spray of a metered dose pump of calcitonin salmon. The medication should be refrigerated between uses.

Important Facts about Calcitonin

Calcitonin salmon has the same metabolic effects as human calcitonin and is very safe.

PARATHYROID HORMONE

The parathyroid gland secretes (PTH) which, in cooperation with calcitonin, regulates calcium blood levels. When blood levels of calcium decrease, PTH acts to release calcium as new bone cell development is reduced, and old bone is dissolved to maintain calcium homeostasis. One PTH drug, **teriparatide** (Forteo), is used to treat osteoporosis in postmenopausal women and men who are at high risk of fractures (see Table 20-2).

CORTICOSTEROIDS/STEROIDS

The adrenal glands are located directly over each kidney and are composed of two parts: an outer portion called the *cortex,* which secretes a number of hormones that are essential for life, including cortisone, hydrocortisone, aldosterone, and deoxycorticosterone; and an inner portion, called the *medulla* (see Figure 20-1), which secretes epinephrine and norepinephrine and is considered part of the sympathetic nervous system. Hormones of the adrenal cortex are activated by ACTH from the anterior pituitary gland. The most important functions of adrenal cortex hormones are regulation of water and salt metabolism, regulation of carbohydrate metabolism, and production of antiinflammatory effects. The terms *adrenocorticosteroids, corticosteroids,* and *steroids* all refer to the same natural or synthetic substances, which may be grouped as mineralocorticoids, glucocorticoids, or mixed steroids.

Adrenal Cortex Hormones

The adrenal cortex has three levels. The outer level secretes **mineralocorticoids,** and the middle level secretes **glucocorticoids** (the inner layer secretes small amounts of male and female sex hormones). Like all tropic hormones, ACTH is regulated by the hypothalamus, which is influenced by the sleep-wake cycle, negative feedback, and stress. More corticotropin is available during the awake period to regulate body metabolism, and negative feedback inhibits the release of corticotropin to keep cortisol levels relatively constant day to day. As body stress rises, corticotropin stimulates secretion of cortisol to increase the body's ability to cope with stress.

Glucocorticoids regulate metabolism of proteins and carbohydrates, particularly when the body is under stress. With therapeutic use, glucocorticoids cause retention of sodium, leading to water retention and possible hypertension. Glucocorticoids, potent agents used in acute and chronic inflammatory processes including organ transplants, may be administered orally, intramuscularly, intraarticularly, intravenously, topically, or by inhalation, for either local or systemic effect. Preparations for intramuscular use have **repository actions** to allow the drug to be released slowly for a longer duration of action. Therapeutic doses vary widely and must be adjusted to meet the patient's needs. Steroids should be used with caution with gastrointestinal ulcers or colitis, renal disease, herpes simplex, and emotional instability and are contraindicated in patients with systemic fungal infections, tuberculosis, and local viral infections. Adverse effects include joint tissue damage to cushingoid symptoms such as fatigue, weakness, edema, "moon face," "pot belly," "buffalo hump," and excessive hair growth. After long-term or high-dose steroid therapy, cessation of steroid use must be tapered off slowly in small decrements. Ocular use over long periods of time may lead to glaucoma and cataracts.

Live virus vaccines may not be effective for the patient who is taking steroids and could even put the patient at risk for developing infections that may advance at an alarming rate because steroids suppress the body's inflammatory response. Drug interactions are numerous and are listed in Table 20-3.

Mineralocorticoids regulate blood levels of sodium and potassium by increasing the reabsorption rate of sodium by the kidneys. The most important mineralocorticoid is aldosterone, which acts on distal tubules of kidney nephrons. Mineralocorticoids are usually administered in conjunction with glucocorticoids for replacement therapy in adrenocortical insufficiency resulting in Addison disease (Table 20-4).

TABLE 20-3 COMMON DRUG INTERACTIONS ASSOCIATED WITH GLUCOCORTICOIDS

INTERACTIVE MEDICATIONS	POSSIBLE RESPONSE
amphotericin B	Potentiates hypokalemia
digitalis	Possible digitalis toxicity
diuretics	Potential for hypokalemia, decreased therapeutic effect of diuretics
antibiotics, macrolides	Increased clearance of corticosteroids from bloodstream, decreased metabolism of steroid
anticoagulants	Increases chance of thrombosis by inhibiting anticoagulant actions
insulin, oral hypoglycemics	Increased requirements of medication for diabetes mellitus because of increased blood glucose levels
isoniazid	Increased doses of isoniazid may be needed
oral contraceptive, estrogen	Increase steroid effect, because drugs inhibit steroid metabolism
phenobarbital, phenytoin, rifampin	Increase steroid effect because of the enhanced metabolism of steroids
antacids	Decreased steroid absorption

TABLE 20-4 SELECT DRUGS USED AS STEROIDS OR CORTICOSTEROIDS*

GENERIC NAME/ TRADE NAME	USUAL ADULT DOSE AND ROUTE	INDICATIONS FOR USE	MAJOR SIDE EFFECTS	DRUG INTERACTIONS
GLUCOCORTICOIDS		Allergies, body stress, replacement therapy, antiinflammatory agents, leukemia, pruritus	Insomnia, mood changes, personality changes	See Table 20-3
cortisone acetate (NTN)	Varies; individualized doses, PO			
hydrocortisone (Cortisol, Cortef)	Varies, PO, topical, IM, IV, enema			
hydrocortisone sodium succinate (Solu-Cortef)	Varies, IM, IV			
prednisolone (Orapred)	Varies, PO			
methylprednisolone (Medrol)	Varies, PO, IM, IV, IA, R (enema)			
methylprednisolone acetate (Depo-Medrol)	Varies, IM	Same as glucocorticoi and bursitis		
methylprednisolone sodium succinate (Solu-Medrol)	Varies, IM, IV, IA			
betamethasone (Celestone)	Varies, PO, IA, IM			
dexamethasone (DexPak)	Varies, PO, IM, IV	Same as glucocorticoids, bursitis, and before radiation, chemotherapy		
prednisone (NTN)	Varies, PO	Same as glucocorticoids and multiple sclerosis		
triamcinolone (Aristocort, Kenacort)	PO, topical, gingival, inhaled	Same as glucocorticoids, oral lesions, asthma		
beclomethasone (Beconase, QVAR)	Intranasal Inhaled	Asthma, bronchitis, allergies		
fluticasone (Flonase, Flovent, Cutivate)	Nasal topical Inhaled Topical	Rhinitis, asthma		
MINERALOCORTICOIDS			Edema, weakness, hypertension	
deoxycorticosterone acetate (DOCA) (Percorten)	Varies, IM	Addison disease		digitalis, diuretics
fludrocortisone (Florinef)	Varies, PO			
INHIBITORS OF CORTICOSTEROIDS		Cushing syndrome	Nausea, headache, fever, drowsiness, dizziness, muscle pain, cardiovascular irregularities, changes in sexual characteristics	dexamethasone
aminoglutethimide (Cytadren)	250 mg PO			
trilostane (Modrastane)	30 mg PO			

IA, Intra-articularly; *IM*, intramuscularly; *IV*, intravenously; *NTN*, no trade name; *PO*, orally; *R*, rectal.
*See Chapter 22 for dermatologic use of steroid agents.

Adrenal steroid inhibitors suppress adrenal cortex function in adrenal gland malignancies or other adrenal hyperplasias. These medications are used temporarily until the radiation therapy to the pituitary gland is effective. Adverse reactions are cardiovascular irregularities and liver dysfunction. Precocious sexual development occurs in males, and females acquire masculine features (see Table 20-4).

ADMINISTRATION TECHNIQUES WITH STEROID THERAPY

Steroids are given in two unique ways:
1. Alternate-day therapy (ADT) is used to reduce or eliminate adverse drug reactions. Short-acting medicine is given every other morning, with its effects persisting into day 2, when the adrenal gland functions by negative feedback. On the following day, the medication is given again. This routine allows the adrenal gland to function with fewer adverse reactions.
2. Declining or decreasing dose so that the body receives a therapeutic dose rapidly, and the doge is then tapered off. Usually the drug is given in 2-day increments, although this may change with individual dosages for specific conditions. Depending on increments and total dosage, the dosage declines by a tablet per day or so until the total dosage has been given.

Table 20-4 lists typical steroid and corticosteroid medications and their drug forms. Some topical steroids used for various conditions are found in Table 20-5. Over-the-counter (OTC) glucocorticoid preparations contain 0.5% to 1% hydrocortisone for topical use. Prescription topical medications are listed in Chapter 22.

TABLE 20-5 EXAMPLES OF OVER-THE-COUNTER STEROID PREPARATIONS

NAME OF PRODUCT	FORM OF MEDICATION
Cortaid	Cream, ointment, lotion, spray
Preparation H with hydrocortisone	Cream
Aloe Gel HC (*Aloe vera* and hydrocortisone)	Gel
Caldecort	Ointment, spray, rectal foam
Gynecort, Cortef, Feminine Itch Cream	Cream
Bactine HC	Cream

Patient Education for Compliance

1. Before medical or dental procedures, the health care professional should be informed when steroids are being taken because of bleeding, altered healing processes, and altered responses to infection.
2. When taking steroids, watch for signs of salt and water retention such as weight gain and edema of the feet and lower legs.
3. Reduce the intake of sodium-rich foods and increase intake of potassium-rich foods when using steroid preparations.
4. Do not stop taking steroid medications abruptly unless directed by prescriber.
5. Nonprescription medications should not be taken with steroids without consulting a physician or pharmacist because of numerous drug interactions.

Important Facts about Corticosteroids and Steroids

- Steroids may be administered orally, parenterally, topically, intranasally, or by inhalation.
- Glucocorticoids influence metabolism of fats, carbohydrates, and proteins as well as affecting the skeletal, muscular, cardiovascular, immune, and central nervous systems.
- Aldosterone, the major mineralocorticoid, acts on kidneys to promote retention of sodium and water and allows excretion of potassium.
- Excessive doses of steroids can cause cushingoid symptoms and Cushing disease.
- When used in low doses for replacement therapy, steroids are therapeutic. Conversely, when used chronically for pharmacologic needs in nonendocrine diseases, these drugs have severe adverse effects.
- Glucocorticoids are used to reduce inflammatory and immune system responses, as in arthritis, allergic disorders, asthma, cancer, and organ transplant rejection.
- When used with nonsteroidal antiinflammatory drugs (NSAIDs), steroids increase the risk of peptic ulcers.
- Steroids can increase the risk of toxic effects from ***digoxin.***

LEARNING TIP

When "HC" follows a drug name, most often it indicates inclusion of hydrocortisone.

DRUGS USED AS ANTIDIABETIC AGENTS

The pancreas secretes two hormones, insulin and glucagon, to regulate metabolism of proteins, fats, and especially carbohydrates. A cluster of pancreatic cells known as the **islets of Langerhans** produces insulin, which acts as the key to opening body cells to glucose. Insulin and glucagon allow cells to receive an adequate supply of glucose for body fuel and to regulate blood glucose levels. Insulin has three distinct purposes: (1) it aids in use of glucose as energy; (2) it prompts liver storage of excess glucose as glycogen; and (3) it is responsible for conversion of glucose to fat. By negative feedback, glucagon stimulates breakdown of glycogen to increase circulating glucose when blood glucose levels are too low.

Diabetes Mellitus

The most common endocrine gland disease involving the pancreas is diabetes mellitus (DM), the sixth leading cause of death in the United States. DM affects about 16 million Americans, with 90% to 95% of cases being type 2 DM (T2DM). In persons with DM, carbohydrate metabolism involves insulin deficiency, insulin resistance, or both, leading to hyperglycemia. Most authorities believe that any abnormal level of pancreatic function may lead to DM, either type 1 DM (T1DM) or T2DM. Patients with T1DM have very little or no **endogenous** insulin so require **exogenous** insulin for survival. These individuals seem to have a genetic abnormality involving autoimmune destruction of beta cells of the islets of Langerhans. T2DM usually is of maturity onset, although recent research shows a rise in this disease in obese children. With T2DM, the patient has some insulin function, but production of secretions of the beta cells is low or insufficient. The disease may be the result of aging, improper diet, or genetic factors leading to insulin resistance. Classic signs of T1DM and T2DM are **polydipsia, polyphagia,** and **polyuria** (Table 20-6).

Obese persons with insulin resistance are prone to metabolic syndrome, a cluster of conditions that occur together for increased risk for heart disease, stroke, and diabetes. Four conditions found in the syndrome are obesity around the waist, hypertension, hyperglycemia, and hyperlipidemia. In combination, the risk is even greater; the person having one factor is more likely to have others. A family history of T2DM with insulin resistance or a history of gestational diabetes increases the likelihood of having the disease. Certain medications increase blood glucose levels and cause hyperglycemia in the prediabetic person. These drugs include glucocorticoids, prednisone, thiazide diuretics, and epinephrine.

Treatment for DM includes medications as well as dietary adjustment to limit ingested carbohydrates and consistent exercise to control glucose. The drugs for DM are in three categories: insulins, oral antidiabetic agents, and drugs that affect glucose absorption or production, including new adjunctive therapy drugs that increase effectiveness of other antidiabetic agents. Insulins and sulfonylureas decrease blood glucose levels. Antidiabetic medications delay dietary glucose absorption and inhibit glucose production in the liver to lower blood glucose levels, especially postprandial blood glucose levels. Persons with T1DM must administer exogenous insulin for life and must adjust their diets and exercise. Patients with T2DM secrete some endogenous insulin, and diet alone may control elevated serum glucose levels for those persons who do not respond to the dietary controls, or diet alone may be insufficient, necessitating an oral antidiabetic drug.

TABLE 20-6 COMPARISON OF TYPES 1 AND 2 DIABETES MELLITUS

	T1DM	T2DM
Former name	IDDM, juvenile-onset diabetes, Type 1 DM	NIDDM, adult-onset diabetes, Type 2 DM
Usual age of onset	Childhood or adolescence	Usually >40 yr
Onset speed	Rapid	Gradual
Family history	Usually negative	Frequently positive
Predominance	5%-10% of people with diabetes	90%-95% of people with diabetes
Etiology	Autoimmune process	Unknown; strongly familial
Primary cause	Loss of insulin secretion	Insulin resistance or decreased insulin
Insulin secreted	None in later stages	Levels may be low, normal, or high (resistance)
Ketosis	Common	Uncommon
Signs and symptoms	Polyuria, polyphagia, polydipsia, weight loss	May be asymptomatic
Body	Thin, undernourished	Frequently obese
Blood glucose levels	Fluctuates in response to body activities and illness	More stable
Treatment	Insulin replacement, diet, and exercise	Exercise and reduced caloric intake; in some cases, oral hypoglycemics or even insulin

IDDM, Insulin-dependent diabetes mellitus; *NIDDM,* non–insulin-dependent diabetes mellitus; *T1DM,* type 1 diabetes mellitus; *T2DM,* type 2 diabetes mellitus.

When too much insulin or insufficient glucagon allows lowering of serum glucose levels, a hypoglycemic reaction (the opposite of DM) may be precipitated. Table 20-7 compares signs and symptoms of **hypoglycemia** and **hyperglycemia.**

TABLE 20-7 COMPARISON OF SIGNS AND SYMPTOMS OF HYPOGLYCEMIA AND HYPERGLYCEMIA

	HYPOGLYCEMIA OR INSULIN SHOCK	HYPERGLYCEMIA OR DIABETIC COMA
Onset	Sudden	Gradual
Skin	Pale, moist	Flushed, dry
Tongue	Moist	Dry
Breath	No change	Fruity odor (acetone smell)
Thirst	None	Intense
Respirations	Shallow	Deep
Vomiting	Rare	Common
Pulse	Fast, bounding	Fast, weak
Urine	No glucose or acetone	Positive for glucose, acetone or both
Serum glucose	↓ 50 mg/dL	↑ 200 mg/dL
Blood pressure	Normal	Low
Abdominal pain	Common, acute	None

Administration of Insulin in Type 1 Diabetes Mellitus

T1DM requires use of injected insulin because insulin is inactivated in the digestive tract with oral administration. The forms of insulin differ with respect to their time and course of action. Insulin is usually given by subcutaneous or intramuscular injection using an insulin syringe. Regular insulin may be administered intravenously in emergencies or circumstances in which immediate insulin action is necessary. Illnesses, trauma, and stress increase blood glucose levels, and thus higher doses of insulin may be required to keep the body in homeostasis. Dosage of insulin is individualized and may change over time depending on lifestyle changes.

Commercial insulin preparations produce similar effects in the body but vary in time for **action onset,** time to **action peak,** and duration. The four groups of insulins that are modified human derivatives are (1) rapid acting (**lispro** [Humalog], aspart [NovoLog] and **glulisine** [Apidra]); (2) short acting (regular, **Humulin, Novolin R**); (3) intermediate acting (**isophane** [NPH] [Humulin N, Novolin N]); and (4) long acting (**glargine** [Lantus] and **detemir** [Levemir], and premixed combinations (Table 20-8).

Two processes have been used to prolong insulin's effects: (1) adding a protein to natural insulin (NPH) and (2) removing an amino acid from a natural insulin (detemir) by altering DNA. A graph of action has been

TABLE 20-8 COURSE OF ACTION OF INSULIN PREPARATIONS

INSULIN TYPE/NAME	LETTER ON BOTTLE	ONSET	PEAK	DURATION
RAPID-ACTING INSULINS				
insulin lispro (Humalog)	H	15-30 min	½-1 hr	3-4 hr
insulin aspart (NovoLog)		10-20 min	1-3 hr	3-5 hr
glulisine (Apidra)		15-30 min	1 hr	3-4 hr
SHORT-ACTING INSULIN				
regular insulin (Humulin R, Novolin R)	R	½-1 hr	2.5-5 hr	up to 6 hr
INTERMEDIATE-ACTING INSULIN				
isophane insulin (NPH) (Humulin N, Novolin N)	N	1-2 hr	4-12 hr	up to 24+ hr
LONG-ACTING INSULINS				
insulin glargine (Lantus)		1-2 hr	No peak identified	≥24 hr
insulin detemir (Levemir)		8 min to 2 hr	Unknown	up to 24 hr
insulin regular concentrated (Humulin R U-500)		½-1 hr		up to 24 hr
COMBINATIONS				
NPH and mixtures, (Humulin, Novolin 70/30, 50/50)		10-20 min	2-4 hr	up to 24 hr
NPL and lispro (Humalog 75/25, 50/50)		72 hr	Dual	10-16 hr
NPA/N and aspart (NovoLog 70/30)		1½-1 hr	Dual	10-16 hr

NPA, Isophane (NPH) and aspart; *NPL,* isophane (NPH) and lispro.

sulfonylureas. These medications have early side effects of flatulence, diarrhea, and abdominal pain that subside with continued use (see Table 20-9).

Biguanides act by lowering cellular resistance to insulin. **Metformin** (Glucophage) decreases production of glucose by the liver while not releasing insulin from the pancreas and does not cause hypoglycemia. It reduces blood glucose levels in patients who no longer produce insulin in adequate quantities to prevent hyperglycemia. Metformin is used for T1DM and T2DM but is not recommended for use by older adults or patients with renal dysfunction (see Table 20-9).

Thiazolidinediones, or glitazones, are a class of antihyperglycemic medications not related to any other oral medications for T2DM. These medications (i.e., rosiglitazone [Avandia]) decrease insulin resistance and improve blood glucose control to be effective in persons with insulin resistance, even those who no longer respond to sulfonylureas. Their action is to increase insulin sensitivity in adipose tissue, muscles, and liver. These agents may be used alone or in combination with metformin or sulfonylureas (see Table 20-9).

Meglitinides, also called *rapid insulin releasers*, are short-acting medications that may be used alone or with other medications to stimulate beta cells to release insulin in an action similar to that of sulfonylureas. These medications can be used with injected long-acting insulin therapy to provide enhanced blood glucose control. Persons who eat carbohydrates and have a subsequent blood sugar spike will most likely benefit from these medications. **Repaglinide** (Pradin) and **nateglinide** (Starlix) should be taken 10 to 15 minutes before meals and should not need to be taken if the meal is skipped (see Table 20-9).

Dipeptidyl peptidase-4 inhibitors (DPP-4), the newest addition to the oral hypoglycemic agents for treating T2DM, may be used alone or in combination with metformin or a thiazolidinedione. Less weight gain and fewer incidences of hypoglycemia occur with these drugs (i.e., **saxagliptin [Onglyza]**) as they work to reduce release of glucagon and increase release of insulin to restore blood glucose levels toward normal after eating (see Table 20-9).

OTHER INJECTABLES FOR TYPE 2 AND TYPE 1 DIABETES MELLITUS

Amylin glucagon-like peptide (GLP)–1 analogues, injectable medications, stimulate secretion of insulin in beta cells when large amounts of glucose are found in the bloodstream, thus promoting beta-cell regeneration. These drugs curb the appetite and control blood glucose levels while minimizing the chance of hypoglycemia by delaying gastric emptying to lower high postprandial blood glucose levels. These drugs may also be used in patients who have undergone islet transplantation.

Incretin mimetics are given subcutaneously to persons whose diabetes cannot be controlled with oral antidiabetic medications and may be used for stand-alone therapy with T2DM. The medication is administered twice a day before the morning and evening meal. **Exenatide** (Byetta), the first drug in this class, and **liraglutide** (Victoza) are available as prefilled pen-injector devices to be used in combination with other medications (see Table 20-9).

Synthetic human amylin, used as adjunct therapy with insulin for uncontrolled T1DM and T2DM, is available in vials for injection. The dose is injected SC before meals and before snacks of 30 g of carbohydrates or more. **Pramlintide** (Symlin) should not be mixed in the same syringe with insulin preparations, and the injection sites must be at least 2 inches apart. Side effects include decrease in appetite with resultant decrease in caloric intake and weight loss.

Patient Education for Compliance

1. When taking insulin, the person should not smoke for 30 minutes after administration because nicotine produces vasoconstriction, which slows the circulation of insulin.
2. Diet and exercise are important in control of diabetes. Persons taking insulin should not skip meals and must exercise routinely. If a meal is skipped, the insulin dose should not be injected.
3. Blood glucose levels should be monitored routinely.
4. Persons with diabetes should wear medical identification at all times.
5. When using lispro insulin, the patient must eat within 15 minutes of medication administration or injection may be given immediately after a meal.
6. Suspensions of insulin, including those used in insulin pens, should be gently rolled between the hands before administration. Vigorous agitation makes the drug frothy, causing an inaccurate dose. Insulin pens should be stored with the needle up.
7. Fast-acting and rapid-acting insulins are clear solutions, not cloudy as suspensions.
8. Injection sites should be rotated with each insulin administration.
9. Unopened vials of insulin should be refrigerated but not frozen. Vials in current use can be stored at room temperature for up to 1 month but must be kept out of heat or direct sunlight.
10. Persons with diabetes should always read labels of OTC medications or check with a pharmacist before buying these medications. Sugar content of OTC medications changes frequently, so the person should check labels each time medication is purchased.
11. Inform patients that reduced food intake, vomiting, diarrhea, excessive alcohol consumption, and excessive exercise may cause hypoglycemia.

Patient Education for Compliance—cont'd

12. Teach patients signs of hypoglycemia—tachycardia, palpitations, sweating, nervousness, headache, confusion, and fatigue.
13. Persons with diabetes should always carry oral carbohydrates to counteract a hypoglycemic reaction, preferably an easily synthesized carbohydrate such as sugar, nondiet soda, or juice. A carbohydrate that is slower in digestion, such as peanut butter or fruit, should immediately follow the rapidly digested carbohydrate.

Important Facts about Antidiabetic Agents

- Diabetes mellitus (DM) is characterized by sustained hyperglycemia. T1DM is insulin dependent, whereas T2DM is not usually insulin dependent but insulin may be needed on some persons. T1DM, an autoimmune disease, represents a complete absence of insulin and must be treated with insulin. T2DM results from a cellular resistance to insulin and may be treated with oral antidiabetic agents and/or insulin, but diet and exercise are also important. Patients with T2DM may not need oral antidiabetic medications after undergoing weight reduction and exercise programs. T2DM requires a change in lifestyle to achieve a good quality of life.
- Four forms of injectable insulin are used in the United States: rapid acting, fast acting, intermediate acting, and long acting. Premixed combinations of these types of insulin are also available.
- Rapid-onset insulins (8-15 minutes) have a very short duration and action.
- Short-acting insulin has a fast onset (approximately 30 minutes) and short duration of action.
- Intermediate-acting insulin has an intermediate onset and duration of action.
- Long-acting insulin has a prolonged onset and duration of action. This group includes insulins that provide a continuous 24-hour supply of insulin, with no plasma peak.
- All insulins should be given subcutaneously, but regular insulin may be administered intramuscularly or intravenously if necessary.
- Many new insulin delivery systems such as pumps are available. Oral and nasal administration and insulin patches are being investigated.
- Some classes of antidiabetic agents do not cause hypoglycemia, including α-glucosidase inhibitors, biguanides, glitazones, and amylin/GLP-1 analogs.
- Oral antidiabetic agents must be evaluated for use in pregnancy, as they cross the placenta and cause hypoglycemia in the fetus, and in lactation, because they are found in breast milk.
- Alcohol should not be used with sulfonylureas.

HYPERGLYCEMIC AGENTS

Hyperglycemic medications that elevate blood sugar level and are antagonists to insulin may be used to treat hypoglycemic reactions or hypersecretion of insulin from the pancreas in diseases such as pancreatic cancer.

Glucagon, produced in alpha cells of pancreatic islets, stimulates the breakdown of glycogen and increases the body's use of glucose, causing blood sugar levels to rise. Glucagon is given parenterally for an insulin overdose in people with T1DM diabetes. It is not effective in starvation-caused hypoglycemia because starvation first depletes glycogen storage, and glucagon must have glycogen to work. Glucagon may also be used with barium in gastrointestinal radiography to relax the gastrointestinal tract.

Diazoxide, (Proglycem) used in patients with inoperable pancreatic cancers, is an oral preparation that produces a prompt increase in blood glucose levels by inhibiting pancreatic insulin release.

Glucose tablets and gels in tubes are available for use in persons with hypoglycemic reactions. These agents are monosaccharides that can be carried for emergency use. Glucose tablets are especially effective for emergency use in children (see Table 20-9).

SUMMARY

The endocrine system has no concrete hands-on physiology because hormones may be either endogenous or exogenous. Hormones are transported mainly in the bloodstream to target cells where the response occurs, and their action is inhibited by negative feedback to the organ of origin. Pathologic conditions result from underproduction or overproduction of hormones. For underproduction, replacement therapy is usually prescribed. For overproduction, medications, surgery, or irradiation may be used.

Pituitary gland medications are used for replacement therapy related to specific disorders, such as GH for children who fail to grow and growth-inhibiting hormone for children with gigantism or adults with acromegaly. Hormones from the posterior pituitary gland are used to treat diabetes insipidus.

The thyroid gland secretes three hormones: thyroxine (T_4), triiodothyronine (T_3), and calcitonin. T_3 and T_4 affect all body cells by increasing metabolism, whereas calcitonin regulates the body's calcium levels. Replacement therapy is necessary for hypothyroidism, to increase circulating hormones and relieve symptoms. Medications are also used in hyperthyroidism to block synthesis of thyroid hormone.

The corticosteroids—glucocorticoids and mineralocorticoids—originate in the adrenal cortex. These steroids have many pharmacologic effects including antiinflammatory action; metabolism of carbohydrates, fats, and proteins; immunosuppression with organ transplantation; and effects related to physiologic and psychologic response to stress. Steroids are given by mouth, parenterally, topically, and via other routes; some are available OTC.

The primary pancreatic hormones are insulin and glucagon. When insulin causes blood glucose levels to decrease, glucagon is released. This allows the use of glycogen stored in the liver, which again increases blood glucose levels. Negative feedback allows more insulin to be released, which maintains homeostasis of carbohydrate metabolism.

The relative absence or deficiency of insulin secretions is the cause of DM, either from insufficient secretions or body resistance to insulin, or both. DM is of two types: T1DM is insulin dependent, and T2DM is considered a non–insulin-dependent condition, although insulin may be needed in some cases of T2DM. Insulins come in several types, depending on their time of onset and duration of action. Different types of injectable insulin may be mixed to provide adequate coverage throughout a day, but dosages of each must be individualized to each patient's needs and physical condition. T2DM is usually treated with dietary management, weight reduction, exercise, and if necessary oral antidiabetic agents.

Oral antidiabetic medications are used by millions of Americans with T2DM. Some of these drugs act by increasing pancreatic insulin secretion; others inhibit carbohydrate metabolism. The newer medications act by increasing the function of glucose metabolism in persons with insulin resistance.

CRITICAL THINKING EXERCISES

Scenario

Josie has been taking steroids for a prolonged period of time as treatment for rheumatoid arthritis. She has gained weight, especially in her face, and notices that her skin is thin and bleeds easily.

1. What do you need to tell Josie about salt and water intake?
2. What about the chance of menstrual irregularities?
3. She is concerned about the increased hair on her face and body. How can you explain this to her?
4. What other symptoms can she expect?
5. After you talk with her, she says she is going to stop taking the medicine at once because she is afraid of the side effects. What do you tell her about abruptly discontinuing these medications?

DRUG CALCULATIONS

1. Order: Humulin R 25 units and Humulin N 30 units
    Available medication:

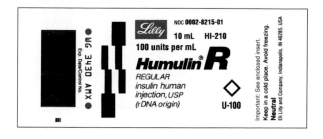 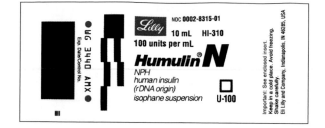

Show the correct amount of insulin on the marked syringes.

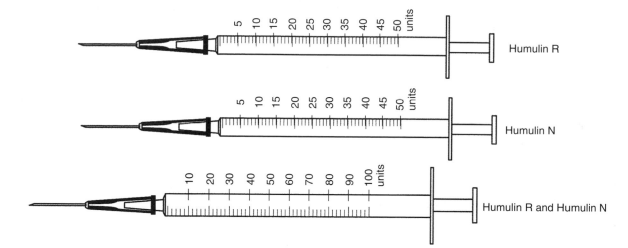

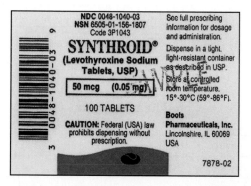

2. Order: Synthroid 0.1 mg
    Available medication:

Dose to be given: _____

REVIEW QUESTIONS

1. What is a hormone and what is its function? _____

    _____

2. What are the two major therapeutic uses of hormones? _____

    _____

3. What hormones are secreted by the thyroid gland? _____
_____

4. What is an adrenocorticoid? A glucocorticoid? A mineralocorticoid? A steroid? _____
_____
_____
_____
_____

5. Steroids are ordered in what two unique ways that are specific to these medications? _____
_____
_____

6. What is the only drug for type 1 diabetes? How is it administered? Why can it not be administered orally?
_____
_____
_____
_____

7. What are the sources for insulin replacement? Which source is most like the body's insulin? _____
_____
_____
_____

8. What is the time to onset, peak time, and time of duration of the different insulin types? Describe these in terms of lispro, regular, isophane, and Lantus insulins. _____
_____
_____
_____
_____
_____

9. What are some of the newest forms of insulin administration techniques being developed to avoid the regular injections? _____
_____

10. How do the sulfonylureas work? Do they produce hypoglycemia? _____
_____
_____
_____

11. How do the biguanides work? Do they cause hypoglycemia? _____
_____
_____
_____

12. Why would insulin need to be administered to a patient who is taking an oral hypoglycemic? _____
_____

CHAPTER 21

Eye and Ear Disorders

OBJECTIVES

After studying this chapter, you should be capable of doing the following:

- Explaining the difference between ophthalmic and otic preparations.
- Recognizing ophthalmic and otic medications and their uses.
- Describing drugs used in the treatment of ototoxicity and vertigo.
- Describing how to store ophthalmic and otic preparations to prevent their being inadvertently interchanged.
- Providing patient education for compliance with medications used to treat diseases and conditions of the eye and ear.

Gene has an inflammation of the cornea of his left eye. He has been prescribed an antiinflammatory solution to use in his eye three times a day. Gene tells you that in the past, Dr. Merry has prescribed the same medication for use in his ears for an infection. The expiration date on the old otic medication has not passed.

Can Gene use the otic solution rather than buy the new ophthalmic medicine?
Why can Gene expect some blurring of vision after instilling the drops?
Where should Gene instill the drops in his eyes?

KEY TERMS

Accommodation
Adrenergic agonist
Anticholinergic agent
Ataxia
Auralgia
Blepharitis
Cataract
Cerumen
Chalazion
Cholinergic agent (or parasympathomimetic)
Closed-angle glaucoma
Conjunctivitis

Cycloplegia
Glaucoma
Hordeolum
Keratitis
Miosis
Miotic
Mydriasis
Myopia
Nystagmus
Open-angle glaucoma
Ophthalmic preparations
Otic preparations

Otitis media
Ototoxicity
Paresthesia
Photophobia
Presbyopia
Sympathomimetic agent
Tinnitus
Tonometry
Tympanic membrane
Uveitis
Vasocongestion
Vertigo

EASY WORKING KNOWLEDGE OF INDICATIONS AND SIDE EFFECTS

Common Symptoms of Ear and Eye Disorders

Eyes
Visual disturbances
Eye redness
Pain or burning in or around the eye

Ears
Loss of hearing
Vertigo or dizziness
Tinnitus
Earache and increased pressure in the ear

Common Side Effects of Medications

Ophthalmic
Changes in intraocular pressure
Burning, stinging, or pain on administration
Blurred vision or diplopia
Photophobia
Headache
Increased tears

Otic
Tinnitus
Burning or itching of ear canal
Dizziness

EASY WORKING KNOWLEDGE OF DRUGS USED FOR EAR AND EYE DISORDERS

DRUG CLASS	PRESCRIPTION	OTC	PREGNANCY CATEGORY	MAJOR INDICATIONS
OPHTHALMIC				
Antiinfectives	Yes	Yes (boric acid)	B, C	Eye infections
Antiinflammatories and corticosteroids	Yes	No	C	Eye inflammation
Irrigating solutions	Yes	Yes	B	Foreign bodies
Antiglaucoma agents	Yes	No	C, X	Glaucoma
Mydriatics, cycloplegics	Yes	No	B, C	Diagnostic studies
Local anesthetics	Yes	No	C	Eye irritation
Immunomodulators	Yes	No	C	Dry eyes
Artificial tears, lubricants	Yes	Yes	N/A	Replace tears
Antiallergics	Yes	Yes	B	Eye allergies
Diagnostic aids	Yes	No	C	Diagnostic studies
OTIC				
Antiinfectives, antibiotics	Yes	No	C	Middle ear and external canal infections
Antiinflammatories and corticosteroids	Yes	No	C	Ear inflammation
Combination preparations	Yes	No	B, C	Infections, inflammations
Ceruminolytics	Yes	Yes	B	Soften ear wax
Ear analgesics	Yes	Yes	B, C	Earache
DRUGS FOR VERTIGO	Yes	Yes	B, C	Vertigo and motion sickness

N/A; Not applicable.

Two sense organs are discussed in this chapter. The eye is responsible for vision, and the ear is necessary for the senses of hearing and equilibrium. Any impairment of these senses causes changes in lifestyle—either temporarily or permanently.

EYE

The eye, one of the most delicate yet most valuable of the sense organs, captures light and transforms it into images in the brain. Any disorder results in visual impairment (Figure 21-1).

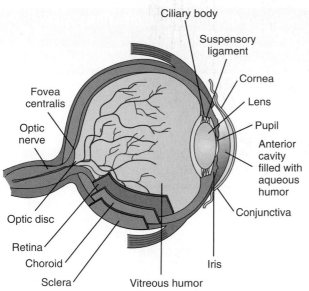

Figure 21-1 Anatomy of the eye. (From Young AP, Proctor DB: *Kinn's the medical assistant: an applied learning approach,* ed 11, St Louis, 2011, Saunders.)

Figure 21-2 Aqueous humor passes into anterior chamber through the pupil, where it is drained away by the ring-shaped canal of Schlemm. (From Thibodeau GA, Patton KT: *Anthony's textbook of anatomy and physiology,* ed 18, St Louis, 2007, Mosby.)

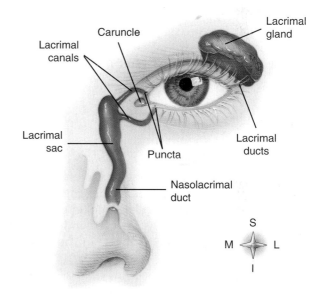

Figure 21-3 Lacrimal apparatus of the eye. (From Thibodeau GA, Patton KT: *Anthony's textbook of anatomy and physiology,* ed 18, St Louis, 2007, Mosby.)

The protective outer layer of the eye consists of the cornea (transparent anterior covering of the eye that allows the entrance of light) and the sclera (a white fibrous continuation of the cornea that maintains the shape of the eyeball). The eye surface has a thin layer of epithelial cells called the *conjunctiva* that is resistant to infection.

The middle layer of the eye consists of the iris, choroid, and ciliary body. The iris surrounds the pupil and has the ability to relax and constrict to control the amount of light that enters the eye. Constriction of the pupil is **miosis;** dilation of the pupil is **mydriasis.** Drugs may be used to produce either of these conditions for ocular examinations or to treat eye diseases.

The lens lies behind the iris to ensure a clear sharp focal image and sends signals for retinal interpretation. On each side of the lens is a ciliary body that changes the shape of the lens for **accommodation.** Accommodation occurs readily in young people, but as the lens loses elasticity with age, the ability to focus on near objects is lost, and the point at which an object is in focus recedes—known as **presbyopia,** usually starting at approximately age 40 to 45. If the lens loses its transparency and becomes cloudy, the condition is called a **cataract.** A paralysis of the ciliary muscle is called **cycloplegia.**

The third layer of the eye consists of the anterior and posterior chambers. The anterior chamber is the space between the cornea and the lens. The *aqueous humor* flows forward between the lens and the iris into the anterior chamber to help maintain the shape and pressure in the anterior eye (Figure 21-2). The posterior chamber lies between the lens and retina and is filled with the colorless, transparent, gel-like *vitreous humor,* which holds the retina firmly against the wall of the eye to help maintain its shape (see Figure 21-1).

The eye is protected by eyelashes to catch foreign materials; blinking to keep the corneal surface free of mucus and moistened by the tears; and tears that are bactericidal, preventing infections and draining into the inner corners of the eyelid into the nasolacrimal ducts (Figure 21-3).

TABLE 21-1 OCULAR SIDE EFFECTS FROM SYSTEMIC MEDICATIONS

DRUG	POSSIBLE SIDE EFFECTS
aspirin	Allergic keratitis and conjunctivitis
Barbiturates	Nystagmus
marijuana	Nystagmus, conjunctivitis, double vision, miosis
clonidine	Miosis
Corticosteroids	Cataracts, increased intraocular pressure
ethyl alcohol	Nystagmus
ibuprofen	Altered color vision, blurred vision
indomethacin	Mydriasis
isoniazid	Optic neuritis
lithium	Exophthalmos
Opiates	Miosis
phenothiazine	Cataracts
phenytoin	Nystagmus
Thiazide diuretics	Transient myopia, yellow color to vision

Modified from Salerno X: *Pharmacology for health professionals,* St Louis, 1999, Mosby.

TABLE 21-2 OPHTHALMIC MEDICATIONS WITH ADVERSE SYSTEMIC EFFECTS

DRUG AND CLASS	ADVERSE EFFECTS
ANTIMICROBIAL	
chloramphenicol	Aplastic anemia
ANTICHOLINERGICS	
atropine	Increased temperature, tachycardia, delirium
cyclopentolate	Convulsions, hallucinations, psychotic reactions
scopolamine	Acute psychosis
ANTIGLAUCOMA MEDICATIONS	
Beta-blocking agents	Bradycardia, syncope, decreased blood pressure, asthma, congestive heart failure, nausea, hallucinations, anorexia, headaches, weakness, depression
Cholinergic agents	Salivation, nausea and vomiting, asthma attacks, low blood pressure
Carbonic anhydrase inhibitors	Diarrhea, headache, nervousness, nausea and vomiting, diuresis, anorexia, paresthesia, weight loss, photosensitivity
Prostaglandin agonists	Upper respiratory tract infection; muscle, back, joint, and chest pain; angina; rash
Osmotic diuretics	Nausea and vomiting, headache, increased thirst, dry mouth, diarrhea, confusion
Anticholinergics	Sweating, flushing, tachycardia, respiratory depression, changes in mental attitude

Medications specifically for use in the eye are called **ophthalmic preparations.** Medications given for systemic diseases may have ocular side effects (Table 21-1). Conversely, medications for eye conditions may cause systemic effects and changes in homeostasis (Table 21-2).

ANTIINFECTIVE AND ANTIINFLAMMATORY AGENTS

As with other infections, ocular infections should be cultured to determine the antibiotic of choice. In many cases, however, treatment is started before culture results are available so the severity of infection is limited; in some cases, systemic medications are used in conjunction with ocular medications.

Most antiinfective agents do not readily penetrate the eye, although some topical agents are absorbed when the mucous membrane has been injured or inflamed. Such ocular infections as **conjunctivitis, hordeolum, chalazion, blepharitis, keratitis,** and **uveitis** are treated with topical agents. To avoid possible sensitization to systemic antiinfectives and to discourage drug-resistant strains, antibiotics for ophthalmic symptoms are usually administered locally. With ophthalmic antiviral medications, for conditions such as viral conjunctivitis caused by the common cold, both eyes are treated to prevent infection spread (Table 21-3).

TABLE 21-3 SELECT DRUGS USED AS OPHTHALMIC AGENTS

GENERIC NAME/ TRADE NAME	USUAL ADULT DOSE, ROUTE, AND FREQUENCY*†	MAJOR SIDE EFFECTS	INDICATIONS FOR USE	DRUG INTERACTIONS
ANTIINFECTANTS AND ANTIINFLAMMATORY AGENTS		Stinging, irritation, tearing	Broad-spectrum antibacterial for superficial ocular infections and gram-positive infections	
triple antibiotic (Neosporin Ophthalmic ointment, solution)	Small amount, CS gtt ī͞i q4h			None identified
ciprofloxacin (Ciloxan solution, ointment)	gtt ī͞i q2-4h Small amount, CS			None identified
polymyxin B (Polysporin [ophthalmic] ointment, solution)	Small amount, CS gtt ī-ī͞i in eye qh until favorable response			None identified
bacitracin ointment	Small amount, CS			None identified
erythromycin ointment	Small amount, CS		Bacteriostatic, neonatal conjunctivitis	None identified
gentamicin (Gentak ointment, solution)	Small amount, CS gtt ī-ī͞i q2-4h		Gram-positive and gram-negative organisms that are drug resistant	None identified
tobramycin (Tobrex solution, ointment) with dexamethasone (TobraDex solution)	gtt q2h, ointment ī͞i-ī͞i͞i qd ¼ to ½ inch in CS gtt ī-ī͞i gtt q4h, ointment q4-6h		Same as for gentamicin Same as for gentamicin	Systemic aminoglycosides
sulfacetamide (Bleph-10, Sulamyd solution)	gtt ī-ī͞i q2-3h		Same as for gentamicin	Must be instilled 30 minutes after ocular anesthetics
moxifloxacin (Vigamox)	gtt ī-ī͞i tid			
ANTISEPTICS			Prophylaxis; treatment of eye infections; many are OTC preparations	None identified
boric acid (Blinx, Collyrium 2% solution, 5%-10% ointment)	gtt ī-ī͞i to eye, CS			
silver nitrate 1% solution	gtt ī both eyes at birth		Neonates after birth for prophylaxis of gonococci	
ANTIFUNGALS			Fungal blepharitis, conjunctivitis, or keratitis	Not systemically absorbed
natamycin (Natacyn)	Individualized, usually gtt ī q4-6h			

CS, Conjunctival sac.
*The route of administration in this table is topical unless otherwise stated.
†Ointments are placed in conjunctival sac; liquids are instilled in eye.
Note: The use of the bar over letters in a dosage indicates that the letter is a roman numeral. The bar is not used consistently in the industry.

Continued

TABLE 21-3 SELECT DRUGS USED AS OPHTHALMIC AGENTS—cont'd

GENERIC NAME/ TRADE NAME	USUAL ADULT DOSE, ROUTE, AND FREQUENCY*†	MAJOR SIDE EFFECTS	INDICATIONS FOR USE	DRUG INTERACTIONS
ANTIVIRALS			Viral infections of eye, herpes simplex, keratitis	None identified
trifluridine (Viroptic solution)	gtt ī q2-4h			
CORTICOSTEROIDS		Burning, tearing, blurred vision, headache, pain	Allergic or inflammatory disorders; used in combinations with antibiotics and mydriatics such as Isopto Cetapred, Medrapred, and Optimyd	May have systemic effects over prolonged periods of use (see discussion of corticosteroids in Chapter 20)
dexamethasone (Maxidex suspension, solution, ointment)	Varies with patient and condition in eye			
polyvinyl alcohol (Liquifilm Tears; Forte) with steroid (Poly-Pred Liquifilm)	gtt ī to īī gtt ī-īī			
prednisolone sodium phosphate (Pred Forte, Omnipred as suspensions and solutions)	Varies			
NONSTEROIDAL ANTIINFLAMMATORY DRUGS				
flurbiprofen (Ocufen solution)	gtt ī q30min for a total of 4 gtt before surgery		Inhibits intraocular miosis	None identified
ketorolac (Acular, Acuvail solution)	gtt ī qid		Prophylaxis; treatment of ocular inflammation	None identified

---

CLINICAL TIPS

- Only ophthalmic preparations should be used in the eye.
- Ophthalmic preparations are sterile and care must be taken to prevent contamination.
- Be sure sulfa preparations have not darkened from their normal light yellow color.
- Action of sulfonamides is inhibited by ophthalmic anesthetics, so the two agents should be administered 30 to 60 minutes apart.
- A good rule for administration of ophthalmic topical medications is to allow time (15 minutes to 1 hour) between administration of different ophthalmic preparations unless prescribed otherwise.
- Sulfonamides are incompatible with thimerosal (a mercurial antiseptic) and silver preparations.

- Silver nitrate, used for gonococcal infections at birth, comes in a collapsible capsule containing five drops. The capsule to be used should be tested with one drop to ensure a liquid state before administration to prevent damage to eyes if the silver nitrate has crystallized.
- When irrigating eyes, turn patient's head toward affected side to prevent cross-contamination of unaffected eye.
- Ophthalmic corticosteroids may have a systemic effect if used over a prolonged time.
- Contact lenses, especially soft lenses, should be removed before administration of ophthalmic preparations to prevent absorption of medication by the lens.

AGENTS FOR GLAUCOMA

Glaucoma is the name for a group of diseases characterized by increased intraocular pressure (IOP) as a result of excessive production of aqueous humor or diminished ocular fluid outflow. Several terms are used to describe glaucoma—*primary* or *secondary, acute* or *chronic,* and **open-angle glaucoma** or **closed-angle glaucoma.** If pressure is persistently high, blindness may occur secondary to optic nerve damage. Primary medications used to treat glaucoma include beta-adrenergic receptor-blocking agents, cholinergics, and sympathomimetics.

The aim of treatment for glaucoma is to decrease IOP, thus decreasing damage to the optic nerve.

Beta-adrenergic receptor blockers (beta blockers), when used for glaucoma, decrease production of aqueous humor to reduce IOP (Table 21-4).

Cholinergic agents (or parasympathomimetics) or **miotics** constrict pupils, causing **myopia,** opening spaces for movement of aqueous humor. Because the pupil cannot accommodate to changes in illumination, end-of-day and nighttime activities are particularly hazardous for individuals using these medications. Other miotics are *cholinesterase inhibitors,* which inhibit destruction of acetylcholine. Cholinesterase inhibitors are

TABLE 21-4 DRUGS USED TO TREAT GLAUCOMA

GENERIC NAME/ TRADE NAME	USUAL ADULT DOSE, ROUTE, AND FREQUENCY*†	MAJOR SIDE EFFECTS	INDICATIONS FOR USE	DRUG INTERACTIONS
BETA-ADRENERGIC BLOCKING AGENTS		*Local*—burning, stinging, eye irritation, visual disturbance, pruritus *Systemic*—bradycardia or tachycardia, confusion, insomnia, weakness, respiratory symptoms, GI disturbances	Glaucoma	Essentially none when used topically
betaxolol 0.25% (Betoptic solution)	gtt ī bid			
carteolol solution (Ocupress solution)	gtt ī bid			
levobunolol 0.25% to 0.5% (Betagan solution)	gtt ī-īī bid gtt ī-īī qd			
metipranolol (OptiPranolol 0.3% solution)	gtt ī bid			
timolol (Timoptic solution, Tomoptic-XE)	gtt ī bid			
CHOLINERGIC (MIOTIC) DIRECT-ACTING AGENTS		*Local*—blurred vision, myopia, eye irritation, headaches; No systemic side effects		
carbachol (Isopto Carbachol solution)	gtt īī tid			None identified
pilocarpine (Isopto Carpine solution) (Ocusert)	gtt īī tid-qid Insert disk in CS			None identified
CHOLINESTERASE INHIBITORS				
echothiophate (Phospholine Iodide)	gtt ī			None identified

CS, Conjunctival sac; *GI*, gastrointestinal; *PO*, orally.
*The route of administration in this table is topical unless otherwise stated.
†Ointments are placed in conjunctival sac; liquids are instilled in eye.
Note: The use of the bar over letters in a dosage indicates that the letter is a roman numeral. The bar is not used consistently in the industry.

Continued

TABLE 21-4 DRUGS USED TO TREAT GLAUCOMA—cont'd

GENERIC NAME/ TRADE NAME	USUAL ADULT DOSE, ROUTE, AND FREQUENCY*†	MAJOR SIDE EFFECTS	INDICATIONS FOR USE	DRUG INTERACTIONS
SYMPATHOMIMETICS		*Local*—same as cholinergic agents; *Systemic*—see Table 21-2		
dipivefrin (Propine solution)	gtt ī qd			None identified
CARBONIC ANHYDRASE INHIBITORS				
acetazolamide (Diamox)	250-500 mg PO bid, IV	Fatigue, ↓ appetite, ↑ urination	Glaucoma	Amphetamines, quinidine, memantine
dorzolamide (Trusopt 2% solution)	gtt ī tid			
PROSTAGLANDIN INHIBITORS		*Local*—blurred vision, burning, stinging, **photophobia**, ↑ brown pigmentation; *Systemic*—see Table 21-2		
latanoprost (Xalatan solution)	gtt ī qd			None identified
travoprost (Travatan 0.005% solution)	gtt ī qd			
bimatoprost (Lumigan 0.03% solution)	gtt ī qd			
MISCELLANEOUS				
apraclonidine (Iopidine 0.5% solution)	gtt ī-īī tid		Glaucoma, to reduce aqueous humor production	No significant interactions identified
brimonidine (Alphagan solution)	gtt ī tid			

usually reserved for people who had no response to other antiglaucoma agents (see Table 21-4).

Sympathomimetic agents mimic the sympathetic nervous system to dilate pupils in patients with open-angle glaucoma. **Dipivefrin** is converted to epinephrine, lowering IOP, decreasing aqueous humor production, and increasing outflow (see Table 21-4).

Oral *carbonic anhydrase inhibitors* are diuretics used to lower IOP by decreasing aqueous production and reducing aqueous humor volume by more than 50% (see Table 21-4). Diuretics are discussed in Chapters 26 and 27.

Prostaglandin agonists approved for topical treatment of glaucoma and ocular hypertension are as effective as beta blockers with fewer side effects. Now considered the first-line medications for glaucoma, these agents reduce IOP by increasing aqueous humor outflow and are usually well tolerated, with the major side effect being irreversible browning of the iris pigment (see Table 21-4).

Osmotic diuretics are used to reduce IOP after surgery or in treatment of acute glaucoma (see Tables 21-2 and 21-4).

MYDRIATICS AND CYCLOPLEGICS

Mydriatics and cycloplegics are used for pupil dilation for ophthalmologic testing and other ophthalmologic conditions.

Adrenergic agonists mimic the sympathetic nervous system to bring about pupillary dilation, or *mydriasis.*

Cycloplegic agents cause paralysis of ciliary muscles or prevent accommodation and are used primarily in diagnosing ophthalmologic disorders, causing dilation of the iris opening to make the pupil larger. The inherent danger is that many of these agents are available over the counter (OTC) to reduce redness in eyes caused by **vasocongestion.** Prescription medications, used to treat glaucoma, produce mydriasis for ocular examinations and relieve ocular vasocongestion (Table 21-5).

Anticholinergic agents block the parasympathetic nervous system, causing dilation, and are used to relax inflamed intraocular muscles to relieve pain with uveitis. Other uses are for accurate measurement of refractive errors and before and after intraocular surgery. Some medications are administered in combinations to produce greater mydriasis (see Table 21-5).

Local Ophthalmic Anesthetic Agents

Ophthalmic anesthetic agents are used to eliminate the blink reflex and pain associated with ophthalmic procedures, **tonometry,** removal of foreign objects, suturing

TABLE 21-5 DRUGS USED AS MYDRIATICS OR CYCLOPLEGICS

GENERIC NAME/TRADE NAME	USUAL ADULT DOSE, ROUTE, AND FREQUENCY*†	MAJOR SIDE EFFECTS	INDICATIONS FOR USE	DRUG INTERACTIONS
MYDRIATICS OR CYCLOPLEGICS		Burning, itching, blurred vision	Glaucoma; mydriasis for ocular surgery	No significant interactions identified
atropine (Isopto Atropine)				
solution 1%	gtt ī			
ointment 1%	Small amt CS			
cyclopentolate (Cyclogyl 0.5% 1% solution)	gtt ī-īī			
homatropine (Isopto Homatropine solution 2%-5%)	gtt ī-īī			
scopolamine (Isopto Hyoscine solution 1%)	gtt ī-īī			
tropicamide (Mydral, Tropicacyl solution 0.5%-1%)	gtt ī-īī			
ADRENERGIC AGONISTS AND ANTICHOLINERGICS		Burning and stinging on initial application	Mydriasis, decrease eye redness	No significant interactions identified
epinephrine (Epifrin, Glaucon‡ 0.5%-2% solution)	gtt ī			
hydroxyamphetamine (Paremyd‡ 1% solution)	gtt ī-īī			
naphazoline (Naphazoline, AK-Con‡ 1% solution, Naphcon, Clear Eyes§ solution)	gtt ī-īī gtt ī			
oxymetazoline (Visine§ solution)	gtt ī			
phenylephrine (AK-Dilate, Altafrin, Neofrin‡ 2.5%-10% solution)	Varies			
tetrahydrozoline (Murine Plus, Visine§ 0.05% solution)	gtt ī			

CS, Conjunctival sac.
*The route of administration in this table is topical unless otherwise stated.
†Ointments are placed in conjunctival sac; liquids are instilled in eye.
‡Prescription medications.
§Over-the-counter medications.
Note: The use of the bar over letters in a dosage indicates that the letter is a roman numeral. The bar is not used consistently in the industry.

or removal of sutures, and radial keratotomy. The eye should be protected until anesthesia wears off because of loss of the blink reflex (Table 21-6).

IMMUNOMODULATORS

An emulsion to increase tear production, *cyclosporine* (Restasis), is considered an immunomodulator or immunosuppressant. Available only as a prescription medication, cyclosporine should not be administered when an individual is wearing contact lenses, nor should it be administered with other topical ophthalmic medications. Before administration, invert several times to restore the medication back into an emulsion (see Table 21-6).

ARTIFICIAL TEARS AND LUBRICANTS

Artificial tear solutions or lubricants are used to produce eye lubrication when tear production and blink reflexes are decreased. Products are normal saline with agents

TABLE 21-6 MISCELLANEOUS OPHTHALMIC PREPARATIONS

GENERIC NAME/ TRADE NAME	USUAL ADULT DOSE, ROUTE, AND FREQUENCY*†	MAJOR SIDE EFFECTS	INDICATIONS FOR USE	DRUG INTERACTIONS
OCULAR ANESTHETICS				
tetracaine (Tetcaine, Altacaine 0.5% solution)	gtt ī-īī	Burning on initial administration	Anesthetizing the eye for ophthalmologic procedures and in cases of eye trauma	No significant interactions identified
proparacaine (Alcaine, Ophthetic, Parcaine 0.5% solution)	gtt ī-īī	Same as for tetracaine	Same as for tetracaine	No significant interactions identified
IMMUNOMODULATORS				Do not use with contact lens in place
cyclosporine (Restasis 0.05% emulsion)	One vial (gtt ī) applied topically bid	Discard any medication left in vial	Increases tear production	
ARTIFICIAL TEARS AND LUBRICANTS		No major side effects because of saline base	Artificial tears, eye lubricants	No significant interactions identified
Most of these agents are OTC medications, with a base of normal saline. A few examples are provided:				
Lacrisert ophthalmic insert	One or two inserts topically			
Lacri-Lube ointment	Ointments are instilled in CS			
Duratears solution, HypoTears, Tearisol	Liquids are instilled in eye			
ANTIALLERGENIC AGENTS			Ophthalmic allergies and allergic conjunctivitis	No significant interactions identified
cromolyn sodium† (Crolom solution)	gtt ī-īī 4-6×/day			

*This medication is applied topically unless otherwise indicated.
†Over-the-counter (OTC) medication.
Note: The use of the bar over letters in a dosage indicates that the letter is a roman numeral. The bar is not used consistently in the industry.

TABLE 21-6 MISCELLANEOUS OPHTHALMIC PREPARATIONS—cont'd

GENERIC NAME/ TRADE NAME	USUAL ADULT DOSE, ROUTE, AND FREQUENCY*†	MAJOR SIDE EFFECTS	INDICATIONS FOR USE	DRUG INTERACTIONS
lodoxamide (Alomide solution)	Varies with age, usually gtt ī-īī qid			
ketotifen 0.025%† (Zaditor solution)	Varies, usually gtt ī bid			No contact lens wear
olopatadine (Patanol solution)	gtt ī bid			None
pemirolast 1% (Alamast solution)	gtt ī-īī qd-bid			No contact lens wear
epinastine (Elestat solution)	gtt ī			No contact lens wear
OCULAR DECONGESTANTS See phenylephrine, naphazoline, oxymetazoline found in adrenergic agonists (see Table 21-5)			Ophthalmic vascular congestion	
tetrahydrozoline† (Visine Allergy Relief solution)			Relief of symptoms of allergies manifest in eyes	
OPHTHALMIC DIAGNOSTIC AIDS fluorescein (Fluorescite solution) (Flu-Glo, Bio Glo, Fluorets ophthalmic strip)	gtt ī-īī Application of strip to eye		Diagnosis of corneal epithelial defects, fittings of contact lens, ophthalmic angiography	Should not be used with soft contact lenses

Major Side Effects: Burning, stinging, staining of contact lens

added to extend eye contact time to lubricate artificial eyes, moisten contact lenses, and remove debris from the eyes. These products are usually used three or four times a day. An artificial tear insert (Lacrisert) and ointment preparations are used for a prolonged effect (see Table 21-6).

OPHTHALMIC ANTIALLERGIC AND DECONGESTANT AGENTS

Agents for allergic eye disorders prevent histamines from producing allergic reactions and relieve tearing, itching, and redness related to allergic eye conditions. Corticosteroids may be used for allergic conjunctivitis, including vernal (spring) conjunctivitis and keratitis. OTC medications should be used only short term (see Table 21-6).

Decongestant agents, weak adrenergic agents that reduce eye redness by acting as topical vasoconstrictors, are available OTC (see Table 21-6).

OPHTHALMIC STAINING AGENTS

Fluorescein sodium, a nontoxic, water-soluble dye, is used to diagnose corneal epithelial defects caused by injury or infection and to locate foreign bodies in the eye. When applied to the cornea, fluorescein stains corneal lesions shown as green, and foreign bodies have a green ring surrounding them. This agent is also used to assess fit of hard contact lens, as a dye for retinal studies, and for ophthalmic angiography (see Table 21-6).

Patient Education for Compliance

1. Care should be taken when using ophthalmic preparations to prevent contamination of medications by the applicator touching the eye.
2. Wear dark glasses with medications that cause photosensitivity and pupil dilation.
3. Consult a physician if eyes do not show improvement after using ophthalmic antifungals for 7 to 10 days.
4. Treatment with antivirals should continue for 3 to 5 days after healing or according to physician's orders.
5. Corticosteroids should be used for only a limited time because systemic effects may occur with long-term use. When using corticosteroids in patients with diabetes, blood glucose levels should be monitored closely for hyperglycemia.
6. Ophthalmic suspensions and emulsions should be placed back into solution by agitation or inversion before administration.
7. When using anticholinergics, be careful to illuminate dark areas because of decreased vision in dim light. With anticholinergics, use care in driving and performing other hazardous activities because of loss of eye accommodation. Close-up visual acuity will be greatly diminished, making reading and other close-up activities difficult.
8. Take carbonic anhydrase inhibitors early in the day for maximum benefit.

Important Facts about Ophthalmic Agents

- Most ophthalmic antiinfective agents do not readily penetrate eyes but are used topically when mucous membranes are inflamed or injured.
- Many ophthalmic solutions cause burning or stinging on application and cause headaches.
- Instill ophthalmic medications in the inner canthus of the eye.
- Before administration of topical ophthalmic medications, removal of contact lens is recommended except when using wetting solutions and lubricants especially manufactured for contact lenses. The lens should not be reinserted for 15 to 30 minutes after medication administration.
- Ophthalmic medications cause systemic effects if used over prolonged time periods, particularly corticosteroids, beta-adrenergic blockers, and cholinergic agents.
- Sympathomimetic agents are used to treat open-angle glaucoma by decreasing aqueous humor production and increasing its outflow.
- Mydriatics and cycloplegics, used as diagnostic aids, paralyze ciliary muscles to dilate the pupil; conversely, miotics constrict the pupil.
- Anticholinergic agents are used to treat inflamed intraocular muscles during procedures to measure refractive errors and before and after intraocular surgery.

Important Facts about Ophthalmic Agents—cont'd

- Many adrenergic agents available OTC act by causing vasoconstriction and optical dilation to reduce eye redness. These agents must be used with care with glaucoma.
- Local ophthalmic anesthetics are used to reduce the blink reflex and eliminate pain associated with ophthalmic procedures.
- Artificial tears or lubricants, used with contact lenses, are basically normal saline solutions to which buffers have been added to prolong their eye contact, thus their effectiveness.
- Antiallergic agents are used to reduce eye itching and redness associated with allergic reactions.

EAR

The ears, the sensory organ of hearing and equilibrium, are important organs carrying countless clues about environment to the brain (Figure 21-4). The eustachian tube connects the middle ear cavity to the pharynx to equalize pressure on both sides of the tympanic membrane. Because the ear canal is a dark, moist channel near the eardrum, bacteria will travel down the canal and cause infections such as swimmer's ear. Bacterial and fungal infections of the ear canal are fairly common, especially in children, as the pediatric ear canal is shorter and straighter than in adults. Likewise, microorganisms can travel up the eustachian tube from the pharynx to cause otitis media, especially in children. Individuals with ear disorders may have auralgia, vertigo, and ataxia. Infections of the inner ear cause hearing impairment and imbalance.

Pain, fever, malaise, pressure, and a sensation of ear fullness, with some hearing loss are common symptoms of ear disorders. External ear conditions seen in ambulatory care settings include infections, ear wax accumulation, and minor trauma. Many ear disorders are minor and easily treated with OTC medications; others are self-limiting. Sometimes hair follicles become infected, causing furuncles. Seborrheic dermatitis, psoriasis, and contact dermatitis may also cause ear inflammation.

OTIC PREPARATIONS

Ear conditions are often treated with systemic medications such as antibiotics. Topical medications, labeled otic preparations, are instilled into the external ear to treat bacterial or fungal infections or as analgesics.

Drying agents, usually combinations of **alcohol, boric acid,** and **hydrogen peroxide,** dry the canal and prevent outer ear infections after activities such as swimming (Table 21-7).

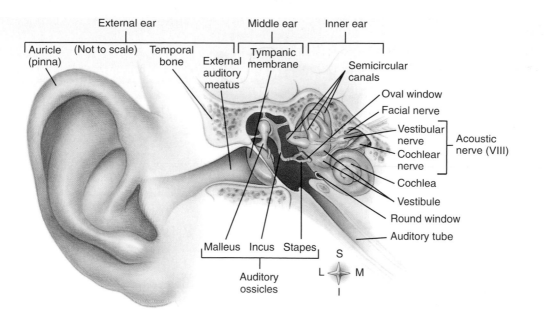

Figure 21-4 Anatomy of the ear. (From Thibodeau GA, Patton KT: *Anthony's textbook of anatomy and physiology,* ed 18, St Louis, 2007, Mosby.)

Antiinfective ear preparations, either instillations or irrigations, inhibit growth of or kill bacteria, thus reducing swelling, relieving pruritus, and promoting drainage of external ear infections (see Table 21-7).

Corticosteroids, used to suppress uncomfortable symptoms associated with ear inflammation, also reduce ear edema and pruritus. Corticosteroids should not be used to treat viral or fungal infections or with a perforated eardrum (see Table 21-7).

Otic preparations are often found in combinations to treat more than one symptom or condition at the same time. Combination medications may contain two or more antibiotics, an antibiotic-benzocaine combination, or an antibiotic-corticosteroid combination (see Table 21-7).

Ceruminolytics soften hardened **cerumen** blocking the external ear canal, a condition common with people wearing hearing aids. Hardened wax can interfere with hearing and block actions of medications instilled into the ear canal. A ceruminolytic is often ordered to soften wax before ear irrigations. Many of these preparations can be bought OTC (see Table 21-7).

Ear analgesics, used to relieve pain, may be warmed mineral oil, sweet oil, or glycerin. Medications with a **benzocaine** base may be prescribed for auralgia (see Table 21-7).

VERTIGO AND OTOTOXICITY

Some patients may think they have ear infections or vertigo when they are actually experiencing **ototoxicity**—a detrimental effect from medication on cranial nerve VIII (auditory nerve that innervates the ear). Ototoxicity

BOX 21-1 SOME MEDICATIONS THAT CAUSE OTOTOXICITY

Antibiotics
amikacin (Amikin)
streptomycin
neomycin
gentamicin (Garamycin)
erythromycin (E-Mycin, Eryc)
kanamycin (Kantrex)
tobramycin (Nebcin)
vancomycin (Vancocin)

Diuretics
acetazolamide (Diamox)
furosemide (Lasix)
bumetanide (Blenoxane)
ethacrynic acid (Edecrin)

Antineoplastic Medications
cisplatin (Platinol-AQ)
bleomycin (Blenoxane)
vincristine (Oncovin)

Many more medications cause ototoxicity but those listed are the more damaging.

can affect hearing, balance, or both. The most common signs are **tinnitus,** vertigo, and difficulty with equilibrium. When ototoxicity occurs, the causative medication should be discontinued. Box 21-1 lists some more common medications that cause ototoxicity.

Patients with Ménière's disease have many of the same symptoms of ototoxicity including vertigo. The patient

TABLE 21-7 DRUGS USED AS OTIC MEDICATIONS

GENERIC NAME/TRADE NAME	USUAL ADULT DOSE, ROUTE, AND FREQUENCY*	MAJOR SIDE EFFECTS	INDICATIONS FOR USE	DRUG INTERACTIONS
DRYING AGENTS		Irritation, swelling, urticaria, overgrowth of nonsusceptible microorganisms	To treat external ear infections, and to dry ear after contact with water	No significant interactions identified
acetic acid solutions (Vo-Sol†)	gtt iv-vi instillation, irrigation			
boric acid solutions (Ear Dry, SwimEar‡)	Fill ear with solution			
isopropyl alcohol (AuraDry‡)	Fill ear with solution			
ANTIBIOTICS		Same side effects as drying agents		
ciprofloxacin otic (Cetraxal solution†)	ī container bid			No significant interactions identified
ofloxacin (Floxin Otic solution†)	gtt x̄ qd-bid			
CORTICOSTEROIDS				
dexamethasone solution†	gtt īīī-īv			No significant interactions identified
fluocinolone (DermOtic†)	gtt īīī-īv			
COMBINATION PRODUCTS				
hydrocortisone–acetic acid (Acetasol HC solution†)	gtt īīī-v̄			No significant interactions identified
+ alcohol (EarSol HC solution†)	gtt īv-vi			
colistin, neomycin, hydrocortisone, thonzonium (Coly-Mycin S Otic suspension†)	gtt īīī			
isopropyl alcohol, glycerin (SwimEar Drops‡)	gtt īīī-īv after swimming			
acetic acid, boric acid, benzalkonium, aluminum acetate (Burrow's Solution‡)	Varies with use as irrigation or instillation			
CERUMINOLYTICS				
carbamide peroxide (Debrox, Murine Ear Drops, Auro Ear Drops‡)	gtt v̄-x̄		Softening and removal of cerumen	No significant interactions identified
EAR ANALGESICS				
glycerin, mineral oil, sweet oil	Fill ear canal with warm solution		Relieve itching and burning in ear	No significant interactions identified
benzocaine-antipyrine† (Auralgan solution)	Fill ear canal		Analgesic	

*All otic medications are instilled topically in the external ear canal.
†Prescription medications.
‡Over-the-counter medications.
Note: The use of the bar over letters in a dosage indicates that the letter is a roman numeral. The bar is not used consistently in the industry.

TABLE 21-8 DRUGS USED FOR VERTIGO

GENERIC NAME/ TRADE NAME	USUAL ADULT DOSE, ROUTE, AND FREQUENCY	INDICATIONS FOR USE	DRUG INTERACTIONS
meclizine (Antivert*)	25-100 mg PO qd in divided doses	Vertigo, motion sickness	CNS depressants
diphenhydramine (Benadryl†)	25-50 mg PO, IM, IV q6-8h		Same as for meclizine
dimenhydrinate (Dramamine†)	50-100 mg PO, IM q4-6h		Same as for meclizine
(Calm-X† chewable tablet)	As directed by manufacturer		
scopolamine (Transderm Scop*)	Apply transdermal patch behind ear as needed q3d		Same as for meclizine

Major Side Effects of Drugs Used for Vertigo: Drowsiness, except with scopolamine

IM, Intramuscularly; *IV,* intravenously; *PO,* orally.
*Prescription medications.
†Over-the-counter medications.

feels that the room is in motion and has a sensation of pressure or fullness in the ear (Table 21-8). The drug of choice to reduce the symptoms of vertigo or ototoxicity is **meclizine** (Antivert).

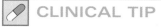

CLINICAL TIP

- To instill medications in a child's ear, gently pull auricle down and back to straighten external canal; in an adult or older child, pull auricle up and back (see Chapter 13 for the correct technique for instilling otic and ophthalmic medications).
- Ear medications should be warmed to room temperature before instillation.
- Otic medications should never be used ophthalmically. Any medications for eye use should be labeled "ophthalmic." In an emergency, ophthalmic medications may be used otically with physician's permission.
- If ear is draining, medications should not be instilled without consulting a physician.
- Never occlude external ear with a tight-fitting plug of any type after instillation of a medication because occlusion may cause eardrum to rupture from increased ear canal pressure. Cotton plugs may be used because these do not increase pressure but allow air to pass through fibers.

Important Facts about Otic Medications

- Pain, fever, malaise, increased pressure, and feeling of ear fullness with hearing loss are common signs of middle ear infections.
- Children often have middle ear infections accompanying pharyngitis because of eustachian tube angle relative to pharynx.
- Ototoxicity may occur from systemic medications including symptoms of tinnitus, loss of balance, and vertigo.

STORAGE OF EYE AND EAR PREPARATIONS

Ophthalmic medications are sterile and are manufactured to be safe when used on a thin eye membrane, whereas otic medications do not require sterility and are administered in a nonsterile ear canal. Ophthalmic and otic liquid preparations are packaged in similar containers and are easily confused. The small bottles are similar in shape, with many of the same names for otic and ophthalmic drugs. Because of these similarities, ophthalmic and otic medications should not be stored in the same area. One way of preventing this potential medication confusion is to place ophthalmic medications on one shelf and otic medications on another. Extreme care should be taken to return medications to their correct place after use. A good rule of thumb where ophthalmic and otic preparations are stored in close proximity is to check the name of the medication and route of administration more than the usual three times to ensure the correct medication has been chosen. While checking accuracy of the preparation, make sure the expiration date has not passed; this is especially important with ophthalmic preparations because of the delicate eye surface tissue.

SUMMARY

Preparations to treat ophthalmic disorders are divided into specific categories. Medications used in eyes should be labeled "ophthalmic" to ensure proper strength and sterility. Many medications used in the eye cause stinging or burning on instillation; some are systemically absorbed. Patients should be aware of medication effects.

Otic medications are agents used to treat ear disorders. Medications are available by prescription and OTC to treat ear infections and ototoxicity.

CRITICAL THINKING EXERCISES

Scenario

Jimmy's mother asks why every time Jimmy, age 2, has a sore throat, he seems to have an earache.

1. What do you expect Dr. Merry to tell her?
2. She wants to know if she should use the ear drops at a cold temperature to relieve the earache. What is the best answer?
3. Can she buy any otic drops OTC to relieve minor pain of an earache and remove excess wax found in Jimmy's ear? If so, which preparations?

DOSAGE CALCULATIONS

1. Order: Pontocaine Ophth Sol 0.5% gtts both eyes stat, then q4h until scratching sensation disappears.
   Interpret the order: _____
   What is the indication for this medication?

   _____

   _____

2. Order: Debrox gtt v AD bid × 4 d
   Interpret the order: _____
   What is the indication for this medication?

   _____

   _____

REVIEW QUESTIONS

1. What does a cycloplegic do? _____

   _____

2. Why is it important to know systemic medications that may cause ophthalmic side effects? _____

   _____

   How would this knowledge be used in prescribing ophthalmic medications? _____

   _____

3. What kind of systemic reactions can occur from use of ophthalmic medications? What is the role of the allied health professional in watching for these reactions? _____

   _____

   _____

4. Why must any medication used in the eye be labeled "ophthalmic"? _____

   _____

5. What do miotics do? What is their use in glaucoma? _____

6. How does fluorescein demonstrate corneal defects from injury and foreign bodies on the cornea? _____

   _____

7. What is a ceruminolytic? _____

   _____

CHAPTER 22

Drugs for Skin Conditions

OBJECTIVES

After studying this chapter, you should be capable of doing the following:

- Describing how topical medications are absorbed into skin.
- Explaining why some topical medications may have systemic effects.
- Discussing various classes of medications used to treat dermatologic conditions.
- Describing general properties of dermatologic preparations, both legend and over-the-counter (OTC), and their indications.

- Defining and naming typical topical keratolytics, acne preparations, ectoparasiticidal agents, and agents for alopecia.
- Providing patient education for compliance with medications used to treat diseases and conditions of the skin.

Johnny fell off his bicycle and skinned his knee. His mother has cleansed the wound with soap and water.

Why is this step in treatment important, other than to remove bacteria?

Dr. Merry wants the medication to go into deeper crevices of the abrasion. Would you expect him to prescribe an ointment or a cream? Why would that be the medication of choice?

How often do you think the bandage will be changed if a standard schedule for antibiotic dressing is used?

What should you tell Johnny's mother about keeping the bandage dry?

Why is it important to obtain a health history of possible allergies even when applying a topical medication?

If Dr. Merry orders an occlusive dressing, what would you expect to place on the abrasion?

KEY TERMS

Acne	Disinfectant or	Keratin	Psoriasis
Actinic keratosis	germicidal agent	Keratolytic agent	Pustule
Antiseptic	Eczema	Liniment	Rubs
Bactericidal agent	Edema	Lotion	Scabicide
Bacteriostatic	Emollient	Nits	Seborrheic dermatitis
agent	Eschar	Occlusive dressing	Sebum
Bath	Furuncle	Papule	Skin cleanser
Carbuncle	Hives	Pediculicide	Ulceration
Comedones	Impetigo	Photosensitivity	Vehicle

EASY WORKING KNOWLEDGE OF INDICATIONS AND SIDE EFFECTS

Common Symptoms of Skin Disorders
Dermatologic lesions or eruptions
Pruritus and **hives**
Inflammation
Edema
Discomfort
Erythema

Common Side Effects of Medications for Skin Disorders
Burning
Pruritus
Skin dryness
Rashes
Thinning of skin
Irritation of skin

EASY WORKING KNOWLEDGE OF DRUGS USED FOR SKIN CONDITIONS

DRUG CLASS	PRESCRIPTION	OTC	PREGNANCY CATEGORY	MAJOR INDICATIONS
ANTIINFECTIVES				
Antibiotics	Yes	Yes	B, C	Skin infections
Antivirals	Yes	Yes	B, C	Herpetic infections, viral infections
Antiinflammatories, corticosteroids	Yes	Yes	C	Inflammatory responses
Antifungals	Yes	Yes	B, C	*Candida,* tinea infections
Acne preparations	Yes	Yes	B, C, D (tetracyclines), X (tazarotene, isotretinoin)	Acne vulgaris
Keratolytics	Yes	Yes	C, X (podophyllum)	Hyperkeratotic skin lesions
Antipsoriatic agents	Yes	No	B	Plaque psoriasis
Shampoos	Yes	Yes	C	Seborrheic dermatitis
Topical anesthetics	Yes	Yes	B, C	Pain, itching
Topical antipruritics	No	Yes	B	Itching
Sulfonamides	Yes	No	B, C	Burns and minor bacterial wound infections
Proteolytic enzymes	Yes	No		Débridement of wounds
PROPHYLACTIC AGENTS				
Sunscreens	No	Yes		Prevent sunburns
Protectives	No	Yes		Protect skin from irritants
Scabicides, pediculicides	Yes	Yes	B	Skin parasites
MISCELLANEOUS				
minoxidil	Yes	Yes	C	Alopecia
fluorouracil	Yes	No	D	Actinic keratosis, superficial basal cell carcinomas

Skin, the body's largest organ, is a complex structure divided into three main layers—the epidermis, composed of a thin layer of epithelial cells that are continuously sloughed and replaced; the dense, fibrous dermis, containing blood vessels, nerve endings, and gland openings within connective tissue; and the subcutaneous layer consisting mainly of loose connective tissue and adipose (fat) tissue such as nail beds, sweat and oil glands, and elastic and fibrous tissues (Figure 22-1).

Skin has six functions: protecting against drying of deeper tissues; providing a mechanical barrier against bacterial infection; regulating body temperature by releasing heat through perspiration for a cooling effect; interacting with the environment through nerve endings of pain, touch, pressure, and temperature to ensure personal safety; excreting minerals and water through perspiration; and preventing absorption of toxic substances while having the ability to absorb desired substances—the function of pharmacologic importance.

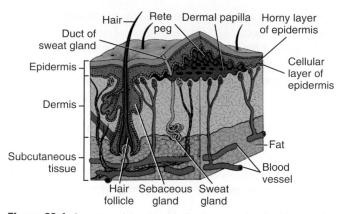

Figure 22-1 Structure of the skin. Medications are absorbed through the epidermis to the dermis and then absorbed into the bloodstream, as well as for local response to pain by nerve fibers. (From Young AP, Proctor DB: *Kinn's the Medical Assistant: an applied learning approach*, ed 11, St Louis, 2011, Saunders.)

Medications may be absorbed through the skin for local effect or they may be slowly absorbed in sufficient quantities for systemic effect. Some medications may be injected into upper skin layers (intradermally) or into subcutaneous tissues for release into the bloodstream for transport throughout the body (see Chapter 14 for parenteral medication administration).

CLASSIFICATION OF DERMATOLOGIC PREPARATIONS

Several kinds of medications, such as antiinfective agents, antiinflammatory agents, enzymatic preparations, and antinauseant medications, have systemic effect when applied transdermally. Rate of medication absorption depends on drug form, size of molecules (smaller molecules are more rapidly absorbed), and medication base (oil- or more readily absorbed water-based **vehicles**). Such medications as hormones, antianginals, antihypertensives, analgesics, and antihistamines may be specifically applied transdermally for prolonged release for systemic therapy. General goals of therapy are to remove causes of skin disorders, find measures to restore and maintain normal skin function, and relieve symptoms such as itching, dryness, pain, or inflammation. Medications, such as transdermal **fentanyl** for analgesia, are discussed in the appropriate chapters for their therapeutic use (Chapter 13 describes proper administration of transdermal medications).

Some systemic medications cause skin diseases such as exfoliative dermatitis and scaling of skin that is eventually sloughed. Patients taking any medications should be evaluated for possibility of adverse skin reactions. Box 22-1 lists types of medications that may produce reactions from erythema to life-threatening responses.

DERMATOLOGIC PREPARATIONS AND ABSORPTION

Many forms of dermatologic preparations—such as liquids, ointments, gels, beads, pastes, plasters, creams, powders, foams, and sprays—are available to treat skin disorders. The selected form depends on the desired therapeutic effect and the ability of the person's skin to absorb medication. Skin **keratin,** when moisturized, provides a waterproof barrier for the body; therefore skin must be hydrated for absorption of water-based drugs.

Some drugs are placed in dressings to trap perspiration and prevent water loss and to assist with hydration and absorption. Water-soluble drugs are more readily absorbed and excreted, whereas fat-soluble drugs in a lipid base have slower excretion rates. In some body areas, such as the eyelids or behind the ears, the thinness of skin allows rapid absorption of medication, whereas areas such as the palms of the hands and soles of the feet are thick, making them almost impenetrable by medications. Some products contain lanolin to smooth skin and apply moisture in a lipid-soluble base. Other products, in alcohol bases, dry skin. Product use dictates the medication base needed, its method and site of application, and ability to be absorbed.

Just as with medications taken by other routes, the patient's medical record should be checked for allergies to medications to prevent skin irritation or other allergic reactions. Skin should be clean and dry for optimal absorption. If medication is for a specific site, such as a topical antiinfectant for an infected wound, it should be applied to the specific site without spreading onto surrounding tissues. If patches are used for systemic medications, sites should be rotated to avoid skin irritation and prevent decreased absorption occurring because of skin sensitization to medication.

TYPES OF PREPARATIONS FOR THE SKIN

Preparations for the skin come in many different forms, dependent on the condition being treated. Many of these preparations are available OTC.

Baths are used to cleanse skin, to lower body temperature, or to apply medications such as use of *povidone-iodine* as an antiseptic to prepare skin for surgery; in some skin conditions even water may not be tolerated. Persons with dry skin should bathe less frequently than those with oily skin and should use an oily lotion to hydrate the skin rather than one with an alcohol base. Baths for soothing irritated skin conditions may have gelatin, oatmeal (Aveeno), or starch added to water. Oils, such as Alpha-Keri, may be added to a tub of water to prevent drying of skin.

A lubricating medication or topical drug product for hydration should be applied immediately after a bath while skin is moist to increase absorption.

Did You Know?

Soaps are made by splitting fats with alkalis, using glycerol and an alkali salt of the fatty acid. Soaps are made from different oils such as olive oil (to make castile soaps), coconut oil, and animal fats.

Soaps are relatively alkaline and can irritate skin. Because of friction needed to cleanse skin with soap, it becomes a mechanical antiseptic, or some may have medications added to make them chemical antiseptics. Some products called soaps are actually **disinfectant** or **germicidal agents.** Soap and water promote healthy skin; however, perfumed or medicated products may cause irritation in a person with hypersensitivities. Because of the drying effect, all soaps should be adequately rinsed off unless otherwise instructed.

Skin cleansers are usually free of soap or are modified soap products used by persons who have sensitive, dry, or irritated skin or who have had an allergic reaction to soap products. Cleansers such as Neutrogena bars are less irritating, may contain an **emollient** to smooth skin, and may have a slightly acidic to neutral pH to be less irritating.

Gels are found in an alcohol base and are drying; therefore gels are appropriate for use on oily skin and weepy or vesicular lesions.

Emollients are fatty or oily substances to smooth or soften irritated skin and mucous membranes and may be used to apply medications; examples of emollients are lanolin, petroleum jelly, and vitamins A, D, and E ointments.

Skin protectants coat minor skin irritations and are used to protect skin from chemical irritants such as **benzoin** and benzoin compounds. Sween Cream is used to protect colostomy and ileostomy patients' skin and to protect pressure point skin of bedridden persons.

Lotions, liquids with an insoluble powder in a suspension, are mildly acidic or alkaline. Others, such as *calamine* or Caladryl lotion, may be used for their soothing effect in contact dermatitis, insect bites, or prickly heat.

Rubs and **liniments** are indicated on *intact* skin, such as the pain associated with muscle aches, neuralgia, rheumatism, arthritis, and sprains or strains, producing heat for relief of aches and pains. Ingredients may include counterirritants such as *camphor* or *methyl salicylate* or analgesics such as salicylate substances with potential to burn or irritate skin. Because of the danger of burning skin or causing severe irritation, external heat such as a heating pad or hot water bottle should not be used with these medications unless so prescribed. Local anesthetics and antiseptics may also be added for relief of pain.

Important Facts about Skin Preparations

- Skin preparations used on a daily basis include soaps, gels, disinfectants, baths, lotions, and sunscreens.
- Soaps and baths are drying to skin.
- Skin protectants should be used to protect skin around pressure ulcers or ostomies to prevent further trauma.
- Rubs and liniments tend to produce vasodilation and heat. External heat should not be applied to skin after a liniment or rub has been applied because of chance of burning skin.

ANTIINFECTIVE AND ANTIINFLAMMATORY TOPICALS

Skin is subject to infections by bacteria, fungi, and viruses. Topical antiinfectives may be used alone as superficial wound therapy. Where wounds have deep infection penetration, systemic antiinfectives may be indicated.

Topical antibiotics, much like systemic antibiotics, are used for the two most common organisms found in skin infections—*Streptococcus pyogenes* and *Staphylococcus aureus*—causes of infections such as folliculitis, **impetigo, furuncles, carbuncles,** and cellulitis (Figure 22-2 shows characteristics of various skin lesions).

Antiinfectives may be **bacteriostatic agents, bactericidal agents,** germicides, disinfectants, or antiseptics. Antiinfectives such as isopropyl alcohol, hexachlorophene, iodine, Lysol, and benzalkonium chloride are discussed in Chapter 17. Table 22-1 lists typical topical antibiotics, both OTC and legend medications.

PRIMARY LESIONS

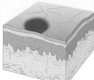

MACULE
Flat area of color change (no elevation or depression)

Example: Freckles

PAPULE
Solid elevation less than 0.5 cm in diameter

Example: Allergic eczema

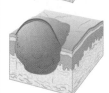

NODULE
Solid elevation 0.5 to 1 cm in diameter. Extends deeper into dermis than papule

Example: Mole

TUMOR
Solid mass—larger than 1 cm

Example: Squamous cell carcinoma

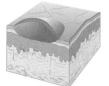

PLAQUE
Flat elevated surface found on skin or mucous membrane

Example: Thrush

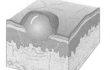

WHEAL
Type of plaque. Result is transient edema in dermis

Example: Intradermal skin test

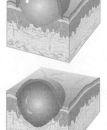

VESICLE
Small blister—fluid within or under epidermis

Example: Herpesvirus infection

BULLA
Large blister (greater than 0.5 cm)

Example: Burn

PUSTULE
Vesicle filled with pus

Example: Acne

SECONDARY LESIONS

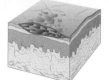

SCALES
Flakes of cornified skin layer

Example: Psoriasis

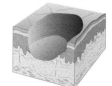

CRUST
Dried exudate on skin

Example: Impetigo

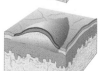

FISSURE
Cracks in skin

Example: Athlete's foot

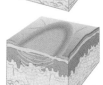

ULCER
Area of destruction of entire epidermis

Example: Decubitus (pressure sore)

SCAR
Excess collagen production after injury

Example: Surgical healing

ATROPHY
Loss of some portion of the skin

Example: Paralysis

Figure 22-2 Characteristics of skin lesions. (From Young AP, Proctor DB: *Kinn's the Medical Assistant: an applied learning approach*, ed 11, St Louis, 2011, Saunders.)

TABLE 22-1 SELECT TOPICAL ANTIINFECTIVES, ANTIVIRALS, ANTIINFLAMMATORY, AND ANTIFUNGAL AGENTS

GENERIC NAME/TRADE NAME	USUAL ADULT DOSE AND ROUTE	INDICATIONS FOR USE
TOPICAL ANTIINFECTIVES*		Skin infections
mupirocin (Bactroban[†] ointment and cream, 2%)	Apply topically	
bacitracin[†‡] ointment and cream	Apply topically	
gentamicin[†] cream, ointment	Apply topically	
neomycin, polymyxin B, bacitracin (Triple Antibiotic[‡], Neosporin[‡] cream, ointment)	Apply topically	
nitrofurazone[‡] soluble dressing	Apply topically	Burns, ulcers, infections
hexachlorophene (Dial soap[‡])	Soap for bathing	Soap; do not use on infants

Side Effects of Topical Antiinfectives:

mupirocin—local irritation and burning; *nitrofurazone*—pruritus, burning, ulceration; *bacitracin, gentamicin, neomycin, polymyxin B*—allergic dermatitis; *nitrofurazone*—pruritus, burning, ulceration; *hexachlorophene*—kills normal bacterial flora

*Topical antiinfectives have no major drug interactions.
[†]Prescription medications.
[‡]OTC medications.

GENERIC NAME/TRADE NAME	USUAL ADULT DOSE AND ROUTE	INDICATIONS FOR USE
TOPICAL ANTIVIRALS		
acyclovir (Zovirax 5%* ointment, powder) with hydrocortisone (Xerese Cream)	Apply topically	Herpetic lesions and other dermatologic viral conditions
penciclovir (Denavir[†] ointment, cream)	Apply topically	Herpetic lesions
docosanol (Abreva[‡] cream 10%)	Apply topically	Cold sores, herpes simplex

*Topical antiinfectives have no major drug interactions.
[†]Prescription medications.
[‡]OTC medications.

GENERIC NAME/TRADE NAME	USUAL ADULT DOSE AND ROUTE	INDICATIONS FOR USE
TOPICAL ANTIINFLAMMATORY OR CORTICOSTEROID AGENTS[§]		
betamethasone (Diprolene[†] cream, ointment, gel, lotion) (Luxiq, foam) (Diprosone[†] cream, ointment, lotion, aerosol)	Apply topically	Inflamed tissue, psoriasis, rashes, insect bites, eczema
clobetasol (Temovate, Clobex, Olux[†] cream, ointment, lotion, gel, foam, shampoo, solution)	Apply topically	
desonide (DesOwen[†] cream, ointment, lotion, gel)	Apply topically	
diflorasone (Apexicon,[†] ointment, Maxiflor[†] cream)	Apply topically	
desoximetasone (Topicort[†] cream, ointment, gel)	Apply topically	
fluocinonide[†] cream, ointment (Lidex[†] gel, solution, ointment, cream)	Apply topically	
halcinonide (Halog[†] cream, ointment, solution)	Apply topically	
triamcinolone[†] cream, ointment, lotion, aerosol (Kenalog[†] and others in the same forms)	Apply topically	
hydrocortisone (Westcort[†] cream, ointment; Cortizone 10[‡] cream, ointment; Cortaid[‡] and other preparations in cream, ointment, lotion, solution[‡])	Apply topically	
dexamethasone (Decaspray [†] aerosol spray; Decadron[†] cream)	Apply topically	
fluocinolone[†] (Derma-Smoothe[†] cream, solution, ointment, oil, shampoo)	Apply topically	

TABLE 22-1 SELECT TOPICAL ANTIINFECTIVES, ANTIVIRALS, ANTIINFLAMMATORY, AND ANTIFUNGAL AGENTS—cont'd

GENERIC NAME/TRADE NAME	USUAL ADULT DOSE AND ROUTE	INDICATIONS FOR USE
mometasone (Elocon cream, ointment, lotion, solution)	Apply topically	
prednicarbate (Dermatop† cream, ointment)	Apply topically	

†Prescription medications.
‡OTC medications.
§No major side effects or drug interactions are found with topical antiinflammatory agents.

TOPICAL ANTIFUNGALS¶

clioquinol (Vioform)	Apply topically	Antibacterial
clotrimazole (Mycelex, Mycelex Troches†, Desenex†, Lotrimin‡ topical cream, solution, lotion)	Use as topical agents	Candidiasis and tinea infections
plus beta metnazone (Lottisone)	apply topically	
(Gyne-Lotrimin‡ vaginal suppository and cream)	Inserted vaginally	
econazole (NTN)	Apply topically	Tinea
itraconazole (Sporanox† 100-mg cap)	Oral dose varies	Tinea
ketoconazole		Tinea capitis and seborrheic dermatitis
(Nizoral† cream)	Apply topically	
(Xolegel gel)	Shampoo	
(Nizoral shampoo)	Oral dose varies	
(Extina foam)	Apply topically	
(Nizoral 200 mg tab)		
miconazole (Micatin†‡, Lotrimin topical cream, spray, powder, ointment)	Apply topically	Candidiasis and tinea infections
(Monistat‡ vaginal suppository)	Insert vaginally	
(Monistat cream)	Apply topically	
oxiconazole (Oxistat† cream, lotion)	Apply topically	Candidiasis and tinea infections
sertaconazole (Ertaczo cream)	Apply topically	Tinea only
undecylenic acid (Desenex, Cruex‡, Caldesene‡, Fungoid‡ in cream, powder, solution, soap, spray, liquid)	Apply topically	Candidiasis and tinea infections and diaper rash
ciclopirox (Loprox† gel, topical suspension, topical solution, shampoo, cream)	Apply topically	Tinea only
tolnaftate (Tinactin‡ powder, cream, solution, spray, gel; Absorbine‡ solution; Aftate, NP-27‡ cream)	Apply topically	Tinea only
terbinafine tablet	250 mg PO qd	Tinea only
(Lamisil cream, gel, solution‡)	Apply topically	
naftifine (Naftin‡ cream, gel)	Apply topically	Tinea only
nystatin (Nystop†)		Candidiasis, diaper rash
tablet	400,000-600,000 units PO tid-qid	
suspension	Swish and swallow	
powder, cream, ointment	Apply topically	
vaginal tablets	Insert vaginally	

Continued

TABLE 22-1 SELECT TOPICAL ANTIINFECTIVES, ANTIVIRALS, ANTIINFLAMMATORY, AND ANTIFUNGAL AGENTS—cont'd

GENERIC NAME/TRADE NAME	USUAL ADULT DOSE AND ROUTE	INDICATIONS FOR USE
terconazole (Terazol)		Candidiasis
vaginal cream	Apply topically	
vaginal suppository	Insert vaginally	
nystatin + triamcinolone	Apply topically	Candidiasis
(Mycolog† cream, ointment)		

Drug Interactions: H₂ blockers, anticholinergics

H_2, histamine₂; *NTN*, no trade name; *PO*, orally
†Prescription medications.
‡OTC medications.
§No major side effects or drug interactions are found with topical antiinflammatory agents.
¶No major side effects are found with topical antifungal agents. Those found include local irritation, pruritus, burning sensation, scaling, dryness, erythema, blistering, peeling, stinging, urticaria.

Topical antivirals are applied several times a day to skin lesions such as herpes and herpes zoster. **Acyclovir** is applied six times a day for 7 days. Multiple OTC preparations are available for treating such viral disorders as cold sores (herpes simplex). Table 22-1 lists medications used as topical antivirals.

Topical antifungal medications, such as **clotrimazole** (Desenex, Cruex) and **tolnaftate** (Tinactin), are used to treat fungal infections of hair, nails, or skin. Because of the dampness and warmth of body areas such as feet, axilla, perineal area, and under breasts, fungal infections seem to thrive in these areas. Most antifungals, by changing the integrity of the fungal cell membrane, are either fungistatic or fungicidal. Topical antifungals are generally used to treat *Candida* and tinea infections. Fungal infections of nails, or onychomycosis (tinea unguium), are difficult to treat and require prolonged therapy with oral and topical medications. Topical antifungal preparations, sprays, lotions, creams, ointments, and powders, are available as both prescription and OTC medications; some, such as betanethazone and clotrimazole (Lotrisone), are combined with corticosteroids. Fungal medications should not come in contact with eyes or delicate mucous membranes. For topical antifungals to be effective, skin should be clean and dry before application. If no improvement occurs with OTC medications in 2 to 3 weeks, a physician should be consulted (see Table 22-1).

Topical corticosteroids are used to relieve inflammation and pruritus of contact dermatitis, insect bites, minor burns, seborrheic dermatitis, **psoriasis,** and **eczema.** These medications contain a drying agent or conversely an emollient and are usually found in creams, ointments, lotions, and gels to facilitate absorption at the site of action. Absorption is high in areas of thin skin, but penetration is poor with thick skin.

These preparations vary widely in strength, with those available OTC being of low potency. Systemic toxicity may be a side effect with long-term therapy using high-potency topical preparations. Site of application influences the medication form choice. Gels and lotions are used in hairy areas. Creams rub easily into tissue if needed for weepy, wet tissue lesions. Lipid-based ointments are more occlusive and moisturizing and are best for application on dry or scaly areas. Apply as a thin film and gently rub into skin (see Table 22-1 and Chapter 20 for systemic corticosteroids.)

CLINICAL TIP

Topical medications should be applied with a finger cot or gloves to prevent transfer of the pathogen to other body sites or people and to avoid effects to the skin on an undesired location. For patients who are self-medicating, hands should be washed immediately after application.

Patient Education for Compliance

1. Topical medications should be applied at regular intervals.
2. Cleanse and dry affected area before applying topical medication; the best time is after a shower, for better absorption. Skin should be dried before application.
3. Use gloves or other protective equipment when applying antiviral medications to herpes lesions to prevent the infection from spreading.
4. Avoid eye contact with antivirals and corticosteroids.
5. Apply a thin film of corticosteroid medication.
6. Do not cover corticosteroid preparations with occlusive dressings or clothing unless directed. Also avoid sunlight on treated areas.
7. Avoid prolonged use of corticosteroids and do not apply to weeping or denuded areas unless specifically prescribed.
8. Do not use tight diapers, diaper covers, or plastic pants when applying corticosteroids on infants. Occlusion increases absorption of the steroids.
9. Use full treatment for fungal infections, even if symptoms improve; therapy is long term. If condition persists or worsens, contact physician.

Acne Preparations

Acne vulgaris, a skin disease with increased sebum and oil production and increased formation of keratin, usually on the face, chest, back, and neck, appears as papules, pustules, and comedones. Treatment includes reduction of sebum and bacteria with many preparations available OTC; others require a prescription.

Oral antibiotics such as tetracycline and erythromycin are used to treat acne concurrently with topical medications.

A drug specific for acne is isotretinoin (Amnesteem, Claravis, Sotret), a derivative of vitamin A, and in pregnancy is category X, with many teratogenic effects. Because of severe side effects caused by isotretinoin, it is reserved for severe disfiguring cases of acne. Physicians prescribing and persons taking the drug must enroll in the iPLEDGE program to ensure that no woman beginning therapy is pregnant nor becomes pregnant while taking the drug. A prescription written for isotretinoin must have a special sticker applied by a physician certified to prescribe the medication before it can be filled because of innate neonate dangers.

Two combination oral contraceptives (Estrostep and Ortho Tri-Cyclin) have been approved for treating women at least 15 years of age who have reached menarche and have not responded to topical medications for acne. Benefits are from estrogen, which suppresses and inactivates sebum production (see Chapter 28 for estrogen preparations).

A few of the available topical preparations for acne are as follows:

Benzoyl peroxide is the ingredient in many prescription and OTC preparations such as Acnomel, Acne-10, Benoxyl, Clearasil, Dryox, Fostex, Neutrogena, and Oxyderm. It promotes peeling of skin and suppresses growth of bacteria by releasing active oxygen.

Topical and systemic antibiotics are used to treat acne; the oral antibiotic of choice usually is tetracycline. The most commonly prescribed topical antibiotics for mild to moderate acne are erythromycin and clindamycin, which work by decreasing sebaceous fatty acid byproducts and preventing formation of new acne lesions (oral antibiotics are discussed in Chapter 17).

Tretinoin (Retin-A, Renova), an irritant, stimulates rapid turnover of epithelial cells followed by skin peeling. It reduces fatty acids within comedones, causing them to be removed while suppressing formation of new plugs. This drug is a pregnancy category X preparation and should not be used by pregnant women or those who may become pregnant. Tretinoin is applied to the face once a day for peeling; therefore it is also used to remove fine wrinkles caused by aging or sun exposure. Risk of sunburn is increased with use of this agent.

Adapalene (Differin) reduces the formation of comedones and may even appear to exacerbate acne before becoming effective. Adapalene is not systemically absorbed, but risk of sunburn is also increased with this agent (Table 22-2).

Azelaic acid (Azelex), an antiinfective, is used for mild to moderate acne to suppress the bacterial growth.

Patient Education for Compliance

1. Keep acne preparations away from eyes, mouth, and other mucous membranes.
2. Expect dryness and peeling of skin with most acne preparations; discontinue with rash or irritations.
3. Water-based cosmetics should be used with acne preparations. Do not countertreat desired dryness resulting from these preparations with emollients.
4. Wait at least 1 hour after applying any other topical medication or cosmetics to apply topical erythromycin.
5. Topical tetracyclines may stain fabrics and may turn skin yellow.
6. Persons using tretinoin are susceptible to sunburn and should wear sunscreen (SPF 15 or greater) and protective clothing. If sunburned, do not apply tretinoin.
7. When tretinoin is used, the skin should be washed and dried 15 to 30 minutes before application and hands should be washed immediately after application. Contact with eyes, nose, or mouth should be avoided.
8. Cosmetics should be removed before tretinoin is used. Treatment may be needed for up to 6 months before a response is seen.

TABLE 22-2 SELECT MEDICATIONS FOR ACNE

GENERIC NAME/ TRADE NAME	USUAL DOSE, ROUTE, AND FREQUENCY	INDICATIONS FOR USE	MAJOR SIDE EFFECTS	DRUG INTERACTIONS
benzoyl peroxide 2.5%-10% (PanOxyl, Desquam, Benzac, Brevoxyl[†] as soap, cream, gel, liquid, lotion, mask, foam, pad)	Apply topically	Acne	Dryness of skin	Usually none with topicals
clindamycin (Cleocin T* solution, gel, foam, lotion, swab; Evoclin)	Apply topically		Dryness, scaling, peeling of skin, stinging and burning, itching, tenderness	
erythromycin (solution, gel, ointment, pledgets)	Apply topically		Same as above	
with benzoyl peroxide (Benzamycin* gel)	Apply topically			
clindamycin 1.2% + tretinoin (Veltin gel) 0.025% gel (Ziana)	Apply topically		Inflammation of throat and nose, dry skin,	Abrasive soaps or cleansers, sun exposure
doxycycline (Oracea 40-mg delayed-release capsule)	40 mg PO qd	Pustules, papules of rosacea	Headaches, dizziness, blurred vision; flulike symptoms; loss of appetite	See doxycycline in Chapter 17
minocycline (Solodyn extended-release tab)	1 mg/kg PO qd	Inflammatory lesions of acne	Lightheadedness, dizziness; do not use before age 12 years because it will darken teeth	See minocycline in Chapter 17
isotretinoin (Sotret, Amnesteem, Claravis*[†])	0.5-1 mg/kg PO daily in 2 divided doses	Acne		carbamazepine
tretinoin (retinoic acid) (Retin-A*)	Apply topically	Acne	Redness, edematous blisters, crusting, stinging	
(Avita gel, cream)	Apply topically			
adapalene (Differin* gel, cream, lotion)	Apply topically		Burning, pruritus, erythema, dryness, scaling	
azelaic acid (Azelex* cream Finacea gel)	Apply topically		Same as adapalene with tingling and depigmentation	

PO, orally.
*Prescription medication.
[†]OTC medication.
[‡]Pregnancy category X drug.

Important Facts about Acne Preparations

- Acne preparations containing benzoyl peroxide are drying. Oil-based creams and cosmetics should not be used after application of these medications.
- Some of the acne preparations are applied to skin to cause peeling. Care should be taken to prevent sun burning.
- Vitamin A preparations should not be used during pregnancy or if possibility of becoming pregnant exists.

Keratolytic Agents

Keratolytic agents or keratin dissolvers are used to soften scales and to promote shedding of the skin's horny layer. Effects range from peeling to extensive skin desquamation. These products are used to treat dandruff, **seborrheic dermatitis,** acne, and psoriasis, as well as warts and corns.

Salicylic acid, resorcinol, and **sulfur** are the drugs of choice, but *benzoyl peroxide* may be also used with these conditions. Salicylic acid, podophyllum resin, and cantharidin may be used for common warts, as well as for venereal warts.

Podophyllum, used for genital warts, is teratogenic with the potential for systemic reactions and is not particularly effective against common warts. These resins should be applied and washed off in 1 to 4 hours at weekly intervals for 4 weeks.

Cantharidin (Cantharon), used to remove common warts, is harmful to normal skin. Normal skin should be cleaned immediately with acetone or alcohol in the event it is accidentally touched (Table 22-3).

TREATMENTS FOR SEBORRHEIC DERMATITIS

Shampoos for seborrheic dermatitis, characterized by inflammation and scaling on the face or scalp, under the arms, on the chest, and in the anogenital region, are available as OTC and prescription items. Seborrheic dermatitis begins on the scalp and is characterized by yellowish, brownish-gray greasy scales. **Ketoconazole,** an antifungal, is used as a shampoo; other medications such as **pyrithione zinc** or **selenium sulfide** are available OTC (Selsun Blue, Head and Shoulders) and by prescription (Selsun, Exsel) because of the stronger strength. These agents may cause skin irritation, alopecia, and hair discoloration (see Table 22-3).

MEDICATIONS FOR PSORIASIS

New medications specific for psoriasis have been recently introduced. **Calcipotriene** (Dovonex) is a foam that is applied topically. **Ustekinumab** (Stelara) is injected subcutaneously at 12 week intervals after the first two doses that are administered 4 weeks apart. However, the medication also lowers the body's immune response to infections including tuberculosis, fungi, bacteria, and viruses, and increases susceptibility to cancers. The

dosage should not be given concurrently with immunizations, with immunosuppressives, and active infections since this medication leaves the body's response to infection greatly diminished. Effectiveness is about 75% for clearance of psoriasis in 12 weeks.

Coal and *pine tars* used for psoriasis (identified by red, raised lesions covered with dry silvery scales), are found in shampoos, soaps, lotions, and creams. In severe cases, chemotherapeutic agents, such as methotrexate, may be used to treat lesions.

Alefacept (Amevive), the first injectable immunosuppressive biologic agent used as therapy for psoriasis, is expensive (approximately $1000 per month) and inconvenient because the need for injections weekly for 12 treatments but produces prolonged remission. However, long-term use may result in malignancies.

TOPICAL ANESTHESIA AND ANTIPRURITICS

Topical anesthetics such as **lidocaine** (Solarcaine, Anbesol) and **dibucaine** (Nupercainal) are used for itching of skin or mucous membranes and for skin desensitization to painful stimuli. These medications are available as OTC preparations and are available for prescription use as **tetracaine** (Pontocaine) and lidocaine (Xylocaine) (see Table 22-3).

Dilute solutions of **phenol** have also been used for anesthesia and pruritus. Lotions of calamine or phenolated calamine are often used for pruritus. A cream with **diphenhydramine** (Benadryl) alone or as a lotion with calamine (Caladryl) may be bought OTC for relief of pruritus. Cornstarch and oatmeal baths (Aveeno) are also used, especially for children with chickenpox (see Table 22-3).

TABLE 22-3 MISCELLANEOUS DERMATOLOGIC PREPARATIONS

GENERIC NAME/TRADE NAME	USUAL DOSE, ROUTE, AND FREQUENCY	INDICATIONS FOR USE	DRUG INTERACTIONS
KERATOLYTICS			
salicylic acid (Compound W, Wart-Off, (Mediplast) plasters, adhesives, cream, solutions, lotions, foam, ointments, gels, shampoo	Tincture—apply topically Plasters—apply topically Solution, foam, creams—topically Shampoo—topically	Hyperkeratotic skin conditions, common or plantar warts, psoriasis, calluses, corns, dandruff	Usually none with topical preparations
resorcinol (found in many OTC and prescription products i.e., shampoos, ointments, lotions, creams)	Apply topically	Acne, eczema, psoriasis, seborrheic dermatitis	
sulfur (found in many OTC and prescription products i.e., lotions, shampoos, soap)	Apply topically	Acne, eczema, psoriasis, seborrheic dermatitis	
cantharidin (Cantharone, Verr-Canth‡ powder)	Apply topically and cover with tape for 24 hr; then remove	Common warts and viral induced skin diseases	
imiquimod (Aldara‡, Zyclara cream)	Apply topically	Venereal warts	
podophyllum (Podocon-25‡ liquid, powder)	Apply topically	Venereal warts	
ammonium lactate (Lac-Hydrin lotion, cream)	Apply topically	Acne, eczema, psoriasis, seborrheic dermatitis	
MEDICATIONS FOR PSORIASIS			
calcipotriene (Dovonex solution, cream, ointment)	Apply topically	Plaque psoriasis	Flammable
ustekinumab (Stelara)	45-90 mg SC q4-12 wks	Moderate to severe psoriasis	BCG vaccine
SELECT TOPICAL ANESTHETICS AND ANTIPRURETICS§			
benzocaine (Benzocaine‡, Orajel, Hurricaine, Zilactin, Benzodent as cream, liquid, gel, ointment, spray, solution, swab; also available in otic drops)	Topically	Anesthesia	None noted
lidocaine (Xylocaine, Anestacon‡, Solarcaine, ointment, solution, aerosol spray, cream, lotion)	Topically	Anesthesia	None noted
lidocaine with prilocaine (EMLA gel)	Topically before venipuncture	For injection site anesthesia	None noted
tetracaine solution, cream, ointment	Topically	Toothache, sunburn, pruritus, oral pain	None noted
dibucaine (Nupercainal* ointment)	Topically	Sunburn, rectal pain, pruritus	None noted
ethyl chloride 2%, ethyl chloride spray	Topically	Freezing before minor surgical procedures, sprains, strains	None noted
calamine lotion with diphenhydramine (Caladryl cream and lotion)	Apply topically	Prutitis	
oleated oatmeal (Aveeno powder)	Mix with bath water as needed for itching	None noted	
benzyl alcohol (Ulesfia)	Apply topically	Allergic or irritant dermatitis	

TABLE 22-3 MISCELLANEOUS DERMATOLOGIC PREPARATIONS—cont'd

GENERIC NAME/TRADE NAME	USUAL DOSE, ROUTE, AND FREQUENCY	INDICATIONS FOR USE	DRUG INTERACTIONS
SCABICIDES AND PEDICULICIDES			
lindane‡ lotion, shampoo	As directed topically	Scabies/pediculosis	
permethrin (Nix*)	One application topically	Head lice, scabies	
(Elimite‡ shampoo, ointment, cream, lotion, liquid)	One application topically	Lice	
malathion (Ovide‡, lotion, A-200*, Rid-X*)	4-48 oz depending on length of hair	Lice	

Drug Interactions: Usually none with topical preparations when used as directed

MEDICATIONS FOR BALDNESS			
minoxidil (Rogaine topical solution)	Apply 1 mL of solution to affected area of scalp	Baldness	
finasteride (Propecia)	1 mg PO qd	Baldness	
MEDICATIONS FOR MISCELLANEOUS DERMATITIS CONDITIONS			
coal tar*‡ (various OTC preparations as shampoo and soaps	Use topically	Psoriasis, seborrheic dermatitis	
fluorouracil (Efudex solution‡ cream, carac, cream)	Apply topically for disintegration of tissues	Actinic keratosis, superficial basal cell carcinomas	
mexoryl SX (Anthelios SX moisturizing cream*)	Apply topically	Sunscreen	

BCG, bacille Calmette-Guérin; *PO,* orally; *SC,* subcutaneously.
*OTC medication.
†Used by medical professionals only; not dispensed.
‡Prescription medication.
§No major side effects are found with topical anesthetics and antipruritics.

TOPICAL TREATMENT OF BURNS AND CHRONIC WOUNDS

Burn treatment is dependent on the type and depth of the burn, as well as the percentage of affected body area. Types of burns include thermal, chemical, and electrical burns, as well as inhalation of smoke. Chronic wounds, including pressure ulcers, diabetic ulcers, and venous ulcers, are wounds that are not completely healed after 4 to 6 weeks of treatment. Emergency and long-term treatment may be accomplished by using dressings such as DuoDERM or OpSite as well as antimicrobials, débriding agents, dressings, and wound cleansers.

Two topical sulfonamides are frequently used with second- and third-degree burns because of their broad spectrum of action against gram-positive and gram-negative bacteria. **Silver sulfadiazine** (Silvadene) is used for prevention of infections and to soften and facilitate **eschar** removal. **Mafenide** (Sulfamylon), also a broad-spectrum bacteriostatic agent, penetrates eschar, even in the presence of pus and serum. This agent rapidly diffuses through burns and is effective against bacterial wound invasion. Mafenide is relatively nontoxic, but some burning, stinging, or pain may occur on application (see Table 22-4).

CLINICAL TIP

Before using silver sulfadiazine, be sure the patient is not allergic to either of the active ingredients—silver and sulfa.

Alginate dressings, made of spun fibers of brown seaweed, absorb serous drainage or exudates to assist with debridement and to keep a moist wound area.

TABLE 22-4 MEDICATIONS USED FOR BURNS AND DÉBRIDEMENT*

GENERIC NAME/ TRADE NAME*	USUAL ADULT DOSE AND ROUTE	INDICATIONS FOR USE	DRUG INTERACTIONS
silver sulfadiazine (Silvadene cream)	Apply topically	Second- and third-degree burns	Proteolytic enzymes
mafenide (Sulfamylon cream, powder for solution)	Apply topically		
collagenase (Santyl ointment)	Apply topically	Débride wounds for eschar, necrotic tissue	Cleansing agents
alginate (spun seaweed) dressing (AlgiDERM, Curasorb, Sorbsan)	Apply topically		
trypsin (Granulex, Xenaderm gel, ointment, spray)	Apply topically		
fibrinolysin (desoxyribonuclease) (Elase ointment)	Apply topically		
dextranomer (Debrisan hydrophilic beads)	Apply topically		
hydrophilic polyurethane foam (Biopatch, Curafoam, Flexzan)	Apply topically		
hydrocolloid dressing and granules (DuoDERM, Curaderm)	Apply topically		
hydrogel (Curasol, Tegaderm, Vigilon)	Apply topically		
polyurethane film dressing (Bioclusive, Carrafilm, Tegaderm HP)	Apply topically		
becaplermin gel (Regranex)	Apply topically		

*All prescription medications.

Collagenase ointments, are sterile enzymatic débriding ointments with the ability to digest collagen in necrotic tissue.

Hydrophilic polyurethane foam, also called *open-cell foam dressing,* are sheets of foamed solutions containing variable sized open cells to hold exudates away from wounds while maintaining a moist environment.

Hydrogels are glycerin-based or water-based dressings for hydrating wounds.

Transparent film dressings, polyurethane sheets that will not adhere to moist surfaces, do not have any absorbent qualities but do allow some transfer of oxygen and water vapor.

Becaplermin gel (Regranex) is a recombinant formulation of platelet-derived growth factor to promote granulation of tissue.

Proteolytic enzymes are used to clean and débride tissues of debris and exudates by dissolving protein found in necrotic tissue. Some of these medications are combined with antibiotics to add bactericidal action (see Table 22-3).

Patient Education for Compliance

1. Burns should be cleaned and débrided before sulfonamides are applied.
2. Burns may be continuously covered with sulfonamides to soften eschar.

Important Fact about Burn Medications

Proteolytic enzymes are used to débride and clean tissues of debris and exudate.

PROPHYLACTIC AGENTS

Sunscreens, which absorb or reflect harmful rays from the sun, are used when extended sun exposure may lead to premature skin aging or to sunburn during leisure activities or occupations requiring outdoor exposure.

Some chemicals and medications such as tetracyclines, sulfonamides, thiazides, phenothiazines, tricyclic antidepressants, and antineoplastic agents, as well as cosmetics, may increase the chance of **photosensitivity.** Skin becomes red and painful and burns, with peak reactions occurring 24 to 48 hours after exposure. Skin damage may result in precancerous or cancerous tissues. Absorbing agents, chemicals that absorb harmful rays into the skin, prevent erythema, burns, and other harmful effects. Reflecting agents are opaque, like pastes such as **zinc oxide** and **titanium dioxide,** and must be applied heavily to be effective.

The Food and Drug Administration (FDA) has classified sun products by their sun protection factor (SPF), the ratio between exposure to ultraviolet radiation (UVR) waves and time required to cause erythema with or without sunscreen, or minimum erythema dose (MED). The best way to choose a sunscreen is by type of skin and length of time in the sun. The general recommendation for use with medications is a minimum SPF of 15. In the tropics, an SPF of 30 is recommended for individuals who will be in the sun for even a brief period of time. Efficacy of a sunscreen is related to its ability to stay on the skin through exercise, sweating, and swimming. Water-resistant sunscreens should remain on the skin for 40 minutes in water; waterproof sunscreens should remain on the skin twice as long. Some protectants have dual SPFs on the label—one for dry conditions and one for use in water.

Skin protectives form a film on skin to prevent maceration of and dryness of the skin. These products will also keep out light, air, and dust. Nonabsorbable powders may not be useful as protectants because they tend to stick to wet surfaces and are difficult to remove. These powders include zinc oxide, **zinc stearate,** bismuth preparations, and talcum powder. **Collodion** (a mixture of alcohol, ether, and pyroxylin) is applied for protection; the ether and alcohol evaporates, leaving a thin, transparent film on the skin. Flexible collodion is collodion mixed with camphor and castor oil to make an elastic, flexible film. Styptic collodion contains tannic acid as an astringent, as well as protectant. These agents protect the skin to allow stimulation of healing and prevent further trauma.

MEDICATIONS FOR SCABIES AND PEDICULOSIS

Scabicides and **pediculicides** are used against animal parasites. Pediculosis is an infestation of lice—pediculosis pubis (pubic lice), pediculosis corporis (body lice), or pediculosis capitis (head lice). Pediculosis corporis is usually found around the waist, collar, or axillary area because after biting the individual the parasite hides in the clothing. The drug for pediculosis is **lindane** in topical creams and lotions applied to affected areas and left on for 12 hours, then thoroughly removed. Shampoo is worked into scalp for 4 minutes, shampooed, and then rinsed. Finally, **nits** are combed from hair shafts. Repeated applications of lindane, a strong insecticide, may cause central nervous system toxicity, especially in children.

Scabies are small parasites that bore into the horny layer of the skin, causing irritation and pruritus. A month after mites burrow under skin, symptoms such as watery blisters between fingers appear. Infestation then spreads around wrists and elbows and onto buttocks. With scabies, lindane lotion is left on the entire body for 8 hours. Other medications such as **crotamiton** (Eurax), **permethrin** (Nix, Elimite), and **malathion** (Ovide) are applied to infested areas. Elimite, a prescription drug for scabies, is applied from the neck down over the body and is left on for 12 hours before removal. Clothing and bed linens must be treated at the same time as skin to destroy mites (see Table 22-3).

Patient Education for Compliance

1. Do not apply scabicides and pediculicides to the face unless specifically instructed by a physician.
2. Wear gloves for application of these medications.
3. Do not apply conditioners to hair after use of medications for lice.
4. Treat all household and sexual contacts for lice concurrently.
5. Because of flammability, avoid open flames around Ovide and other malathion derivatives. Do not use hair dryers and do not smoke.

Important Facts about Scabicides and Pediculicides

- Medications for scabies and pediculosis are found in prescription and OTC forms.
- The insecticides malathion and lindane can be absorbed, causing systemic reactions if used too often.

OTHER DERMATOLOGIC PREPARATIONS

Minoxidil (Rogaine) in different strengths may be used for alopecia in men and women by applying 1 mL of solution to thinning areas of the hair twice a day.

Did You Know?

Minoxidil was originally produced as an antihypertensive, but excessive hair growth was seen to be a persistent side effect, and the FDA approved its use for alopecia.

Another hair stimulant for use in men, *finasteride* (Propecia), an androgen inhibitor, is a category X medication in women because handling of the medication or contact with semen may be teratogenic to the male fetus.

Fluorouracil (Efudex), used for **actinic keratosis** and superficial basal cell carcinoma, works by causing a mild inflammation that progresses to severe inflammation with burning, stinging, and vesicle formation. This reaction is followed by tissue disintegration, necrosis, erosion, **ulceration,** and finally healing (see Table 22-3).

Patient Education for Compliance

Use gloves or a cotton-tip applicator when applying fluorouracil, and apply only to affected areas. Protect surrounding areas by encircling lesion with Vaseline.

SUMMARY

Many preparations for treating skin disorders exist. Many of them may be bought OTC and may be the same medications as prescription drugs but of weaker strength. Many topical preparations such as soaps, baths, and skin protectants are used on a daily basis.

Antiinfectives and antiinflammatories are some of the same medications with the same indications as described in Chapter 17 but are in topical forms for dermatologic uses. When used under normal conditions, topical antiinfectives do not have systemic effects or dangers of drug resistance that are found with systemic preparations. Dermatologic therapeutic agents cover a wide range of medications, including preparations for acne, psoriasis, seborrheic dermatitis, burns, baldness, itching, and parasites. Many patients use OTC medications for warts, contact dermatitis, itching, sunburn, or lesions caused by diseases such as chickenpox. Protective agents such as sunscreens and skin protectants around colostomies or pressure sores are important in prophylaxis against further skin trauma.

CRITICAL THINKING EXERCISES

Scenario

James plays football and has a problem with athlete's foot. He does not want to go to the dermatologist with the problem but wants to use a product that can be bought OTC.

1. Is an OTC product a possible answer for his problem? Explain.
2. What forms of medication can be obtained OTC for fungal infections?
3. What OTC medication would you think that James might try?
4. James also wants to know how long he can use this medicine if it does not seem to help his fungal infection before he must see a physician. How would you answer?

DRUG CALCULATIONS

1. Order: Tetracycline 250 mg qid
   Available medication: Tetracycline 0.25 g caps
   Dose to be administered: _____

   _____
   _____
   _____

2. Order: Lindane Shampoo, Wash hair hs and rep in 1 wk. Comb hair p̄ washing
   Interpret the order: _____

   _____
   _____
   _____

REVIEW QUESTIONS

1. How are the form and size of the chemical molecule related to absorption of medications through the skin?
   _____
   _____

2. What is the difference between a soap and a cleanser? _____
   _____
   _____

3. What are the modes of action for topical antiinfectives used for such conditions as impetigo, carbuncles, and furuncles? _____
   _____

4. What are indications for topical corticosteroids? _____
   _____
   _____

5. What are the many forms of antifungals? Why are all of these forms necessary? _____
   _____
   _____
   _____
   _____

6. What is the leading ingredient in acne preparations, and how does it act on the skin? _____
   _____
   _____

7. How are topical anesthetics used? _____
   _____
   _____

8. What antiinfective class of medications is used for burns? How do these preparations facilitate burn treatment?
   _____
   _____
   _____

CHAPTER 23

Musculoskeletal System Disorders

OBJECTIVES

After studying this chapter, you should be capable of doing the following:

- Describing causes and symptoms of joint and muscle pain.
- Discussing therapy for osteoporosis.
- Explaining classes of medications used to treat musculoskeletal conditions.
- Describing how muscle relaxants affect the body and appropriate patient education needed for patient safety.
- Identifying medications used for arthritis.
- Providing patient education for compliance with medications used to treat diseases and conditions of the musculoskeletal system.

Ms. Werner is approaching menopause and cannot drink milk because of allergies. She comes to Dr. Merry for a regular office visit and asks if she needs to be concerned about her lack of calcium intake. Dr. Merry suggests Ms. Werner use Tums as a calcium substitute. As she is leaving the office, Ms. Werner questions use of an over-the-counter (OTC) preparation that is indicated for gestric disturbances.

What is your response concerning the use of Tums?
A few weeks later Ms. Werner calls to say that she has heard of an OTC product for calcium that is eaten as candy. What would be your response if she asks for the product name?
Should she use Tums with this candy-like preparation?

KEY TERMS

Ankylosing spondylitis
Ankylosis
Arthritis
Articulate
Bursitis
Crepitus
Disease-modifying antirheumatic drug (DMARD)

Exacerbate
Fibromyalgia
Fusion
Hyperuricemia
Immunomodulator
Immunosuppressant
Kyphosis
Muscle spasm

Muscle spasticity
Myasthenia gravis
Nonsalicylate
Nonsteroidal antiinflammatory drug (NSAID)
Osteoarthritis

Osteoporosis
Pannus
Purine
Salicylate
Tumor necrosis factor (TNF)

EASY WORKING KNOWLEDGE OF INDICATIONS AND SIDE EFFECTS

Common Symptoms of Musculoskeletal Disorders
Joint stiffness, pain, inflammation, swelling
Weight loss
Bone mass loss, bone deformities
Fatigue, malaise, weakness, fever
Tenderness and swelling of joints and bones
Loss of motion, immobility

Common Side Effects of Medications Used for Musculoskeletal Disorders
Nausea and vomiting
Pain in abdomen
Drowsiness, dizziness, orthostatic hypotension
Headache
Constipation and diarrhea
Visual changes

EASY WORKING KNOWLEDGE OF DRUGS USED FOR MUSCULOSKELETAL CONDITIONS

DRUG CLASS	PRESCRIPTION	OTC	PREGNANCY CATEGORY	MAJOR INDICATIONS
OSTEOPOROTIC MEDICATIONS				Prevention and treatment of osteoporosis
Bisphosphonates	Yes	No	C	
Bone resorptive inhibitors	Yes	No	X	
Calcitonin	Yes	No	C	
Calcium carbonate	Yes	Yes	Not categorized	
Parathyroid hormone	Yes	No	C	
ANTIRHEUMATIC AND ANTIARTHRITIC MEDICATIONS				
Nonsteroidal Antiinflammatory Drugs				
Salicylates	Yes	Yes	C	Antiinflammatory agents, analgesics
Nonsalicylates	Yes	Yes	B, C, D	
Disease-Modifying Antirheumatic Drugs				
Immunosuppressants	Yes	No	D	Relieve symptoms of rheumatoid arthritis
Immunomodulators	Yes	No	B	
TNF factor blockers	Yes	No	B	Moderate to severe rheumatoid arthritis
Gold salts	Yes	No	C, D	
Antimalarials	Yes	No	B, C, D	
OTHER AGENTS FOR MUSCULOSKELETAL CONDITIONS				
Antigout medications	Yes	No	C, D	Relieve symptoms of gouty arthritis
Skeletal muscle relaxants	Yes	No	B, C	Reduce muscle spasms and spasticity
Anticholinesterase agents	Yes	No	C	Increase muscle tone

The musculoskeletal system is really two different systems that work closely together for body mobility and stability. The two systems include a sturdy collection of connective tissue, muscles, and bones to allow change of position and give the body height and form (Figures 23-1 and 23-2).

The muscular system includes muscles, which are slightly contracted at all times, and specialized connective tissue such as tendons and ligaments. Tendons connect muscle to bone, whereas ligaments are strong fibrous tissues binding bones together to facilitate motion. Muscles require electrical impulses from nerves for stimulation that cause muscle contraction and relaxation to produce movement; these actions are the basis on which muscle relaxants work with the peripheral and central nervous systems. Muscle relaxants relieve the pain of muscle spasms by relaxing muscle contractions. Several disease processes, among them myasthenia

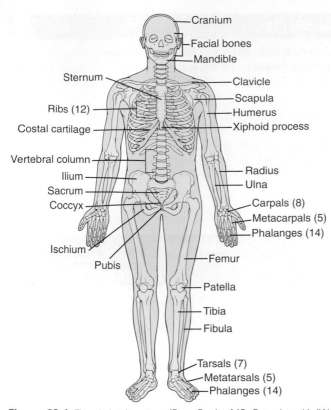

Figure 23-1 The skeletal system. (From Frazier MS, Drzymkowski JW: *Essentials of human diseases and conditions,* ed 4, St Louis, 2008, Saunders.)

gravis, fibromyalgia, muscle spasticity, multiple sclerosis, and spinal cord diseases or injuries, result in inability of muscles to contract and relax properly.

The skeletal system consists of bones that **articulate** in joints that are covered with cartilage to allow the body to be mobile and flexible. The capsule surrounding the joint, called a *bursa,* is lined with a synovial membrane filled with synovial fluid. Diseases of the joints are considered **arthritis** or **bursitis,** of which there are many different types. Bone mass reduction is called *osteoporosis.*

OSTEOPOROSIS AND MEDICATIONS FOR TREATMENT

Osteoporosis, a metabolic musculoskeletal disease, is characterized by a porous appearance of bone mass. In older adults, especially postmenopausal women, the resorption of existing bone begins to exceed formation of new bone, causing deterioration in bone mass and density. First signs of bone mass loss may be fractures without causative trauma. Most fractures occur in vertebrae, hips, and wrists, especially dorsal and lumbar vertebral fractures and thus leading to height loss, chronic back pain, and spinal deformities such as **kyphosis.** To prevent osteoporosis, adults need to maximize bone

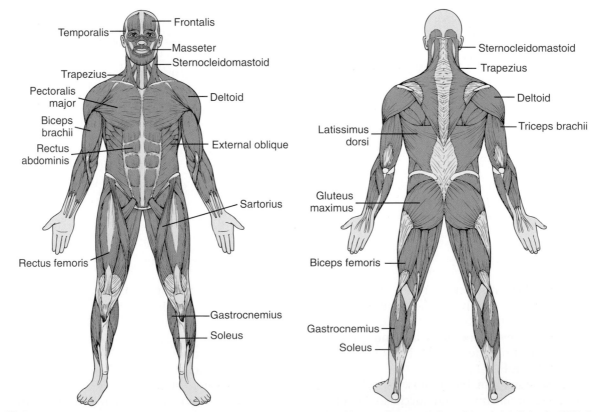

Figure 23-2 Muscles of the body. (From Frazier MS, Drzymkowski JW: *Essentials of human diseases and conditions,* ed 4, St Louis, 2008, Saunders.)

strength by ensuring sufficient intake of calcium and vitamin D throughout life and by promoting lifestyle measures such as regular exercise. Calcium may be obtained from milk and milk products or through calcium carbonate supplements such as Tums or Viactiv, an OTC chewable supplement in a candy-like form.

Medications include agents to decrease bone resorption and promote bone formation. Antiresorptives include bisphosphonates as preferred treatment and calcitonin for those who cannot tolerate bisphosphonates.

Estrogen therapy may be added, although this is not a Food and Drug Administration (FDA)–approved use (Table 23-1) and is not recommended for long-term therapy because of the increased risk of certain cancers, blood clots, and cardiovascular disease. Bisphosphonates are approved for osteoporosis and are safe for prevention of fractures. ***Alendronate*** (Fosamax) and ***risedronate*** (Actonel) are available in a weekly administration regimen, whereas ***ibandronate*** (Boniva) is administered monthly. For these medications to be

TABLE 23-1 MEDICATIONS USED TO PREVENT AND TREAT OSTEOPOROSIS

GENERIC/TRADE NAME	USUAL DOSE, ROUTE, AND FREQUENCY	INDICATIONS FOR USE	DRUG INTERACTIONS
RECOMBINANT PARATHYROID HORMONE		Osteoporosis	
teriparatide acetate (Forteo)	20 mcg SC qd		digoxin
Major Side Effects:			
Leg cramps, nausea, dizziness, headaches, orthostatic hypotension, tachycardia			
BISPHOSPHONATES			
alendronate (Fosamax*)	5-10 mg PO daily dose		Basically none
with vitamin D (Fosamax 70 + D)	1 tab PO weekly dose		
(Fosamax-70*)	70 mg PO weekly dose		Basically none
risedronate (Actonel)	5 mg PO daily dose or 35 mg PO weekly		Antacids, NSAIDs
ibandronate (Boniva)	150 mg PO monthly		Dietary supplements, antacids, NSAIDs
Boniva injection	3 mg IV q3mo		
etidronate (Didronal)	5-15 mg/kg PO qd		warfarin, calcium
pamidronate (Aredia)	15-90 mg IV		
Major Side Effects:			
alendronate—headache, GI symptoms; *risedronate*—arthralgia, rash; *ibandronate*—dysphagia, bone pain, heartburn, gastric ulcers, dyspepsia, chest pain, myalgia, numbness; *etidronate and pamidronate*—same as with other bisphosphonates			
CALCIUM PREPARATIONS		Osteoporosis	
calcitonin salmon (Miacalcin*)	1 spray in nostril qd		
calcium carbonate (Tums, Viactiv chews, Os-Cal-D†)	1000-1500 mg Ca qd		
SELECTIVE ESTROGEN RECEPTOR MODULATORS		Prevention and treatment of osteoporosis	
raloxifene (Evista)	60 mg PO qd		ampicillin, estrogen replacement preparations, anticoagulants
Major Side Effects of Selective Estrogen Receptor Modulators:			
Hot flashes, flulike symptoms, arthralgia, sinusitis, insomnia			

GI, Gastrointestinal; *IV,* intravenously; *NSAIDs,* nonsteroidal antiinflammatory drugs; *PO,* orally; *SC,* subcutaneously.
*Prescription medication.
†OTC medication.

effective, an adequate intake of calcium and vitamin D is necessary. Bisphosphonates should be taken on an empty stomach on arising, with 6 to 8 ounces of plain water; the patient should not lie down or eat for 30 to 60 minutes after administration.

To decrease bone resorption, *raloxifene* (Evista), a selective estrogen receptor modulator (pregnancy category X), is prescribed to both prevent and treat osteoporosis in postmenopausal women. It can be taken without regard to meals.

Calcitonin salmon nasal spray (Miacalcin), for treatment of osteoporosis and not a prophylactic agent, inhibits bone resorption to decrease bone loss. It is safe when sprayed into alternating nostrils daily.

Teriparatide (Forteo), a parathyroid hormone, has been approved to stimulate new bone formation (see Chapter 20).

Men are also treated for osteoporosis. The decline in bone mass in men begins at approximately age 50 and occurs at the same rate as in women. An exception in women is the accelerated rate of bone loss during menopause. The same drugs are used for treatment of men as for women, except testosterone is substituted for estrogen (see Table 23-1).

Patient Education for Compliance

1. Calcium preparations must have vitamin D (from sunlight or other sources) to be effective.
2. Bisphosphonates must be taken on an empty stomach with a full 8-oz glass of water at least 30 to 60 minutes before breakfast to be effective and may cause esophagitis if they become lodged in the esophagus. Patient should remain in an upright position for at least 30 to 60 minutes after administration.
3. Calcium carbonate, preferably with vitamin D, should be taken with or after meals to promote absorption.
4. Calcium and tetracycline should be taken at least 1 hour apart.
5. When using intranasal calcitonin salmon, nostrils should be alternated on a daily basis.

Important Facts about Drugs for Osteoporosis

- Preferred drugs for osteoporosis prevention are bisphosphonates.
- Calcitonin salmon mimics body chemicals to inhibit bone resorption.
- Calcitonin is safest drug for osteoporosis but is not as effective as bisphosphonates or as preventive as estrogens.

JOINT DISEASES AND THEIR TREATMENT

Arthritis is characterized by joint pain and limitation of joint movement. The most common type of arthritis is osteoarthritis, a degenerative noninflammatory disease that causes destruction of bones and joints from constant wear and tear. It has an insidious onset in large weight-bearing joints. Joint cartilage gradually becomes thinner and loses its ability to keep pace with the need for its replacement. The disease is characterized by dull, aching pain with joint soreness and stiffness with little limitation of movement. With disease progression, deformity may occur, with crepitus on movement, progressive loss of joint stability, decreased range of motion, and increased pain as bone enlarges and deforms the joint, necessitating joint replacement surgery in some instances (Figure 23-3).

Rheumatoid arthritis, an autoimmune disease, can manifest in numerous forms. Beginning with stiffness and fatigue and progressing to ankylosis or permanent joint fusion, it can be found in all age groups but usually peaks between ages 20 and 50. The condition of the joints becomes progressively worse; the joints become red, swollen, tender, and warm, with considerable pain and limitation of movement. Synovitis with resultant pannus formation also occurs, permitting tissue overgrowth, which eventually converts to scar tissue, causing joint stiffness. With prolonged illness, scar tissue replaces bony tissue and further ankylosis occurs. Replacement surgery may also be performed when joints are sufficiently deformed to prevent movement (Figure 23-4).

Bursitis, an inflammation of the bursa, occurs when the joint is traumatized, overused, or infected or when deposits of calcium accumulate. Common sites of bursitis are the shoulder, knee, and elbow; common signs are tenderness on movement and inability to flex or extend the joint. With chronic inflammation, calcification may occur in the affected joint.

No cure for arthritis currently exists, just alleviation of symptoms. Goals of arthritis therapy are threefold: (1) to relieve pain, inflammation, and stiffness; (2) to maintain joint function and range of motion; and (3) to prevent joint deformity. These objectives are achieved through physical therapy, surgery, and pharmacotherapy. Patient education must stress that excessive rest of a joint causes stiffness and that, conversely, excessive use causes intensification of inflammation and pain. Medications are only part of the necessary treatment with exercise therapy and surgery as needed.

Antiarthritic medications are used to treat all rheumatoid conditions and may be used for conditions such as osteoarthritis, inflammatory conditions, and other joint diseases. Medications such as corticosteroids (see Chapter 20) and analgesics (see Chapter 15) have already been discussed. More commonly used salicylates and

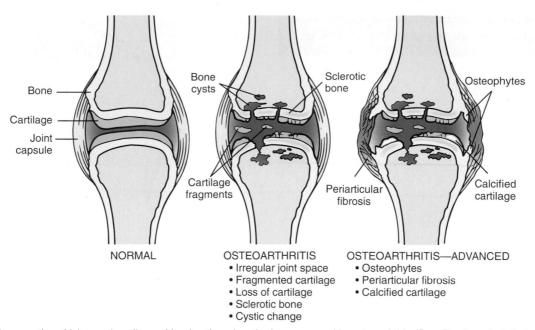

Figure 23-3 Degeneration of joints and cartilage with sclerotic and cystic changes caused by osteoarthritis. (From Damjanov I: *Pathology for the health professions*, ed 4, St Louis, 2012, Saunders.)

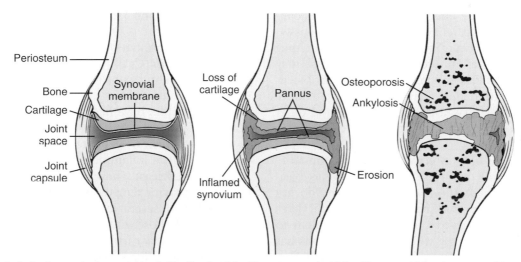

Figure 23-4 Pathologic changes in rheumatoid arthritis. The first joint illustrates a typical joint. The second joint shows synovitis and loss of articular space caused by pannus formation. The third joint is ankylosed owing to rheumatoid arthritis and osteoporosis. (From Damjanov I: *Pathology for the health professions*, ed 4, St Louis, 2012, Saunders.)

nonsteroidal antiinflammatory drugs (NSAIDs), which are not used primarily for analgesic effects, are briefly discussed here to assist in understanding their use as musculoskeletal agents. Antiarthritic medications, used for long-term symptomatic relief, may produce short-term disease remission. Rarely does remission continue, and eventually the disease becomes **exacerbated,** with further progression of symptoms and increased debilitation.

Antiarthritic medications usually fall into three major categories: NSAIDs, **disease-modifying antirheumatic drugs (DMARDs),** and glucocorticosteroids. NSAIDs may be further subdivided into **salicylate** and **nonsalicylate** medications. Safer than the other types of medications, these drugs give relief of symptoms but do not prevent disease progression. DMARDs, more toxic and with a slower onset of action, necessitate regular monitoring, but they do delay disease progression.

BOX 23-1 TYPICAL PROGRESSION OF MEDICATIONS FOR ARTHRITIS

Mild Symptoms
1. Salicylate NSAIDs (aspirin)
   ↓
2. Nonsalicylate NSAIDs (ibuprofen, naproxen)
   ↓
Moderate Symptoms
3. Add DMARDs
   ↓ ↑
   May be prescribed together
4. Glucocorticosteroids (short term)

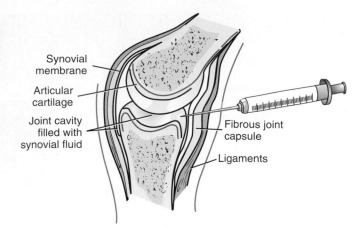

Figure 23-5 Intraarticular injections of glucocorticosteroids may be used with patients with inflammatory joint disease.

Glucocorticosteroids provide rapid symptom relief, do not prevent disease progression, and are toxic with long-term use. Therefore steroids are indicated only for short-term, acute therapy. Progression of therapeutic agents is found in Box 23-1. In some instances, NSAIDs and DMARDs are used together in an effort to delay joint degeneration.

Salicylate NSAIDs are effective, fast-acting, and, considering their ability to relieve symptoms, inexpensive. Their actions are generally antiinflammatory, but they also provide analgesia. Enteric-coated medications may reduce the chance of gastric symptoms and gastric bleeding. Medication compliance may be difficult to achieve because the patient may not believe ***aspirin*** and other OTC salicylates can be effective for arthritic symptoms (Table 23-2).

Nonsalicylate NSAIDs, effective as antiinflammatory and analgesic agents, are more expensive and act basically as salicylate medications do. Patients who do not respond to salicylates may respond to nonsalicylates and may respond better to one nonsalicylate than to another. Short-term therapy with these medications has less of a tendency to cause gastrointestinal (GI) upset; however, when used long-term, nonsalicylate NSAIDs may cause GI ulceration and should be taken with meals or food. At present, many of these medications are on the market to treat not only arthritis but bursitis and tendonitis. Patients who are hypersensitive to aspirin may be hypersensitive to these aspirin-like medications. Contrary to some patients' beliefs, ***acetaminophen*** (Tylenol), an analgesic, is *not* effective for inflammatory or arthritis-like symptoms. ***Meloxicam*** (Mobic), an antiinflammatory, analgesic, and antipyretic, is specific for osteoarthritis and should not be taken with other NSAIDs (see Table 23-2).

Late in 2010, a new group of drugs to relieve osteoarthritis, rheumatoid arthritis, and other musculoskeletal diseases such as **ankylosing spondylitis,** while decreasing the risk of development of gastric ulcers from NSAIDs, was introduced by combining medications for arthritis with proton pump inhibitors. The first medication in the group, available in two strengths, is ***naproxen*** combined with ***esomeprazole,*** a protein pump inhibitor (see Chapter 24 and Table 23-2).

Cyclooxygenase-2 (COX-2) inhibitors are used to suppress joint inflammation while causing minimal side effects. ***Celecoxib*** (Celebrex) is indicated for osteoarthritis and rheumatoid arthritis but should not be used by people with sulfa allergies (see Table 23-2). The other COX-2 inhibitors have been removed from the market because of the toxic cardiovascular effects.

Glucocorticosteroids (Chapter 16), powerful medications that reduce inflammatory responses, are useful in treating joint disease. These medications palliate arthritis but do not provide remission or halt disease progression. For people with several joints involved, oral steroids may be prescribed; those with only one or two joints involved may be given intraarticular medications with lower toxicity and greater effectiveness and that allow more dramatic increases in mobility (Figure 23-5). With steroids, joints that were previously immobile may become mobile; however, these medications should be reserved for short-term therapy in those who have not responded to other medications or for treatment of an exacerbation of the disease.

DMARDs are used with moderate to severe rheumatoid arthritis when NSAIDs have not been effective. These include gold salts, **immunosuppressant** agents, **immunomodulators,** and antimalarials. Many of these medications have black box warnings.

Gold salts are expensive but seem to reduce synovitis seen with rheumatoid diseases. Used since 1930 to relieve joint stiffness and pain, these medications may even halt progression of joint degeneration. They do not

TABLE 23-2 MEDICATIONS USED FOR JOINT CONDITIONS

GENERIC/TRADE NAME	USUAL DOSE, ROUTE, AND FREQUENCY	INDICATIONS FOR USE	DRUG INTERACTIONS
SALICYLATES		Antiinflammatory, analgesic agents for osteo- and rheumatoid arthritis	Antacids, corticosteroids, ACE inhibitors, beta blockers, methotrexate, anticoagulants, probenecid, sulfinpyrazone, sulfonylurea, alcohol, penicillin, naproxen, valproic acid, oral hypoglycemics, ibuprofen
aspirin (Ecotrin, Bayer, Bufferin*)	650 mg PO q4h		
choline magnesium salicylate (NTN)	3000 mg PO daily divided in 2-3 doses		
magnesium salicylate (Magan, Mobidin, Doan's Pills*)	tab ī PO q4h		
salsalate (NTN)	1000-1500 mg bid/qid		
NONSALICYLATES		Analgesic, antiarthritis, antiinflammatory	
diclofenac (Voltaren, Cataflam)	25-50 mg PO bid/qid		ACE inhibitors, lithium, warfarin, aminoglycosides
with misoprostol (Arthrotec)	50/200 mg PO tid		
diflunisal (Dolobid)	125-500 mg PO bid		digoxin, furosemide, methotrexate, warfarin
etodolac (NTN)	1200 mg PO divided bid/tid		
fenoprofen (Nalfon)	300-600 mg PO tid/qid		
flurbiprofen (Ansaid)	200-300 mg PO in 2-4 divided doses		
ibuprofen (Motrin*†, Rufen, Advil*†)	200-800 mg tid/qid (max 3200 mg/d)		
indomethacin (Indocin)	25-50 mg PO bid/tid	Gout and arthritic conditions	Not for use by children younger than age 14 years or pregnant or lactating women
ketoprofen (Orudis, plain and extended-release)	50-100 mg PO tid	Analgesic, anti-inflammatory, arthritis	See all above
meloxicam (Mobic)	15 mg PO qd		
nabumetone (NTN)	1000-2000 mg PO qd		
naproxen (Naprosyn†)	250-500 mg PO bid		
naproxen sodium (Anaprox, Aleve*)	275-550 mg PO bid		
	220-440 mg PO bid		
oxaprozin (Daypro)	600-1200 mg PO qd		
piroxicam (Feldene)	10-20 mg PO bid/qd		
sulindac (Clinoril)	150-200 mg PO bid		
tolmetin (NTN)	200-400 mg PO tid		

ACE, Angiotensin-converting enzyme; *COX,* cyclooxygenase; *ER,* extended release; *IA,* intraarticularly; *IM,* intramuscularly; *IV,* intravenously; *NSAIDs,* nonsteroidal antiinflammatory drugs; *PO,* orally; *PPI,* protein pump inhibitor; *RA,* rheumatoid arthritis; *SC,* subcutaneously.
*OTC medication.
†Prescription medication.

Continued

TABLE 23-2 MEDICATIONS USED FOR JOINT CONDITIONS—cont'd

GENERIC/TRADE NAME	USUAL DOSE, ROUTE, AND FREQUENCY	INDICATIONS FOR USE	DRUG INTERACTIONS
COX-2 INHIBITORS		Antiinflammatory, analgesic for arthritis	
celecoxib (Celebrex)	100-200 mg PO bid		lithium, cannot be used by persons allergic to sulfa medications
IMMUNOSUPPRESSANTS			
methotrexate (Rheumatrex)	7.5-20 mg PO, IM, IA, IV qwk	RA	Vaccines, NSAIDs, probenecid, sulfinpyrazone, trimethoprim-sulfamethoxazole
azathioprine (Imuran)	1-2.5 mg/kg PO qd		Allopurinol
TUMOR NECROSIS FACTOR INHIBITORS			
adalimumab (Humira)	40 mg SC q2wk	Moderate to severe RA	Live virus vaccines
infliximab (Remicade)	3-5 mg/kg IV q4-8wk		Live virus vaccines
certolizumab pegol (Cimzia)	200-400 mg SC q2-4wk		etanercept
golimunab (Simponi)	50 mg SC qmo		etanercept
INTERLEUKIN-6 INHIBITOR			
tocilizumab (Actemra)	4-8 mg/kg IV q4wk		etanercept
IMMUNOMODULATORS			
abatacept (Orencia)	500-1000 mg IV q2-4wk then qmo	Antirheumatic agent	Vaccines, corticosteroids
anakinra (Kineret)	100 mg SC qd	Moderate to severe RA	None
etanercept (Enbrel)	50 mg SC qwk	Osteoarthritis, RA	None
leflunomide (Arava)	20 mg PO qd	RA	methotrexate, rifampin
gold sodium thiomalate	10-50 mg IM q2wk	Antirheumatic, antiinflammatory	None noted
auranofin (Ridaura)	6 mg PO qd	RA	See literature
ANTIMALARIAL			
hydroxychloroquine (Plaquenil)	400-600 mg PO qd	RA	None noted
COMBINED NSAIDS AND PPIS			
naproxen + esomeprazole (Vimovo)	375 mg/20 mg bid	Osteoarthritis, RA	Similar to naproxen, esomeprazole separately
(Vimovo-ER)	500 mg/20 mg bid		
MISCELLANEOUS			
glucosamine chondroitin	1200-1500 mg PO	Natural supplement for arthritis	Possibly heparin
hyaluronate (Hyalgan)	Weekly × 3 or 5 IA	Osteoarthritis of knee	No other medications in knee

reverse any previous joint damage. Oral gold preparations cause fewer toxic effects, but when taken orally, gold preparations can cause GI distress (see Table 23-2).

Immunosuppressants, also used as antineoplastics, may be used therapeutically for rheumatoid conditions by reducing the autoimmune response to the body's own tissues. These agents have to be taken for several weeks to be effective. **Methotrexate** (Rheumatrex), also a chemotherapeutic agent (see Chapter 18), is the fastest acting of the DMARDs and is first choice in this group.

Immunomodulators are used to alter immune response to inhibit production of antibodies in response to an antigen and therefore have many black box warnings against such diseases as tuberculosis, human immunodeficiency virus (HIV), and fungal disorders. **Abatacept** (Orencia), **etanercept** (Enbrel), and **adalimumab** (Humira) are typical of these drugs.

Tumor necrosis factor (TNF) inhibitors are a rapidly increasing group of medications that are used to block the immune response in autoimmune diseases such as rheumatoid arthritis. Because the immune system is suppressed, the danger of use of these drugs is infections, either acute or chronic. **Infliximab** (Remicade), a typical drug, is administered intravenously with methotrexate for rheumatoid arthritis therapy. **Certolizumab** (Cimzia) and **golimumab** (Simponi) may be administered by the patient using the route established by the physician. These drugs may be administered with DMARDs and methotrexate (see Table 23-2).

LEARNING TIP

Many TNF inhibitors end in "mab".

CLINICAL TIP

Patients starting most immunomodulators and TFN inhibitors should have a tuberculin skin test as a base-line before treatment.

Antimalarials, such as **hydroxychloroquine** (Plaquenil), may produce remission of rheumatoid arthritis but are usually reserved for patients who have not responded to other antiarthritic treatment. Several months may be required to produce a therapeutic effect, and NSAIDs should be used during this interval.

Other miscellaneous medications used for joint conditions such as arthritis include **penicillamine** (Cuprimine), which can produce remission of rheumatoid arthritis. It should not be used unless arthritis does not respond to more conventional therapy. With a slow onset of action, the drug may not produce therapeutic effects for several months. **Glucosamine chondroitin,** a combination of glucosamine (a form of amino sugar) and chondroitin (a large protein molecule), is not available by prescription but rather is considered a nutritional supplement. Glucosamine is extracted from crab, lobster, and shrimp shells, whereas chondroitin is from animal cartilage. Effectiveness has not been determined, although studies have shown pain relief at NSAID level, but cartilage damage from osteoarthritis may be slowed. Because glucosamine is an amino sugar, persons with diabetes mellitus should check blood sugar levels more frequently. Combined with anticoagulant agents, chondroitin may cause bleeding because this supplement is similar in chemical structure to **heparin** (see Table 23-2).

Patient Education for Compliance

1. In susceptible persons, salicylates may cause asthma attacks.
2. Many nonsalicylate nonsteroidal antiinflammatory drugs (NSAIDs) may not be taken with aspirin because of the similarity of the drug after metabolism. The patient should be told which drugs may or may not be taken together.
3. Patients taking **diclofenac** (Voltaren) should undergo liver function tests regularly and should report any signs of jaundice, nausea, or fatigue.
4. Because of their antiinflammatory or analgesic properties, NSAIDs may mask signs of infection.
5. Ibuprofen (Motrin) may cause visual problems, including diminished vision and changes in visual color.
6. NSAIDs should be taken with food, milk, or a full glass of water to reduce gastric upset. Alcohol should not be consumed with NSAIDs because of the increased risk of gastrointestinal bleeding.

Important Facts about Medications for Joint Disorders

- Three objectives of arthritis therapy are to reduce pain, inflammation, and stiffness; to prevent joint deformity; and to maintain joint function.
- Three classes of drugs are used to treat rheumatoid conditions: nonsteroidal antiinflammatory drugs (NSAIDs), disease-modifying antirheumatic drugs (DMARDs), and glucocorticosteroids.
- NSAIDs suppress inflammation and relieve mild to moderate pain found with rheumatoid disease.
- NSAIDs and steroids quickly relieve symptoms of arthritis, whereas DMARDs take longer.
- NSAIDs and steroids do not slow progression of rheumatoid diseases, but DMARDs slow progression.
- Aspirin is the least expensive treatment for arthritis, but it is associated with gastrointestinal distress when taken over a prolonged period of time.
- Nonsalicylate NSAIDs are more expensive than salicylates.

GOUTY ARTHRITIS

Gouty arthritis, or gout, is associated with an inborn error in uric acid metabolism, a byproduct of **purine** metabolism, causing **hyperuricemia.** With gout, uric acid accumulates and crystals are deposited in tissues and joints, producing acute pain, swelling, redness, warmth, and tenderness of joints, especially of the big toe, ankle, instep, knee, and elbow. Treatment goals are to end the attack as soon as possible, prevent recurrence of the acute condition, and decrease the possibility of

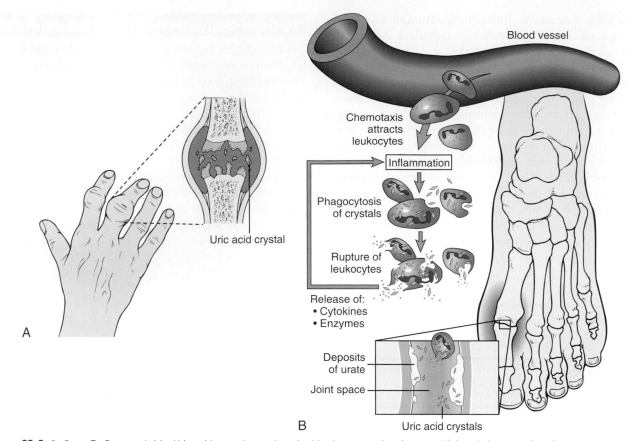

Blood vessel

Chemotaxis attracts leukocytes

Inflammation

Phagocytosis of crystals

Rupture of leukocytes

Release of:
• Cytokines
• Enzymes

Uric acid crystal

Deposits of urate

Joint space

A

B

Uric acid crystals

Figure 23-6 A, Gout. **B,** Gouty arthritis. Uric acid crystals are deposited in the connective tissue and joints. It is most often found in the joint of the great toe. (A from Frazier MS, Drzymkowski JW: *Essentials of human diseases and conditions,* ed 4, St Louis, 2008, Saunders; B from Damjanov I: *Pathology for the health professions,* ed 4, St Louis, 2012, Saunders.)

complications. Patient education includes giving specific information about avoiding foods high in purines, such as oatmeal, cheese, red meat, tomatoes, alcohol, shellfish, and fatty foods (Figure 23-6).

Medications used to treat acute gout include colchicine, NSAIDs, corticosteroids, and *febuxostat* (Uloric), approved in 2009. A derivative of the autumn crocus, *colchicine* is not an analgesic but an antiinflammatory agent specific for gout. It is ineffective for any other disease and is used to treat acute attacks, to reduce incidence of chronic gout attacks, and to abort a possible attack. It should be used with care by older patients because of dangers of GI, renal, hepatic, and cardiac diseases. For chronic gout symptoms, *allopurinol* (Aloprim or Zyloprim), *probenecid* (Benemid), and *sulfinpyrazone* (Anturane) decrease uric acid production and are indicated in prophylaxis and treatment of chronic gouty arthritis. Probenecid has no antiinflammatory or analgesic effects and cannot be given during an acute gout attack and may even precipitate an acute attack at initiation of medication therapy. Sulfinpyrazone (Anturane) is used for chronic gout attacks. Febuxostat (Urolic) is specific for hyperuricemia, with major side effects being liver function abnormalities, nausea, joint pain, and rashes. Urolic, a *xanthine* oxidase inhibitor, is used for chronic management of hyperuricemia of gout. This drug acts by lowering serum uric acid levels but may initially increase gout flares. These flares may require the initial concurrent use of NSAIDs or colchicine. A new medication, *pegloticase* (Krystexxa), is a biological agent for the treatment of chronic gout for persons who have not responded to conventional gout medications. It may produce a gout flare in some persons so use of colchicine or an NSAID should be given for 7 days before treatment (Table 23-3).

Important Facts about Medications for Gout

• Colchicine is a gout-specific antiinflammatory and is not an analgesic, so it does not relieve pain of gout.
• Allopurinol reduces blood uric acid levels and may be used as prophylaxis for gout.
• Probenecid is used for relief of symptoms from chronic gouty arthritis conditions.
• Febuxostat and pegloticase are specific drugs for chronic gout.
• Pegloticase is the first biological agent specific for gout.

TABLE 23-3 ANTIGOUT AGENTS

GENERIC/ TRADE NAME	USUAL DOSE, ROUTE, AND FREQUENCY	INDICATIONS FOR USE	DRUG INTERACTIONS
colchicine (Colcrys)	0.5-0.6 mg/day PO prophylactically; 0.5-1.2 mg PO q2h for acute attack	Gout	None noted
allopurinol (Zyloprim)	200-800 mg PO qd		Anticoagulants
probenecid (NTN)	250-500 mg PO bid		indomethacin and other NSAIDS, aspirin and other salicylates, heparin
febuxostat (Uloric)	40-80 mg PO qd	Hyperuricemia	azathioprine, mercaptopurine, or theophylline
pegloticase (Krystexxa)	8 mg IV q2wk	Chronic gout	None noted

NSAIDs, Nonsteroidal antiinflammatory drugs; *TNT,* no trade name; *PO,* orally.

DISEASES INVOLVING MUSCLES

When the central nervous system neuromuscular junction has interruptions in normal transmission of nerve stimuli, skeletal **muscle spasms** and **muscle spasticity** occur.

Skeletal muscle spasms cause pain with a decreased level of functioning. Most muscle spasms are caused by local injury, but others may result from mineral deficiencies or diseases that cause seizures. Each spasm must be treated according to its cause. Skeletal muscle injuries are usually self-limiting and are treated with rest, physical therapy, and possibly antiinflammatory medications. Centrally acting skeletal muscle relaxants are used for spasms that do not respond quickly to other therapy, but these agents are not always effective.

The exact way centrally acting skeletal muscle relaxants, such as **carisoprodol** (Soma), **methocarbamol** (Robaxin), and **tizanidine** (Zanaflex), work is not completely understood. They are used to treat localized spasms resulting from muscle injury by decreasing local pain and tenderness, increasing range of motion, and causing sedation. No studies have shown that one medication is better than others or whether these muscle relaxants are more effective than NSAIDs and other analgesic antiinflammatory agents. Choice of a medication is usually determined by physician's preference and patient response to medication.

Diazepam (Valium) and **baclofen** (Lioresal) are the only medications that are effective as central muscle relaxants and for muscle spasticity caused by neuromuscular disorders (Table 23-4).

Patient Education for Compliance

1. Skeletal muscle relaxants cause central nervous system depression, so hazardous activities such as driving should be avoided until the patient can evaluate the effects of the medication.
2. Effects of opioids and other analgesics are intensified by skeletal muscle relaxants.
3. Alcohol should be avoided when taking skeletal muscle relaxants because of synergistic actions.

Important Facts about Skeletal Muscle Relaxants

- Skeletal muscle relaxants give relief for muscle injuries, but a side effect is depression of the central nervous system.
- Skeletal muscle relaxants are chosen according to physician's preference and patient response, as effectiveness of drugs seems to be the same.
- Diazepam (Valium) and baclofen (Lioresal) are the only centrally acting muscle relaxants useful with spasticity from neuromuscular diseases and other muscular conditions such as localized muscle spasms.

Diseases with Muscle Spasticity

Muscle spasticity is caused by muscle stimulation from either the spinal cord or the brain in patients with central nervous system injuries or strokes, as well as in diseases such as multiple sclerosis and cerebral palsy. Centrally acting and direct-acting muscle relaxants, accompanied by physical therapy, are the drugs of choice

TABLE 23-4 MEDICATIONS USED TO TREAT MUSCLE DISORDERS AND MISCELLANEOUS DISORDERS

GENERIC/TRADE NAME	USUAL DOSE, ROUTE, AND FRREQUENCY	INDICATIONS FOR USE	DRUG INTERACTIONS
CENTRALLY ACTING MUSCLE RELAXANTS		Muscle spasms and muscle spasticity	Other CNS depressants and MAOIs
baclofen (Lioresal)	15-20 mg PO tid		
carisoprodol (Soma)	350 mg PO tid-qhs		
chlorzoxazone (Paraflex, Parafon Forte, Remular-S)	250-500 mg PO tid-qid		
cyclobenzaprine (Flexeril)	10 mg PO tid		
diazepam (Valium, Zetran)	2-10 mg PO, IM, IV	May also be used as a peripheral muscle relaxant	
metaxalone (Skelaxin)	800 mg PO tid-qid		
methocarbamol (Robaxin)	1000 mg PO qid		
tizanidine (Zanaflex)	4-8 mg PO bid-tid		CNS depressants, phenytoin, alcohol, antihypertensives
orphenadrine (Norflex)	60 mg IM q12h; 100 mg PO bid		
dantrolene (Dantrium)	25-100 mg PO, IV qid		
CHOLINESTERASE INHIBITORS			
ambenonium (Mytelase)	5-25 mg PO tid-qid	Myasthenia gravis	
neostigmine (Prostigmin)	150 mg PO in divided doses		
pyridostigmine (Mestinon)	600 mg PO daily in divded doses; 2 mg IM, IV q2-3h		
ER tabs	180-540 mg PO qd-bid		
MISCELLANEOUS MEDICATIONS			
milnacipran (Savella)	50-100 mg PO bid	Fibromyalgia	SNRIs and SSRIs, clonidine

Major Side Effects: constipation, hot flashes, hyperhidrosis, vomiting, palpitations, increased heart rate, dry mouth, hypertension; suicidal tendencies, increased depression

CNS, central nervous system; *ER*, extended release; *IM*, intramuscularly; *IV*, intravenously; *MAOI*, monoamine oxidase inhibitor; *PO*, orally; *SNRI*, serotonin-norepinephrine reuptake inhibitor; *SSRI*, selective serotonin reuptake inhibitor.

for relief of muscle spasticity. **Diazepam** (Valium) and **dantrolene** (Dantrium) are drugs of choice as peripheral or direct-acting skeletal muscle relaxants (see Table 23-4).

Myasthenia gravis, characterized by skeletal muscle weakness and fatigue, is a progressive, incurable auto-immune disease caused by loss of acetylcholine receptors that block spinal cord nerve stimulation to prevent muscles from overresponding to stimuli. Cholinesterase-inhibiting agents such as **neostigmine** (Prostigmine) and **pyridostigmine** (Mestinon) block cholinesterase and allow acetylcholine to accumulate, increasing muscle strength and function. Dosages of these medications vary greatly based on disease severity (see Table 23-4).

Patient Education for Compliance

1. For evaluation of drug effectiveness as treatment progresses, patients taking medications for myasthenia gravis should record time medications are taken and when signs and symptoms recur after medication administration.
2. Cholinesterase inhibitor dosage for myasthenia gravis is variable and lifelong. Patients must be taught to recognize the need for more or less medication and to adjust dosage as needed.

Important Facts about Medications for Muscle Spasticity

- Spasticity is treated with four medications: baclofen (Lioresal), diazepam (Valium), tizanidine (Zanaflex), or dantrolene (Dantrium).
- Myasthenia gravis is treated with cholinesterase inhibitors to increase muscle strength.

Fibromyalgia

Fibromyalgia is a painful, debilitating syndrome that causes chronic pain in muscles and soft tissues surrounding joints. Symptoms include aching of muscles throughout the body, stiffness, fatigue, disturbed sleep, depression, and specific tender points that are indicative of the syndrome. Excessive stimulation by bright lights, odors, and loud noises makes symptoms worse. Treatment includes NSAIDs (see Table 23-2), analgesics such as *pregabalin* (Lyrica), and physical therapy.

SUMMARY

The musculoskeletal system is composed of two distinct systems that are often discussed together because of their interdependency, which allows the body to remain upright and provides mobility. Daily wear and tear on these systems takes its toll, and disease processes such as arthritis and muscle injuries become more prevalent with aging. Also, softening and decrease in bone mass (osteoporosis) may occur, especially in postmenopausal women. The treatment of osteoporosis centers on increasing bone mass. Bisphosphonates are drugs specific for osteoporosis. For therapy to be successful, vitamin D and calcium must also be present.

Pain, a common symptom of all musculoskeletal conditions, is treated on a short-term basis for acute conditions or on a long-term basis for the person with chronic lifelong arthritic conditions. NSAIDs and DMARDs are used to treat arthritic conditions. NSAIDs may be changed based on patient tolerance. DMARDs are more toxic and are used as rheumatoid symptoms increase, although some therapeutic protocols suggest using these medications early in the disease process to prevent deformities of joints. A new group of drugs, TFN inhibitors, are used for moderate to severe rheumatoid arthritis by blocking the immune response to prevent inflammatory responses in joints. The natural OTC supplements glucosamine and chondroitin are used for osteoarthritis.

Gout is a painful joint inflammatory condition caused by hyperuricemia. Colchicine is specific for acute gout attacks; other medications may be given long term to decrease uric acid production. All antigout medications tend to cause GI distress. The first biological agent to treat chronic gout is pegloticase.

Skeletal muscle spasms and spasticity may occur from muscle injury or from such diseases as multiple sclerosis, strokes, or cerebral palsy. These conditions may be treated with centrally acting or peripherally acting muscle relaxants, which tend to decrease pain and tenderness and increase range of motion. Patients taking muscle relaxants should be warned against engaging in hazardous activities because of possible central nervous system depression.

Myasthenia gravis, a progressive, incurable disease related to the diminished release of acetylcholine or the excessive release of cholinesterase, is treated with neuromuscular blocking agents or cholinesterase inhibitors to increase muscle strength and reduce muscle flaccidity. Dosage of these drugs varies greatly and depends on level of the disease.

Fibromyalgia, a painful disease that causes lethargy and fatigue, is treated with physical therapy, NSAIDs, and analgesics such as pregabalin.

CRITICAL THINKING EXERCISES

Scenario

Mr. Quan has been diagnosed with osteoarthritis and has been taking aspirin, but he believes there must be a better product for his condition and the pain.

1. What do you tell him about aspirin therapy for osteoarthritis?
2. Mr. Quan returns to the office 2 months later complaining of ringing in his ears and stomach pain. What suspicions come to mind?
3. What suggestions can you give Mr. Quan to relieve the stomach discomforts caused by the NSAID now prescribed?
4. If he wants to take aspirin now that the ringing has stopped, what type of aspirin would you expect the physician to suggest?

DRUG CALCULATIONS

1. Order: dexamethasone 6 mg IM
   Available medication:

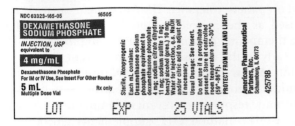

2. Order: indomethacin 50 mg
   Available medication:

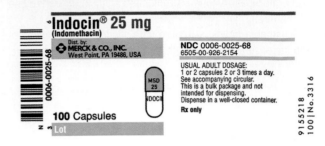

Dose to be given: _____
Show the amount on the syringe below.

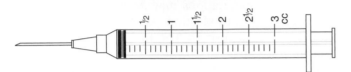

Dose to be given: _____

REVIEW QUESTIONS

1. What are the specific preferred drugs for osteoporosis? Gouty arthritis? _____
   _____
   _____

2. What are the three types of medications used to treat arthritic symptoms? Which are usually used first? Which are fast acting? Which are the slowest? _____
   _____
   _____
   _____
   _____

3. What are some of the side effects of aspirin or salicylate therapy? _____
   _____
   _____

4. Why is it safer to use steroid preparations intraarticularly than systemically? _____
   _____
   _____

5. How do immunosuppressants work in the treatment of arthritis? What are their dangers? _____
   _____
   _____

6. How do gold preparations have therapeutic effect in arthritis therapy? _____
   _____
   _____

7. Why would a medication for hyperuricemia be important in the treatment of gout? _____

_____

_____

8. What symptoms do skeletal muscle relaxants relieve? _____

_____

_____

CHAPTER 24

Gastrointestinal System Disorders

After studying this chapter, you should be capable of doing the following:

- Describing how medications move through the gastrointestinal (GI) tract to be absorbed for the body's use.
- Discussing medications used for prophylaxis in mouth and tooth disorders and as therapeutics for mouth diseases.
- Explaining actions of medications used for stomach and gallbladder conditions.
- Describing agents used for treatment of hepatitis B and C.
- Describing actions of pancreatic enzymes, antiflatulents, antidiarrheals, carminatives, cathartics, and laxatives.

- Describing how antiinflammatory agents are used with large bowel conditions.
- Discussing preparations used for anorectal disorders.
- Explaining proper choice and use of medications for intestinal parasites, including the needed prophylaxis to prevent recurrence.
- Discussing drugs used for appetite suppression and their side effects.
- Providing patient education for compliance with medications used to treat diseases and conditions of the gastrointestinal system.

Kim is flying to Europe in 2 weeks. She has had motion sickness on previous air trips and does not want to be nauseated on this long flight. She asks Dr. Merry if there is a medication she can take to prevent nausea.

What medications could Dr. Merry prescribe?
Can Kim expect these drugs to make her sleepy?
Are all these medications taken by mouth, or are other methods available? (Do not consider injections.)

Acid rebound	**Antispasmodics**	**Effervescence**	**Masticate**
Adsorbent	**Antiviral**	**Emesis**	**Palliative**
Anorectal	**Astringent**	**Expectorate**	**Peristalsis**
Anthelmintics	**Caries**	**Gastroesophageal**	**Prokinetic agent**
Anticholinergics	**Carminative**	reflux disease	**Proton pump**
Antidiarrheal	**Cathartics**	(GERD)	**Regurgitation**
Antiemetic	**Cholelithiasis**	**Gingivitis**	**Stomatitis**
Antiflatulent	**Defecation**	**Halitosis**	**Ulcer**
Antisecretory agent	**Dentifrice**	**Laxative**	**Viscosity**
Antiseptic	**Diaphoresis**	**Magaldrate**	

EASY WORKING KNOWLEDGE OF INDICATIONS AND SIDE EFFECTS

Common Symptoms of Gastrointestinal Disorders
Loss of appetite and weight loss
Abdominal pain
Nausea and vomiting
Change in bowel habits (diarrhea, constipation)
Flatulence
Blood or mucus in feces
Fever
Heartburn, indigestion, difficulty swallowing
Diaphoresis

Common Side Effects of Gastrointestinal Medications
Antacids
Constipation or diarrhea
Electrolyte imbalances

Laxatives
Electrolyte imbalances
Habituation

Other Gastrointestinal Medications
Headache, dizziness, confusion, vertigo, drowsiness
Rash
Abdominal pain or cramping
Diarrhea or constipation
Blurred vision
Dry mouth

EASY WORKING KNOWLEDGE OF DRUGS USED FOR GASTROINTESTINAL CONDITIONS

DRUG CLASS	PRESCRIPTION	OTC	PREGNANCY CATEGORY	MAJOR INDICATIONS
Oral preparations				
Mouthwashes, gargles	Yes	Yes		Antiseptic and anesthetic
Fluoride preparations	Yes	Yes		Fluoridating agents
Oral antifungals	Yes	No	B, C	Oropharyngeal candidiasis
Saliva substitutes	No	Yes		Replace salivary secretions
Oral antiviral agents	Yes	Yes	B, C	Herpes simplex infections
Oral topical anesthetics	Yes	Yes	C	Mouth lesions and irritations
Antacids and related drugs	Yes	Yes	B (sucralfate), C	Reduce gastric acids
Antiulcer and GERD agents				
Antibiotics	Yes	No	B	Treat *Helicobacter pylori*
Anticholinergic agents	Yes	No	C	Treat ulcers by reducing secretions
H$_2$-receptor antagonists	Yes	Yes	B, C	Treat ulcers and GERD by blocking histamine
Proton or gastric pump inhibitors	Yes	Yes	B, C	Inhibit gastric secretions and protect gastric mucosa
Prostaglandin analogues	Yes	No	X	Inhibit gastric secretions and protect gastric mucosa
Antispasmodics	Yes	No	B, C	Reduce gastric spasm and slow gastric motility
Prokinetic agents	Yes	No	C	GI stimulant
Hepatitis B and C agents	Yes	No	C	Treat hepatitis B and C
Pancreatic enzymes	Yes	No	C	Pancreatic enzyme replacement
Gallstone solubilizing agents	Yes	No	B (ursodiol)	Dissolve gallstones
Antiemetics	Yes	Yes	B, C	Stop vomiting

GERD, Gastroesophageal reflux disease; *GI*, gastrointestinal.

Continued

EASY WORKING KNOWLEDGE OF DRUGS USED FOR GASTROINTESTINAL CONDITIONS—cont'd

DRUG CLASS	PRESCRIPTION	OTC	PREGNANCY CATEGORY	MAJOR INDICATIONS
Agents for large intestines				
Antiflatulents	No	Yes	C	Relief of GI gas
Laxatives, cathartics	Yes	Yes	C, X (castor oil)	Relief of constipation and in preparation for gastric diagnostic testing
Antidiarrheals	Yes	Yes	B, C, D (Pepto-Bismol)	Relieve symptoms of diarrhea
GI antiinflammatories	Yes	No	B, C	Inflammatory and irritative colon disorders
Anorectal preparations	Yes	Yes	C	Rectal fissures and hemorrhoids
Antiinfectives, anthelmintics	Yes	Yes	C	Intestinal parasites
Anorexiants	Yes	Yes	B, C, X	Appetite suppression and weight loss

Some medications discussed in this chapter are easily recognized over-the-counter (OTC) drugs used daily for such common disorders as gastritis, indigestion, and constipation. Many drugs relieve symptoms rather than control or cure gastrointestinal (GI) tract diseases or disorders. These same medications may cause electrolyte imbalances when absorbed systemically.

GASTROINTESTINAL SYSTEM AND HOW DRUGS ACT

The process of converting food into chemical substances that can be used by the body, primary digestion, begins with intake of large food particles to be chewed (or **masticated**) then broken down by saliva in the mouth to complex molecules that can be absorbed and used by the body. Once swallowed, the bolus of food mixes with enzymes and other fluids from the gastric mucosa to be further broken down and digested by churning action into a semisolid mixture called chyme. **Peristalsis** moves chyme through the stomach toward the pyloric sphincter. If the mixture passes through the stomach too slowly, the rate at which nutrients are digested and absorbed is diminished; if the mixture passes too rapidly, gastric juices are not allowed to mix and the food's absorbability may be decreased. Passage of chyme into the small intestine is the first step in nutrient absorption by villi. Accessory organs—gallbladder, liver, and pancreas—add secretions of mucus and enzymes to further aid in the breakdown of food substances for use. Residue from digestion passes into the large intestine, where digestion does not continue; rather, the large intestine absorbs

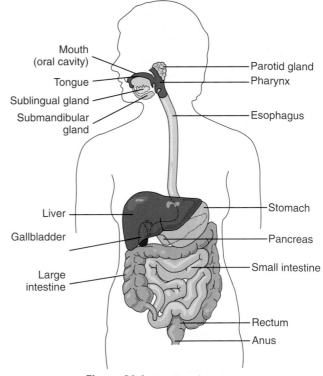

Figure 24-1 The digestive system.

electrolytes and excess fluids to maintain fluid balance. Remaining residue becomes fecal material and is pushed to the rectum for expulsion from the body. The digestion process is also important for breakdown and absorption of medications (Figure 24-1).

Many drugs for GI disorders work in three ways on muscular tissue and glandular tissue either directly or through the influence of the autonomic nervous system: (1) increase or decrease function of the GI tract by changing muscle tone, and change secretions of or into the GI tract; (2) increase or decrease emptying time as food passes through the stomach, or change the rate of peristalsis; or (3) replace enzyme deficiencies. Through these actions, medications counteract hyperacidity or flatulence, induce or prevent vomiting, and help the GI tract diagnose disorders (e.g., agents used in radiology). Oral medications and agents, including anesthetics, are also used for the GI tract, including drugs for parasites and antibiotics.

DRUGS USED IN THE MOUTH

Good oral hygiene is essential in maintaining homeostasis. Trauma, nutritional deficiencies, chemotherapy, infections, and dental disorders may cause mouth disorders, and systemic diseases may cause stomatitis. Symptoms such as blistering of the tongue and mucous membranes of the mouth and gums, as well as mouth pain and inflammation, may occur. Most systemic medications generally have little oral effect, but systemic drugs may be administered buccally or through oral cavity mucous membranes.

Agents Used for Mouth Conditions

Most oral agents are OTC preparations used to relieve sore gums and remove plaque (e.g., mouthwashes), lip balms, and agents to treat toothaches, gingivitis, or gum irritation from dental appliance irritation. These products should be used only as adjunctive care to proper brushing and flossing of teeth.

The American Dental Association classifies mouth rinses as follows:

1. Anesthetics, such as Chloraseptic, or antibacterials, such as Peridex, to be used twice a day.
2. Cosmetics, such as Lavoris and Scope, used as often as needed to mask mouth odors.
3. Fluorides, such as Reach with fluoride, used daily to prevent caries.
4. Oxygenating agents, such as Permax and Peroxyl, used to loosen debris in inaccessible mouth areas.
5. Phenolic compounds, such as Listerine, are antibacterial, and prebrushing rinses, such as Plax, aid in the removal of plaque.

Mouthwashes, such as those containing **alcohol** (Cepacol and Listermint), are used for halitosis and as gargles for sore throats. Gum and mouth diseases, the most common cause of halitosis, cannot be treated with mouthwashes. Sore throats are usually caused by bacterial or viral infections, and gargling with mouthwash cannot reach the infection site, which most often is deep in the throat.

Topical anesthetic agents may be used for temporary relief of oral lesions while proper treatment for a systemic disease or condition becomes effective. Adults who have gum irritation caused by dental appliances and teething infants may use these **phenol** or topical anesthetic preparations for relief. Topical anesthetics come in gels, ointments, aerosol sprays, and rinses. Lozenges, pastes, and film-forming gels are formulated for prolonged pain relief. OTC lozenges and sprays such as benzocaine-containing anesthetics (e.g., Chloraseptic or Spec-T) may also be used for oral pain and sore throats.

Hydrogen peroxide, an oxygenating agent and a weak antibacterial agent, works by effervescence to loosen tissue debris and reduce bacteria orally. Rinses such as OxyGel are available for oral irritations, and a gel (Peroxyl), available for minor mouth irritation, is applied, allowed to work, and then expectorated after use. These agents should not be swallowed.

Fluoride products are available in the form of mouthwashes, toothpaste, tablets, and solutions to prevent dental caries by hardening tooth enamel. Mouthwashes should be used for a 1-minute gargle daily after brushing teeth. Nothing should be taken by mouth for 30 minutes after use. Fluoride products, as tablets and drops, are used by children for the prevention of dental caries in areas where water is not adequately fluorinated.

Dentifrices, or toothpastes, are mild abrasives with a foaming agent and flavorings, in paste, gel, or powder form, to clean teeth and reduce most plaque buildup with daily use. Many types of toothpaste have fluoride added for daily **fluorine** contact. Some dentifrices for hypersensitive teeth contain **potassium nitrate** as a desensitizing ingredient to reduce the pain associated with heat or cold.

Whitening agents containing **carbamide peroxide** are OTC products used to bleach teeth discolored by tobacco, coffee, tea, alcohol, and the like. These agents should be used according to manufacturers' directions to prevent permanent tooth damage.

Oral antifungals (see Chapter 17) such as **clotrimazole** (Mycelex lozenges) and **ketoconazole** (Nizoral) are used for oropharyngeal candidiasis (thrush). Lozenges should be dissolved, not chewed, to ensure coverage of the affected area during a 15- to 30-minute period. These medications bind to the oral mucosa and remain for therapeutic action for up to 3 hours.

Saliva replacements are natural therapeutics to be used when saliva is absent or secretions are minimal. Water is frequently used but is a poor substitute because it lacks ions and lubricants needed. Artificial saliva products have chemical and physical properties that are similar to those of saliva and are cellulose derivatives with flavoring agents and antibacterials included to increase **viscosity.** Most saliva products come in sprays, although lozenges are available. Agents must be administered repeatedly throughout the day to be prophylactically effective; they may also be used therapeutically in chronically ill persons who need mouth moisture.

Antivirals may be prescribed for either systemic or local use for oral viral infections. Treatment is **palliative** for herpes zoster and herpes simplex infections, varicella, and HIV lesions. One topical medication, ***docosanol*** (Abreva), has been approved by the Food and Drug Administration (FDA) for OTC use. ***Acyclovir*** (Zovirax) is used for symptomatic relief of oral mucosal shedding, local pain, and encrusted lesions caused by these diseases (see Chapter 17). To prevent disease spread, care should be taken to avoid contact with lesions while treatment is in progress (Table 24-1).

Patient Education for Compliance

1. Local topical anesthetics are only temporary relief agents for toothaches, lesions from ill-fitting dentures, or disease. Care should be taken with oral topical anesthetics to prevent injury to local tissues because of loss of sensation. Patients using topical oral anesthetics should not eat or drink while mouth and throat are desensitized.
2. If stored in a glass container, fluoride drops may cause etching of glass.
3. Following use of fluoride products, food and drink should be avoided for 30 minutes.
4. Dentifrices, if used once a day, should be used at night to reduce buildup of plaque. Dentifrices with fluoride added are helpful in caries prevention.
5. Directions on whitening agents should be followed to prevent tooth damage.

Important Facts about Oral Preparations

- Many oral preparations are OTC medications used to relieve mouth lesions caused by local or systemic diseases. Good oral hygiene is essential to prevent oral lesions and maintain homeostasis.
- Fluoride products are used in areas where water fluoridation is not adequate to protect teeth.

DRUGS USED FOR GASTRIC CONDITIONS

As food enters the stomach, it is mixed with hydrochloric acid and the enzymes pepsin, rennin, and lipase in the stomach's acidic environment. Sometimes the acid becomes so strong that it actually eats away the stomach wall. Stress and anxiety seem to increase the stomach secretions, causing **ulcers** and sloughing of gastric tissue.

Antiulcer medications fall into five distinct categories: antacids, mucosal protectants (forming barriers to ulcers), antibiotics, anticholinergic **(antisecretory) agents,** and **antispasmodics** to reduce pain and progression of gastric ulcers. However, antibiotics together with antisecretory agents and **proton pump** inhibitors (PPIs) work to eradicate the microorganism *Helicobacter pylori* while also reestablishing an intact stomach lining through neutralization of hydrochloric acid.

Because of ready availability, OTC medications, including antisecretory medications, are often the first-used therapeutic agents for gastric conditions. These agents relieve the burning sensation (heartburn) that occurs with acid reflux into the esophagus. If therapy is not started during the early stages of gastric discomfort, peptic ulcers may occur, making treatment more difficult.

Antacids, alkaline compounds used to neutralize hydrochloric acid, are mainstays of peptic ulcer therapy. Newer medications are available as prophylaxis for stress-induced ulcers and to relieve symptoms of **gastroesophageal reflux disease (GERD)** by neutralizing acid to protect the intestinal mucosa. With the exception of ***sodium bicarbonate*** (baking soda), these agents are poorly absorbed and do not alter systemic pH when used as directed. However, overuse of antacids may actually interfere with proper digestion. To be most effective, antacids should be taken on a regular basis, not just to relieve pain when discomfort occurs; however, effectiveness is limited by the short duration of action, approximately 30 minutes on an empty stomach. Food acts as a buffer for antacids, continuing activity for 2 to 3 hours. Chronic use of antacids produces **acid rebound,** thus neutralizing the effects of the drug. Usual dosage is seven times a day: before meals, 1 to 2 hours after meals, and at bedtime. Because these medications are inconvenient to take so frequently and tend to have an unpleasant taste, administration usually occurs with the onset of pain rather than on a dosage schedule. Antacids come in liquids (which must be placed back into a suspension before administration) and chewable tablets (which should be followed by a glass of water after chewing thoroughly).

Families of antacids are classified by chemical formulation as aluminum, magnesium, calcium, and sodium compounds. Each family has a different effect on bowels

TABLE 24-1 ORAL PREPARATIONS

GENERIC/TRADE NAME	USUAL DOSE, ROUTE, AND FREQUENCY	INDICATIONS FOR USE	DRUG INTERACTIONS
TOPICAL ANESTHETICS		Mouth lesions and irritations	Usually none
benzocaine*			
(Hurricaine aerosol)	1 spray topically		
(Orajel, Num-Zit gel)	Apply gel topically		
(Cepacol lozenges)	Dissolve 1 lozenge PO q2h		
(Chloraseptic spray)	1 spray topically		
(Benzodent, Anbesol ointment)	Apply ointment topically		
lidocaine (Xylocaine† ointment or spray)	Apply or spray topically		
ORAL ANTISEPTICS		Antiseptic, anesthetic, caries prevention	
Mouthwashes* (e.g., Cepacol, Listerine, Scope, Lavoris)	Swish as directed or desired		
hydrogen peroxide (Paramax,* Peridex¹ as mouthwash) (Peroxyl* mouthwash or gel)	Apply or swish bid	Relieves mouth irritation and removes debris	Usually none
FLUORIDE PREPARATIONS† Fluor-a-day tablets (Luride) (TheraFlur, Gel Kam)	5-10 mL solution PO apply topically qd	Prevent dental caries	Usually none
ANTIFUNGALS clotrimazole (Mycelex lozenges, troches)	Dissolve 10 mg PO qid	Oropharyngeal candidiasis	None indicated
ketoconazole	200-400 mg PO qd		astemizole, terfenadine
nystatin (Mycostatin, Nilstat)			None indicated
lozenges/troches	Dissolve 1 or 2 lozenges PO qid		
suspension	4 mL suspension, swish and swallow		
ORAL ANTIVIRALS		Herpes lesions and varicella lesions of mouth	Usually none
acyclovir (Zovirax†)			
tablet	200 mg PO q4h		
ointment	Apply topically		
penciclovir (Denavir†)	Apply topically		
docosanol (Abreva*)	Apply topically		
SALIVA SUBSTITUTES Selected saliva substitutes*		Replace saliva	None None
(Entertainer's Secret, Salivart, Salix, Moi-Stir, Swabsticks)	Spray topically Lozenges topically Swabs		
Cholinergic Agonist cevimeline† (Evoxac)	30 mg PO tid	Increases saliva output	None

PO, Orally.
*Over-the-counter medication.
†Prescription medication.
Note: A prescription is required for all oral antifungals except docosanol.

TABLE 24-2 CAUSATIVE PROPERTIES OF ANTACID COMPOUNDS

ANTACID	CONSTIPATION	DIARRHEA
Aluminum compounds	Yes	No
Magnesium compounds	No	Yes
Calcium compounds	Yes	No
Sodium compounds*	No	No

*Should not be used routinely because routine use changes systemic pH of body.

BOX 24-1 LIFESTYLE TIPS TO IMPROVE GASTROINTESTINAL CONDITIONS

Certain foods will increase the secretions of stomach acids, among them tomato, orange, and grapefruit juices; alcohol; colas; coffee; fried or fatty foods; chocolate; peppermint; and spices.

Diet itself plays only a minor role in ulcer treatment; eating five or six small meals will be helpful in treatment by reducing fluctuations in stomach acidity to facilitate healing.

Do not overeat. Watch weight. Weight gain contributes to stomach problems.

Avoid eating within 2 hours of bedtime.

Do not smoke.

Elevate head of bed 6 to 8 inches so gravity helps in emptying stomach.

and systemic pH. Sodium bicarbonate, a household chemical used indiscriminately as an antacid, is very dangerous because of systemic absorption, changing the entire body's acid-base balance. Calcium preparations, such as Tums, are frequently used for gastric symptoms and as calcium supplements for prevention of bone mass loss with osteoporosis. Aluminum and magnesium salts are mixed to form **magaldrate** compounds, used to prevent diarrhea and constipation occurring with use of the chemical compounds alone. Added ingredients include **simethicone** (an **antiflatulent**), mineral oil, saccharin, or **sorbitol** (an osmotic laxative) (Table 24-2).

Other uses of antacids include replacement therapy for some needed minerals. Aluminum compounds may be used for hyperphosphatemia. Magnesium deficiency from alcoholism and other medical conditions may be treated with **magnesium hydroxide.**

Thus antacids must be chosen with care to suit each patient's needs and should not be taken for prolonged periods of time. The indication for continued use is relief of acute symptoms of GERD, heartburn, and hyperactivity (Table 24-3).

Patient Education for Compliance

1. Alcohol consumption exacerbates ulcer symptoms. Certain foods such as colas, acid juices, coffee, chocolate, and spices aggravate stomach and gallbladder conditions.
2. Chewable antacids should be taken seven times a day and followed by a glass of water or milk to improve absorption.
3. Liquid suspensions need shaking before administration and should not be followed by any liquids that will dilute the medication.
4. Antacids and histamine₂ (H₂)-receptor blockers should be taken at least an hour apart, with antacids taken first.
5. Antacids should not be taken routinely with other medications because the stomach's acid content may be necessary for absorption of some drugs.
6. Patients should be aware that dark, tarry stools and "coffee-ground" vomitus are signs of gastrointestinal bleeding.

Important Facts about Antacids

- Because antacids interfere with absorption of many medications, especially antibiotics, other medications should not be given with antacids.
- The ideal time to give antacids is 2 hours after meals when acid rebound occurs.

Other Medications for Peptic Ulcers

Optimal antiulcer therapy requires drug therapy and changes in lifestyle (Box 24-1). The goal of ulcer treatment should be to alleviate symptoms, promote healing of the ulcer, prevent complications, and prevent recurrence. *H. pylori* has been found in 85% of cases of duodenal ulcer disease and 70% of gastric ulcers and is believed to be an opportunistic infection at the ulcer site.

Mucosal protectants, used to protect the mucosa from acid secretions and irritating medications, should be taken on an empty stomach to be effective. **Sucralfate** (Carafate), a nonsystemic complex of aluminum hydroxide and sulfated sucrose with a local soothing effect in the GI tract, promotes healing of peptic ulcers by adhering to the gastric ulcer, forming a mechanical protectant against hydrochloric acid and digestive enzymes. Unlike antacids, no potential for altering pH is usually seen. When used over prolonged periods of time, sucralfate may cause deficiencies in fat-soluble vitamins (Table 24-4).

Histamine₂ (H₂)-receptor antagonists (antisecretory agents) decrease gastric fluid secretions. Gastric mucosa histamine receptors mediate secretion of gastric acid and pepsin with ulcers and GERD. The H₂-receptor antagonists **cimetidine** (Tagamet) and **ranitidine** (Zantac) inhibit interaction of H₂ at its receptors and are available

TABLE 24-3 ANTACIDS AND RELATED DRUGS

GENERIC/TRADE NAME	USUAL DOSE, ROUTE, AND FREQUENCY	INDICATIONS FOR USE	DRUG INTERACTIONS
SELECTED ANTACIDS*		Reduce stomach acid	tetracyclines, quinidine, morphine, penicillin, pseudoephedrine, INH, aspirin, dicumarol, digoxin, allopurinol, anticholinergics, corticosteroids, H_2-receptor antagonists, thyroid hormones, salicylates, corticosteroids, chlorpromazine
Sodium Compounds			
sodium bicarbonate or baking soda	Not advised, but indiscriminately used at home		
with acetaminophen granules (Bromo—Seltzer)	1 packet in water PO q4h		
with aspirin as effervescent tablets (Alka-Seltzer)	1 tab in water PO q4h		
Aluminum Compounds			
aluminum hydroxide (AlternaGEL, Amphojel)	10-30 mL PO q3-6h		
Magnesium Compounds			
magnesium hydroxide* (Phillips chewable tablets)	1 or 2 tablets PO qid		
(Milk of Magnesia, Maalox)	10-30 mL PO qid		
magaldrate + simethicone (Maalox Plus, Riopan)	10-30 mL PO qid		
magnesium + aluminium (Gaviscon, Gelusil)	1 or 2 chewable tabs PO qid		
Calcium Compounds		Also used with prevention of osteoporosis	
calcium carbonate* (Tums, Rolaids)	1 or 2 chewable tabs PO q3-6h		

H_2, Histamine$_2$; *INH*, isoniazid; *PO*, orally.
*Medications in this table are OTC products.
Note: Medications under drug interactions apply to the entire table.

OTC and by prescription at different strengths. Not affected by food, these medications may be taken with meals. Well tolerated for short-term and chronic maintenance therapy, antacids and H_2-receptor antagonists should not be taken at the same time (see Table 24-4).

LEARNING TIP

Many antisecretory agents end in "dine."

Proton pump inhibitors (PPIs) (also called *gastric pump inhibitors*) work by inhibiting chemicals essential for production of hydrochloric acid. **Omeprazole** (Prilosec), **lansoprazole** (Prevacid), **esomeprazole** (Nexium), and **rabeprazole** (AcipHex), chief medications in the class, are used for the short-term treatment of benign gastric ulcers and GERD. When used in combination with antibiotics for *H. pylori*, these drugs promote ulcer healing and prevent recurrence. All PPIs are used for active duodenal ulcers, erosive esophagitis, or pathologic hypersecretory conditions. Prolonged use of PPIs for benign

TABLE 24-4 MEDICATIONS FOR TREATING AND PREVENTING GASTRIC DISORDERS

GENERIC/TRADE NAME	USUAL DOSE, ROUTE, AND FREQUENCY	INDICATIONS FOR USE	DRUG INTERACTIONS
PROTECTIVE BARRIERS			
sucralfate* (Carafate)	1 g PO qid	Protect against ulcer formation; protect gastric mucosa	magnesium antacids, caffeine, antacids, calcium channel blockers, cisapride, carbamazepine, and many others
ANTISECRETORY OR H₂-RECEPTOR ANTAGONISTS		Reduce histamine secretions in stomach	
cimetidine (Tagamet,*† Tagamet HB†)	200-400 mg PO qd		
famotidine (Pepcid,* Pepcid AC†) with antacid (Pepcid Complete)	20-40 mg PO bid 1 or 2 tabs PO qd		
ranitidine (Zantac*†)	150-300 mg PO bid		
nizatidine (Axid*†)	150-300 mg PO qd		
PROTON PUMP INHIBITORS*		Short-term treatment of ulcers and GERD; reduce gastric acid production and lower esophagitis	
omeprazole (Prilosec*†)	10-40 mg PO qd	Same as for PPIs	Oral anticoagulants, diazepam, phenytoin
lansoprazole (Prevacid*)	15-30 mg/day PO qd		ketoconazole, iron salts, ampicillin, digoxin, sucralfate
rabeprazole (AcipHex*)	20 mg PO‡ qd		
esomeprazole (Nexium*)	20-40 mg PO‡ qd		ampicillin, clarithromycin
pantoprazole (Protonix*)	20-40 mg PO qd		No significant interactions noted
dexlansoprazole (Kapidex, Dexilant)	60 mg PO qd		
COMBINATION PROTON PUMP INHIBITORS AND ALKALINES			
sodium bicarbonate with omeprazole (Zegerid*)	1100 mg/20- to 40-mg cap packet mixed in water, PO qd		
PROSTAGLANDIN ANALOGUE			
misoprostol* (Cytotec)	100-200 mcg PO qid	Prevention of NSAID-induced gastric ulcers	magnesium antacids, caffeine, antacids, calcium channel blockers, cisapride, carbamazepine, and many others

GERD, Gastroesophageal reflux disease; *IV*, intravenously; *IM*, intramuscular; *NSAID*, nonsteroidal antiinflammatory drug; *PO*, orally.
*Prescription medication.
†Over-the-counter medication.
‡Must be swallowed whole.

TABLE 24-4 MEDICATIONS FOR TREATING AND PREVENTING GASTRIC DISORDERS—cont'd

GENERIC/TRADE NAME	USUAL DOSE, ROUTE, AND FREQUENCY	INDICATIONS FOR USE	DRUG INTERACTIONS
SELECTED ANTICHOLINERGICS*		Peptic ulcers, spasms, intestinal and biliary colic	Usually none
belladonna			
with phenobarbital (Donnatal)	1 or 2 tabs PO tid-qid		
hyoscyamine	0.125-0.25 mg PO q4h prn		
(Anaspaz, Levbid, Levsin)	0.375 mg PO (timed release) q12h		
glycopyrrolate (Robinul, Robinul Forte)	1-2 mg PO tid/qid		
dicyclomine (Bentyl)	10-20 mg PO qid		None indicated
Major Side Effects:			
Dizziness, headache, insomnia, drowsiness, visual disturbances, changes in heart rhythm			
PROKINETIC AGENT			
metoclopramide* (Reglan)	5-10 mg PO, IV, IM qid ac	GERD; also may be used for vomiting with chemotherapy for cancer	alcohol
(Metozolv)	5-10 mg po dissolving tab qid ac		
Major Side Effects:			
Diarrhea, abdominal pain, headache, restlessness, drowsiness, fatigue, insomnia, headaches, dizziness			

disease will lead to a decrease in body fluids (see Table 24-4).

LEARNING TIP

Many PPIs end in "zole."

Prostaglandin analogues, indicated for nonsteroidal antiinflammatory drug (NSAID)–induced gastric ulcers, have as a typical agent **misoprostol** (Cytotec) to inhibit gastric secretions and protect against irritant effects of medications. Aspirin and other NSAIDs may irritate the stomach. Taken with food to suppress acid secretions and increase cytoprotective mucus in the GI tract, this medication is for use with those who are susceptible to medication-induced gastric irritation. It must be used with care in women of childbearing age because of category X pregnancy classification.

Muscarinic antagonists (**anticholinergics**), such as **dicyclomine** (Bentyl), are also called *antispasmodics* because they decrease secretions and slow peristalsis and spasms that occur with irritable bowel syndrome,

ulcerative colitis, diverticulitis, ulcers, and biliary spasm by blocking acetylcholine at muscarinic receptors. These agents should be taken 30 minutes before meals and at bedtime to reduce heartburn frequency and allow healing of irritated tissue. These medications may cause visual disturbances, increased confusion in demented patients, and changes in heart rhythm; therefore they should not be used by patients with glaucoma, urinary retention, or obstructive bowel syndrome (see Table 24-4). Anticholinergics are also used for urinary incontinence (see Chapter 27).

Antibiotics are common therapy for *H. pylori*. Treatment includes two antibiotics (to reduce the risk of drug resistance), usually in combination with **bismuth salts** (Pepto-Bismol) to prevent the bacteria from attacking the stomach wall. Antibiotics of choice are **amoxicillin, tetracycline, metronidazole** (Flagyl), and **clarithromycin** (Biaxin) (Table 24-5) (see Chapter 17 for antibiotics and antifungals). Some physicians prefer to add a PPI or an antisecretory agent to the regimen. Some medications come in blister packs containing medications such as bismuth salicylate tablets, metronidazole tablets, and antibiotics, for a dosage of one or two blister packs per day for 2 weeks (see Table 24-4).

TABLE 24-5 COMBINATION OF MEDICATIONS FOR *H. PYLORI**

SHORT-TERM THERAPY	DOSE
Helidac (bismuth subsalicylate [Pepto-Bismol] with metronidazole [Flagyl] and tetracycline)	1 pack PO qid

LONG-TERM THERAPY	DOSE
Prevpac	
lansoprazole (Prevacid)	30 mg PO bid
amoxicillin (Trimox)	2000 mg PO bid
clarithromycin (Biaxin)	500 mg PO bid

*These medications come in a package that is a single dose. All medications should be taken at one time.

Prokinetic agents, such as **metoclopramide** (Reglan), are used to stimulate GI motility by lowering esophageal sphincter pressure, accelerating gastric emptying and movement of food through intestines. These agents are used to treat symptoms of GERD when lifestyle changes and diet have not been effective (see Table 24-4).

Patient Education for Compliance

1. Sucralfate, a protective barrier, should be taken on an empty stomach 1 hour before meals and not within 2 hours of any other medication.
2. Patients with peptic ulcer disease should eat five or six small meals a day to decrease fluctuation of gastric acidity.
3. H_2-receptor antagonists or blockers may be taken once a day (at bedtime), or twice a day, without regard to meals. Acid secretions peak during sleeping hours, so H_2-receptor blockers should always be administered at bedtime.
4. Cigarette smoking decreases the effects of H_2-receptor antagonists and increases the amount of acid the stomach produces.

Important Facts about Medications to Treat or Prevent Peptic Ulcers

- Goals of peptic ulcer disease therapy are to alleviate symptoms, promote ulcer healing, prevent complications, and prevent disease process recurrence.
- Lifestyle changes related to smoking, alcohol, and carbonated beverages may be required for treatment of gastrointestinal symptoms. Stress relief and dietary changes are essential in ulcer treatment.
- H_2-receptor antagonists block gastric H_2 to suppress gastric acid secretion.
- Proton pump inhibitors, or gastric pump inhibitors, inhibit H^+ and K^+ ions, needed for production of gastric acids.

DRUGS USED TO TREAT HEPATITIS B AND HEPATITIS C

Viral hepatitis is the most common liver disease, with millions of Americans affected. Immunization with hepatitis B vaccine is the best resource for prevention of hepatitis B disease. Acute hepatitis lasts for about 6 months or less and is characterized by liver inflammation and jaundice. Chronic hepatitis is caused by hepatitis B and C. Hepatitis C is treated with **interferon alfa-2a** (Pegasys), **peglyted interferon** (peginterferon), and **peginterferon alfa-2b** (PEG-Intion) for 12 months. Unfortunately, half of the people relapse after treatment is stopped. Adverse reactions include flulike symptoms, depression, fatigue, alopecia, and GI symptoms. In some cases, oral **ribavirin** (Rebetrol), an antiviral, may be combined with parenteral (subcutaneous) interferon alfa for more intense treatment.

Acute hepatitis B is decreasing owing to immunization with hepatitis B virus (HBV) vaccine. However, as chronic hepatitis B develops, cirrhosis, hepatitis failure, and hepatocellular carcinoma occur. Treatment is much like that for chronic hepatitis C without the use of peginterferon alfa-2b. The medications are more effective when used with nucleoside analogues such as **lamivudine** (Epivir HBV), **adfovir** (Hepsera), and **entercavir** (Baraclude), also antivirals, which are administered by mouth. Side effects are basically the same as with drugs for chronic hepatitis C (Table 24-6).

DRUGS USED AS PANCREATIC ENZYME REPLACEMENTS

The pancreas produces four main digestive enzymes—lipase, amylase, chymotrypsin, and trypsin—to aid in digestion of fats, carbohydrates, and proteins. Pancreatic enzyme replacements must be taken with every food intake and are available in two basic preparations—**pancreatin** (Pancreatin) and **pancrelipase** (Cotazym, Pancrease MT)—from animal sources. The capsules contain enteric-coated microspheres and antacids to protect inactivation of the medication by gastric juices. The dosage is individualized due to patient needs (Table 24-7).

DRUGS USED WITH GALLBLADDER DISEASE

The gallbladder is the only site for excretion of cholesterol from the body. Most cholelithiasis is from cholesterol stones alone that cannot be seen on radiographs, whereas calcium stones are observable. When symptoms of cholelithiasis occur, oral radiopaque drugs

TABLE 24-6 DRUGS FOR HEPATITIS B AND C

GENERIC NAME/ TRADE NAME	USUAL DOSE, ROUTE, AND FREQUENCY	INDICATIONS FOR USE	DRUG INTERACTIONS
INTERFERON-LIKE DRUGS			
interferon alfa-2b (Intron A)	Varies with patient, SC	Hepatitis B and C	aminophylline, warfarin, zidovudine
peginterferon alfa-2a (Pegasys)	180 mcg SC once wkly	Hepatitis B and C	lithium
interferon alfacon-1 (Infergen)	9 mcg SC 3×/wk	Hepatitis C	None indicated
peginterferon alfa-2b (PEG-Intron)	1 mcg/kg SC once wkly	Hepatitis C	Same as peginterferon alfa-a
ribavirin (Rebetol, Copegus)	Based on body weight, PO varies	Used with peginterferon alfa for hepatitis C	Other antivirals
ANTIVITALS			
lamivudine (Epivir HBV)	100 mg PO qd	Hepatitis B	TMP-SMZ, zidovudine
adefovir (Hepsera)	10 mg PO qd	Hepatitis B	Multiple interactions, see literature
entecavir (Baraclude)	Based on renal function, PO varies	Hepatitis B	None indicated
telbivudine (Tyzeka)	600 mg PO qd	Hepatitis B	antivirals, HMG-CoA reductase inhibitors, penicillamine, cyclosporine, erythromycin, niacin, corticosteroids, hydroxychloroquine

PO, orally; *SC,* subcutaneously; *TMP-SMZ,* trimethoprim-sulfamethoxazole.

TABLE 24-7 DRUGS FOR PANCREATIC AND GALLBLADDER DISEASE

GENERIC NAME/TRADE NAME	USUAL DOSE, ROUTE, AND FREQUENCY	INDICATIONS FOR USE	DRUG INTERACTIONS
PANCREATIC ENZYMES		Aid in digestion	antacids, iron supplements
pancreatin (Pancreatin)	Individualized, PO varies		
pancrelipase (Creon, Pancrease, Zenpep)	Individualized, PO varies		
DRUGS FOR GALLBLADDER DISEASE		Dissolve gallstones	
chenodiol (Chenodal)	250 mg, PO tid		Usually none
ursodiol (Actigall, Urso, Urso Forte)	8-10 mg/kg, PO divided qd		aluminum antacids, cholestyramine, colestipol, oral contraceptives, estrogens

Major Side Effects:
Absence of taste, biliary pain, diarrhea, nausea, vomiting with chenodiol

PO, orally.
Note: All of the drugs listed in this table require a prescription.

to aid in visualizing the stones, such as Telepaque or Bilopaque, may be given to the patient before radiographic gallbladder studies are performed. The dose is based on patient weight. After a low-fat evening meal, tablets are taken at 5-minute intervals until all ordered tablets have been taken; then nothing including water should be taken by mouth until the test has been performed.

In patients who are asymptomatic but have been shown to have gallstones, medications to dissolve gallstones may be used, with best results occurring in women with small stones. Therapy may take as long as 2 years. The preferred medication for reducing cholesterol in bile is ***ursodiol*** (Actigall) because it is well tolerated. Usual prolonged treatment is one tablet in the morning and evening, 12 hours apart (see Table 24-7).

Chemotherapy may cause severe nausea and vomiting; these side effects may even be the reason why patients discontinue chemotherapy. Vomiting may be anticipatory emesis (occurring before receipt of anticancer drugs and triggered by memories of previous severe nausea and vomiting), acute emesis (occurring shortly after chemotherapy is administered), or delayed emesis (occurring a day or two after chemotherapy). For emesis prevention, a medication may be administered before chemotherapy. For the patient receiving chemotherapy that causes emesis, a combination of medications may be required, using drugs from several antiemetic drug classes to be effective.

DRUGS FOR EMESIS

Antiemetics are used to suppress nausea and vomiting. **Emesis,** or **regurgitation,** may activate the vomiting reflex via either (1) signals from the stomach or small intestines or (2) direct action of compounds that cause vomiting, such as anticancer medications or opiates used for pain (see Box 24-2 for an explanation of emesis occurring with chemotherapy). Antiemetic drugs are separated into several classes, depending on how they act on the body (Table 24-8).

Serotonin antagonists are the most effective drugs for suppressing nausea and vomiting caused by antineoplastic medications. The side effects include diarrhea and headache. The two typical drugs are **ondansetron** (Zofran) and **granisetron** (Kytril, Granisol).

Dopamine antagonists, a major category of antiemetics, are divided into three groups: phenothiazines, butyrophenones, and a group of other medications. These medications suppress vomiting by blocking dopamine-2 receptors. Phenothiazines such as **promethazine** (Phenergan) are used orally, parenterally, or rectally for nausea and vomiting of chemotherapy, surgery, and toxic poisoning. These medications are also used with psychiatric disorders (see Chapter 30).

Benzodiazepines such as **lorazepam** (Ativan) and **diazepam** (Valium) are also given for chemotherapy patients. Both provide sedation and suppress anticipation of emesis while producing some amnesia of emesis (see Chapter 30).

Anticholinergics, used to treat motion sickness, block acetylcholine and histamine. **Scopolamine** is a cholinergic antagonist used for prevention and treatment of motion sickness through oral, subcutaneous, or transdermal administration. Transdermal patches are changed every 3 days. Box 24-3 has an explanation of vomiting from motion sickness.

TABLE 24-8 MEDICATIONS FOR EMESIS

GENERIC NAME/ TRADE NAME	USUAL DOSE, ROUTE, AND FREQUENCY	INDICATIONS FOR USE	MAJOR SIDE EFFECTS	DRUG INTERACTIONS
SEROTONIN ANTAGONISTS*		Postchemotherapy nausea	Diarrhea, headache	Usually none
ondansetron (Zofran)	4-8 mg PO bid, IV			
granisetron (Kytril, Granisol)	1 mg PO, IV 1 hr before chemotherapy			
(Sancuso patch)	T patch transdermal q3-4d			
dolasetron (Anzemet)	100 mg PO, IV 1 hr before chemotherapy			
palonosetron (Aloxi)	0.5 mg PO 1 hr before chemotherapy, 0.25 mg IV 1 hr before chemotherapy			
DOPAMINE ANTAGONISTS*		Nausea and vomiting from various causes, including motion sickness		alcohol, lithium, tricyclic antidepressants, monoamine oxidase inhibitors, hypotensive agents, antithyroid agents
chlorpromazine	10-25 mg PO q4-6h; 25-50 mg IM, IV q4-6h			

CNS, Central nervous system; *IM,* intramuscularly; *IV,* intravenously; *PO,* orally; *SC,* subcutaneously.
*Prescription medication.

TABLE 24-8 MEDICATIONS FOR EMESIS—cont'd

GENERIC NAME/ TRADE NAME	USUAL DOSE, ROUTE, AND FREQUENCY	INDICATIONS FOR USE	MAJOR SIDE EFFECTS	DRUG INTERACTIONS
perphenazine	8-16 mg PO, IM, IV qd in divided doses			
prochlorperazine (Compazine) (Compro)	5-10 mg PO q12h, IM, IV 25 mg rectal suppository			
promethazine (Phenergan)	12.5-25 mg PO q4-6h, IM, IV, rectal suppository			
Butyrophenone haloperidol (Haldol)	1-2 mg PO qd, IM, IV			alcohol, CNS depressants, lithium
Other Dopamine Antagonists		Nausea and vomiting with chemotherapy	Dizziness, headache, restlessness, dry mouth, hypotension	
metoclopramide (Reglan)	10-15 mg PO qid; 1-2 mg/ kg IV 30 min before chemotherapy			alcohol
ANTICHOLINERGICS *Antihistamines*		Motion sickness, nausea and vomiting from various causes		No significant interactions noted
dimenhydrinate*† (Dramamine)	50-100 mg PO q4-6h, IM, IV			
diphenhydramine*† (Benadryl)	12.5-50 mg PO tid-qid, IM, IV			
hydroxyzine* (Atarax, Vistaril)	25-100 mg PO single dose, IM			
meclizine*† (Bonine,† Antivert*)	25-50 mg PO qd			
(Dramamine Less Drowsy†)	25 mg PO 1hr before travel			
scopolamine*	0.4-0.8 mg PO, 0.6-1 mg SC, IM, IV			
(Transderm Scop)	0.5-mg transdermal patch			
MISCELLANEOUS AGENTS		Nausea and vomiting from various causes		
phosphorated carbohydrate solution† (Emetrol and others)	15-30 mL PO single dose			
trimethobenzamide* (Tigan)	300 mg PO tid-qid; 200 mg IM			CNS depressants
aprepitant (Emend)	125 mg PO on morning of chemotherapy, 80 mg PO on days 2 and 3 after chemotherapy	Nausea and vomiting with chemotherapy		terfenadine, cisapride, astemizole, warfarin

†OTC medication.

Phosphorated carbohydrate solution (Emetrol), a dextrose, fructose, and phosphoric acid combination, works by reducing hyperactivity of smooth gastric wall muscles. Because of its sugar base and its availability OTC, patient education for persons with diabetes mellitus should include the danger of medication use and increased blood glucose levels.

Another popular antiemetic, *trimethobenzamide* (Tigan), may be administered by mouth, injection, or rectal suppository. Because parenteral administration is painful, the Z-track method is the preferred route (see Chapter 14 for methodology for Z-track injection).

Patient Education for Compliance

1. Medications for motion sickness should be taken 30 to 60 minutes before travel.
2. Transdermal scopolamine is a 72-hour patch that is placed behind the ear for continual release of medication for motion sickness or nausea.

Important Fact about Drugs for Emesis

A combination of medications may be necessary to prevent emesis from chemotherapy.

DRUGS USED FOR INTESTINAL CONDITIONS

Drugs for intestinal conditions include **antiflatulents,** and laxatives or **cathartics.** Both groups of drugs are often used with OTC preparations and have names that are commonly recognized.

Antiflatulents

Some people have excess gas production and require relief of gastric and intestinal distention. Medications, including some antacids used as antiflatulents or **carminatives,** are bought OTC, with *simethicone* being the most common active ingredient (e.g., Phazyme, Gas-X, Mylanta). Simethicone disperses and prevents gas pocket formation in the GI tract. Antiflatulents are used to relieve gas; however, patients with excess gas should avoid gas-forming foods such as cabbage, onions, and beans and avoid using straws when drinking liquids (Table 24-9).

Laxatives and Cathartics

Bowel function is a major concern in the elderly (constipation) and young children (diarrhea). Constipation is related to the hardness of stools rather than to their frequency. Laxatives should be used for constipation and hard, dry stools, not for soft, hydrated stools. If a laxative is necessary, it should be used for only a short time in conjunction with dietary changes and exercise. The elderly have increased constipation leading to bowel obstruction or habituation of laxatives because of multiple chronic illnesses, polypharmacy, and decline in body function. Constipation is common in children, with contributing factors such as emotions, new environments, dietary changes, and fever. *Glycerin* suppositories for children are the most appropriate treatment for constipation in children age 10 years and younger. Diarrhea in children may cause rapid electrolyte imbalances, and early treatment is necessary to maintain homeostasis.

Laxatives and cathartics are used to induce **defecation.** Laxatives result in leisurely production of a soft-formed stool over a period of 1 to 2 days. These medications may be abused and/or cause dependency, especially in the elderly, because of preconceived ideas concerning daily bowel evacuation. Cathartics produce a prompt, fast, intense fluid evacuation from the bowel and are used most often for diagnostic testing. Some of these medications may alter the color of stools (Table 24-10).

The advertising for OTC laxatives tends to encourage habitual self-medication when these agents are not actually needed. Unnecessary use of a laxative may perpetuate the patient's perception that a laxative is again necessary. After purging the intestinal tract, the patient will need 2 to 5 days to refill the bowel, during which time the habitual laxative user will take another laxative because a daily bowel movement has not occurred. Over a period of time, the body becomes reliant on the laxative for a bowel movement, leading to pathologic changes such as heart irregularities. Cardiac arrest may even occur from loss of potassium.

Laxatives may be used with patients who have a loss of abdominal and gastric muscle tone. With **anthelmintic** therapy, laxatives are used to obtain stool specimens, empty the GI tract before medication administration, and to expel dead parasites. These medications are also indicated before diagnostic and surgical procedures.

TABLE 24-9 DRUGS USED FOR INTESTINAL CONDITIONS

GENERIC NAME/ TRADE NAME	USUAL DOSE, ROUTE, AND FREQUENCY	INDICATIONS FOR USE	DRUG INTERACTIONS
ANTIFLATULANTS†		Flatulence, including that caused by radiographic studies	
simethicone (Mylicon, Phazyme)	80-160 mg PO tid		Usually none
OSMOTIC LAXATIVES†		Relieve constipation	
polyethylene glycol (MiraLAX)	1 Tbsp PO in 8 oz water PO qd		
lactulose (Constulose, Enulose, Kristalose)	15-60 mL PO qd		
sodium phosphate (Fleet liquid, enema)	1½ oz in 8 oz water PO qd 1 bottle rectal		
Magnesium Compounds			
magnesium hydroxide			
(Milk of Magnesia)	30-60 mL PO qd		
(Phillip's chewable)	300-600 mg qd		
magnesium citrate			
(Citrate of Magnesia)	1 8-oz glass PO as a single dose		
(Citroma)	5-10 oz PO qd		
magnesium sulfate (Epsom salts)	2-4 g in 8 oz water PO qd		
BULK-FORMING LAXATIVES†			
methylcellulose (Citrucel)	1 tbsp in 8 oz water PO qd-tid		K-sparing diuretics, salicylates, digoxin
polycarbophil (FiberCon, Mitrolan, Fiberall)	2 tabs PO qd-qid		
psyllium hydrophilic (Konsyl Perdiem, Metamucil, Serutan)	1 tsp in 8 oz water PO qd-tid		
STIMULANT LAXATIVES†			
bisacodyl (Dulcolax)	10-15 mg PO or 1 rectal suppository	For diagnostic testing	
cascara sagrada (NTN)	1 tab or 1 tsp PO qd, dose may vary		
senna (Senokot, Ex-Lax, Black Draught, Fletcher's Castoria)	10-15 mL or 1 or 2 tabs PO bid		
castor oil	15-60 mL PO qd		
LUBRICANT LAXATIVES†			
mineral oil (Kondremul, Fleet Enema)	15 mL PO qd 1 bottle rectally	Relieve constipation	
olive oil	15 mL PO qd		

CNS, Central nervous system; *MAOI,* monoamine oxidase inhibitor; *PO,* orally.
†OTC medication.

Continued

TABLE 24-9 DRUGS USED FOR INTESTINAL CONDITIONS—cont'd

GENERIC NAME/ TRADE NAME	USUAL DOSE, ROUTE, AND FREQUENCY	INDICATIONS FOR USE	DRUG INTERACTIONS
STOOL SOFTENERS AND MOISTENING AGENTS			
docusate sodium (Colace) with senna (Peri-Colace, Senokot-S)	1 or 2 gel caps PO prn	Relieve constipation, ease defincation	
docusate calcium	1 or 2 tabs PO prn		
glycerin	1 rectal suppository prn		
CATHARTICS AND BOWEL EVACUANTS*		Bloating, nausea, abdominal fullness, diagnostic testing	
polyethylene glycol electrolyte solution (PEG-ES) (GoLytely, CoLyte, NuLytely, MiraLax)	4 L PO (240 mL every 10 min until all consumed)		

Major Side Effects:

Osmotic laxatives—generally none except abdominal cramping; *sodium phosphate*—abdominal cramping; *bulk-forming laxatives*— flatulence and bulky stools, abdominal cramping; *stimulant laxatives*—abdominal cramping, nausea, diarrhea, flatulence

ANTIDIARRHEALS‡		Relieve symptoms of diarrhea	
cholestyramine* (Questran)	2-4 g PO bid-qid		Anticoagulants, digoxin, thiazides, penicillins tetracyclines, propranolol, thyroid replacement, folic acid
bismuth subsalicylate† (Pepto-Bismol)	15 mL PO or 2 tabs PO prn		Anticoagulants, oral hypoglycemics
activated charcoal† (CharcoCaps)	2 caps PO prn		
loperamide (Imodium A-D,† Imodium†)	2-4 mg PO tid prn		
SYNTHETIC OPIOIDS			
diphenoxylate and atropine*† (Lomotil) (Schedule V)	2 tab stat then 1 tab PO prn q		alcohol, CNS depressants, MAOIs

Major Side Effects of Synthetic Opioids:

loperamide—Dizziness, dry mouth, depresses CNS; *diphenoxylate and atropine*—same as loperamide plus agitation, tachycardia, numbness of hands and feet, drowsiness

GASTROINTESTINAL ANTIINFLAMMATORY AND ANTIIRRITANT AGENTS*		Irritable and inflammatory bowel disease Crohn disease Ulcerative colitis	
mesalamine (Rowasa)	Enema; rectal suppository 800-mg mg PO tid		digoxin, mesalamine
controlled release (Pentasa)			
sulfasalazine (Azulfidine)	1 g PO q8h		oral hypoglycemics, warfarin
olsalazine (Dipentum)	500 mg PO bid		None
balsalazide (Colazal)	2.25 g PO tid		warfarin, varicella vaccine
alosetron (Lotronex)	0.5 mg PO bid		fluvoxamine

*Prescription medication.

‡Antidiarrheals are administered as directed until cessation of diarrhea.

TABLE 24-9 DRUGS USED FOR INTESTINAL CONDITIONS—cont'd

GENERIC NAME/ TRADE NAME	USUAL DOSE, ROUTE, AND FREQUENCY	INDICATIONS FOR USE	DRUG INTERACTIONS

Major Side Effects:

mesalamine—abdominal pain, cramping, headache, weakness, dizziness; *sulfasalazine*—nausea, fever, joint pain, rashes; *olsalazine*—abdominal cramping, diarrhea, dyspepsia, joint pain, anorexia; *alosetron*—constipation, bloody diarrhea, heartburn, nausea and vomiting

ANORECTAL PREPARATIONS

dibucaine† (Nupercainal ointment or suppositories) with cortisone (Nupercainal HC)	Apply topically, rectally tid/qid	Hemorrhoids, rectal fissures	None noted

Note: OTC medication. Cortisone suppositories and ointments may also be used; some require a prescription, and others do not.

ANTHELMINTICS

mebendazole*	100 mg PO bid	Roundworms, pinworms	None
pyrantel*† (Pin-X†)	PO based on body weight	Roundworms, pinworms, hookworms	
praziquantel* (Biltricide)	PO based on body weight	Tapeworms, flukes	
thiabendazole*	PO based on body weight	Threadworms, roundworms	
albendazole* (Albenza)	PO based on body weight	Pork and dog tapeworms	

Major Side Effects:

mebendazole and pyrantel—abdominal cramping, diarrhea; *praziquantel*—headaches, drowsiness, abdominal discomfort; *thiabendazole and albendazole*—abnormal cramping, anorexia, nausea and vomiting, dizziness, drowsiness

MISCELLANEOUS INTESTINAL MEDICATIONS

lubiprostone (Amitiza)	8-24 mcg PO bid	Idiopathic, chronic constipation	

MISCELLANEOUS

tegaserod (Zelnorm)	2-6 mg PO bid	Increased GI motility; peristalic agent	None

Major Side Effects:

tegaserod maleate—headaches, diarrhea; *lubiprostone*—occasional diarrhea

Types of Laxatives

Laxatives, mostly OTC preparations, are classified by their source, site of action, degree of action, or mechanism of action (Figure 24-2).

Osmotic saline laxatives increase the amount of water in large intestine so the fecal mass swells, stretching the intestinal wall and increasing peristalsis. Low doses of these medications work in 6 to 12 hours; large doses work in 2 to 6 hours, but a large dose can cause considerable abdominal cramping. Osmotic saline laxatives can cause a substantial water loss, and its replacement is necessary to keep the body in homeostasis. Therefore these drugs should not be used with patients with hypertension, heart failure, or edema because of possible electrolyte changes. Milk of magnesia is the mildest of saline laxatives and the preferred laxative in this category for children. Cephulac, another osmotic saline laxative, contains fructose and lactose; thus it should be used with care in people with diabetes mellitus.

Did You Know?

Milk of magnesia (MOM) may be used as an antacid in low doses.

Bulk-forming laxatives, among the least harmful of laxatives, stimulate peristalsis by swelling, increasing bulk, and modifying consistency of stools to stimulate the intestinal tract. Natural or semisynthetic cellulose derivatives such as **methylcellulose** (Citrucel) and **poly-carbophil** (Fiber-Con) are active ingredients in bulking agents. Bulk-forming agents are laxatives of choice with pregnancy. Patients must take sufficient fluids for these medications to work. Onset of action occurs in 12 hours to 3 days. Prunes and bran have similar effects as these laxatives (see Table 24-9).

TABLE 24-10 MEDICATIONS THAT MAY CHANGE THE COLOR OF STOOLS

DRUG	POSSIBLE COLOR CHANGE
Antacids with aluminum salts (e.g., Maalox, Mylanta)	White specks or white discoloration of stools
Anticoagulants, such as those containing warfarin	Red-orange to black due to intestinal bleeding
Bismuth or iron salts (including Pepto-Bismol)	Black
Laxatives with phenolphthalein	Red
Laxatives containing senna	Yellow to orange to brown
phenazopyridine (Pyridium)	Orange to red
rifampin	Red to orange or brown

Stimulant laxatives are from botanical sources except for **bisacodyl** (Dulcolax). These laxatives, absorbed to stimulate peristalsis, act in 6 to 8 hours and are habit forming. When intestinal motility is increased, water has less time for absorption in large intestines, resulting in watery stools. *Senna, cascara sagrada*, and *aloe* in this group cross into breast milk. Bisacodyl, a relatively non-toxic agent that acts by stimulating peristalsis in the colon, is often used before diagnostic testing. Because of possible stomach irritation, these tablets should not be crushed or chewed, nor should they be taken with milk or antacids because of interference with absorption. *Sennosides* such as Ex-Lax are the mildest of these laxatives and may discolor urine to pink, red, or brown. *Castor oil*, obtained from the seeds of castor beans, passes rapidly through the stomach unchanged, causing small intestine irritation. Rapid movement into the small intestines and colon is the basis for effectiveness. Castor oil is not recommended for pregnant or lactating women (see Table 24-9).

Lubricant laxatives (mineral oil and olive oil) allow water to penetrate the fecal mass, usually acting in 6 to 8 hours. Laxatives do not increase bulk, but oily agents coat the stool surface and soften stool to ease defecation. Large doses of these laxatives tend to cause leakage of oil from the rectum. Glycerin suppositories, another lubricant laxative that is usually effective in 15 minutes to an hour, increase peristalsis in all age groups (see Table 24-9).

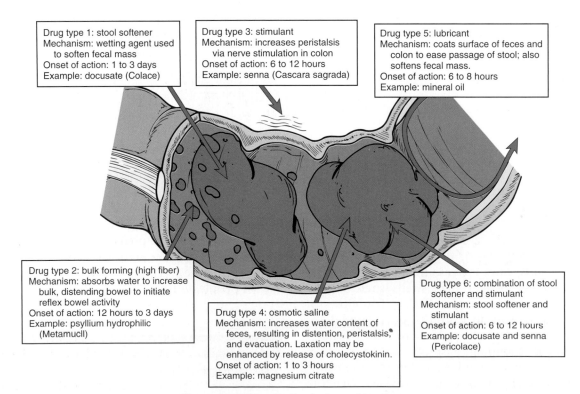

Drug type 1: stool softener
Mechanism: wetting agent used to soften fecal mass
Onset of action: 1 to 3 days
Example: docusate (Colace)

Drug type 3: stimulant
Mechanism: increases peristalsis via nerve stimulation in colon
Onset of action: 6 to 12 hours
Example: senna (Cascara sagrada)

Drug type 5: lubricant
Mechanism: coats surface of feces and colon to ease passage of stool; also softens fecal mass.
Onset of action: 6 to 8 hours
Example: mineral oil

Drug type 2: bulk forming (high fiber)
Mechanism: absorbs water to increase bulk, distending bowel to initiate reflex bowel activity
Onset of action: 12 hours to 3 days
Example: psyllium hydrophilic (Metamucil)

Drug type 4: osmotic saline
Mechanism: increases water content of feces, resulting in distention, peristalsis, and evacuation. Laxation may be enhanced by release of cholecystokinin.
Onset of action: 1 to 3 hours
Example: magnesium citrate

Drug type 6: combination of stool softener and stimulant
Mechanism: stool softener and stimulant
Onset of action: 6 to 12 hours
Example: docusate and senna (Pericolace)

Figure 24-2 Site of action for types of laxatives.

Stool softeners, or fecal moistening agents, decrease the consistency of stools by reducing surface tension. Stool softeners with a wide margin of safety and few potential adverse reactions work by absorbing water into the stool, lubricating the rectum, and increasing stool bulk. ***Docusate*** (Colace) acts as a detergent, permitting water and fatty substances to penetrate and mix with fecal material. These medications usually take 1 to 3 days to be effective, especially for patients who should avoid straining for bowel movements. They may be combined with laxatives with such medications as Peri-Colace and Doxidan to soften stools while enhancing stool evacuation (see Table 24-9).

Bowel evacuants (cathartics) such as ***polyethylene glycol*** (GoLytely) are bowel-cleansing solutions of mixtures similar to body fluids so that water and electrolytes are not absorbed. These agents are safer for patients who are sensitive to electrolyte imbalance because water is not lost and electrolyte balance is more likely maintained. When these agents are used before diagnostic testing, the patient must drink large amounts of these fluids (about a gallon) within 2 to 3 hours; bowel movements begin about an hour after administration is started. If rectal excretions become clear, the laxative may be stopped. Oral medications should not be given within an hour of starting solutions because medicine may be flushed from the GI tract (see Table 24-9).

Miscellaneous agents, including ***lubiprostone*** (Amitiza), increase intestinal fluid secretions to soften stools, increase motility in the intestines, and promote spontaneous bowel movements, reducing bloating and straining associated with chronic idiopathic constipation. Amitiza produces results within 1 week. ***Tegaserod*** (Zelnorm), another miscellaneous agent, is indicated to trigger peristalic reflex in such conditions as irritable bowel syndrome and chronic constipation.

Patient Education for Compliance

1. Health care professionals should obtain a full history of laxative use and possible misuse because these medications interfere with absorption and metabolism of other medicinal items.
2. Patient education should include the need for dietary change by avoiding such constipating foods as cheese and sugar, having adequate fluid intake, and eating high-fiber diet. Patients should avoid indiscriminate use of laxatives but rather should try adding dietary fruits, vegetables, and fluids for all ages.
3. Use of laxatives to force evacuation may initiate laxative abuse.
4. Laxatives should not be used by patients with abdominal pain, nausea, and abdominal cramping or known intestinal disease unless specifically ordered by a physician.

Patient Education for Compliance—cont'd

5. *Constipation* refers to consistency of stools, not frequency, an important fact with geriatric patients.
6. Bulk-forming laxatives and surfactants should be taken with a full glass of water.
7. Castor oil should be mixed with juice to improve taste and should not be administered at night or to someone who has difficulty swallowing.
8. When given in small doses, osmotic laxatives soften stools but cause watery evacuation with large doses.
9. Glycerin suppositories are the safest treatment for constipation in all age groups.

Important Facts about Laxatives and Cathartics

- Laxatives promote defecation.
- Laxatives and stool softeners should be used for legitimate reasons only, such as for diagnostic tests, before surgical procedures, or for medical conditions that prevent straining required for evacuation of bowel movements.
- Elderly patients should be taught to avoid constipating foods such as cheese and sugar and to have adequate fluid intake with a high-fiber diet.
- Bulk-forming laxatives should be given with water.
- Stimulant laxatives should be used with discrimination.
- Osmotic laxatives require an increased intake of fluids to prevent dehydration.
- Stimulating laxatives and osmotic laxatives should not be given at bedtime because of rapid onset of action.

DRUGS USED FOR RELIEF OF DIARRHEA

Antidiarrheal agents are used to treat diarrhea, a symptom of bowel disorders and not a disorder itself. Diarrhea consists of stools of excessive volume and fluidity with increased frequency of defecation and is associated with cramping pain because of rapid passage of intestinal contents. Management of diarrhea depends on finding the underlying cause, replacing water and electrolytes as needed, reducing cramping, and reducing the number of stools. Diarrhea is usually self-limiting and resolves without further effects. Chronic diarrhea needs evaluation for cause and treatment. Diarrhea in children may become a medical emergency in as little as 24 hours because of loss of electrolytes. Antidiarrheal agents may be classified as adsorbents and opioid or synthetic opioid medications.

Adsorbents act by coating the walls of the GI tract, absorbing toxins or bacteria that are causing diarrhea, and excreting these agents with stools. Medications given while adsorbents are being used may not be absorbed at expected levels. OTC medications include activated charcoal, bismuth salts, kaolin, pectin, attapulgite, and the prescription drug *cholestyramine* (Questran), are usually taken after each loose bowel movement until the diarrhea is controlled. Constipation may follow use of large amounts of these products. Pepto-Bismol may be used as an antidiarrheal, antacid, or antiulcer medication; it absorbs irritants of the GI tract (see Table 24-9).

Synthetic opioid medications are prescription drugs that inhibit GI motility, decrease hyperperistalsis, and slow passage of intestinal contents to allow for reabsorption of water and electrolytes, thus slowing stool frequencies. *Loperamide* (Imodium) is a prescription medication but is also found as Imodium AD, an OTC preparation for acute nonspecific and chronic diarrhea. *Diphenoxylate with atropine* (Lomotil) is a Schedule V synthetic opioid that inhibits the propulsion of food through the GI tract (see Table 24-9).

Patient Education for Compliance

1. Antidiarrheals are available OTC and by prescription.
2. Pepto-Bismol, the drug of choice for diarrhea, acts as an **antiseptic** and antidiarrheal to soothe the gastrointestinal tract.

LOWER GI ANTIINFLAMMATORY AGENTS

Antiinflammatory medications for ulcerative colitis are available as rectal suppositories, enemas, and oral tablets. *Mesalamine* (Rowasa), specifically for management of ulcerative colitis and Crohn disease, is administered as oral tablets three times a day, suppositories twice a day, or an 8-hour retention enema at bedtime.

Sulfasalazine (Azulfidine), a member of the sulfonamide family, is indicated only for irritable bowel syndrome. *Olsalazine* (Dipentum) is a salicylate derivative used for ulcerative colitis and other chronic inflammatory bowel diseases; *balsalazide* (Colazal), also a salicylate, has the same indications for chronic inflammatory bowel disease (see Table 24-9).

Important Facts about Lower GI Antiinflammatory Agents

- Medications for lower gastrointestinal tract are primarily used to restore a normal bowel pattern.
- Inflammatory bowel disease may be treated with salicylates, sulfasalazine, glucocorticoids, and immunosuppressants.

ANORECTAL PREPARATIONS

Anorectal preparations are used to provide symptomatic relief from the discomfort of anorectal disorders, such as hemorrhoids. Some contain topical anesthetics—for example, *benzocaine* and *dibucaine,* found in Preparation H and Nupercainal ointment—whereas other preparations contain *hydrocortisone* to reduce swelling, suppress inflammation, and relieve itching and stinging. Acting as *emollients* to lubricate the rectum and reduce irritations, some preparations contain lanolin or mineral oil. **Astringents** such as *witch hazel* are used to reduce swelling, inflammation, and irritation. Nupercainal, Preparation H, and Anusol are medications that come in several forms: suppositories, creams, ointments, foams, and pads. In Table 24-9, Nupercainal is shown as a typical anorectal medication.

Important Fact about Anorectal Preparations

Anorectal preparations containing topical anesthetics are found as OTC preparations. When hydrocortisones are added, many then become prescription medications.

DRUGS USED FOR INTESTINAL PARASITES

Anthelmintics are used to treat commonly found intestinal parasitic worms. Early infestations are asymptomatic, but severe medical problems arise as the infection progresses. Most common types of parasitic worms are pinworms, flukes, roundworms, and tapeworms. Dosages of medications for parasites are based on weight, with most of the dose excreted in feces. *Mebendazole* (Vermox) is relatively slow acting for the treatment of roundworms and pinworms. *Pyrantel* (found in Antiminth, Pin-X, and other anthelmintics), an OTC preparation, acts by killing the parasite; therefore the entire dose must be taken at one time. *Praziquantel* (Biltricide) is absorbed by the helminth, causing the worms to detach from the host's body tissues. *Thiabendazole* (Mintezol) has analgesic, antipyretic, and antiinflammatory actions, providing relief of the abdominal cramping that comes with treatment of parasites. Many of the anthelmintic agents are enhanced when given with fatty food to slow drug distribution. Also, tablets may be chewed or crushed to increase their absorption (see Table 24-9).

TABLE 24-11 ANOREXIANTS

GENERIC NAME/ TRADE NAME	USUAL ADULT DOSE, ROUTE, AND FREQUENCY	INDICATIONS FOR USE	DRUG INTERACTIONS
diethylpropion (Schedule IV)	25 mg PO tid	Weight loss, obesity	
phentermine (Adipex-P) (Schedule IV)	37.5 mg PO qd		
orlistat (Xenical) (OTC) (Alli)	120 mg PO tid 60 mg PO tid		pravastatin, Vitamins A, D, E, K
dextroamphetamine (Dexedrine) (Schedule II)	5-10 mg PO tid		MAOIs
benzphetamine (Didrex) (Schedule III)	25-50 mg PO qd		

CNS, Central nervous system; *MAOI*, monoamine oxidase inhibitor; *PO*, by mouth.
Note: All of the drugs listed in this table require a prescription except Alli.

Patient Education for Compliance

When treating for intestinal parasites, the entire household should be treated. Strict hygiene is essential to prevent reinfection—disinfect toilets, launder undergarments and linens, wash hands before and after eating and after using toilet, and take showers instead of baths.

CLINICAL TIP

Allied health professionals should obtain an accurate body weight for all family members when antihelmintic medication is indicated.

DRUGS USED TO SUPPRESS APPETITE

About 50% of Americans are obese, a state in which an individual's total body weight consists of a greater amount of fat than normal (25% over the ideal weight for men, and 35% for women). Obesity in children and teens is considered one of the leading health problems in the United States today. Genetics, anxiety, stress, and poor self-image are some of the most common reasons for this condition. Obese persons tend to have a greater incidence of cardiovascular disease and a higher incidence of type 2 diabetes mellitus (T2DM).

Anorexiant drugs, or appetite suppressants, include a wide variety of medications that act on the brain as weak stimulators to suppress the appetite center in the hypothalamus and to mimic the sympathetic nervous system.

Most of these prescription medications are controlled substances, subject to regulations governing scheduled drugs (Table 24-11).

Amphetamines and amphetamine-like substances such as *dextroamphetamine* (Dexadrine) are Schedule II drugs because of the danger of habituation. Other prescription drugs that are used as anorexiants are either Schedule III, such as *benzphetamine* (Didrex), or Schedule IV medications, such as *diethylpropion* (Tenuate) and *phentermine* (Fastin, Adipex-P). Bulking agents such as *methylcellulose* (Fiber Trim) and *psyllium hydrophilic mucilloid* (Metamucil) may be used to give a feeling of fullness and reduce craving for food.

Anorexiants have a number of limitations and should be used only short term as an adjunct to behavior modification, diet, and exercise, because medication tolerance may occur in just a few weeks. Short-acting anorexiants usually work for 3 to 4 hours and should be taken about 30 to 60 minutes before meals. Long-acting medications last for about 12 hours and should be taken 12 hours before sleep to prevent insomnia (see Table 24-10).

Important Facts about Anorexiants

- Anorexiants are for short-term treatment of obesity because of danger of habituation. Behavior modification, diet, and exercise should be added to drug therapy for long-term treatment of obesity.
- Anorexiants that stimulate central nervous system may cause insomnia, nervousness, and related side effects.
- Prescription anorexiants are scheduled drugs controlled by the Drug Enforcement Administration.

SUMMARY

Many products used for the GI tract are available OTC and have easily recognizable names. Mouthwashes, gargles, and dentifrices contain fluorides for tooth care and dental caries prevention. Fluoride replacement is especially important in children who do not live where fluorine has been added to water. Dental therapeutics are important to retain teeth for chewing food and to prevent gum diseases.

Saliva is necessary for lubrication of food as it passes through the mouth into the GI tract. Replacement of saliva requires multiple applications daily for needed moisture.

Oral antifungals are used for thrush by coating the mouth.

Antivirals, used for symptomatic relief of herpes simplex, varicella, and HIV infections of the mouth, should be applied using techniques that will not spread lesions during treatment. Viral lesions and lesions from dental work, antineoplastics, or disease processes may be relieved with topical anesthetics.

Gastric conditions are treated with many types of medications to relieve hyperacidity, ulcers, spasms, nausea, and vomiting. Digestants are used to assist with food digestion. Antacids are used either to decrease acid secretions or to neutralize the secreted hydrochloric acid in the stomach when hyperacidity occurs. Antacids have aluminum and magnesium as bases, with each having the opposite effect on bowels; magnesium causes diarrhea, aluminum causes constipation. To prevent side effects, some antacids, known as *magaldrates*, contain both compounds. Calcium carbonate, an antacid, is also effective as a calcium substitute in osteoporosis prevention. Sodium bicarbonate should be avoided as a routine antacid because it interacts with body fluids to change electrolyte levels.

Optimal antiulcer therapy requires drug and lifestyle changes. Antibiotic therapy, using at least two antibiotics to prevent the chance of forming drug-resistant strains of microorganisms, is used for *H. pylori* bacterial ulcers. H_2-receptor antagonists are effective in inhibiting histamine secretions of the gastric mucosa to decrease acid secretions. When antacids and antisecretory agents are to be used therapeutically, agents should be given at least 1 hour apart to be effective. PPIs decrease hydrogen and potassium, chemicals essential for formation of hydrochloric acid in the stomach. Some antiulcer medications protect the gastric wall by coating it to reduce gastric irritations.

Symptoms of GERD may be reduced by using antispasmodics to decrease secretions and slow gastric motility. Prokinetic medications stimulate gastric motility and lower esophageal sphincter pressure. These agents are also used for the treatment of nausea caused by chemotherapy and may be used for GI disorders when lifestyle changes have not been effective.

Viral hepatitis B and C, the main causes of liver disease, may be acute or chronic. Both types of chronic hepatitis are treated with parenteral interferon alfa and peginterferon alfa-2b for 12 months with limited success after treatment is stopped.

Digestive enzyme supplements are specifically for fat digestion in persons who produce insufficient pancreatic enzymes. Cholesterol gallstones may be dissolved by medications, but this is a long process, taking up to 2 years.

Antiemetics work in several ways to suppress vomiting. Some drugs are used with chemotherapy and surgery, whereas others are used to treat motion sickness or hyperactivity of the stomach associated with ingested toxins. Some antiemetics for nausea of travel sickness are available OTC and should be taken 30 to 60 minutes before the beginning of a trip, whereas others are available by prescription for prolonged transdermal application.

Because of ease of obtaining laxatives, these drugs may be the most misused of all medications, especially by the elderly. Rebound constipation occurs when a person depends on laxatives for bowel action. Laxatives work several ways, so the chosen type should be matched to the constipation cause.

Antidiarrheals classified as synthetic opioids are available either by prescription or OTC and should be taken with care. One of the most effective treatments for diarrhea is Pepto-Bismol, which coats the intestinal tract and is bacteriostatic in the stomach.

Irritable bowel syndrome is treated with salicylates and antibiotics. Some preparations for the disease are retention enemas that are used at bedtime.

Anorectal preparations, most being OTC preparations, are topical anesthetics, hydrocortisone, or a combination of both agents for anal discomforts may require a prescription. Emollients are used to lubricate the rectum, whereas astringents are used to decrease swelling, inflammation, and irritation.

Anthelmintics, used to treat intestinal parasites, are enhanced when given with fatty foods. When one member of a family is treated for intestinal parasites, the entire household should be weighed and treated.

Anorexiants, used for treatment of obesity, should be used only short term, with behavioral modification and diet used in the long term. These drugs, which cause central nervous system irritability, are scheduled medications because of their habit-forming nature.

CRITICAL THINKING EXERCISES

Scenario

Sally comes to the medical setting stating she has heartburn on a daily basis. She states that she has also been constipated.

1. What formula for an antacid should she take?
2. How often and at what time of day should she take the antacid?
3. How should she space her routine medications with the antacid?
4. What suggestions would you make if Sally begins to have diarrhea?
5. What lifestyle changes might help Sally's bowel and gastric conditions?

DRUG CALCULATIONS

1. Order: Surfak 100 mg PO hs
   Available medication:

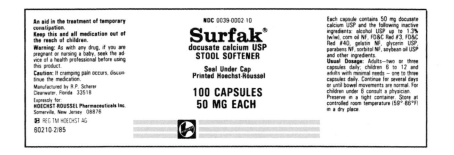

An aid in the treatment of temporary constipation.
Keep this and all medication out of the reach of children.
Warning: As with any drug, if you are pregnant or nursing a baby, seek the advice of a health professional before using this product.
Caution: If cramping pain occurs, discontinue the medication.
Manufactured by R.P. Scherer
Clearwater, Florida 33518
Expressly for:
HOECHST-ROUSSEL Pharmaceuticals Inc.
Somerville, New Jersey 08876
REG TM HOECHST AG
60210-2/85

NDC 0039-0002-10
Surfak®
docusate calcium USP
STOOL SOFTENER
Seal Under Cap
Printed Hoechst-Roussel
**100 CAPSULES
50 MG EACH**

Each capsule contains 50 mg docusate calcium USP and the following inactive ingredients: alcohol USP up to 1.3% (w/w), corn oil NF, FD&C Red #3, FD&C Red #40, gelatin NF, glycerin USP, parabens NF, sorbitol NF, soybean oil USP and other ingredients.
Usual Dosage: Adults—two or three capsules daily; children 6 to 12 and adults with minimal needs — one to three capsules daily. Continue for several days or until bowel movements are normal. For children under 6 consult a physician.
Preserve in a tight container. Store at controlled room temperature (59°-86°F) in a dry place.

Dose to be given: _____

2. Order: Zantac 37.5 mg IM stat
   Available medication:

NDC 0173-0363-00
Glaxo Pharmaceuticals
**Zantac®
(ranitidine
hydrochloride)
Injection**
25 mg/mL*
40-mL Pharmacy Bulk Package—
Not for Direct Infusion
Sterile
Caution: Federal law prohibits dispensing without prescription.

Contents should be used as soon as possible following initial closure puncture. Discard any unused portion within 24 hours of first entry.
* Each 1 mL of aqueous solution contains ranitidine 25 mg (as the hydrochloride); phenol 5 mg as preservative; monobasic potassium phosphate and dibasic sodium phosphate as buffers.
See package insert for Dosage and Administration and directions for use of Pharmacy Bulk Package.
Store between 4° and 30°C (39° and 86°F). Protect from light. Store vial in carton until time of use.
Zantac® Injection tends to exhibit a yellow color that may intensify over time without adversely affecting potency.
Glaxo Pharmaceuticals, Division of Glaxo Inc.
Research Triangle Park, NC 27709
Manufactured
in England
4/93

4043014

Dose to be given: _____
Show the volume of medication on the syringe provided.

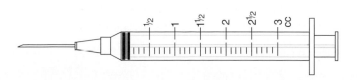

REVIEW QUESTIONS

1. What is the indication for using fluoride products? In what forms are they available? _____

   _____

2. What are the indications for antacids? _____

   _____

3. What bacterium has been found to cause peptic ulcers? What are two antibiotics used in the treatment of bacterial peptic ulcers? _____

   _____

4. What is an antiemetic? What are the classes of antiemetics? How do medications for motion sickness work?

   _____

   _____

   _____

5. What two special groups of patients must be watched closely with the use of laxatives? Why do these populations need special considerations? _____

   _____

   _____

6. Why are laxatives and cathartics used? What is the difference between laxatives and cathartics? _____

   _____

   _____

   _____

7. How do adsorbent antidiarrheals work? Opioid and synthetic opioid antidiarrheals? _____

   _____

   _____

   _____

8. What is the purpose of anthelmintics? What are some of their side effects? _____

   _____

   _____

CHAPTER 25

Respiratory System Disorders

OBJECTIVES

After studying this chapter, you should be capable of doing the following:

- Briefly discussing the respiratory tract as a source for internal and external respirations.
- Describing the effects of antihistamines and decongestants and the use of nasal preparations with respiratory conditions.
- Briefly explaining the need for corticosteroids in acute and chronic respiratory tract diseases and associated side effects of long-term therapy.

- Discussing mucolytics, expectorants, and antitussives and their effects on respiratory secretions.
- Explaining medicinal inhibition of influenza.
- Describing medications for respiratory syncytial virus.
- Providing patient education for compliance with medications used to treat diseases and conditions of the respiratory system.

Mac, age 2, has a cough and congestion because of an upper respiratory infection (URI). Mac visits Dr. Merry because he has begun to wheeze. Mac's mother is concerned that Mac might have asthma and might need corticosteroids. Dr. Merry checks Mac and finds that he also has otitis media.

Would you expect Mac to have an earache with a URI?
Dr. Merry prescribes a decongestant. What side effects would Dr. Merry tell Mac's mother may occur?
Why would Dr. Merry prescribe a decongestant rather than an antihistamine?

KEY TERMS

Anomaly	Dysphonia	Leukotriene	Rale
Anosmia	Dyspnea	Mucokinetic agent	Rebound congestion
Antihistamine	Emphysema	Mucolytic	Rhinitis
Antitussive	Epistaxis	Mucus	Rhinorrhea
Asthma	Expectorant	Nebulizer	Sputum
Atelectasis	Expectoration	Nonproductive cough	Stomatitis
Bronchiectasis	Extrapyramidal	Palliative	Tenacious
Coryza	symptoms	Patent	Tenacious cough
Decongestant	Hemoptysis	Productive cough	

EASY WORKING KNOWLEDGE OF INDICATIONS AND SIDE EFFECTS

Common Symptoms of Respiratory System Disorders
Pain in respiratory tract including chest pain and sore throat
Dyspnea, wheezing, **rales**—leading to cyanosis
Acute or chronic cough, productive or nonproductive cough
Dysphonia
Fatigue and malaise
Chills, fever, and headaches
Hemoptysis and epistaxis

Common Side Effects of Medications for Respiratory System Conditions
Dry mouth
Tachycardia
Sleeplessness and nervousness
Nausea, vomiting, and anorexia
Stomatitis
Drowsiness
Hypotension
Decreased coordination
Hoarseness

EASY WORKING KNOWLEDGE OF DRUGS USED TO TREAT RESPIRATORY SYSTEM DISORDERS

DRUG CLASS	PRESCRIPTION	OTC	PREGNANCY CATEGORY	MAJOR INDICATIONS
Antihistamines	Yes	Yes	B, C	Treatment of histamine-caused allergies such as rhinitis
Decongestants	Yes	Yes	C	Relief of nasal and upper respiratory congestion, including colds and influenza
Nasal sprays and drops	Yes	Yes	C	Relief of nasal membrane edema, as decongestants, and for seasonal allergic rhinitis
Combination decongestant products	Yes	Yes	C	Common cold
Antitussives	Yes	Yes	B, C	Relief of cough, especially nonproductive cough
Mucolytics	Yes	Yes	B	Decrease viscosity of respiratory secretions
Expectorants	Yes	Yes	C	Promote coughing and expectoration of mucus and sputum
Bronchodilators	Yes	Yes	B, C	Dilate bronchial tree to increase O_2-CO_2 exchange
Glucocorticoids	Yes	No	C, D	Relieve acute and chronic asthma
Asthmatic prophylactic agents	Yes	Yes	B	Prevention of an asthma attack
Agents for treating influenza A and B and prophylactic agents	Yes	No	C	Prevention of influenza symptoms
Agents for treating respiratory syncytial virus (RSV)	Yes	No	X (ribavirin), C	Treatment of RSV infection

The respiratory tract carries oxygen to and removes carbon dioxide from the lungs—external respiration. The circulatory system carries oxygen to body cells, where it is exchanged with carbon dioxide at the cellular level or cellular (internal) respiration. These two components of oxygen exchange maintain body pH and homeostasis, with any change in the respiratory system affecting all body systems. Other disease processes increase the work of the respiratory system, and impaired oxygen–carbon dioxide exchange must be treated before other system disorders can be addressed.

HOW RESPIRATION CONTROLS BODY FUNCTIONS

The respiratory tract is divided into upper and lower respiratory tracts and is reliant on accessory organs such as chest wall skeletal muscles and the diaphragm to function (Figure 25-1). In cardiopulmonary resuscitation, *A*, or airway, and *B*, or breathing, are the first steps for maintenance of life, followed by *C*, or circulation (cardiac function), to send needed oxygen to body cells for

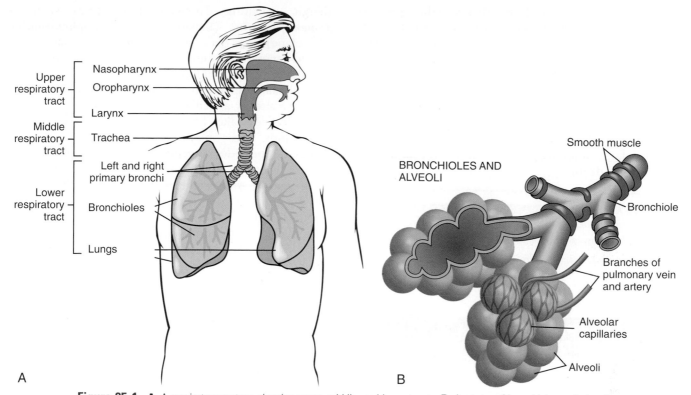

Figure 25-1 **A,** A respiratory system, showing upper, middle, and lower tracts. **B,** Anatomy of bronchioles and alveoli.

homeostasis. Respirations regulate the functionality of body systems, adjusting to any changes in a person's metabolic state.

Keeping the respiratory tract patent with the presence of needed secretions and their tenacity determine respiratory tract efficiency. When **anomalies,** diseases, or injuries occur, medications are used as treatment to ensure flow of air through respiratory passages into body cells for a constant supply of oxygen and continuous removal of carbon dioxide.

Respiratory tract secretions produce thick mucus that bathes the upper tract to protect against toxins. These secretions, together with cilia, prevent pathogens from entering the lower respiratory tract. Watery fluids in the lower respiratory tract coat lung epithelium as protectants. If these secretions become **tenacious,** the cilia are ineffective and have difficulty removing secretions for expulsion. Moisture in the respiratory tract then cannot keep secretions thin, resulting in difficulty breathing. Secretions collect because of excessive amounts of mucus.

The tracheobronchial tree, innervated by the autonomic nervous system, allows smooth muscles to work to improve ventilation. Basic respiratory rhythm and control come from the brain's medulla. Chemoreceptors and baroreceptors in carotid and aortic blood vessels lead to respiratory center stimulation when control of breathing is necessary. Thus respiratory centers control blood pH, and vice versa. Fear, pain, stress, exercise, blood pressure, body temperature, and blood oxygen levels modify the respiratory centers and control of the rhythm and depth of respiration. Although the respiratory system may be affected by voluntary controls, final control is involuntary.

OXYGEN THERAPY

Oxygen therapy is used to treat inadequate oxygen intake resulting from pathologic respiratory conditions that decrease pulmonary gas exchanges, such as found with chronic obstructive pulmonary disease (COPD). Oxygen is ordered by prescription and administered by inhalation through various delivery systems. Oxygen should be available in medical settings such as physicians' offices for emergency use. Allied health professionals should know proper and competent use of available equipment and should ensure it is always in working condition.

In disease processes such as COPD, low doses of oxygen are administered to promote respiratory gas exchange. Effectiveness of oxygen therapy depends on blood carbon dioxide content and response by involuntary respirations. Because oxygen–carbon dioxide exchange is impaired in individuals with chronic respiratory diseases, carbon dioxide content of the blood tends to rise. Also, because carbon dioxide levels are chronically increased with decreased blood oxygen levels as seen with COPD, the respiratory center of the brain is relatively insensitive to carbon dioxide stimulation, decreasing involuntary respiratory response. Therefore these patients are usually prescribed very low doses of oxygen (1 to 2 L/min) to stimulate respirations. Larger doses of oxygen will further suppress involuntary respirations.

Recognizing oxygen toxicity is difficult. Some early signs of high oxygen levels are mental confusion, sternal aching or burning, and dry, hacking cough. Respiratory distress, nausea, vomiting, restlessness, twitching, loss of feeling, and tremors in any order may follow. Excessive oxygen intake for a long period of time can lead to convulsions and death.

Patient Education for Compliance

Oxygen should not be used near an open flame or when there is a possibility of sparks because of the danger of explosion.

UPPER RESPIRATORY TRACT CONDITIONS

The upper respiratory tract consists of the nasal cavity, sinuses, pharynx, larynx, trachea, and mouth. The symptoms of the upper respiratory tract conditions such as **rhinitis** are sneezing, **epistaxis**, runny nose, **dysphonia**, itching, and congestion. Allergic rhinitis is caused by histamine release, whereas nonallergic rhinitis is often a symptom of the common cold. Histamine, a chemical found in body tissue, protects from environmental factors that produce allergic and inflammatory reactions. The principal action of histamine is vascular dilation and contraction of smooth muscles of the bronchial tree and gastrointestinal tract. For the person who is sensitized to histamine release in the respiratory tract, sneezing, increased nasal secretions, itching and watery eyes, and bronchoconstriction may result, leading to **dyspnea** and airway obstruction.

TREATMENT OF NASAL CONGESTION

Several medication classes are used to treat rhinitis, among them antihistamines, decongestants, cromolyn, and intranasal glucocorticoids. All may be used to treat allergic rhinitis; decongestants are used to treat nonallergic rhinitis, **coryza**, or the common cold.

Antihistamines

Hypersecretion of nasal fluids because of allergies may necessitate use of **antihistamines** to block histamine$_1$ (H$_1$)-receptor sites and to prevent histamine from causing edema, inflammation, and itching. Antihistamines have their greatest therapeutic effect on nasal

allergic reactions. First-generation drugs such as **diphenhydramine** (Benadryl) and **brompheniramine** (Dimetane) have been available for many years; newer second-generation drugs include **cetirizine** (Zyrtec) and **loratadine** (Claritin) (Table 25-1).

Antihistamines are not effective against histamines that have already attached to receptor sites, so drugs are most effective if taken before contact with allergy-causing compounds. These medications are palliative because they do not provide protection over a long period of time and are more likely to be effective at the beginning of allergy season. Antihistamines fail to reduce the **asthma** that frequently accompanies seasonal allergic responses such as hay fever.

First-generation antihistamines are nonselective in their effects on peripheral and systemic histamine receptors, although these agents produce the same degree of therapeutic response to histamine. The main difference in specific medications is in their variable degree of sedation and their antihistamine activity.

Did You Know?

Chlorpheniramine (Chlor-Trimeton) may cause insomnia in the elderly. In acute conditions, diphenhydramine (Benadryl) is still the medication of choice for allergies.

The second-generation antihistamines, with equal or better antiallergic effects, are not as sedating or drying and seem to act more selectively on the peripheral histamine receptors. These medications do not cross the blood-brain barrier easily and so are safer for use with central nervous system (CNS) depressants.

Dozens of antihistamines are available for use, and tolerance to them can develop. Antihistamines may be used interchangeably to find the most effective agent to relieve the symptoms, matching drug to patient and his or her tolerance. When choosing from among available antihistamine products, evaluation must include factors such as potency, duration of action, and incidence of side effects such as drowsiness. Often several medications may be tried before the appropriate drug for the person is found.

Because histamine also causes motion sickness, over-the-counter (OTC) antihistamines may be used to relieve these symptoms, as well as vertigo, hay fever, allergic coughs, allergic rhinitis, and allergies to insect bites and contact dermatitis. These products are also used as sedatives because of the major side effect of sedation. Many OTC drugs contain antihistamines as sleeping aids (e.g., Nytol). Oral absorption of these agents is good, with most having an onset of action within 15 to 60 minutes.

When antihistamines are given for nasal secretions of a common cold, the resultant thickening of bronchial

TABLE 25-1 ANTIHISTAMINES

GENERIC NAME/TRADE NAME	USUAL DOSE, ROUTE, AND FREQUENCY	INDICATIONS FOR USE	DRUG INTERACTIONS
FIRST-GENERATION DRUGS		Acute and chronic allergic reactions including allergic rhinitis, dermatitis, and hay fever	alcohol, anticholinergics, MAOIs
brompheniramine* (Bromax)	11 mg PO bid		
chlorpheniramine* (Chlor-Trimeton, and others) SR	4 mg PO q4-6h 8-12 mg PO q8-12h		
dimenhydrinate* (Dramamine)	50-100 mg PO q4-6h		
diphenhydramine*† (Benadryl)	25*-50† mg PO q4-6h		
meclizine*† (Antivert,*† Bonine*, Dramamine Nondrowsy)	25-100 mg PO daily in divided doses		
SECOND-GENERATION DRUGS		Same as for first-generation drugs	Same as for first-generation drugs
cetirizine*† (Zyrtec)	5-10 mg PO qd		
fexofenadine*† (Allegra)	60-180 mg PO qd		
loratadine* (Claritin, Alavert)	10 mg PO qd		
desloratadine† (Clarinex)	5 mg PO qd		
SECOND-GENERATION DRUGS WITH DECONGESTANT*		Same as for first-generation drugs	Same as for first-generation drugs
cetirizine + pseudoephedrine* (Zyrtec-D)	120 mg PO qd		
fexofenadine + pseudoephedrine* (Allegra-D)	60 mg/120 mg PO qd		
loratadine + pseudoephedrine* (Claritin-D, Alavert-D)	5 mg/120 mg- 10 mg/240 mg PO qd		
NASAL SPRAY ANTIHISTAMINE			
azelastine† (Astelin, Astepro)	1-2 sprays each nostril twice daily	Environmental irritants and seasonal allergic rhinitis	None indicated

D, decongestant; *MAOI*, monoamine oxidase inhibitor; *ND*, non-drowsy; *PO*, orally.
*OTC medication.
†Prescription medication.

secretions may cause airway obstruction, especially in patients with COPD. More antihistamines and antihistamine-decongestant combinations are being sold OTC with a reduced dosage rather than on a prescription-only basis. Care should be taken with patients who have glaucoma, ulcers, or urine retention because of the drying effects of antihistamines and the resultant buildup of pressure in the eye. **Extrapyramidal symptoms** such as tremors, dystonia, and Parkinson-like symptoms should be reported immediately.

Patient Education for Compliance

1. Care should be taken when using antihistamines and operating machinery because of the sedating effects. The patient should evaluate his or her state of alertness before operating machinery or driving a car.
2. Antihistamines are drying; frequent sips of water, a piece of hard candy, or chewing gum may temporarily provide relief.
3. When antihistamines are taken for motion sickness, the dose should be taken approximately 30 minutes to 1 hour before travel departure.
4. Patients with benign prostatic hypertrophy or cardiovascular disease, especially hypertension, should not use antihistamines without a physician's supervision.
5. Alcohol should not be used with first-generation antihistamines because of synergistic effects.
6. When using medications for allergic rhinitis, allergens such as pollution and smoke should be avoided.
7. Because many cold and cough preparations contain antihistamines, patients should not mix cold and cough preparations without professional advice.

Important Facts about Antihistamines

- Allergic rhinitis, most common of all allergic disorders, is treated with antihistamines.
- Antihistamines decrease histamine secretions throughout the body and may cause dizziness, drowsiness, photosensitivity, and headaches.
- Antihistamines relieve coughs and colds as well as motion sickness.
- Antihistamines relieve rhinorrhea, sneezing, and itching but do not relieve nasal or chest congestion.
- Sedation, a common side effect of first-generation antihistamines, has been reduced to basically no problem in second-generation agents.

Decongestants

Decongestants, used to relieve nasal congestion, are vasoconstricting agents that shrink the swollen mucous membranes of nasal passages, with a resultant decrease in nasal drainage (Table 25-2). These agents come as both oral and nasal preparations. Most oral agents are adrenergic medications or medications that mimic the effects of the sympathetic nervous system. Label warnings on OTC preparations instruct patients with hypertension, hyperthyroidism, diabetes mellitus, or ischemic heart disease to use these drugs with care.

Decongestants and antihistamines are often combined, but care should be taken to keep the dosage within a safe range. Two agents, phenylephrine and pseudoephedrine, are considered safe as decongestants when used as the label indicates. Medications containing these agents cause vasoconstriction and shrinking of swollen membranes. Phenylephrine, the most widely used of decongestants, is administered topically in the nose alone or as an active ingredient in combination with other preparations. When decongestants such as **oxymetazoline** (Afrin) and **phenylephrine** (Neo-Synephrine) are used topically, action is rapid, whereas oral medications such as **pseudoephedrine** (Sudafed and Contac) have delayed and prolonged responses. Pseudoephedrine has a high incidence of CNS stimulation and is not as widely used as phenylephrine. Persons taking *Ephedra* as an herbal supplement should be extremely careful when using decongestants because of synergistic actions.

Decongestants, topical and oral, are for short-term use, with **rebound congestion** occurring with just a few days of constant use. The patient may develop habituation with use on a prolonged regular basis. With topical nasal agents, the possibility of rebound congestion becomes greater as the effect of nasal spray wears off. To overcome this, patients tend to use larger medication doses more frequently. This cycle of escalating congestion followed by increased doses of medication will become progressively worse unless the patient stops using topical decongestants completely. Discontinuation of topical sprays often produces severe congestion for several days until mucous membranes adjust to lack of medication. Therefore topical decongestants are inappropriate for patients with chronic rhinitis symptoms. Because of the danger of rebound congestion, the time limit for using topical decongestants on a regular basis should be 5 days.

Did You Know?

Because of abuse potential and use with illicit drug manufacturing, pseudoephedrine now is a medication that has a restriction on the amount that may be purchased at a time.

Important Facts about Decongestants

- Decongestants should be used only on advice of physician by patients with heart disease, glaucoma, and prostate cancer. Self-medication using OTC preparations should be avoided, as these may cause tachycardia, nervousness, restlessness, insomnia, blurred vision, and nausea and vomiting.
- Overuse or continued use of nasal sprays causes rebound congestion, making symptoms worse and having inherent danger of side effects from increasing medication use.
- Topical decongestants (e.g., nasal sprays) act rapidly and produce minimal systemic effects; although oral decongestants work slowly, producing central nervous system stimulation, no rebound congestion occurs, so these should be used for therapy lasting longer.

TABLE 25-2 DECONGESTANTS

GENERIC NAME/TRADE NAME	USUAL DOSE, ROUTE, AND FREQUENCY	INDICATIONS FOR USE	DRUG INTERACTIONS
NASAL DECONGESTANTS		Nonallergic rhinitis, such as common cold	MAOIs
epinephrine 0.1% (AsthmaHaler Mist, Bronkaid Mist, Primatene Mist) (Adrenalin)	1 or 2 inhalations		
naphazoline 0.05% (Allerest, Privine)	2 drops or sprays topically in nostril		
oxymetazoline 0.05% (Afrin, Dristan)	2 sprays topically in nostril bid		
phenylephrine 0.125%-1% (Neo-Synephrine, Sinex)	Several drops in nostril, 1 or 2 nasal sprays q4h		
tetrahydrozoline 0.05-0.1% (Tyzine)	2-4 drops in topically in nostril q4-8h		
xylometazoline 0.1% (Otrivin, Triaminic)	2-3 drops topically in nostril; 2 or 3 nasal sprays q8-10h		
ORAL DECONGESTANTS			
pseudoephedrine (Sudafed) (Sudafed 12 HR/Sudafed 24 HR)	60 mg PO q4-6h 120 mg (sustained-release) /240 mg PO q12h		
COMBINATION DECONGESTANTS			
guaifenesin + pseudoephedrine (Guaifenex PSE, Mucinex, Triaminic, Robitussin PE)	60 mg/120 mg PO q12h		
chlorpheniramine + pseudoephedrine (Sudafed Plus, Chlor-Trimeton D)	1 tab PO q12h		
dextromethorphan + pseudoephedrine (in combination with acetaminophen) (Allerest, Contac, many OTC combinations)	1 tab PO q12h		
ZINC PREPARATIONS			
zirconium glucosamine (Zicam,* Cold-Eeze)	1 dose as nasal spray or nasal gel applied locally	Common cold	Usually none

MAOI, Monoamine oxidase inhibitor; *PO*, orally.
*Zicam is available in several different formulas and forms.
Note: All the drugs listed in this table are available OTC.

Cromolyn Sodium

Intranasal **cromolyn sodium** (Nasalcrom) relieves allergic rhinitis by preventing release of histamine after allergen exposure, so it is more effective if used before the onset of allergic symptoms caused by histamines. Approximately a week is needed for cromolyn to be effective, so this medication should be used throughout allergy season. Cromolyn provides no relief for nonallergic rhinitis. If nasal congestion is present, a topical nasal decongestant may be used before cromolyn.

Glucocorticoids

Nasal glucocorticoids, such as **fluticasone** (Flonase) and **triamcinolone** (Nasacort), should be used at times when prolonged effectiveness for seasonal and perennial rhinitis is needed. These agents suppress symptoms

TABLE 25-3 MISCELLANEOUS NASAL PREPARATIONS

GENERIC NAME/TRADE NAME	USUAL DOSE, ROUTE, AND FREQUENCY*	INDICATIONS FOR USE	DRUG INTERACTIONS
cromolyn sodium, intranasal (Nasalcrom)	1 nasal spray q4-6h	Allergic rhinitis	Usually none
INTRANASAL GLUCOCORTICOIDS		Allergic rhinitis	Usually none
beclomethasone (Beconase)	1 puff in nostril bid		
budesonide (Rhinocort aqua)	2-4 nasal puffs qd		
flunisolide	2 nasal puffs bid		
fluticasone (Flonase, Veramyst)	2 nasal puffs qd		
triamcinolone (Nasacort AQ)	1 or 2 nasal puffs qd		
mometasone (Nasonex)	1 spray in nostril qd		
ciclesonide (Omnaris)	2 sprays in each nostril bid		

*All of the drugs in this table are topical application to nasal cavity.
Note: All the drugs listed in this table are prescription drugs.

TABLE 25-4 DIFFERENCES AMONG ALLERGIC RHINITIS, COLDS, AND INFLUENZA

SIGNS AND SYMPTOMS	ALLERGIC RHINITIS	COMMON COLD	INFLUENZA
Fever	No	Occasionally	Common, with temperatures of 102°-104° F with sudden onset
Aching, pain	No	Very occasionally	May be severe
Sneezing	Yes	Yes	Infrequent
Itching	Yes	No	No
Cough	Occasionally	Usually	Yes
Occurrence	Seasonal	Anytime	Anytime
Headache	Maybe	Infrequent	Usually
Cause	Allergens	Viral	Viral

Modified from Salerno E: *Pharmacology for health professionals*, St Louis, 1999, Mosby.

of allergic rhinitis—congestion, **rhinorrhea**, sneezing, itching, and erythema. Unlike corticosteroids used for other conditions, these drugs have minimal systemic effects with topical nasal use, but their use should be limited to 1 month at a time (Table 25-3).

OTC Products for Upper Respiratory Conditions

U.S. citizens spend billions of dollars yearly on OTC medications, with approximately one third being used for upper respiratory tract conditions, such as colds, cough, allergies, and related symptoms. Table 25-4 compares signs and symptoms of allergies, influenza, and the common cold.

Many forms of OTC medications are available for upper respiratory conditions; these agents are the most commonly purchased OTC medications, as shown in Tables 25-1 and 25-2. Some are combinations of decongestants or antihistamines with **antitussives** or analgesics. In most cases, the OTC medication dosage has been reduced from that found in prescription medications. Other, newer OTC medications such as Cold-Eeze and homeopathic medications such as Airborne have zinc bases.

Combination OTC Products

Combination OTC products should be carefully selected because multidrug formulas have some drugs unnecessary for specific disorders. Decongestants, antitussives, and analgesics are used to relieve obvious cold symptoms of rhinorrhea, cough, sneezing, sore throat, headache, malaise, and aching, whereas antihistamines will suppress secretion of mucus through anticholinergic action. Because no single medication relieves all cold symptoms, the pharmaceutical industry has formulated various combination products to relieve multiple symptoms. A cold is self-limiting because of its viral nature, but symptoms should be addressed for patient comfort. Disadvantages of combination medications are subtherapeutic levels found with some dosages and excessive levels of chemical agents that are not needed. If the patient has only one symptom to relieve, then a single-entity preparation should be used. If an adverse reaction occurs with use of combination medications, the offending medication may not be identified. For safety, if an analgesic-antipyretic is necessary, it should be selected and given separately. These combinations should be avoided in most viral infections to prevent missing a diagnosis of a secondary bacterial infection that may be present.

Under Food and Drug Administration (FDA) regulations, a brand-name product may be reformulated and sold under the previous name. Thus, unless they are extremely careful to read medication labels with each purchase, patients may buy a product that lacks agents contained in the same product purchased previously.

Zinc-Based OTC Products

In recent years, zinc-based products such as Cold-Eeze and Zicam have been used for common cold symptoms. Some products are available as zinc gluconate lozenges that have an unpleasant taste. Other items are available as *zinc gluconate glycine* (Zicam) in the form of dose spoons, nasal sprays, swabs, gels, and tablets that melt in the mouth and may cause loss of smell and taste. Zinc-based chemicals are also found in combination with decongestants and antihistamines for relief of symptoms (see Table 25-2).

Herbal Cold Prophylactic Products

Airborne is a unique blend of herbal extracts, vitamins, electrolytes, and amino acids for a boost to the immune system. It is to be used for prophylaxis against the common cold. This product is available as an effervescent tablet and a lozenge.

Did You Know?

Airborne was created by a teacher who was constantly exposed to germs in the classroom and wanted some agent for prophylaxis.

Patient Education for Compliance

1. Nasal stinging and burning may occur with topical nasal products. Zinc-based sprays may cause **anosmia.**
2. Applicators for topical nasal decongestants (nose drops and nasal sprays) should be cleaned after each use.
3. Nasal spray tip should not touch nasal mucosa, and container of medication should not be shared with anyone.
4. Nasal drops should be administered in a lateral head-low position to allow spread over nasal mucosa.

DRUGS USED FOR COUGHS

Coughing is a reflex beneficial for removing foreign matter from the respiratory tract, clear airways, and remove excess secretions from the bronchial tree. Cough preparations are used to suppress cough intensity and frequency while allowing secretions to be eliminated. Coughs that prevent sleep or cause discomfort related to upper respiratory tract infections (URIs) should be treated. A dry nonproductive cough should be treated because it can be exhausting, painful, and detrimental to the circulatory system and the elasticity of the respiratory system. When coughing is prolonged or spastic, **hemoptysis** may occur. However, a **productive cough** from COPD should not be suppressed.

Antitussives

The two major groups of antitussives are opioid and nonopioid. The opioid cough suppressants, Schedule III medications, that contain hydrocodone require a prescription. Codeine cough suppressants are Schedule V medications and may not require a prescription, depending on the laws of each state. Nonopioid antitussives may require a prescription, but some are available OTC (Table 25-5).

Opioid Cough Suppressants

Codeine and codeine-like products are the most effective prescription cough suppressants for routine prescription use. Codeine suppresses both cough frequency and intensity by elevating the cough threshold. Given orally, doses remain low (approximately one tenth of that needed to relieve pain), so the chance of physical dependence is low when taken as directed. Most cough mixtures are Schedule III, IV, or V medications. In some states, Schedule V medications may be bought OTC if the patient signs a roster showing receipt of the medication.

TABLE 25-5 ANTITUSSIVES

GENERIC NAME/TRADE NAME AND CONTROLLED DRUG SCHEDULE	USUAL DOSE, ROUTE, AND FREQUENCY	INDICATIONS FOR USE	DRUG INTERACTIONS
OPIOIDS			
codeine*†‡ (Various preparations in various schedules)	10-20 mg PO q3-6h	Suppression of dry, irritating coughs of upper respiratory diseases	See under *Analgesics* in Chapter 15
hydrocodone (Hydromet, Tussignon)	5-10 mg PO q4-6h		alcohol
with chlorpheniramine (Tussionex)	1-2 tsp PO q		
NONOPIOIDS		Cough suppression	
dextromethorphan†§ with guaifenesin (Sucrets, Benylin DM,	10-30 mg PO q4-6h		MAOIs
Robitussin DM, Romilar CF)	one lozenge q4-6h		
(Benylin DM)	10 mL q4-6h		
	10-20 mg PO q4h		
diphenhydramine† (Benadryl)	25 mg PO q4-6h		Basically none
benzonatate* (Tessalon)	100 mg cap PO tid		Basically none

*Prescription medication.
†OTC medication.
‡Codeine cough preparations are by prescription, although some preparations that are Schedule V drugs may be bought OTC, depending on the amount of codeine present and state regulations. Customer must sign for OTC medications to show proof of receipt.
§When "DM" follows cough preparations, in most cases dextromethorpan is found in the medication.

BOX 25-1 COMMON OTC PREPARATIONS CONTAINING DEXTROMETHORPHAN

Children's Nyquil
Cheracol D
Multisymptom Tylenol Cold
Naldecon DX
Novahistine DMX
Nyquil Nighttime Cold Formula
Robitussin CF
Tylenol Cold
Vicks Formula 44D and 44M

Nonopioid Cough Suppressants

Nonaddicting nonopioid cough suppressants do not have the gastrointestinal side effects found with codeine preparations.

Dextromethorphan, one of the most effective nonopioid cough medicines, does not suppress respirations. Used in recommended doses, it is just as effective as codeine except for severe acute coughs. Dextromethorphan should not be taken with monoamine oxidase inhibitors (MAOIs) because of the chance of excitability, sedation, and severe hypertension (see Box 25-1 for common dextromethorphan OTC preparations).

Diphenhydramine (Benadryl), an active ingredient in many OTC preparations and in some prescription medications, has an antitussive dose of 25 mg every 4 to 6 hours. The cough suppression comes with sedation as a side effect.

Benzonatate (Tessalon), related to **tetracaine** (a local anesthetic), relieves coughing by peripherally anesthetizing cough receptors. These gelcaps should be swallowed intact to prevent anesthesia in the mouth. This drug may affect the gag reflex but has no major systemic effects or interactions with other medications. Onset of action is about 15 to 20 minutes, with a duration of action of approximately 8 hours (see Table 25-5).

Patient Education for Compliance

1. If a cough produces significant amounts of sputum, care should be taken in using cough suppressants because coughing may be needed to expel sputum.
2. All OTC labels should be read carefully before OTC drugs are taken.
3. If a cough persists for more than 10 days with high fever or chest pain, consult a health care provider.
4. Antitussives should be taken only in specified dosages.
5. Avoid irritants such as smoking and dust to decrease throat irritation.
6. Chew gum, drink frequent sips of water, or suck on sugarless hard candy to diminish coughing. However, sugarless products may produce flatulence.

Important Facts about Cough Suppressants

- Coughing is necessary to clear respiratory tract secretions. Antitussives should be used when coughing is nonproductive, interrupts daily activities, or is excessive.
- Cough preparations containing codeine or codeine-like medications cause drowsiness and should be taken with care when machinery is being operated.
- Codeine and codeine-like preparations are the most effective cough suppressants. Only small doses are necessary for effective treatment. Many antitussives are Schedule III drugs.
- Dextromethorphan is the most effective nonopioid cough suppressant available.

UNDERSTANDING LOWER RESPIRATORY TRACT DISORDERS

The lower respiratory tract consists of the bronchial tree and lungs, which must be kept patent for the flow of air. Smooth muscles regulate the size of the passage lumen, and cartilage gives support to keep the passages open. When lower respiratory tract diseases occur, exchange of oxygen and carbon dioxide cannot occur in the single-layered capillaries of alveoli, resulting in serious alterations of blood gases. Acute conditions may include pneumonia and acute asthmatic attacks. Chronic conditions such as COPD (an irreversible disease) and emphysema may lead to bronchiectasis and atelectasis. Symptoms of lower respiratory diseases include dyspnea, wheezing, tenacious sputum, and chest congestion and discomfort. COPD and emphysema eventually lead to a gas exchange problem with a resultant chronic cough, susceptibility to infection, and difficulty in engaging in physical activity. Bronchodilators and mucolytic agents are used, along with breathing exercises and oxygen therapy, to assist in palliatively relieving the respiratory symptoms, but the damage to the lungs is irreversible. Treatment of these diseases includes maintenance of airways using bronchodilators, mucokinetic agents, and expectorants. Chronic conditions may be treated using corticosteroids to reduce the swelling of the bronchial tree and sympathomimetics to reduce the edema and to stimulate vasodilation and bronchodilation. Cigarette smoking and toxic fumes lead to chronic bronchial tree irritation, causing increased and thickened pulmonary secretions.

Asthma is a condition caused by an antigen-antibody reaction resulting in wheezing, shortness of breath, and a feeling of suffocation from constriction of bronchioles. This disorder may be caused by many factors such as irritants, exercise, infections of the respiratory tract, allergies, gastroesophageal reflux disease, and salicylates. The airway becomes inflamed with edema and mucous plugs, with bronchial tree hyperactivity adding to symptoms. During asthmatic attacks, when bronchiole constriction and increased secretions are present, bronchodilators are used for relief. Also used for chronic and acute relief are antiinflammatory agents such as glucocorticoids and cromolyn. Most medications for asthma are administered by inhalation to achieve more rapid therapeutic effects in an acute attack and to deliver the medication directly to the site where it is needed and with minimized systemic effect.

DRUGS FOR CONDITIONS OF THE LOWER RESPIRATORY TRACT

Mucokinetic Agents

Patients with chronic respiratory diseases have excessively thick, tenacious sputum that must be thinned for expectoration. Mucokinetic agents, or mucolytics, are drugs that react with mucus to make it more watery. Thus the cough is more productive, sputum is easier to expectorate, and mucus retention is prevented. When using these drugs, the patient must increase fluid intake. Mucus is a normal secretion from the mucous membranes of the respiratory tract, whereas sputum is an abnormal secretion originating in the lower respiratory tract. Sputum may contain pathologic microorganisms because thick mucus tends to remain in place longer, allowing normal flora to become pathologic.

Hypertonic saline solution and acetylcysteine are used for their mucolytic actions. *Hypertonic saline (1.8% sodium chloride)* stimulates a cough by irritating the respiratory mucosa while attracting water to the secretions to assist with expulsion. *Acetylcysteine* (Mucomyst), a prescription mucolytic, is used as an inhalation agent to make mucus less viscous, but as an undesireable effect this drug has an unpleasant, musty odor (Table 25-6).

CLINICAL TIP

Hypertonic saline may be used for relief as a home remedy by using table salt and water as a gargle or as an inhalation through mists or in a room humidifier. If a humidifier is not available, table salt in boiling water for inhalation as a vapor will assist with removal of thick, tenacious mucus of respiratory diseases.

Expectorants

Expectorants, which render coughs more productive by stimulating respiratory tract secretions to decrease the viscosity of mucus, are relatively safe drugs. The drug with greatest evidence of safety and effectiveness is

TABLE 25-6 MUCOLYTICS EXPECTORANTS

GENERIC NAME/ TRADE NAME	USUAL DOSE, ROUTE, AND FREQUENCY	INDICATIONS FOR USE	DRUG INTERACTIONS
acetylcysteine*	3-5 mL of 20% solution; 6-10 mL of 10% solution, inhaled	Thin viscous mucus	Usually none
guaifenesin*† (Robitussin,* Mucinex*)	100-400 mg PO q4h	Increases output of respiratory tract fluids	
(guaifenesin XR, Organdin NB)	600-1200 mg PO q12h		
dornase alfa† (Pulmozyme)	2.5 mg inhaled qd	Expectorant for cystic fibrosis	

*OTC medication.
†Prescription medication.
Note: Guaifenesin is available in several formulas based on presenting symptoms and use, such as Robitussin DM, which contains a decongestant with the expectorant.

guaifenesin. Expectorants are often combined with other medications for respiratory conditions such as antihistamines, decongestants, and antitussives to help remove mucus. Most have no significant contraindications.

A specific expectorant for cystic fibrosis, **dornase alfa** (Pulmozyme), digests extracellular DNA to improve pulmonary function and reduces risk of respiratory infections. The drug works within 3 to 7 days after the patient starts taking it (see Table 25-6).

Inhalation Medications Used As Bronchodilators

Three devices for inhalation administration are *metered dose inhalers* (MDIs), *nebulizers*, and *dry powder inhalers* (DPIs), each of which provides a different medication form to give a more rapid response. Using these methods of delivery provides local effects, minimizing systemic absorption (see Chapter 13 for inhalation administration).

MDIs deliver a fine mist of medication that is usually accomplished with one or two puffs from a hand-held pressurized device. Medications delivered by this method include **albuterol** (Ventolin) and **terbutaline** (Brethaire). Approximately 10% of medications administered by an MDI reach the lungs. Eighty percent is swallowed in the mouth and pharynx, possibly causing stomatitis with long-term use. Patients must be taught to use this device correctly with hand-lung coordination. Correct administration is difficult, but use of a spacer will aid with appropriate administration.

DPI medications, such as **tiotropium** (Spiriva), deliver a given amount of medication into the lungs in the form of dry powder. DPIs are breath activated and easier to use than MDIs. Some medications are available in both DPI and MDI administration forms.

A nebulizer uses a small machine to convert a solution into a mist, using such medications as **epinephrine** (Primatene) and **isoetharine** (Bronkometer). Mist droplets are inhaled either through a face mask or through a mouthpiece. Not used as frequently today, nebulizers have a degree of effectiveness that depends on the size of medication droplets as they reach the lungs and on the responsiveness of the patient's respiratory system.

Patient Education for Compliance

1. When medication is administered via MDI in two puffs, a full minute should elapse between puffs.
2. Patients should gargle after use of medications delivered by MDIs and DPIs to prevent throat irritation and possible stomatitis.

Epinephrine, Ephedra, and Beta₂-Adrenergic Drugs

The major drugs used to treat asthma and other congestive obstructions of airways include sympathomimetic medications and xanthine derivatives (Table 25-7).

Nonselective adrenergic medications such as epinephrine and ephedrine stimulate body cells to produce vasoconstriction and reduce edema, whereas other medications stimulate vasodilation and bronchodilation. **Epinephrine** (Adrenalin) and **ephedrine,** with a rapid onset of action, are indicated to prevent bronchospasm and for treatment of bronchial asthma and bronchitis. Duration of action is 1 to 3 hours when used by inhalation or 1 to 4 hours when given parenterally. Ephedrine, not as potent as epinephrine, is useful when taken orally, with a longer duration of action, but causes nervousness and stimulation of the heart and nervous system.

Beta-adrenergic (beta₂) drugs such as **metaproterenol** (Alupent) and **albuterol** (Proventil) work as both cardiac

TABLE 25-7 BRONCHODILATORS

GENERIC NAME/ TRADE NAME	USUAL DOSE, ROUTE, AND FREQUENCY	INDICATIONS FOR USE	DRUG INTERACTIONS
epinephrine*[†] (Adrenalin,* Bronkaid,[†] Medihaler Ep,[†] Primatene[†])	0.3 mg by injection, 2.25% in NEB inhaled; 10 drops of 1% solution by inhalation	Dilation of bronchial tree	Anesthetics, tricyclic depressants, beta blockers, digitalis, cardiac glycosides, ergotamine and its derivatives
ephedrine[†] (Vicks inhaler)	Inhaled topically		Same as for epinephrine

Major Side Effects of Epinephrine and Ephedrine:
Increased heart rate, tachycardia, palpitations, muscle tremors, CNS stimulation, nervousness, anorexia

BETA-ADRENERGIC AGENTS		Same as for epinephrine	Same as for epinephrine
formoterol (Foradil)	1 cap DPI inhaled in aerolizer bid		
levalbuterol (Xopenex)	0.63 mg-1.25 mg inhaled in NEB q6-12h MDI		
(Xopenex HFI)	45 mcg as MDI q6-12h		
albuterol* (Ventolin)	2-4 mg tab PO tid-qid		Beta blockers, amitriptyline, MAOIs
(Proventil HFA*, Ventolin HFA)	2 puffs inhaled (DPI) q4-6h		
	1-2 puffs inhaled (DPI) q4-6h		
pirbuterol* (Maxair)	2 puffs inhaled (MDI) q4-6h		None indicated
terbutaline*	2.5-5 mg PO tid		albuterol
	0.25 mg SC		
metaproterenol* (Alupent)	2 or 3 inhalations NEB, q4h aerosol		Same as for albuterol
salmeterol* (Serevent Diskus)	1 inhalation (DPI) bid		None indicated
arformoterol (Brovana)	2 NEB doses q12h	COPD, including bronchitis and emphysema	aminophylline, theophylline, diuretics

Major Side Effects of Beta-Adrenergic Agents:
Increased heart rate, tachycardia, palpitations, muscle tremors, CNS stimulation, nervousness, anorexia, nervousness
In addition: *formoterol*—tremors, muscle cramps, insomnia, headache; *eformoterol*—pain, headache, nervousness, hypokalemia

METHYLXANTHINES			Caffeine, cimetidine, fluoroquinolone, antibiotics, rifampin, phenobarbital, phenytoin
theophylline, aminophylline* (Elixophyllin)	Varies by immediate and sustained-release factors		
dyphylline* (Dylix, Lufyllin)	15 mg/kg PO q6h		

Major Side Effects of Methylxanthines:
Nausea, anxiety, restlessness, gastric upset, GERD, headache, insomnia, tachycardia, nervousness

CNS, central nervous system; *COPD*, chronic obstructive pulmonary disease; *DPI*, dry powder inhaler; *GERD*, gastroesophageal reflux disease; *MAOIs*, monoamine oxidase inhibitors; *MDI*, metered dose inhaler; *NEB*, nebulizer; *PO*, orally; *UTI*, urinary tract infection.
*Prescription medication.
[†]OTC medication.

Continued

TABLE 25-7 BRONCHODILATORS—cont'd

GENERIC NAME/ TRADE NAME	USUAL DOSE, ROUTE, AND FREQUENCY	INDICATIONS FOR USE	DRUG INTERACTIONS
ANTICHOLINERGIC AGENTS		None	Basically none
ipratropium* (Atrovent)	2-4 puffs inhaled (MDI) qd		
tiotropium (Spiriva)	1 puff inhaled (DPI) qd		
Major Side Effects of Anticholinergics: Dry mouth, plus sinusitis, UTI, dyspepsia, tiotropium with rhinitis			
COMBINATION BRONCHODILATORS*		Dilation of bronchial tree	None
fluticasone + salmeterol		Used in chronic asthma, emphysema	
(Advair Diskus)	1 powder dose inhaled (DPI) q12h		
(Advair HFA aerosol)	1 dose inhaled (MDI) q12h		
ipratropium + albuterol* (Combivent, Duonebs)	2 or 3 puffs inhaled (MDI) q12h		
Major Side Effects of Combination Bronchodilators: Dry mouth with fluticasone + salmeterol			

and respiratory agonists. Their main action is on the smooth muscle of the bronchial tree and on the heart. Beta$_2$-receptor medications, the most effective medications to reduce acute and exercise-induced bronchospasms, suppress lung histamine release, provide bronchodilation, and increase ciliary mobility to move mucus. Because beta$_2$ agents are selective, these medications have replaced older, less selective sympathomimetics such as epinephrine in treating asthma and other chronic congestive conditions. Beta$_2$ agonists relieve ongoing asthmatic attacks and may be used prophylactically and for necessary relief of breakthrough symptoms. Short-acting agents begin to work almost immediately; their effect peaks in 30 to 60 minutes and lasts 3 to 5 hours. Long-lasting preparations have a slow onset of action, but their effects persist for 12 hours. *Salmeterol* (Serevent) is preferred for prophylaxis but it is not effective in aborting an attack because of action slowness. These drugs may be administered by inhalation and may also be given orally or by injection.

Xanthine Derivatives

Xanthine derivatives relax the smooth muscles of the bronchial tree and stimulate cardiac muscle and the CNS. These drugs include *theophylline* and *aminophylline* (Slo-Phyllin, Elixophyllin), used for prevention and treatment of bronchial asthma and for treatment of emphysema, COPD, and bronchitis. Some states do not allow generic product substitutions because release time for action varies between generic and trade name drugs. Theophylline, the basic active ingredient of xanthines, is available in oral standard or sustained-release formulas, with forms effective for up to 24 hours. Because theophylline has a narrow therapeutic range and because beta$_2$ agonists are safer and more effective, xanthines are not used as frequently today. Patients with congestive heart failure, coronary heart disease, hypothyroidism, convulsive disorders, and acute pulmonary edema cannot use these derivatives (see Table 25-7).

Anticholinergic Medications

Anticholinergic (atropine-like) medications, used for asthma, act by drying mucous membranes in patients who cannot use other bronchodilators. With asthma, anticholinergic medications offer some relief of asthma symptoms. *Ipratropium* (Atrovent) is used in patients with chronic asthma, has a rapid onset of action (30 seconds), and reaches maximum effect in 3 minutes; and effects last for 6 hours (see Table 25-7).

Glucocorticoids

Glucocorticoids, effective as antiasthmatic medications, are usually administered by inhalation with either a DPI or an MDI but may be given orally or by injection. These medications are safe and highly effective with glucocorticoid adverse reactions being minor when used for a short period of time with acute pulmonary diseases. However, long-term systemic use has severe adverse effects (see Chapter 20). With asthma, these medications suppress inflammation and reduce bronchial tree hypersecretions. Prophylactic administration in chronic asthma is preferably given by inhalation to prevent systemic side effects, whereas oral use is effective in severe asthma. Inhaled doses are given on a daily basis, at a lower dose, and not on an as-needed basis because of slowness in development of therapeutic effects (Table 25-8).

Patient Education for Compliance

Patients using inhaled glucocorticoids should rinse their mouths after inhaling medications to prevent possibility of oral candidiasis.

Prophylactic Medications for Asthma

Cromolyn (Intal and Nasalcrom) and **nedocromil** (Tilade) are used to prevent asthma attacks but are not useful for ongoing attacks (Table 25-9). Cromolyn suppresses inflammation but does not dilate the bronchial

TABLE 25-8 GLUCOCORTICOIDS USED IN TREATING ASTHMA

GENERIC NAME/ TRADE NAME	USUAL DOSE, ROUTE, AND FREQUENCY	INDICATIONS FOR USE	DRUG INTERACTIONS
beclomethasone (Beclovent, Vanceril, QVAR)	2 puffs (MDI) bid	Chronic or acute asthma attacks	See Chapter 20
budesonide		Same as for beclomethasone	Same as for
(Pulmicort Flexhaler)	1-4 puffs (MDI)	For ages 12 and younger	beclomethasone
(Pulmicort Respules)	NEB Inhaled bid		
fluticasone (Flovent HFA)	2-4 puffs (MDI)		
prednisone	5-60 mg tab PO qid		
prednisolone (Prelone)	40-60 mg PO qd		

MDI, metered dose inhaler; *PO*, orally.
Note: All the drugs listed in this table are prescription medications.

TABLE 25-9 ASTHMATIC PROPHYLACTICS

GENERIC NAME/ TRADE NAME	USUAL DOSE, ROUTE, AND FREQUENCY	INDICATIONS FOR USE	DRUG INTERACTIONS
cromolyn (Nasalcrom)	nasal spray nebulizer	Prophylaxis in chronic asthma	None
zafirlukast (Accolate)	20 mg PO bid		aspirin, warfarin, glucocorticoids, phenytoin, cyclosporine, astemizole, theophylline
montelukast (Singulair)	5-10 mg PO qd		None

PO, orally.
Note: All the drugs listed in this table are prescription medications.

tree; rather, it inhibits release of histamines, acting as an antiallergenic. Cromolyn is the prophylactic drug of choice for moderate allergic asthma, especially in children, because of its safety and efficacy. It has no therapeutic effect in acute asthma attacks. The most common side effects are wheezing and coughing on administration. Nedocromil, also antiinflammatory and antiallergic, has an unpleasant taste.

Leukotrienes contribute to inflammation associated with asthma. Leukotriene antagonists block bronchoconstriction, production of mucus, and inflammation occurring with asthma. *Zafirlukast* (Accolate), the first medication in this new antiinflammatory class, is used as maintenance therapy for patients with chronic asthma. It has few side effects but has multiple drug interactions. *Zileuton* (Zyflo) is rapidly absorbed, but its place in asthma therapy is not completely understood, although it is used for prophylaxis and treatment of chronic asthma in persons older than 12 years. *Montelukast* (Singulair), a bronchodilator, respiratory stimulant, and leukotriene receptor antagonist, should be given at night for maximum effectiveness for prophylactic use. If short-acting bronchodilators are needed more frequently while the patient is on montelukast, the physician should be notified.

Patient Education for Compliance

1. Cromolyn is for prophylaxis of asthma and should be administered 30 minutes before exercise.
2. Beta$_2$ agonists taken for long-term therapy should be taken on a regular schedule and not only as needed but may be used for short-term therapy as needed.
3. If symptoms of asthma become worse, patients should not change doses or self-medicate without physician's direction.
4. A patient with thick lung secretions should drink six to eight glasses of water per day to decrease viscosity of bronchial secretions.
5. OTC and prescription medications for respiratory disorders should not be mixed because of the chance of multiple doses of similar drugs, especially sympathomimetic drugs.
6. Colas, coffee, chocolate, and charbroiled foods should be avoided when taking xanthine preparations such as theophylline and its derivatives.

Important Facts about Medications for Asthma

- Many beta$_2$ agonists are inhaled forms to be delivered by metered dose inhaler (MDI), dry powder inhaler (DPI), or nebulizer, rarely causing systemic side effects.
- Asthma and chronic obstructive pulmonary disease (COPD) are chronic diseases causing inflammation of airways, hyperactivity of bronchial secretions, and bronchospasm. Allergies may be the underlying cause of asthma.

Important Facts about Medications for Asthma—cont'd

- COPD and asthma are treated with antiinflammatory agents and bronchodilators. Correct use of MDIs, DPIs, and nebulizers is tricky, and patient education is essential.
- Inhaled beta$_2$ antagonists are the most effective medications to relieve acute bronchospasm and exercise-induced bronchospasm attacks.
- Inhaled salmeterol, used to prevent COPD and asthma, has a delayed onset and extended duration of action.
- Glucocorticoids, are used orally for acute asthma attacks for preventive short-term therapy in respiratory tract. These drugs suppress inflammation of bronchial asthma.
- Inhaled glucocorticoids used for long-term prophylaxis are relatively safe, with oropharyngeal candidiasis and dysphoria being major side effects.
- Cromolyn, a nebulized antiinflammatory medication, is used for prophylaxis.
- Theophylline and xanthines relieve COPD and asthma by bronchodilation, although xanthines have been replaced with newer drugs because of narrow therapeutic range and danger of use with some diseases.

INFLUENZA A AND B

Influenza, a serious disease causing morbidity and mortality throughout the world, is caused by influenza viruses, of which two types are more prevalent: *influenza A virus* and *influenza B virus*. Influenza A virus causes more infections than type B, but these viruses are constantly undergoing evolution and changes. The virus enters the body through highly contagious droplets from sneezing and coughing, but its replication takes place within the respiratory tract.

Influenza is best managed by yearly prophylactic influenza vaccines that change from year to year depending on the expected virus of the current year. However, drugs are available for secondary treatment of the illness. These drugs fall into two distinct categories: adamantanes are active against only influenza A, whereas the newer drugs, neuraminidase inhibitors, can be used with either influenza A or B virus.

Medications for Inhibition of Influenza

Some newer medications are used to lessen or inhibit signs and symptoms of influenza, but these products are not substitutes for influenza vaccine administered to prevent or attenuate symptoms. Rather, they are for patients who, for medical reasons (such as elderly patients with severe chronic medical conditions) or personal reasons, need prophylaxis against the disease after exposure to the virus. These medications are relatively expensive and are not widely used (Table 25-10).

TABLE 25-10 DRUGS USED FOR INHIBITION OF INFLUENZA VIRUS

GENERIC NAME/ TRADE NAME	USUAL DOSE, ROUTE, AND FREQUENCY	INDICATIONS FOR USE	DRUG INTERACTIONS
ADAMANTANES			
rimantadine (Flumadine)	100 mg PO bid	Prophylaxis of influenza	acetaminophen, aspirin, cimetidine
amantadine	100-200 mg PO bid		anticholinergics
NEURAMINIDASE INHIBITORS			
oseltamivir (Tamiflu)	75 mg PO bid		None
zanamivir (Relenza)	2 inhalations (5 mg) bid for treatment, qd for prophylaxis		

Note: All the drugs listed in this table are prescription medications.

TABLE 25-11 DRUGS USED FOR RESPIRATORY SYNCYTIAL VIRUS

GENERIC/TRADE NAME	USUAL DOSE, ROUTE, AND FREQUENCY	INDICATIONS FOR USE	DRUG INTERACTIONS
ribavirin (Virazole)	20 mg inhaled NEB over qd12-18h	RSV	Nucleoside analogues
palivizumab (Synagis)	15 mg/kg IV once monthly	RSV	None

IV, Intravenously; *RSV*, respiratory syncytial virus.

The adamantanes, not recommended by the Centers for Disease Control and Prevention (CDC) because of the fast development of resistance, are **rimantadine** (Flumadine) and **amantadine** (Symmetrel), used in the prophylaxis and treatment of influenza A infections. These should be used only in the documented presence of an influenza A virus epidemic.

The newer medications, neuraminidase inhibitors, are fairly expensive but are more effective and better tolerated. **Oseltamivir** (Tamiflu) is indicated for the treatment of uncomplicated influenza infections (including avian and swine flu) with symptoms present for less than 2 days. **Zanamivir** (Relenza) is for patients who have had symptoms for more than 2 days. This medication is administered by using a Diskhaler and a 5-mg blister pack that is inhaled twice a day for 5 days, with the doses approximately 12 hours apart. Inhaled bronchodilators should be used to open the airways before use of zanamivir. Safety in patients with COPD has not been established, and a question has arisen concerning safety in coronary patients.

Patient Education for Compliance

New antiviral influenza medications must be used within 2 days of the onset of symptoms to be effective.

Important Facts about Influenza Medications

- Vaccination against influenza A and B should be the first line of defense. Disease treatment should be used only when necessary.
- Amantadines are used with care in the elderly for prophylaxis and treatment of influenza A infections.
- Neuraminidase inhibitors are used with influenza A and B infections.

MEDICATIONS FOR RESPIRATORY SYNCYTIAL VIRUS INFECTION

Respiratory syncytial virus (RSV) is a major lower respiratory tract infection in the young, the elderly, and those with cardiac, respiratory, or immune system diseases. Like influenza it is seasonal. Two drugs are approved for use against this disease, although neither is really effective: ribavirin is in inhaled or oral form, and palivizumab is injectable. **Ribavirin** (Virazole), also used for hepatitis C, is a broad-spectrum virustatic antiviral drug. Expense (over $1300 per day) with minimal benefits necessitates selective use of the medication. **Palivizumab** (Synagis) is used with children and those with chronic respiratory diseases. This medication, which should be given before and through RSV season, is given intramuscularly and costs about $7000 seasonally (Table 25-11).

SUMMARY

Effectiveness of the respiratory system affects the body's ability to function in homeostasis. The respiratory tract is necessary for inspiration of oxygen and expiration of carbon dioxide. Oxygen is essential to sustain life. Because of flammability, the need for safety with therapeutic oxygen around flames should be explained during patient teaching.

Antihistamines are used to relieve allergic reactions and are also used frequently to relieve rhinorrhea and allergic bronchitis. Allied health professionals must know symptoms of allergic conditions versus common colds versus influenza to be sure that an antihistamine is the correct medication for use. If congestion is from colds, a decongestant is more appropriate, to relieve thickened mucus.

Cough-suppressing preparations are indicated for dry, nonproductive coughs that interrupt daily activities. If a cough is productive, suppression is not appropriate and an expectorant may be administered to help expel secretions. For thick phlegm or sputum, mucolytics may be prescribed to decrease the secretions' viscosity. Many preparations are available OTC, so a working knowledge of indications for each is important.

Because topical nasal preparations are readily available, an explanation of the dangers of rebound congestion when used for more than short-term therapy, usually no longer than a week, is important. Cromolyn may be used prophylactically for asthma over a long period of time.

Bronchodilators for smooth muscle relaxation are used to ease breathing in the treatment of asthma, COPD, and chronic bronchitis. Some agents, such as epinephrine and beta$_2$ agonists, are used in acute respiratory attacks. Others include leukotriene agonists, for long-term therapy; albuterol, for exercise-induced asthma; and cromolyn. Glucocorticoids, relatively safe for short term use with bronchoconstriction and to liquefy thick mucous secretions, are administered by inhalation to achieve local respiratory tract effects.

COPD and asthma should be treated on an individualized basis, as should allergic conditions. In treatment of these conditions, especially with antihistamines, drug tolerance occurs and medications may need changing regularly. For persons with seasonal allergies, prophylaxis by avoiding allergens is indicated; for chronic allergic reactions, cromolyn may be indicated for long-term prophylaxis.

Two groups of medications to prevent or reduce symptoms of influenza A and B are available as nasal or oral preparations. Because of the expense, these drugs are not used routinely. The best prophylaxis for influenza remains the annual immunization with influenza vaccine.

RSV is a major disease in the elderly and children. Two drugs are available to treat this disease, but treatment is very expensive and should begin before and continue throughout the disease season.

CRITICAL THINKING EXERCISES

Scenario

Smokey has COPD, and his breathing has become progressively more difficult. His physician has prescribed sympathomimetic bronchodilators for his condition. Smokey wants to know how these will help his condition when he is administering the medications by breathing them through the mouth rather than taking a tablet.

1. How would you explain the actions, safety, and prolonged use of the medicines to Smokey?
2. He also tells you that the prescribed low dose of oxygen does not seem to help him at all, and he wants to increase the flow to 6 L/min, rather than the prescribed 2 L/min as ordered. How would you explain the dangers of this change?
3. What questions should the allied health professional ask about bronchial secretions and the ability to expel these secretions?

DRUG CALCULATIONS

1. Order: guaifenesin ER 600 mg q12h
Available medication:

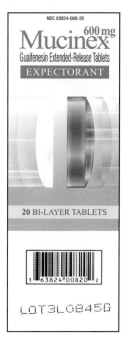

Dose to be administered: _____
_____

2. Order: diphenhydramine 60 mg
Available medication:

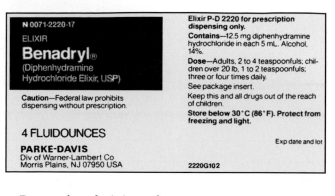

Dose to be administered. _____
_____

What amount of medication would be administered
using household utensils? _____

REVIEW QUESTIONS

1. Why do we use antihistamines? Decongestants? _____
_____
_____

2. What is the indication for topical nasal glucocorticoids? What is the safety factor in using these medications?
_____
_____

3. When would you expect the physician to order a cough suppressant? A mucolytic? An expectorant? _____
_____
_____
_____

4. What is the common medication found in nonopioid cough suppressants? What are the expected side effects?
_____
_____

5. What do bronchodilators do? _____
_____

6. What are the three inhalation devices used to deliver medications as topical bronchodilators? How does each one work? _____

_____

_____

_____

7. Glucocorticoids are generally discouraged for long-term oral therapy. Why are the topical agents for asthma considered reasonably safe for long-term use? _____

_____

8. What medications are available for the prophylaxis of influenza? _____

_____

_____

9. Why must the prophylactic agents for asthma be taken on a regular basis rather than prn? _____

_____

_____

CHAPTER 26

Circulatory System and Blood Disorders

Ms. Ellory, age 67, has a history of angina pectoris for which Dr. Merry has prescribed nitroglycerin patches. Ms. Ellory knows she should change the patch daily, leaving it off for several hours during the day.

What else does Ms. Ellory need to know about the placement of patches?

What does she need to know about administration of the nitroglycerin tablets that Dr. Merry has also prescribed?

After the container has been opened, how long will these sublingual tablets maintain their strength?

Should Ms. Ellory carry this medication with her at all times? Why or why not?

Can she put some tablets in another clear medicine bottle with other medications? Why or why not?

KEY TERMS

Aggregation
Angina pectoris
Arrhythmia
Arteriosclerosis
Atherosclerosis
Automaticity
Chronotropic effect
Digitalization
Dromotropic effect
Dysrhythmia

Ectopic beats
Embolus
Glycoside
Hemostasis
High-density lipoprotein (HDL)
Hypertension
Inotropic effect
Intermittent claudication
Ischemia

Low-density lipoprotein (LDL)
Myocardial infarction (MI)
Necrosis
Orthostatic hypotension
Paresthesia
Peripheral vascular resistance

Point of maximum impulse (PMI)
Sympatholytic agent
Thromboembolism
Thrombus
Triglycerides
Vasoconstrictors
Vasodilators
Very-low-density lipoprotein (VLDL)

EASY WORKING KNOWLEDGE OF INDICATIONS AND SIDE EFFECTS

Common Symptoms of Circulatory Disorders

Chest pain
Dyspnea, tachypnea
Fatigue and weakness
Palpitations, tachycardia
Bradycardia
Pallor, cyanosis
Edema
Syncope
Unusual sweating
Nausea, vomiting, anorexia
Headache
Anxiety

Common Side Effects of Circulatory Medications

Orthostatic hypotension
Urinary frequency
Headaches, dizziness, lightheadedness
Anorexia
Nausea, diarrhea, or constipation
Fatigue and weakness
Bradycardia

EASY WORKING KNOWLEDGE OF DRUGS USED TO TREAT CIRCULATORY DISORDERS

DRUG CLASS	PRESCRIPTION	OTC	PREGNANCY CATEGORY	MAJOR INDICATIONS
Antianginal agents	Yes	No	B, C, X (amyl nitrate)	Relieve angina pectoris
Cardiac glycosides	Yes	No	C	Treat congestive heart failure
Antiarrhythmic agents	Yes	No	B, C, D	Treat dysrhythmias and disorders of cardiac rhythm
Diuretics	Yes	Yes (e.g., caffeine)	B, C	Treat edema of congestive heart failure and hypertension
Antihypertensives	Yes	No	B, C, D (ACE inhibitors)	Treat hypertension
Peripheral vasodilators	Yes	No	C (cilostazol)	Treat peripheral vascular disease
Hypolipidemics	Yes	No	B, C, X (statins)	Treat elevated serum lipoproteins
Anticoagulants	Yes	No	B, C, X (oral anticoagulants)	Prevent venous thrombi
Thrombolytics	Yes	No	B, C	Dissolve thrombi
Antiplatelet medications	Yes	Yes	C, D (aspirin in the third trimester)	Prevent aggregation of platelets and prevent arterial thrombi
Topical hemostatics	Yes	No		Provide topical hemostasis
Hematopoietics, erythropoietics	Yes	No	C	Increase production of blood cells

ACE, Angiotensin-converting enzyme.

According to American Heart Association statistics, cardiovascular disease is the leading cause of death in the United States, with one out of every five deaths directly related to such diseases. More than 60 million Americans have some type of heart condition. Major advances have been made in knowledge and treatment of heart disease, and with this knowledge have come major changes in pharmacologic treatment of heart conditions.

FUNCTION OF THE CIRCULATORY SYSTEM

The circulatory system, composed of the heart and blood vessels, has two primary functions: (1) delivery of oxygen, nutrients, hormones, and other essential body substances in blood to cells throughout body and (2) removal of waste products from cells. Pulmonary

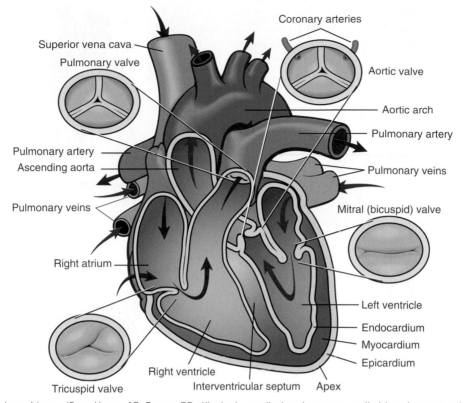

Figure 26-1 Internal view of heart. (From Young AP, Proctor DB: *Kinn's the medical assistant: an applied learning approach,* ed 11, St Louis, 2011, Saunders.)

circulation is responsible for oxygen and carbon dioxide exchange by carrying blood to lungs to receive inhaled oxygen and removing carbon dioxide by exhalation. Coronary circulation promotes nutrition and health of heart muscle itself. Systemic circulation delivers blood and its components to all tissues except lungs and myocardium.

A strong muscle about the size of a fist, the heart is in the thorax between the lungs. Two thin-walled atria are essentially receiving and holding chambers for blood before it enters two thick-walled ventricles to be pumped to lungs or body. Pumping of the heart forces blood from the heart into either pulmonary or systemic circulation. The pulse created by the heart can be felt beating at the **point of maximum impulse (PMI);** this landmark is used to take an apical pulse before cardiac medications are administered (Figure 26-1).

How Drugs Affect the Cardiac Electrical Conduction System

Blood flow through coronary arteries (Figure 26-2) and systemically depends on the heart contraction's force. When myocardial function is decreased, the heart's ability to contract is also decreased. Drugs that work on the heart's contraction force, an action referred to as **inotropic effect,** are the cardiac **glycosides.**

The heart's electrical conduction system consists of specialized tissues. The heart sets its own rhythm at the sinoatrial (SA) node, the pacemaker of the heart, found on the posterior wall of the right atrium near the entrance of the vena cava. The atrioventricular (AV) node, on the floor of the right atrium near the interatrial septum, continues impulses to the bundle of His, or AV bundle. From this point, conduction spreads to the left and right sides of the heart through bundle branches to Purkinje fibers, or conduction myofibers (Figure 26-3). Conduction of the regularly spaced electrical impulses through the cardiac muscle produces normal rhythm. When the heart does not beat in a regular rhythm, antidysrhythmics, or drugs that have a **dromotropic effect,** may be ordered. If the heart rate is too fast or too slow, medications may be prescribed to either increase or decrease the rate or to convert the rhythm to normal sinus rhythm (i.e., drugs with a **chronotropic effect**). Calcium channel blockers and antianginal medications act on coronary arteries to lessen heart work. Table 26-1 summarizes the pharmacologic effects of cardiac medications on heart action.

Coronary artery disease (CAD) caused by **arteriosclerosis** occurs when insufficient blood flows through hardened and narrowed coronary arteries, causing

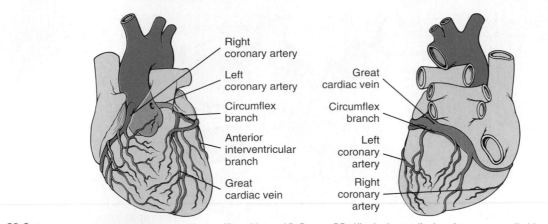

Figure 26-2 Coronary arteries affected by vasodilators. (From Young AP, Proctor DB: *Kinn's the medical assistant: an applied learning approach,* ed 11, St Louis, 2011, Saunders.)

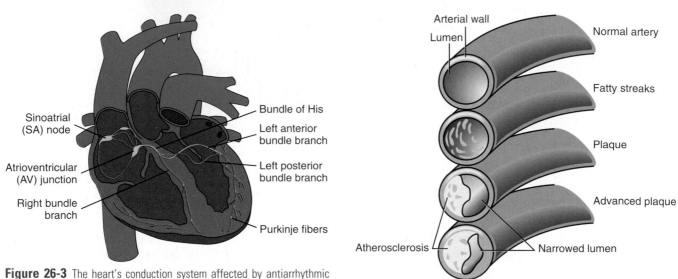

Figure 26-3 The heart's conduction system affected by antiarrhythmic agents. (From Young AP, Proctor DB: *Kinn's the medical assistant: an applied learning approach,* ed 11, St Louis, 2011, Saunders.)

Figure 26-4 Atherosclerosis and narrowing of artery lumen.

TABLE 26-1 HOW CARDIAC MEDICATIONS AFFECT HEART ACTION		
DRUG GROUP	**HEART TISSUE**	**PHARMACOLOGIC ACTION**
A—Cardiac glycosides	Myocardium	Positive inotropic (increases force of myocardial contraction)
B—Antidysrhythmics	Cardiac conduction	Positive and negative dromotropic (increases and decreases conduction of electrical impulses through heart muscle)
		Positive and negative chronotropic (increases and decreases heart rate to convert to normal sinus rhythm)
C—Calcium channel blockers	Coronary arteries	Vasodilation of coronary arteries
Antianginal medications	Coronary arteries	Lessens work of heart

decreased blood flow to the heart itself. Narrowing of arteries may also occur when plaque from fatty deposits develops in the arteries—**atherosclerosis,** a form of arteriosclerosis (Figure 26-4).

The first symptom of a **myocardial infarction (MI),** or heart attack, is often **angina pectoris** or spasms of the cardiac muscle caused by **ischemia.** When a heart area is deprived of blood supply, the result is myocardial cell **necrosis** or an MI occurs. Because damaged cells of the myocardium will not regenerate, contractility is permanently reduced; depending on the infarct site, the conduction system may also be affected, causing permanent damage. Medications are directed toward establishing sufficient myocardial contractility to force blood through the body.

DRUGS FOR ANGINA PECTORIS

Angina pectoris, or cardiac muscle spasms, is temporary interference with the flow of blood, oxygen, or nutrients to the heart, resulting in coronary ischemia. Drug therapy is based on relaxation of coronary smooth muscle to bring about vasodilation and therefore improve blood flow to the heart, using nitrates to produce temporary relief.

Stable, or *exertional, angina* is often triggered by physical activity or stress and is related to arteriosclerosis. The goal of therapy for stable angina is to reduce intensity and frequency of anginal attacks to decrease cardiac oxygen demand. Three types of medications are used for treating stable angina: nitrates, beta blockers, and calcium channel blockers. These drugs only relieve symptoms; they do not affect underlying diseases.

Variant, or *vasospastic, angina* is caused by coronary artery spasms restricting myocardial blood flow. The goal of treatment of vasospastic angina is to reduce the number and severity of attacks by increasing cardiac oxygen. Calcium channel blockers and nitrates are used to dilate heart vessels.

The third type of angina is *unstable angina.* This medical emergency is treated in a hospital situation and only rarely in an ambulatory care setting.

Nitrates

Nitrates, the oldest and most frequently used antianginal medications, are not true coronary artery dilators as previously thought because coronary arteries are already dilated by arteriosclerotic vascular disease. Nitrates dilate systemic vessels to reduce cardiac work and oxygen consumption and relax vascular smooth muscle when converted to nitric oxide. A decrease in venous return to the heart causes a decrease in blood pressure, reducing the heart's workload. Nitrates are used during attacks of angina to relieve intense pain and are used prophylactically to prevent attacks. The most common route of administration is sublingual, with almost immediate onset of action (within minutes) but short duration of action (<30 minutes) (Table 26-2).

Nitroglycerin (NTG), the most widely used nitrate, is effective, fast acting, and inexpensive; it acts directly on vascular smooth muscle to dilate blood vessels. Nitrate preparations decrease cardiac oxygen demand in stable angina, whereas in variant angina they relax the spasms and increase oxygen supply. Initial use produces a severe headache that can be relieved with mild analgesics such as **acetaminophen.** Patients on high doses of

TABLE 26-2 ONSET AND DURATION OF ACTION OF NITRATES

DRUG AND FORM	TIME TO ONSET OF ACTION	DURATION OF ACTION
Nitroglycerin		
Sublingual	1-3 min (R)	30-60 min (B)
Translingual spray	2-3 min (R)	30-60 min (B)
Oral capsules or tablets, SR	20-45 min (S)	3-8 hr (L)
Transdermal patches	½-1 hr (S)	24 hr (L)*
Topical ointment	½-1 hr (S)	2-12 hr (L)*
Isosorbide mononitrate		
Oral tablets	½-1 hr (S)	6-10 hr (L)
Oral tablets, SR	½-1 hr (S)	7-12 hr (L)
Isosorbide dinitrate		
Sublingual or chewable tablets	2-5 min (R)	1-3 hr (L)
Oral tablets	20-40 min (S)	4-6 hr (L)
Oral tablets or capsules, SR	30 min (S)	6-8 hr (L)
Amyl nitrite	30 sec (ultra R)	3-5 min (B)

B, brief acting; *L,* long acting; *R,* rapid onset; *S,* slow onset; *SR,* sustained-release.
*Should not be used for more than 12 hours, to prevent tolerance.

nitroglycerin or those who have continuous therapy over a length of time may develop drug tolerance. To prevent tolerance, the lowest effective doses of daily nitroglycerin preparations should be given. Long-acting formulas should be used on an intermittent basis, allowing the patient to be drug free at some time during the day (usually at night). Acquired tolerance is reversible when nitrates are withheld for short periods of time. Nitroglycerin preparations are available in a variety of routes to produce similar responses; time of onset and duration of action differ. Some preparations are rapidly effective (1 to 5 minutes) and last for about an hour, whereas for others the effect is slower in onset but lasts for several hours (see Table 26-2).

The most commonly used form of nitroglycerin is **sublingual nitroglycerin** (Nitrostat), an ideal preparation for acute anginal pain that works rapidly and lasts for about an hour. Medication administration should begin as soon as pain begins and should not be delayed until pain is severe, or medication may be given prophylactically when exertion is anticipated. If one tablet is not sufficient, one or two additional tablets should be taken at 5-minute intervals. For persistent pain, emergency medical attention should be obtained to rule out MI. **Transdermal nitroglycerin** (Transderm Nitro), available as a patch, contains a reservoir of drug that is slowly released for absorption daily through skin. The site should be rotated daily to prevent local irritation. To avoid development of tolerance to nitroglycerin, the patch should not be worn for more than 10 to 12 hours per day; usually it is applied in the morning and removed in the evening. Patches result in a slow onset and are not effective for an ongoing anginal attack. ***Topical nitroglycerin ointment*** must be measured on a paper provided with medication to ensure proper dosage. Topical ointment sites should also be rotated. ***Nitroglycerin spray*** (Nitrolingual) is especially useful in patients who have decreased dexterity. Each container holds 200 immediately absorbed sprays, providing quicker relief than other forms of nitroglycerin. The mist may be sprayed into the mouth every 5 minutes for three doses; each dose contains nitroglycerin 0.4 mg. This medication form is more stable and not sensitive to heat, light, or moisture.

If nitroglycerin is discontinued, this action should take place over a period of time. Abrupt discontinuation of long-acting preparations may cause angina and vasospasms (Table 26-3).

Patient Education for Compliance

Patient education for using nitroglycerin spray should include priming of container by pointing nozzle away and depressing until a click is heard. This should be repeated every 6 weeks if container is not used. To use spray, remove cap and do not shake. Hold bottle as close to mouth as possible to release spray into mouth (under tongue is not necessary). *Do not inhale spray.* No food or drink should be taken for 5 to 10 minutes after administration.

 CLINICAL TIP

Sublingual tablet is to remain under tongue until it dissolves. Because nitroglycerin is chemically unstable and loses its effectiveness over a period of time, the medication bottle should not be opened until needed. Shelf-life is longer in a dark, tightly closed container. After container is opened, drug is effective for approximately 6 months, and the date on which it was opened should be written on container. Six months after opening, medication should be discarded and replaced with a new bottle.

Beta-Adrenergic Blockers

Used for several cardiovascular disorders, betaadrenergic blockers (beta blockers) reverse sympathetic heart stimulation caused by exercise, stress, or physical exertion, including increased heart rate, increased force

of contraction, and increased oxygen use. These drugs decrease the heart's rate and force of contraction, lowering oxygen use to prevent myocardial ischemia and pain. Beta blockers are used for chronic management of angina by lessening frequency of attacks, delaying onset of pain during exercise, allowing increased heart work capacity, and allowing increased exercise tolerance. (Other uses for beta blockers, such as antihypertensive and antidysrhythmic applications, are discussed later in this chapter.)

Propranolol (Inderal) is used alone or in combination with nitrates for angina control. The goal of administration is to reduce the pulse to 50 to 60 beats/min at rest and 100 beats/min during exercise. Beta blockers should be avoided with asthma and may mask hypoglycemia in patients with diabetes mellitus (see Table 26-3).

Calcium Channel Blockers

Calcium channel blockers interfere with movement of calcium ions through cell membranes to treat anginal pain. Because vascular smooth muscle contraction is dependent on calcium movement from extracellular to intracellular sites, inhibition of calcium prevents this contraction, allowing vasodilation to occur. Calcium blockers also dilate larger coronary arteries to increase blood flow to the heart. These medications are indicated for vasospastic angina.

Verapamil (Calan) and ***diltiazem*** (Cardizem) have a primary use as antidysrhythmics but are used for their vasodilating properties in the treating of angina. These medications also decrease heart rate, thus decreasing the heart's work. ***Nifedipine*** (Adalat), ***nicardipine*** (Cardene), ***amlodipine*** (Norvasc), ***felodipine*** (Plendil), and ***isradipine*** (DynaCirc), used as antihypertensives (see later in this chapter), are also used for angina because their properties cause vasodilation and relaxation of coronary artery spasms with minor effect on decreasing heart rate.

 LEARNING TIP

Many of the calcium channel blockers have names that end with "pine."

Combining the Medications for Angina

Combinations of nitrates, beta blockers, and calcium channel blockers may be used for anginal treatment. The goal is to reduce frequency and intensity of angina attacks without overly suppressing cardiac action. Before administering calcium channel or beta blockers, it is important to take blood pressure and pulse to ensure both are within normal range.

TABLE 26-3 ANTIANGINAL AGENTS

GENERIC NAME/ TRADE NAME	USUAL DOSE, ROUTE, AND FREQUENCY	INDICATIONS FOR USE	MAJOR SIDE EFFECTS	DRUG INTERACTIONS
		Angina pectoris, MI, CHF	Headache, hypotension, tachycardia, lightheadedness, dizziness, burning sensation in mouth with spray	Use with care with hypotensives, beta blockers, verapamil, diltiazem, sildenafil, alcohol
nitroglycerin (Nitrostat)	0.3-0.6 mg SL q5min × 3 doses			
(NitroMist)	1 or 2 translingual sprays q5min × 3 doses			
(Nitroglycerin SR, Nitro-Time)	2.5-6.5 mg PO* bid			
(Transderm Nitro, Nitro-Dur, Nitro-Disc, Minitran)	1 patch qd; remove after 12-14 hr			
(Nitro-Bid IV)	5 mcg/min IV to desired response			
(Nitro-Bid, Nitrol ointment)	1-2 inches topically qd			
isosorbide mononitrate (Monoket)	20 mg PO* qid			
(Imdur SR)	30-120 mg PO bid			
isosorbide dinitrate	2.5-10 mg SL, PO qid			
(Isordil Titradose)	5-40 mg PO* q8-12h			
(Dilatrate-SR)	40 mg q8-12h			
amyl nitrite	0.18-0.3 mL inhaled			
BETA-ADRENERGIC BLOCKERS			Insomnia, depression, bizarre dreams	
propranolol (Inderal) (See Table 26-8 for other beta blockers)	20-80 mg PO bid-qid	In combination with nitrates for angina pectoris		theophylline, calcium channel blockers, reserpine, cimetidine, phenytoin, alcohol
CALCIUM CHANNEL BLOCKERS (See Table 26-5 for class III agents and Table 26-11 for other calcium channel blockers used with angina)		Angina pectoris	Fatigue, headache, flushing, dizziness, hypotension, GI disturbances, constipation	
MISCELLANEOUS ANTIANGINAL MEDICATIONS				
ranolazine (Ranexa)	500-1000 mg PO bid	Antianginal, antiischemic	GI symptoms, headache, dizziness, nausea, weakness, indigestion	quinidine, sotalol, ketoconazole, HIV medications, macrolide, antibiotics, diltiazem, verapamil, grapefruit

CHF, Congestive heart failure; *GI*, gastrointestinal; *HIV*, human immunodeficiency virus; *IV*, intravenously; *MI*, Myocardial infarction; *PO*, orally; *SL*, sublingually; *SR*, sustained release.

*To avoid tolerance, the doses should allow the patient to be medication free at some time during the day.

Ranolazine (Ranexa) is a medication specified as an antianginal with an unknown mode of action. Used with chronic stable angina, this medication should be used in combination with other antianginals such as nitrates and beta-blockers.

Patient Education for Compliance

1. Nitroglycerin sublingual tablets should be carried at all times in an easily accessible, dark container.
2. Transdermal nitroglycerin is for prophylaxis of angina. To prevent tolerance to nitroglycerin patches, they should be rotated on a daily basis and should not be worn more than 10 to 12 hours per day.
3. A nitroglycerin sublingual tablet should not be swallowed but should be placed under the tongue until it has fully dissolved. The mouth should be moist for absorption of sublingual nitroglycerin tablets.
4. Medical evaluation for possible myocardial infarction (MI) is necessary if acute anginal pain has not been relieved after three sublingual nitroglycerin tablets have been taken.
5. Long-acting nitroglycerin should not be discontinued abruptly but must be tapered off because vasospasm may occur.
6. Nitroglycerin ointment should be measured on paper supplied by manufacturer and applied in 1- to 2-inch strips as directed by physician but should be removed at some point, usually at night, to prevent tolerance.
7. Changes in lifestyle—diet, smoking cessation, and weight control—are important with use of medications for angina pectoris.
8. Headaches caused by nitroglycerin will gradually diminish with long-term use and may be relieved by nonsteroidal antiinflammatory drugs.
9. Patients using nitroglycerin should avoid alcohol and medications for erectile dysfunction.
10. Patients taking these medications should move slowly from a lying position to a sitting or standing position because of the chance of **orthostatic hypotension.**

Important Facts about Medications for Angina Pectoris

- Angina pectoris occurs when the heart's oxygen supply is insufficient to meet its oxygen demands.
- Three types of angina exist: (1) chronic stable, or exertional, angina, caused by coronary atherosclerosis; (2) variant, or vasospastic, angina, caused by coronary artery spasm; and (3) unstable angina, which requires immediate medical care.

Important Facts about Medications for Angina Pectoris—cont'd

- Drugs that increase myocardial oxygen flow will decrease anginal pain. Cardiac oxygen needs are determined by heart rate, heart contractility, venous return to the heart, blood pressure, and heart pressure.
- Drugs for stable angina relieve pain by decreasing venous return to lower the heart's oxygen demand, not by increasing oxygen supply.
- Drugs for variant angina increase oxygen supply but do not decrease oxygen demand. Nitroglycerin further dilates atherosclerotic veins to relieve stable angina.
- Three common side effects of nitroglycerin are headache, orthostatic hypotension, and tachycardia.
- Continuous use of nitroglycerin results in tolerance. To prevent tolerance, the lowest possible effective dose should be used and administration should be on an intermittent schedule, with the patient being drug free for at least 8 hours a day.
- Nitroglycerin with a rapid onset should be used for anginal attacks or for prophylaxis before exertion. Nitroglycerin preparations with a long duration of effect are for protection against anginal attacks and should be administered on a fixed schedule.
- Beta blockers prevent stable angina by decreasing heart rate and heart contractility, thus reducing cardiac oxygen need.
- Calcium channel blockers relieve pain of stable angina by reducing heart's oxygen demand.

CONGESTIVE HEART FAILURE AND ITS TREATMENT

Congestive heart failure (CHF) affects more than two million Americans, with almost half a million cases, primarily in elderly individuals, added each year. Symptoms such as tiredness, fatigue, shortness of breath, rapid heart rate, and peripheral edema occur when heart contractility is decreased and less blood is pumped than it receives. With blood accumulating in heart chambers, less blood circulates, leading to retention of electrolytes, including sodium, to allow fluids to remain in intracellular spaces, a condition called *edema.*

CHF is a progressive disease characterized by reduced cardiac output, ventricles that do not contract efficiently, and accumulation of fluids or congestion in tissues and lungs. Of all factors, depressed heart contractility is a major cause of heart failure. Principal drugs for heart failure change the force of contraction and the heart rate. Overall therapeutic goals are to correct the underlying cause and gain the patient's compliance in pharmacologic treatments and nonpharmacologic care such as

TABLE 26-4 CARDIAC GLYCOSIDES

GENERIC/TRADE NAME	USUAL DOSE, ROUTE, AND FREQUENCY	INDICATIONS FOR USE	DRUG INTERACTIONS
digoxin (Lanoxin)	0.125-0.25 mg PO qd	Congestive heart failure, arrhythmias, and to control ventricular rate	See Box 26-1

decreasing dietary sodium, limiting alcohol, increasing exercise, and lowering stress levels.

Medications for Treating Congestive Heart Failure

Three major classes of drugs for CHF are (1) vasodilators, to reduce symptoms; (2) diuretics, to reduce edema in the peripheral vessels and to reduce blood volume overload; and (3) cardiac glycosides, to reduce the symptoms in chronic heart failure.

The *cardiac glycosides* (digitalis group or digoxin) are the oldest medicinal agents for CHF and are obtained from digitalis plant leaves. After treatment with cardiac glycosides, heartbeats are more forceful within a shorter period of time to increase the volume of blood pumped from the heart, improving circulation and decreasing congestion without increasing oxygen consumption. With edema reduction, weight is lost and blood volume is reduced. Normal blood circulation is restored and kidney function is increased. Digoxin produces improvement of exercise tolerance and reduces fatigue. However, even with improvement of symptoms, this medication does not alter the disease process and does not prolong life.

Because cardiac glycosides slow heart rate, patients must be taught to count the pulse before taking medication, being sure the pulse rate is above 60. If the pulse is below 60, the medication should not be taken without a physician's permission (Table 26-4 and Box 26-1).

Did You Know?

Digitalis works much like a spark plug in an automobile—it makes the heart work on all cylinders.

Digitalization is administration of therapeutic glycosides at a rapid rate to produce a blood digitalis level that subsequently is maintained. Dosages of digoxin are highly individualized, and each patient

BOX 26-1 DRUGS THAT INTERACT WITH DIGOXIN

Drugs That Decrease Digoxin Levels
cholestyramine
kaolin/pectin (aluminum salts)
neomycin (and other aminoglycosides)
sulfasalazine
antacids

Drugs That Increase Digoxin Levels
aminoglycosides
erythromycin
omeprazole
tetracycline
alprazolam
amiodarone
diltiazem
nifedipine
propafenone
quinidine
verapamil

Drugs That Increase the Incidence of Dysrhythmias
Thiazide and loop diuretics
amphotericin
Glucocorticoids

Drugs That Decrease Heart Rate and Contractility
Beta blockers
verapamil
diltiazem

Drugs That Increase Heart Rate and Contractility
Sympathomimetics

should be carefully evaluated until an effective dose has been established, after which monitoring is generally not necessary. The difference between therapeutic and toxic levels with digitalis is slim, and patients must be watched closely for signs of toxicity (Box 26-2).

BOX 26-2 SIGNS AND SYMPTOMS OF DIGITALIS TOXICITY

Confusion
Loss of appetite
Headaches, malaise, fatigue
Nausea, vomiting, diarrhea
Palpitations or bradycardia
Irregular pulse
Visual changes (unusual)—halos or rings of light around objects or seeing lights or bright spots
- Changes in color perception
- Blind spots or blurred vision

Decreased urinary output
Excessive nocturnal urination
Swelling
Decreased consciousness
Difficulty breathing when lying down

Patient Education for Compliance

1. Patients should be warned not to double up on missed doses of digoxin.
2. Switching among brands and formulations of digoxin may lead to altered responses, as bioavailability differs with different brands.
3. Patients should monitor pulse for rate and rhythm daily before taking digoxin. Pulse rate should be above 60 and below 90 before medication is taken.

Important Facts about Drugs for Congestive Heart Failure

- Therapy for heart failure relieves pulmonary and peripheral edema, increases quality of life, and prolongs life expectancy.
- Cardiac glycosides increase heart muscle contraction force to increase cardiac output.
- Oral cardiac glycosides are relatively safe for long-term use with congestive heart failure (CHF). However, digoxin has a narrow therapeutic dose range before causing side effects and adverse reactions.
- By increasing cardiac output, digoxin can reverse the manifestations of heart failure by increasing cardiac output, decreasing heart rate, and decreasing heart size while decreasing vasoconstriction, blood volume, and pulmonary and peripheral edema and reversing water retention to decrease weight and increase exercise tolerance.
- Digitalization is done when quick therapeutic levels are necessary.
- Diuretics, angiotensin-converting enzyme (ACE) inhibitors, and beta blockers are used with cardiac glycosides to treat CHF.

CARDIAC DYSRHYTHMIAS AND THEIR TREATMENT

Medications used to treat disorders of cardiac rhythm, or **arrhythmias,** are called *antidysrhythmics* or *antiarrhythmics*. Although *arrhythmia*, meaning loss of rhythm, is most often used, perhaps **dysrhythmia** is a better way to denote abnormal heart rhythm. Dysrhythmia is actually a deviation from normal rhythm that may be from CAD, electrolyte imbalances, cardiac conduction abnormalities, or even thyroid disease, as well as chronic drug therapy. Some dysrhythmias may have only a mild effect on cardiac output, whereas others may cause severe compromise of cardiac pumping.

Dysrhythmia is caused by an electrical impulse alteration and is treated with medication to regulate rhythm. Any change in the normal, automatically-controlled heartbeat may be caused by electrical impulses not interpreted into normal heart rhythm by the heart cells, producing *ectopic beats*. When severe dysrhythmia occurs, especially in ventricular disorders, patients may be experiencing a medical emergency and need hospital care. This section focuses on medications used in ambulatory care.

Therapeutic effects of antidysrhythmics lie in the ability to restore the ions of the heart to normal or to improve the heart's ability to pump blood. Antidysrhythmic medications, found in four distinct groups by effect, do not cure dysrhythmia, but they do attempt to restore normal cardiac function.

Class I drugs bind to sodium channels and interfere with sodium ion movement during heart excitation, lowering heart excitability. Medications also slow conduction velocity, prolong the heart's refractory period, and decrease **automaticity** of the heart's action. Quinidine is used to treat supraventricular arrhythmias, such as atrial flutter and fibrillation and some ventricular dysrhythmias. The myocardium's conduction system is depressed, decreasing contractile heart force and slowing heart rate. **Procainamide** (Pronestyl or Procan SR), related to procaine (an anesthetic), depresses cardiac muscle excitability and slows conduction to increase the refractory period. **Disopyramide** (Norpace), a cardiac depressant, is another medication to decrease cardiac excitability. Two medications chemically and therapeutically related to lidocaine, **mexiletine** (Mexitil) and **tocainide** (Tonocard), have been modified for oral administration for ambulatory care with ventricular arrhythmias (Table 26-5).

Class II antidysrhythmic medications are beta-adrenergic blockers that decrease heart rate, heart excitability, conduction velocity, and automaticity, particularly of the ventricles to mimic the sympathetic nervous system. **Propranolol** (Inderal), **metoprolol** (Toprol SL), and **atenolol** (Tenormin) are common beta blockers

TABLE 26-5 CARDIAC ANTIDYSRHYTHMICS

GENERIC NAME/TRADE NAME	USUAL DOSE, ROUTE, AND FREQUENCY	INDICATIONS FOR USE	MAJOR SIDE EFFECTS	DRUG INTERACTIONS
CLASS I AGENTS				
quinidine polygalacturonate (NTN)	300-600 mg PO q6h 200-400 mg IV	Treatment of supraventricular and ventricular dysrhythmias	Nausea, vomiting, diarrhea, fatigue, weakness, tinnitus, hypotension, severe headache, blurred vision, dizziness	beta blockers, digitalis, potassium, nifedipine, procainamide
gluconate (Quinaglute [SR])	324-648 mg PO q8-12h			
sulfate (Quinidex [SR])	300-600 mg PO q8-12h			
procainamide (NTN)	IV dose varies with dysrythmia		Same as for quinidine	pimozide, neuromuscular blockers, quinidine, alcohol, cimetidine
disopyramide (Norpace [CR, SR])	400-800 mg PO q12h		Dry mouth, constipation, visual disturbances, urinary retention	pimozide, other antidysrhythmics
mexiletine (NTN)	200 mg PO q8h		GI distress, dizziness, lightheadedness, tremors	urinary acidifiers, metoclopramide, phenytoin, rifampin
phenytoin (Dilantin)	50-100 mg IV every 10-15 mins as needed			
flecainide (Tambocor)	100-400 mg PO bid			Same as for disopyramide
propafenone (Rythmol)	150-300 mg PO q8h			propranolol, digoxin, warfarin
CLASS II AGENTS				
propranolol (Inderal, Inderal LA)	10-30 mg PO tid-qid 60-100 mg PO qd	Depress depolarization	Rashes, mental confusion	diuretics, NSAIDs, hypotensives, xanthines
acebutolol (Sectral)	600-1200 mg PO in divided doses daily			
CLASS III AGENTS				
		Depress depolarization, atrial fibrillation	Dizziness, nausea, vomiting, anorexia, bitter taste, weight loss, paresthesia of hands and feet, weakness	
amiodarone (Cordarone, Pacerone)	200-400 mg PO qd, IV	Life-threatening ventricular arrhythmia		cardiac glycosides, anticoagulants
dofetilide (Tikosyn)	Individualized PO for the elderly; dose varies based on response			None identified
CLASS IV AGENTS	(see Table 26-11)			

CR, Continuous release; GI, gastrointestinal; IV, intravenously; LA, long acting; NSAIDs, nonsteroidal antiinflammatory drugs; NTN, no trade name; PO, orally; SR, sustained release.

used as antidysrhythmics. Besides having beta-blocking effect, they also cause quinidine-like depression of cardiac muscle excitability to delay ventricular repolarization. The most common cardiovascular adverse reactions are hypotension and decreased heartbeat (see Table 26-5).

✐ LEARNING TIP

Most of the beta blockers have names that end in "lol."

Class III antidysrhythmic medications interfere with outflow of potassium during repolarization, prolonging the potential contraction duration of Purkinje fibers and ventricular muscle fibers to decrease the heart failure frequency. **Amiodarone** (Cordarone) decreases automaticity, prolongs AV conduction, and blocks exchange of sodium and potassium. This action can cause serious side effects, and amiodarone is used only for life-threatening dysrhythmias not responding to other medications (see Table 26-5).

Class IV agents, referred to as *calcium channel blockers*, decrease entry of calcium into heart cells and blood vessels. The SA and AV nodes require calcium for normal activity and normal sinus rhythm. Reducing calcium decreases SA node rate and AV node conduction velocity to treat supraventricular tachycardia. These calcium antagonists may also decrease the heart's ability to produce forceful contractions, leading to CHF. Useful with angina and for **hypertension,** these medications also relax smooth muscles and cause vasodilation. **Verapamil** (Calan, Isoptin) decreases SA node activity to decrease heart rate and AV node conduction. Verapamil is contraindicated with known SA or AV node disorders or with CHF. **Diltiazem** (Cardizem) is less potent in decreasing heart rate but has greater potency as a vasodilator; therefore it is used mainly as an antihypertensive agent (see Table 26-11 for calcium channel blockers.)

Patient Education for Compliance

1. Antidysrhythmic medications must be taken at prescribed levels and must not be skipped unless instructed by a physician.
2. Patients should take no OTC medications with antidysrhythmics without obtaining permission from a physician.
3. Avoid alcohol and nicotine with antidysrhythmics.

Important Facts about Antidysrhythmics

- Dysrhythmias result from electrical impulse alteration beginning at SA node. Antidysrhythmics control cardiac rhythm by correcting or compensating for altered rhythm.
- All antidysrhythmic medications can worsen existing conditions and generate new rhythm disorders.
- Class I antidysrhythmic medications block cardiac sodium channels, slowing impulse conduction. Quinidine blocks sodium channels and delays ventricular repolarization.
- Class II medications are beta blockers, which decrease SA automaticity, AV velocity, and myocardial contractility.
- Class III antidysrhythmics block potassium channels, prolonging ventricular repolarization.
- Class IV antidysrhythmics are calcium channel blockers, which reduce SA node automaticity, AV node conduction, and myocardial contractility.

HYPERTENSION AND ITS TREATMENT

Hypertension is a chronic cardiovascular disorder affecting millions of Americans: 25% of the U.S. population has hypertension. Effects of hypertension kill 2500 Americans every day, and two of every five deaths in the United States are related to hypertension and cardiovascular disease. In approximately 90% of cases, no cause is apparent, and, more important, over one third of those affected have no idea they have hypertension, making the disease a silent killer. Hypertension with an unknown etiology is referred to as *essential* or *primary hypertension.* Generally in adults, blood pressure above 120/80 is considered prehypertensive, with 140/90 being hypertensive. When either systolic or diastolic pressure or both are above baseline for an extended period of time, hypertension should be suspected. Diagnosis of hypertension should not be made based on a single blood pressure reading. Unless blood pressure poses an immediate danger, readings should be taken on at least two subsequent visits, a week to several weeks apart. Two readings should be taken at each visit and averaged.

Risk factors for hypertension include family history, stress, obesity, smoking, sedentary lifestyle, diabetes mellitus, and excessive lipid blood levels. When hypertension is not properly treated, risk of stroke, cerebral hemorrhage, coronary heart disease, and CHF increases. Renal failure is increased during hypertension because blood flow through kidneys is reduced.

Blood pressure is controlled by complex interactions among nervous, hormonal, and renal systems. When blood pressure drops, information activates the sympathetic nervous system. Epinephrine increases heart rate and force of heart contractions to elevate cardiac output and blood pressure. At the same time, the renin-angiotensin-aldosterone (RAA) mechanism helps regulate blood pressure by increasing or decreasing renal blood flow. Increase in blood volume from retention of water and sodium causes blood pressure increase. The RAA mechanism therefore functions in maintenance of blood volume and blood pressure (see Box 26-3 for a review of RAA mechanism).

Blood pressure responds to changes in arterial blood flow. **Peripheral vascular resistance** in blood vessels as well as blood volume and viscosity are factors in arterial wall pressure exerted. Atherosclerosis, with reduced arterial diameter, will necessitate more force when blood is pushed through vessels to increase blood pressure. Finally, cardiac output and the heart's ability to pump blood proficiently affect blood pressure.

BOX 26-3 REVIEW OF RENIN-ANGIOTENSIN-ALDOSTERONE MECHANISM

1. Decreased blood pressure stimulates kidneys to secrete renin.
2. Renin changes plasma protein angiotensinogen (synthesized by the liver) to angiotensin I.
3. Angiotensin I is converted to angiotensin II by enzymes found primarily in lung tissue.
4. Angiotensin II causes vasoconstriction and stimulates adrenal cortex to secrete aldosterone to increase blood pressure.

Antihypertensive Therapy

Antihypertensive therapy is often a difficult area for obtaining patient compliance because the patient is asked to comply with therapy for a disease that is basically asymptomatic. Long-term therapy is necessary to prevent the morbidity and mortality associated with uncontrolled hypertension; noncompliance leads to a poor prognosis, whereas compliance with an individualized regimen is associated with a good prognosis.

Antihypertensive Therapy and Lifestyle Changes

The basic approach for antihypertensive therapy begins with changes in lifestyle (Figure 26-5). If desired effects are not produced, medication may be started to lower blood pressure. Treatment begins with one drug. If this drug fails to produce desired effects, another medication may be added. Before a second medication is added, evaluation of patient's compliance in taking the first medication and with lifestyle changes should be undertaken to determine whether an adequate dosage of the first medication was prescribed. If treatment with two medications is not successful, after further close evaluation, a third medication may be added (Figure 26-6).

Adding Medications for Treatment of Hypertension

Initial drugs used in treatment of hypertension are usually either diuretics or beta blockers. Alternatively, angiotensin-converting enzyme (ACE) inhibitors, calcium

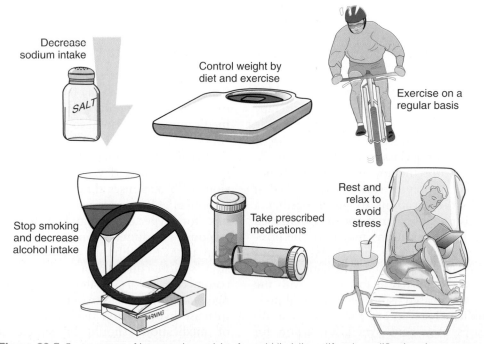

Decrease sodium intake

Control weight by diet and exercise

Exercise on a regular basis

Stop smoking and decrease alcohol intake

Take prescribed medications

Rest and relax to avoid stress

Figure 26-5 For treatment of hypertension, striving for multidisciplinary lifestyle modifications is necessary.

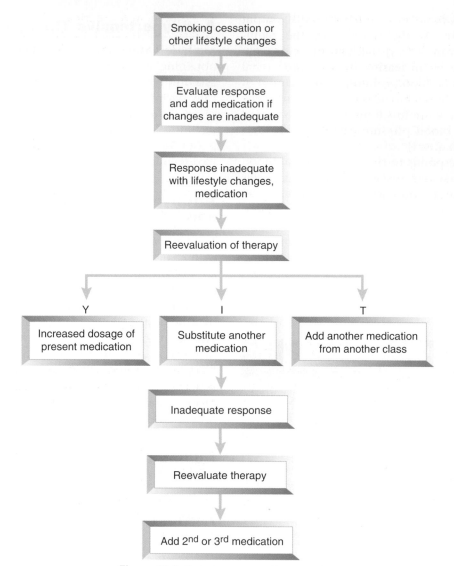

Figure 26-6 Typical treatment of hypertension.

channel blockers, alpha-adrenergic blockers, or alpha-beta–adrenergic blockers may be used for initial therapy if needed.

When medications are added, each medication is chosen from a different drug class with a different mechanism of action. Multidrug therapy increases the chance of success, with several receptor sites being attacked at the same time. When medications are given together, a lower dose of each is possible than if one drug were used alone. Using multiple medications may have the positive effect of reducing side effects and adverse reactions that occur with higher doses of one medicine. Finally, medications are usually started at low doses, with the dose then gradually increased as needed for blood pressure control. Medicinal treatment for concurrent illnesses and diseases may have synergistic action for treatment of both diseases; for example, hypertensive

patients with angina may use calcium channel blockers to treat both conditions. However, antihypertensive medications may also have antagonistic effects on some conditions.

Patients from some ethnic and cultural groups may react in unexpected ways to medicines for hypertension, with responses different from routinely expected responses. African American patients are at increased risk for hypertension and generally have a better response to diuretics and calcium channel blockers than to ACE inhibitors and beta blockers. Hypertension is more common in women who have taken oral contraceptives for 5 years than in those who have not. Age, smoking, and estrogen replacement therapy also increase hypertension risk. In the elderly, lower doses of medications should be started at less frequent intervals because of the aging body's sensitivity to fluid depletion and because of impaired cardiovascular reflexes.

If hypertension has been controlled for a year, the medication dose may be decreased, but all lifestyle modifications must continue. If drug dosage is lowered slowly, disease control may be achieved with less medication. In reducing dosage, the patient must continue to follow the prescribed regimen faithfully and must continue to undergo regular follow-up evaluations to detect any return of elevated blood pressure.

CATEGORIES OF ANTIHYPERTENSIVE MEDICATIONS

Antihypertensive medications are classified into five major categories: (1) diuretics, (2) centrally and peripherally acting adrenergic inhibiting agents, (3) ACE inhibitors and angiotensin II receptor antagonists, (4) calcium channel blockers, and (5) vasodilators. The adrenergic-inhibiting agents include such groups of medications as beta-adrenergic blockers, *Rauwolfia* derivatives, and alpha-adrenergic blockers. Types of medications used to treat hypertension are found in Box 26-4. Each medication has a specific indication, with treatment becoming more aggressive with each level.

Diuretics

Diuretics block reabsorption of sodium and chloride, allowing more water to be excreted. Increase in urinary output is directly related to blocking of resorption of sodium and chloride. Diuretics work early in the nephron to block the greatest amount of sodium and chloride solutes and produce the greatest diuresis with resultant acid-base imbalance and electrolyte level disturbances.

Diuretics are mainstays of hypertensive therapy and may be used alone or in combination with other antihypertensives. The four major categories of diuretics are (1) high-ceiling (loop) diuretics, (2) thiazide diuretics, (3) osmotic diuretics, and (4) potassium-sparing agents.

High-ceiling (loop) diuretics, the most effective diuretics available, produce greater loss of fluids and electrolytes by acting on the loop of Henle (Figure 26-7). Not used routinely for hypertension, these medications are used when diuresis is necessary to reduce blood volume to decrease blood pressure and to promote vasodilation. Because of electrolyte loss, potassium replacements are necessary with these drugs. **Furosemide** (Lasix) is the most frequently prescribed loop diuretic, acting on the ascending loop of Henle. See Table 26-6 for the loop diuretics.

Thiazide diuretics, most commonly used as antihypertensive agents, reduce blood volume, produce initial reduction in blood pressure, and reduce arterial resistance for long-term antihypertensive effects. These agents increase excretion of sodium, chloride, potassium, and water while raising uric acid and glucose levels but have lower diuresis capability than loop diuretics. Potassium may be replaced by medication or by eating potassium-rich foods such as bananas, greens, meats, and apricots. Hydrochlorothiazide is the most widely used thiazide diuretic. These agents work in the early segment of distal

---

BOX 26-4 TYPES OF MEDICATIONS USED TO TREAT HYPERTENSION

Angiotensin-converting enzyme (ACE) inhibitors act by dilating arterial blood vessels and decreasing blood volume.

Angiotensin II receptor antagonists act by blocking angiotensin II, causing vasoconstriction.

Alpha-beta–adrenergic blockers dilate blood vessels by working on alpha and beta cells to decrease norepinephrine formation.

Antiadrenergic drugs (centrally acting) work on alpha and beta receptors of sympathetic nervous system to dilate blood vessels.

Beta-adrenergic blockers cause heart to beat less frequently and prevents blood vessel constriction.

Calcium channel blockers relax smooth muscle of blood vessels to cause dilation.

Vasodilating agents block calcium movement into smooth muscle of blood vessels to cause relaxation and dilation.

Diuretics cause excretion of sodium and water to decrease blood volume and blood pressure.

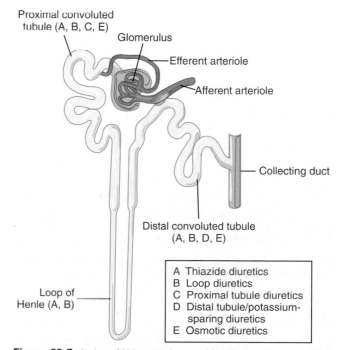

Figure 26-7 Action of kidney nephron and its relationship to diuretics.

TABLE 26-6 DIURETICS*

GENERIC NAME/ TRADE NAME	USUAL DOSE, ROUTE, AND FREQUENCY	INDICATIONS FOR USE	MAJOR SIDE EFFECTS	DRUG INTERACTIONS
LOOP DIURETICS			Loss of potassium, dehydration, elevated blood sugar and uric acid levels, hearing loss	
furosemide (Lasix)	20-80 mg PO qd, IM, IV	Hypertension, congestive heart failure, renal disease		digoxin, NSAIDs, aminoglycosides, potassium-sparing diuretics, lithium
torsemide (Demadex)	5-20 mg PO qd, IV			Other antihypertensives, NSAIDs, digoxin, anticoagulants, lithium, amphotericin, heparin
bumetanide (NTN)	0.5-2 mg PO qd, IV			Same as for ethacrynic acid
THIAZIDE DIURETICS		Hypertension, edema, diabetes insipidus	Loss of potassium, dehydration	digitalis, lithium, cholestyramine, colestipol
chlorothiazide (Diuril)	500 mg PO bid-qd			
hydrochlorothiazide (Hydrodiuril, Microzide)	25-50 mg PO qd			
THIAZIDE-LIKE DIURETICS		Same as for thiazide diuretics	Same as for thiazide diuretics	
chlorthalidone (Thalitane)	25-100 mg PO qd			
metolazone (Zaroxolyn)	5-20 mg PO qd			
indapamide (Lozol)	1.25-5 mg PO qd			
methyclothiazide (NTN)	5 mg PO qd			
DISTAL TUBULE OR POTASSIUM-SPARING DIURETICS		Congestive heart failure, hypertension	Nausea, vomiting, dizziness	anticoagulants, NSAIDs, lithium, ACE inhibitors, potassium-containing diuretics, potassium-containing supplements
amiloride (Midamor)	5-20 mg PO qd			
spironolactone (Aldactone)	25-100 mg PO qd			
triamterene (Dyrenium)	50-100 mg PO bid			

ACE, angiotensin-converting enzymes; *IM*, intramuscularly; *IV*, intravenously; *NSAIDs*, nonsteroidal antiinflammatory drugs; *NTN*, no trade name; *PO*, orally.
Note: All diuretics may cause orthostatic hypotension and dry mouth.
*For combination diuretics and antihypertensives, see Table 26-7.

convoluted tubules (see Figure 26-7) and are not effective in patients with impaired renal function. Also included in this group of medications used for hypertension are four drugs that are thiazide-like, being similar in function and structure: **chlorthalidone** (Hygroton), **indapamide** (Lozol), **metolazone** (Zaroxolyn), and **quinethazone** (Hydromox) (see Table 26-6).

Potassium-sparing diuretics produce a modest increase in urinary output and decrease in potassium excretion. These diuretics are seldom used alone with hypertension but are frequently added to primary agents, because loss of potassium with thiazides and loop diuretics is counteracted. Potassium replacement is not indicated, and potassium-rich foods should be avoided. **Spironolactone** (Aldactone), typical of potassium-sparing diuretics, blocks aldosterone use in the distal nephron, causing retention of potassium and excretion of sodium (see Figure 26-7). Care should be taken with ACE inhibitors (see discussion of ACE inhibitors later in this chapter).

Combination diuretics include thiazide diuretics combined in single-dose medications with potassium-sparing diuretics as well as calcium channel blockers and ACE inhibitors. Fixed-dose combinations may provide diuretic activity and decrease potassium depletion. In addition, diuretics may be combined with other antihypertensives to provide simple compliance after hypertension has been stabilized through medication and lifestyle changes (Table 26-7).

TABLE 26-7 FREQUENTLY PRESCRIBED COMBINATION MEDICATIONS FOR HYPERTENSION

	CONSTITUENT MEDICATIONS	
TRADE NAME	DIURETIC	POTASSIUM-SPARING DIURETIC
Aldactazide	HCTZ	spironolactone
Dyazide, Maxzide	HCTZ	triamterene
	DIURETIC	**ANTIHYPERTENSIVE**
Micardis HCT	HCTZ	telmisartan
Vaseretic	HCTZ	enalapril
Diovan HCT	HCTZ	valsartan
Lopressor HCT	HCTZ	metoprolol
Ziac	HCTZ	bisoprolol
Lotensin HCT	HCTZ	benazepril
Avalide	HCTZ	irbesartan
Hyzaar	HCTZ	losartan
Zestoretic	HCTZ	lisinopril
Prinzide	HCTZ	lisinopril
Combipres	chlorthalidone	clonidine
Tenoretic	chlorthalidone	atenolol
	ACE INHIBITOR	**CALCIUM CHANNEL BLOCKER**
Lotrel	benazepril	amlodipine
Tarka	trandolapril	verapamil
Lexxel	enalapril	felodipine

HCTZ, Hydrochlorothiazide.

Patient Education for Compliance

1. Frequent sips of water or chewing gum may relieve dry mouth occurring with diuretics.
2. Diuretics should be taken in mornings for once-a-day regimens and at 8 AM and 2 PM for twice-a-day regimens to prevent interference with sleep.
3. Furosemide should be taken with food if gastrointestinal upset occurs.
4. Postural hypotension may occur with diuretics.
5. Patients record weight on a regular basis, weighing at same time of day.
6. Patients taking thiazide or loop diuretics should avoid excess exposure to sunlight and ultraviolet light.
7. Patients with diabetes mellitus who take loop diuretics should test blood glucose levels more frequently.
8. Patients taking potassium-sparing diuretics should avoid foods high in potassium and salt substitutes containing potassium.
9. Patients taking diuretics, especially elderly patients, should drink adequate fluids.

Important Facts about Diuretics and Hypertension

- Some vasodilators work on arterial blood flow, some on venous blood flow, and some on both types of vessels.
- Hypertension is systolic pressure above 140 mm Hg or diastolic pressure above 90 mm Hg, whereas a prehypertensive state is blood pressure of 120/80 or above.
- Primary hypertension, most common type of hypertension, has no identifiable cause.

Continued

- Management of prehypertension and hypertension begins with lifestyle changes.
- Thiazide diuretics and loop diuretics reduce blood volume and lower arterial resistance.
- Most diuretics act by blocking active reabsorption of sodium and chloride, thus preventing reabsorption of water to reduce blood volume.
- Drugs acting early on nephrons create greatest diuresis by blocking greatest amount of water reabsorption.
- Loop diuretics block absorption of sodium and chloride in loop of Henle to produce greatest diuresis, causing dehydration through excessive fluid loss.
- Loop diuretics may cause hearing loss.
- Thiazide diuretics produce less diuresis than loop diuretics.
- Potassium-sparing diuretics produce only modest diuresis.

Adrenergic-Inhibiting Agents

Adrenergic-inhibiting agents or **sympatholytic agents** include groups of medications such as beta blockers, *Rauwolfia* derivatives, and alpha-adrenergic agents. The heart, blood vessels, and kidneys influence arterial blood pressure by increasing the heart rate and force of myocardial contractions, by arteriole and venule constriction, and by release of renin in the kidneys. Adrenergic-inhibiting agents are effective to lower blood pressure and prevent serious cardiovascular complications by acting as **vasoconstrictors.** Some of these medications are also used for migraine headaches as seen in Chapter 29 (Table 26-8).

Beta blockers such as **nadolol** (Corgard) and **propranolol** (Inderal) decrease cardiac output, inhibit renin secretion, and interfere with the RAA mechanism, thereby lowering blood pressure (see Box 26-3). These medications are also used with angina and acute MI.

Aldosterone receptor antagonists, such as **eplerenone** (Inspra), block binding of aldosterone in RAA mechanism absorption to lower blood pressure and may be used separately or may be given with thiazide diuretics.

Alpha-beta blockers such as **labetalol** (Normodyne) are similar to beta blockers and are used for severe hypertension. Alpha-receptor blockade causes vasodilation and decreased peripheral vascular resistance when added to beta-blocking mechanisms.

Centrally acting adrenergic inhibitors such as **clonidine** (Catapres) are effective, especially when given with a diuretic. With sympathetic nerves functioning at a higher than normal level, these medications reduce blood pressure, pulse rate, and cardiac output.

Peripherally acting adrenergic inhibitors such as **doxazosin** (Cardura) and **prazosin** (Minipress) are powerful antihypertensives that either interfere with release of norepinephrine from nerve endings or block receptors in vascular smooth muscle. These agents act by decreasing vascular tone, primarily in veins, followed by effects in arteries.

> **LEARNING TIP**
>
> Many of the peripherally acting adrenergic inhibiting agents end with "sin".

Angiotensin II receptor antagonists are used alone or with diuretics to treat hypertension. These medications such as **irbesartan** (Avapro) and **olmesartan** (Benicar) are also used in treatment of MI and CHF in people who cannot tolerate ACE inhibitors. The action is to inhibit binding of angiotensin II in vascular smooth muscle so blood pressure cannot be raised. Because vasoconstriction is blocked, side effects similar to those of ACE inhibitors, such as orthostatic hypotension, occur (see Table 26-8).

> **LEARNING TIP**
>
> Angiotensin II receptor antagonists in most cases have names that end in "tan."

ACE inhibitors such as **benazepril** (Lotensin) and **enalapril** (Vasotec) slow angiotensin II formation, lowering blood volume and blood pressure. Most frequently used with CHF and diabetes, ACE inhibitors are used for treatment of severe hypertension. These drugs result in peripheral vasodilation, renal vasodilation, and suppression of aldosterone-mediated volume expansion. ACE inhibitors are usually associated with the desirable effect of increased renal blood flow while having less interference with mental and physical performance. Consequently, the better quality of life afforded by ACE inhibitors should lead to better compliance (Table 26-9).

> **LEARNING TIP**
>
> Ace inhibitors tend to have names that end with "pril."

Vasodilators

Vasodilators relax or dilate vessels throughout the body—veins or arteries or both. These drugs relax the smooth muscle of peripheral arterioles, thus decreasing peripheral resistance to stimulate the sympathetic nervous system to increase heart rate and cardiac output. Because of this effect, a beta blocker may also be given to inhibit sympathetic response, and a diuretic may be used to alleviate sodium and water retention. **Minoxidil** (Loniten) is usually given with a beta blocker to prevent reflux tachycardia (Table 26-10).

TABLE 26-8 ADRENERGIC-INHIBITING (SYMPATHOLYTIC) AGENTS

GENERIC NAME	USUAL ADULT DOSE, ROUTE, AND FREQUENCY	INDICATIONS FOR USE	DRUG INTERACTIONS
BETA BLOCKERS		Hypertension, angina, cardiac arrhythmias, acute myocardial infarction	Diuretics, xanthines, hypoglycemics, NSAIDs, amiodarone, ampicillin, antacids, digoxin, epinephrine, tacrine, phenylephrine, sympathomimetics
acebutolol (Sectral)	200-800 mg PO qd		
atenolol (Tenormin)	25-100 mg PO qd		
betaxolol (Kerlone)	5-20 mg PO qd		
bisoprolol (Zebeta)	2.5-10 mg PO qd		
metoprolol (Lopressor, Toprol-XL)	25-200 mg PO qd		
nadolol (Corgard)	40-80 mg PO/day every 2-14 days		
penbutolol (Levatol)	10-80 mg PO qd		
pindolol	10-30 mg/day PO in divided doses		
propranolol (Inderal)	160-480 mg PO/day in divided doses		
sotalol (Betapace)	80 mg PO bid		
timolol	10-30 mg PO bid		
ALDOSTERONE RECEPTOR ANTAGONISTS			
eplerenone (Inspra)	25-50 mg PO qd	Hypertension	NSAIDs, lithium, ACE inhibitors
ALPHA-BETA BLOCKERS			
labetalol (Trandate)	100-400 mg PO bid, IV	Severe hypertension	Same as beta blockers plus MAOIs
carvedilol (Coreg CR)	3.125-50 mg PO bid	Hypertension	Same as beta blockers plus MAOIs
CENTRALLY ACTING ADRENERGIC INHIBITORS			
clonidine (Catapres)	0.1-0.8 mg PO qd, transdermal patch	Hypertension	beta blockers, tricyclic antidepressants
guanfacine (Tenex)	1.52 mg PO qd		None
methyldopa	500-2000 mg PO daily in divided doses, IV		MAOIs, sympathomimetics
PERIPHERALLY ACTING ADRENERGIC INHIBITORS			
doxazosin (Cardura)	1-16 mg PO qd	Hypertension	NSAIDs, estrogen
prazosin (Minipress)	1-20 mg PO qd		NSAIDs, verapamil, beta blockers
reserpine (Serpalan)	0.1-0.25 mg PO qd		MAOIs
terazosin (Hytrin)	1-20 mg PO qd		ACE inhibitors, NSAIDs, propranolol
ANGIOTENSIN II RECEPTOR ANTAGONISTS		Hypertension, vasodilation	cimetidine, phenobarbital, rifampin, lithium, ketoconazole, troleandomycin
losartan (Cozaar)	25-100 mg PO qd		
valsartan (Diovan)	80-320 mg PO qd		
irbesartan (Avapro)	150-300 mg PO qd		
olmesartan medoxomil (Benicar)	20-40 mg PO qd		herbal supplements
eprosartan (Teveten)	400-800 mg PO qd		herbal supplements
telmisartan (Micardis)	20-80 mg PO qd		warfarin, digoxin

ACE, angiotensin-converting enzyme; *IV*, intravenously; *MAOI*, monoamine oxidase inhibitor; *NSAIDs*, nonsteroidal antiinflammatory drugs; *PO*, orally.

TABLE 26-9 ANGIOTENSIN-CONVERTING ENZYME (ACE) INHIBITORS USED FOR HYPERTENSION

GENERIC NAME/ TRADE NAME	USUAL DOSE, ROUTE, AND FREQUENCY	INDICATIONS FOR USE	DRUG INTERACTIONS
benazepril (Lotensin)	5-40 mg PO qd	Hypertension	alcohol and diuretics
captopril (Capoten)	25-100 mg PO bid-tid		
enalapril (Vasotec)	5-40 mg PO daily in divided doses		
fosinopril (Monopril)	10-40 mg PO qd		
lisinopril (Prinivil, Zestril)	10-40 mg PO qd		
moexipril (Univasc)	7.5-30 mg PO qd		
quinapril (Accupril)	10-80 mg PO qd		
ramipril (Altace)	2.5-20 mg PO qd		
trandolapril (Mavik)	1-4 mg PO qd		alcohol and diuretics
perindopril (Aceon)	2-8 mg PO qd	For use with thiazides	None identified

Major Side Effects:

Dry nonproductive cough, headaches, diarrhea, constipation, loss of taste, weakness, dizziness, joint pain, upper respiratory infections; *trandolapril*—dyspepsia, cough, syncope, myalgia

TABLE 26-10 VASODILATORS

GENERIC NAME/ TRADE NAME	USUAL DOSE, ROUTE, AND FREQUENCY	INDICATIONS FOR USE	DRUG INTERACTIONS
hydralazine	10-50 mg PO bid-qid, IM, IV	Hypertension	diuretics
minoxidil	5-80 mg PO qd		NSAIDs, nitrates, guanethidine

Major Side Effects:

Headaches, anorexia, constipation, dizziness, nasal congestion

IM, intramuscularly; *IV*, intravenously; *NSAIDs*, nonsteroidal antiinflammatory drugs; *PO*, orally.

Did You Know?

A side effect of minoxidil is increased body hair growth, leading to its primary use in treating baldness.

LEARNING TIP

Many of the calcium channel blockers end in "pine" or "il".

Calcium Channel Blockers

Calcium channel blockers are used to treat angina, cardiac dysrhythmia, and hypertension by interfering with influx of calcium in vascular and smooth muscles. Of most concern in blood pressure treatment is action on the muscle of peripheral arterioles because peripheral vasodilation or decreased peripheral vascular resistance lowers blood pressure during rest and exercise. Calcium channel blockers approved by the Food and Drug Administration (FDA) for treatment of hypertension are listed in Table 26-11. Special considerations for use in the elderly are described in Box 26-5.

BOX 26-5 SPECIAL CONSIDERATIONS FOR USE OF CALCIUM CHANNEL BLOCKERS IN THE ELDERLY

Elderly patients are more susceptible to calcium channel blocking agents and have an increased occurrence of side effects such as weakness, dizziness, fainting, and falls.

Smoking and nicotine should be avoided; they reduce effectiveness of these medications.

Use of alcohol may lead to hypotensive episodes.

Gradual withdrawal is recommended when stopping calcium channel blocking agents.

Patient Education for Compliance

1. Antihypertensives are lifelong medications to control but not cure hypertension.
2. Patients should report signs of peripheral edema when taking calcium channel blockers.
3. Antihypertensives may cause drowsiness, dizziness, or lightheadedness.

TABLE 26-11 CALCIUM CHANNEL BLOCKERS USED TO TREAT HYPERTENSION

GENERIC NAME/TRADE NAME	USUAL DOSE, ROUTE, AND FREQUENCY	INDICATIONS FOR USE	DRUG INTERACTIONS
amlodipine (Norvasc)	2.5-10 mg PO qd	Hypertension and angina pectoris	beta blockers (both systemic and ophthalmologic), digitalis, disopyramide, potassium-depleting medications, quinidine, procainamide
with benazepril (Lotrel)	2.5/10-5/20 mg PO qd		
diltiazem (Cardizem, Tiazac)	varies by product		
felodipine (Plendil)	5-10 mg PO qd		
nicardipine (Cardene)	20-40 mg PO tid		
nifedipine (Procardia, Adalat)	30-90 mg PO qd		
nisoldipine (Sular)	8.5-40 mg PO qd		
verapamil (Calan, Isoptin, Calan SR, Isoptin SR, Verelan)	80-120 mg PO q8h		
	180-480 mg PO qd		

Important Facts about Antihypertensives

- Lack of patient compliance is the major cause of treatment failure in antihypertensive therapy because therapy often causes negative feelings as the body adjusts to the medication. Medication and lifestyle compliance is difficult to achieve because hypertension is a silent disease that progresses slowly but requires lifelong, expensive treatment.
- Beta blockers and diuretics are the preferred drugs for the initial therapy of hypertension.
- Beta blockers reduce blood pressure primarily by reducing peripheral vascular resistance and cardiac output.
- Diuretics increase urinary output to decrease blood volume thus lowering blood pressure.
- Vasodilators and calcium channel blockers reduce blood pressure by promoting dilation of arterioles.
- When a combination of drugs is used for hypertension, each drug should have a different mechanism of action.
- Angiotensin-converting enzyme (ACE) inhibitors are used to treat hypertension, congestive heart failure, and myocardial infarction.
- Calcium channel blockers cause vasodilation, which is useful in hypertension and angina.
- Calcium channel blockers and beta blockers have similar therapeutic effects.

DISEASES OF THE BLOOD VESSELS AND THEIR TREATMENT

Peripheral vascular disease, with extremities becoming cold or numb, with **intermittent claudication** and ulcers, is common among elderly. Usually caused by either atherosclerosis or hyperlipidemia, arteriosclerosis reduces blood flow to tissues, blood viscosity is elevated because of fat content, and blood flow to tissues is diminished. Red blood cells are less flexible, and lack of oxygen causes limitation of blood flow and oxygen and carbon dioxide cell exchange with exercise, resulting in ischemia and pain. Peripheral vasodilators are used to smooth skeletal muscles of the peripheral arterial walls while having little effect on cutaneous blood flow. *Isoxsuprine* (Vasodilan) may relieve these symptoms (Table 26-12).

Hemorrheologic agents are also used to improve blood flow and lower blood viscosity in peripheral tissues. *Pentoxifylline* (Trental) is a hemorrheologic agent used to improve blood flow through rigid blood vessels to improve microcirculation. *Cilostazol* (Pletal) is the second medication in this category, used to reduce the intermittent claudication that comes with walking distances by platelet aggregation (see Table 26-12).

HYPERLIPIDEMIA AND ITS TREATMENT

Some cholesterol and **triglycerides,** necessary in formation of cell membrane and nerve tissue, are found in plasma proteins. Excessive dietary intake of lipids is stored as fat in adipose tissue to be reserved for energy use. Cholesterol is also stored in the gallbladder as a part of bile acids. Lipids do not circulate freely in the bloodstream but instead bind to plasma proteins (albumin and globulin) to form lipoproteins. Excessive circulation of lipids leads to hyperlipidemia, which is associated with atherosclerosis, leading to obstruction of blood

TABLE 26-12 DRUGS USED WITH PERIPHERAL VASCULAR DISEASES

GENERIC NAME/ TRADE NAME	USUAL DOSE, ROUTE, AND FREQUENCY	INDICATIONS FOR USE	DRUG INTERACTIONS
PERIPHERAL VASODILATORS			
isoxsuprine	10-20 mg PO tid-qid	Peripheral vascular disease	None
bosentan (Tracleer)	62.5 mg PO bid		cyclosporine, glyburide

Major Side Effects of Peripheral Vasodilators:
Orthostatic hypotension, flushing, dizziness, weakness, nausea, palpitations, tachycardia

HEMORRHEOLOGIC AGENTS			
pentoxifylline (Trental)	400 mg PO tid	Decrease blood viscosity	Other antihypertensives
cilostazol (Pletal)	100 mg PO bid	Platelet aggregation	erythromycin, diltiazem, omeprazole, ketoconazole

Major Side Effects of Hemorrheologic Agents:
Dizziness, headache, abdominal distress, nausea, vomiting

flow and CAD. The large- and medium-sized arteries are usually the ones involved with these degenerative changes.

Lipoproteins are classified by their density. The three primary groups are **very-low-density lipoproteins (VLDLs), low-density lipoproteins (LDLs),** and **high-density lipoproteins (HDLs).** VLDL particles are secreted by the liver, becoming smaller as the triglycerides are removed. LDLs, considered to be most harmful, contain the major portion of blood cholesterol. HDLs, the smallest and most dense of the lipoproteins, transport cholesterol from the peripheral cells to liver for metabolism and excretion. Because HDL is a transport aid to rid the body of lipoproteins, the higher the HDL level, the more beneficial with regard to preventing accumulation of lipids in arterial walls.

Adults should undergo periodic cholesterol testing because of the clear relationship between LDL and atherosclerosis. An HDL level below 35 mg/dL is considered to put a person at risk for CAD. The decision to provide medications to lower blood cholesterol is based on LDL levels, with levels below 130 mg/dL considered desirable. When the level is above 130 mg/dL, the person should be treated therapeutically, especially when other risk factors such as hypertension, diabetes, and low HDL levels have been found. Familial history and aging may necessitate interventions such as medications when dietary and lifestyle change are not adequate.

Treatment of Hyperlipidemia

Medications are used only if diet modifications, weight loss, smoking cessation, and exercise programs fail to reduce LDL to acceptable levels. When these lifelong medications are initiated, diet therapy must continue. For optimum therapy, LDL levels are reduced without reducing HDL levels. LDL will return to high levels if these drugs are discontinued. The treatment is prophylactic—preventing and retarding arteriosclerosis rather than causing regression of a disease process that has occurred.

Hypolipidemics or *antihyperlipidemics* are used as adjuvant therapy to reduce elevated cholesterol levels with hypercholesteremia and high LDL levels. Two major categories are bile acid sequestrants and HMG-CoA reductase inhibitors or statins. Other combination medications are used for various effects on lipoproteins, including combinations of medications to treat more than one condition (Table 26-13).

Bile acid sequestrants such as ***cholestyramine*** (Questran) are nonabsorbable, cholesterol-lowering medications effective because cholesterol is the major bile acid precursor. To reduce LDL and serum cholesterol levels, these medications bind bile acids in the intestine to prevent their absorption and for excretion in feces. Bile acid–sequestrant medications, used for primary hypercholesterolemia, must be used with care by patients with pancreatitis, hypothyroidism, gallstones, CAD, or hemorrhoids. Because of the binding and loss of fats, deficiencies in fat-soluble vitamins A, D, K, and E may occur.

HMG-CoA reductase inhibitors, or statins, are the most effective agents for lowering LDL and cholesterol levels and cause few adverse reactions. Agents such as ***atorvastatin*** (Lipitor) and ***simvastatin*** (Zocor) are widely used. Statins reduce the liver enzyme HMG-CoA reductase, necessary in cholesterol production. Responses for lowering elevated levels of LDL cholesterol are dose

TABLE 26-13 HYPOLIPIDEMICS

GENERIC NAME/ TRADE NAME	USUAL DOSE, ROUTE, AND FREQUENCY	INDICATIONS FOR USE	DRUG INTERACTIONS
BILE ACID SEQUESTRANT		Hyperlipidemia; reduction of LDL and cholesterol	
cholestyramine (Questran, Prevalite)	4-6 g powder in water-based liquid PO 1-2× daily		anticoagulants, digoxin, thiazides, penicillin, propranolol, aspirin, tetracyclines, folic acid, thyroid hormones
colestipol (Colestid)	15-30 g granules PO bid-qid		

Major Side Effects of Bile Acid–Sequestrant:
Constipation, indigestion, abdominal pain, nausea and vomiting, dizziness, headache, gallstones

HMG-CoA REDUCTASE INHIBITORS STATINS			
atorvastatin (Lipitor)	10-80 mg PO qd		alcohol, niacin, cyclosporine, digitalis, erythromycin, rifampin, anticoagulants, oral contraceptives, propranolol
fluvastatin (Lescol)	20-40 mg PO qd		
lovastatin (Mevacor)	20-80 mg PO qd		
pitavastatin (Livalo)	1-4 mg PO qd		
pravastatin (Pravachol)	10-40 mg PO qd		
simvastatin (Zocor)	10-40 mg PO qd		
rosuvastatin (Crestor)	5-10 mg PO qd		

Major Side Effects of Statins:
Headache, flatulence, constipation, abdominal pain, cramping, dyspepsia

MISCELLANEOUS HYPOLIPIDEMICS		Elevated cholesterol or triglyceride levels	
nicotinic acid, niacin (Slo-Niacin)	1-2 g PO qd in 2-3 divided doses		statins, alcohol
gemfibrozil (Lopid)	600 mg PO bid		statins, anticoagulants
ezetimibe (Zetia)	10 mg PO qd		cyclosporine, bile acid sequestrants
fenofibrate (Tricor, Lofibra)	48-145 mg qd		warfarin, bile acid sequestrants, cyclosporine
fenofibric acid (Trilipix)	135 mg PO qd		cyclosporine, warfarin, diuretics, hormones, beta blockers

Major Side Effects of Miscellaneous Hypolipidemics:
nicotinic acid—flushing, itching, nausea, vomiting, diarrhea; *gemfibrozil*—GI symptoms, dizziness, blurred vision, muscle pain and weakness; *clofibrate*—headache, diarrhea, skin rash; *ezetimibe*—fatigue, arthralgia, myalgia, dizziness, headache, diarrhea; *fenofibrate*—fatigue, arthralgia, headache, insomnia, dyspepsia, rash, pruritus; *fenofibric acid*—stomach pain related to gallbladder disease, nausea, vomiting, jaundice, pain or swelling of legs, chest pain, sudden cough, wheezing, rapid breathing and heart rate

COMBINATION HYPOLIPIDEMICS			
ezetimibe + simvastatin (Vytorin)	10/10-10/40 mg PO qd	Familial hyperlipidemia	Antifungals, erythromycin, clarithromycin, amiodarone, verapamil
amlodipine + atorvastatin (Caduet)	5/10-10/80 mg PO qd	Hyperlipidemia, hypertension	

Major Side Effects of Combination Hypolipidemics:
Headache, gallstones, myalgia

GI, Gastrointestinal; *LDL*, low-density lipoprotein; *PO*, orally.

dependent. Low doses provide a smaller decrease; large doses may reduce production of the enzyme up to 60%. These medications must be continued for life to reduce progression of CAD, decrease number of cardiac problems, and decrease mortality (see Table 26-13).

✎ LEARNING TIP

Because medications in this family have -*statin* in the generic names, they are referred to as "statins."

Nicotinic acid (Nicobid) reduces LDL and VLDL levels and raises HDL levels, but use is limited by side effects such as flushing and tingling sensations. Side effects diminish after several weeks of use and can be lessened by taking aspirin 30 minutes before nicotinic acid administration. Triple therapy consisting of nicotinic acid plus a bile acid–binding resin and a statin may decrease LDL cholesterol levels by 70% or more (see Table 26-13).

Fibric acid derivatives are used to lower triglycerides and raise HDL levels. *Gemfibrozil* (Lopid) inhibits breakdown of fats into triglycerides and decreases hepatic production of triglycerides. This drug, preferred for patients with hypertriglyceridemia when triglyceride levels exceed 1000 mg/dL (normal is 10 to 190 mg/dL), may be used together with other hypolipidemic drugs (see Table 26-13).

With all hypolipidemics and associated medications, patient compliance is essential. For long-term benefit of cholesterol and LDL reduction and prevention of CAD, dosage calculation and scheduling of medications should be individualized to each patient because of possible adverse effects. Serum levels of lipoproteins and liver enzymes should be assessed regularly to be sure the desired effect is being obtained without adverse effects.

Patient Education for Compliance

1. Diet modifications should be carefully followed before using hypolipidemics. Drug therapy alone will not significantly lower blood lipoprotein levels.
2. Cholestyramine (Questran or Prevalite) powder must be mixed with 4 to 6 ounces of water or a noncarbonated beverage. The powder should not be ingested in dry form.
3. Colestipol (Colestid) granules will not dissolve in thin liquids and so should be mixed with thick liquids for ingestion.

Important Facts about Hypolipidemics

- Low-density lipoproteins (LDLs) transport cholesterol to peripheral tissue; high-density lipoproteins (HDLs) transport cholesterol to liver.
- Diet modification is primary method for reducing LDL and cholesterol levels. Drugs are used only if diet modification is unsuccessful.
- Statins, the most effective drugs for lowering LDL and cholesterol levels, cause the fewest side effects.
- Bile acid sequestrants prevent bile acid reabsorption in intestines, causing constipation and other gastrointestinal effects.
- Other oral medications should be given 1 hour before bile acid sequestrants or 4 hours after, to allow for absorption without interference by hypolipidemics.

MEDICATIONS THAT AFFECT COAGULATION

Clot formation to prevent further loss of blood from wounds is necessary for survival with injuries or surgery. **Hemostasis** is necessary for homeostasis. Occasionally the body will form clots or thrombi that jam blood vessels, causing a **thromboembolism**. A **thrombus** is a blood clot within a blood vessel, whereas an **embolus** is a mass of undissolved matter in a vessel moving through the circulatory system (Figure 26-8). Anticoagulants are used to prevent venous clotting in patients with thrombohemolytic disorders. Anticoagulants disrupt the coagulation process and suppress fibrin formation. Thrombolytic medications promote dissolution of thrombi.

Antiplatelet drugs are used to keep platelets from clumping (or aggregating). Antiplatelet medications are most effective in preventing arterial thrombi formation, whereas anticoagulants are used to prevent venous thrombi formation.

Anticoagulants

Anticoagulants may be given parenterally, as heparin, or orally, as **warfarin** (Coumadin). If not given intravenously, heparin must be given by subcutaneous injection because administration into muscle will cause muscle bleeding. Safe for use in pregnancy because it does not cross the placenta, heparin has an almost immediate onset but a short duration of action. Therefore it is usually used in inpatient situations or in intravenous tubing where blood clotting is a possibility, such as during dialysis. Other injectable anticoagulants, including **enoxaparin** (Lovenox) and **dalteparin** (Fragmin), are similar to heparin and are used more often in ambulatory care.

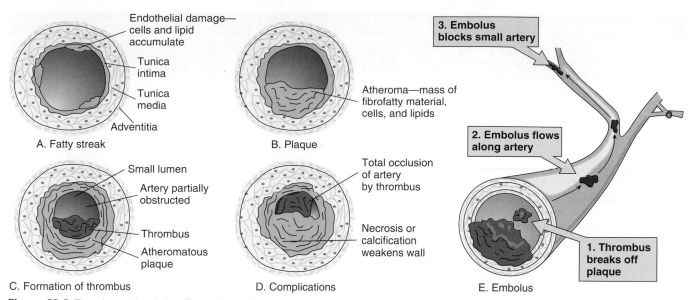

Figure 26-8 Thrombus and embolus. (From Young AP, Proctor DB: *Kinn's the medical assistant: an applied learning approach,* ed 11, St Louis, 2011, Saunders.)

TABLE 26-14 **ANTICOAGULANTS**			
GENERIC NAME/ TRADE NAME	**USUAL DOSE, ROUTE, AND FREQUENCY**	**INDICATIONS FOR USE**	**DRUG INTERACTIONS**
heparin	Individualized IV, deep SC	Prophylaxis of venous thrombi	antiplatelet medications, NSAIDs, diuretics, thrombolytics, antacids, allopurinol, cimetidine, tricyclic antidepressants, antibiotics, estrogen, oral hypoglycemics, barbiturates
warfarin (Coumadin)	0.25-10 mg PO, individualized dependent on prothrombin time		
enoxaparin (Lovenox)	Individualized SC		
dalteparin (Fragmin)	Individualized SC		

GI, Gastrointestinal; *IV,* intravenously; *NSAIDs,* nonsteroidal antiinflammatory drugs; *PO,* orally; *SC,* subcutaneously.

Oral anticoagulants, used to prevent thrombi, have a delayed onset of action; therefore they are not appropriate in emergency situations. Rather, these agents are used prophylactically for deep vein thrombosis or to prevent thrombus formation in such conditions as atrial fibrillation, to prevent pulmonary embolus, and in heart valve replacement surgery.

Warfarin

The oldest and most used anticoagulant medication is warfarin, an antagonist to vitamin K, which is needed for clotting factors to work. Medication levels peak a few days after initiation of treatment, and the drug remains in the body for 2 to 5 days after discontinuation. Prothrombin times are necessary to evaluate dosage safety. Patients must be carefully watched for bruising, bloody stools, bleeding gums, and blood in urine. An overdose

is treated with vitamin K. A long list of interactions is shown in Table 26-14.

> **Did You Know?**
>
> Warfarin was first found in spoiled silage that caused cattle to bleed. When first developed it was used to kill rats, and it is still one of the most widely used products for eliminating rodents.

> 🖉 **LEARNING TIP**
>
> Anticoagulants tend to end in "in".

TABLE 26-15 ANTIPLATELET DRUGS

GENERIC NAME/ TRADE NAME	USUAL DOSE, ROUTE, AND FREQUENCY	INDICATIONS FOR USE	DRUG INTERACTIONS
aspirin* (Bayer and others)	81-325 mg PO daily in divided doses	Prevention of arterial thromboses by preventing platelet aggregation	oral anticoagulants, ACE inhibitors, diltiazem
ticlopidine[†] (Ticlid)	250 mg PO bid		None indicated
dipyridamole[†] (Persantine)	50-100 mg PO qid		
clopidogrel[†] (Plavix)	75 mg PO once daily		NSAIDs, phenytoin, warfarin, tamoxifen, tolbutamide, torsemide

ACE, angiotensin-converting enzyme; *NSAIDs*, nonsteroidal antiinflammatory drugs; *PO*, orally.
*OTC medication.
[†]Prescription medication.

Antiplatelet Medications

Antiplatelet drugs are used to suppress aggregation of platelets. The most frequently used antiplatelet medication is aspirin, proven effective in preventing MIs and strokes. Dosage is low, with increased doses offering no further therapeutic advantage. *Clopidogrel* (Plavix), used in patients who have recently had an MI, a stroke, or have established peripheral vascular disease, is also used as secondary prevention of further disease processes, complications, or deaths with atherosclerosis. Dentists or surgeons should be informed if a person is taking this medication, to prevent excessive bleeding. *Ticlopidine* (Ticlid), which is more expensive than aspirin, is no more prophylactic. *Dipyridamole* (Persantine) also decreases platelet aggregation and is used in combination with aspirin in heart valve replacement surgery (Table 26-15).

Thrombolytic Medications

Thrombolytic medications, used to dissolve already formed blood clots, or thrombi, are effective for treating MIs if given within 6 hours of chest pain onset. Five thrombolytic drugs are available: *streptokinase* (Streptase), *alteplase* (Activase), *urokinase* (Abbokinase), *reteplase* (Retavase), and *anistreplase* (Eminase). These medications are given in a hospital setting by health care providers experienced in caring for patients with thrombi.

 LEARNING TIP

Note that the names of thrombolytic medications tend to end in "ase," indicating that these are enzymes.

Topical Hemostatics

Topical hemostatics are gelatin or cellulose sponges employed to absorb excess blood and fluids and to control bleeding during oral, ophthalmic, or prostate surgery. These agents expand on contact with wounds to absorb large amounts of blood and permit clotting to occur along surfaces. These hemostatics are ultimately absorbed. Oxidized cellulose cannot be used for permanent implants because it interferes with bone regeneration and may produce cyst formation. *Absorbable gelatin foam* (Gelfoam), *absorbable gelatin film* (Gelfilm), and *absorbable gelatin powder* (Gelfoam powder) are specially prepared nonantigenic preparations available in either strips or powders for complete absorption in 2 to 5 days when applied to skin and 4 weeks to 5 months when applied to surgical wounds. These agents should be moistened with isotonic saline solutions or thrombin solutions before being applied to a wound. *Oxidized cellulose* (Oxycel, Surgicel) is surgical gauze or cotton that exerts a hemostatic effect. Chief uses are in removal of nasal polyps and other minor surgical procedures. The agent should not be used as a surface dressing because it inhibits growth of epithelial tissue and dressing material is not premoistened.

Thrombin (Thrombinar, Thrombostat), a sterile powder obtained from bovine prothrombin, is used topically to treat capillary bleeding.

Patient Education for Compliance

1. Patients taking anticoagulants and antiplatelet drugs must be careful to avoid injury, including using a soft bristled toothbrush and an electric razor.
2. Prothrombin levels should be regularly evaluated when using anticoagulant therapy.

TABLE 26-16 HEMATOPOIETIC AND ERYTHROPOIETIC STIMULANTS

GENERIC NAME/ TRADE NAME	USUAL DOSE, ROUTE, AND FREQUENCY	INDICATIONS FOR USE	DRUG INTERACTIONS
HEMATOPOIETIC AGENTS		Stimulate neutrophil production	
filgrastim (Neupogen)	5 mcg/kg SC, IV once daily		Concomitantly with antineoplastics
pegfilgrastim (Neulasta)	6 mg SC with chemotherapy		lithium

Major Side Effects of Hematopoietic Agents:
Fever, nausea and vomiting, skeletal pain

ERYTHROPOIETIC AGENTS		Stimulate erythropoiesis, antianemics	
darbepoetin alfa (Aranesp)	0.45 mg/kg SC		androgens
epoetin (Epogen, Procrit)	100-150 units/kg SC		None of significance

Major Side Effects of Erythropoietic Agents:
darbepoetin alfa—seizure, stroke, CHF, MI, diarrhea, nausea, fatigue, fever, bone pain, myalgia, dyspnea; *epoetin*—seizure, coldness, sweating, hypertension, bone pain, headache

CHF, Congestive heart failure; *IV,* intravenously; *MI,* myocardial infarction; *SC,* subcutaneously.

Important Facts about Medications That Affect Coagulation

- Hemostasis occurs with formation of platelet plug followed by coagulation.
- Arterial thrombi are best prevented with antiplatelet drugs; venous thrombi are prevented with anticoagulants.
- Heparin is administered subcutaneously and intravenously.
- Warfarin, prototypes for oral anticoagulants, act by blocking biosynthesis of vitamin K.
- Aspirin and other antiplatelet drugs suppress thrombus formation.
- Topical hemostats have no significant drug interactions.

MEDICATIONS USED AS HEMATOPOIETICS AND ERYTHROPOIETICS

Hematopoietic stimulants are given to increase white blood cell levels by stimulating bone marrow to produce more leukocytes, especially neutrophils. By increasing neutrophil levels, the body is better able to fight infections after administration of chemotherapy or with diseases or therapy causing decreased cell formation. On the other hand, erythropoietin stimulators cause bone marrow to produce more erythrocytes and reduce the need for blood transfusions after hemodialysis or therapy that produces anemia. Anemia may be the result of decrease of erythropoietin, a protein produced by kidneys. These medications are administered parenterally and are expensive treatment options. Doses can be adjusted as needed to meet patient needs (Table 26-16).

SUMMARY

Cardiovascular disease is the leading cause of death in the United States. Some medications are effective on the myocardium itself, whereas others are effective on blood. The three actions of medications on cardiac muscle are *inotropic* (force of myocardial contraction), *dromotropic* (conduction of electrical impulses through heart muscle), and *chronotropic* (heart rate). Other medications cause vasodilation, to lessen the heart's work. As CAD occurs (e.g., arteriosclerosis or atherosclerosis), medications are used to increase circulation by increasing myocardial contractions to adequately pump blood through the body.

Vasodilators such as nitrates increase blood vessel size to improve blood circulation. Nitrates are used as antianginal agents. Beta blockers and calcium channel blockers are also used for long-term management of angina, by slowing the heart and interfering with calcium movement through cell membranes of vascular smooth muscle. The therapeutic goal of angina treatment is to reduce frequency and intensity of attacks.

Cardiac glycosides, or digitalis preparations, are used to increase force of myocardial contractions in CHF, increase strength of contractions, slow heart rate, and slow conduction of electrical impulses to the heart. Heart efficiency is increased without increasing oxygen consumption. Glycosides tend to decrease heart rate; therefore patient education should include taking the pulse daily before taking digitalis preparations. If the pulse is below 60, the physician should decide if the patient's medication should be taken.

Antidysrhythmics are used to treat disorders of cardiac rhythm occurring from CAD, electrolyte imbalances, cardiac conduction abnormalities, or even endocrine diseases such as thyroid disorders. Dysrhythmias may have little effect on cardiac output or may cause severe compromise of cardiac pumping action. Medications change heart electrophysiologic properties by regulating calcium, sodium, and potassium ions flowing into heart muscle.

Antihypertensive medications, including diuretics, ACE inhibitors, beta blockers, sympatholytic agents, and vasodilators, are used only when lifestyle changes have not adequately lowered elevated blood pressure. Combinations of medicines may be required, and each new drug should come from a different therapeutic category. Patients must be aware that treatment for hypertension is lifelong, including lifestyle changes, medications, or both.

For peripheral vascular diseases, vasodilators have a relaxing effect on the smooth muscles of peripheral arterial walls to alleviate symptoms of atherosclerosis or hyperlipidemia. Hemorrheologic agents are used to improve blood flow through rigid arteriosclerotic blood vessels and through microcirculation of arterioles, venules, and capillaries. To reduce the circulating lipoproteins and to alleviate hypercholesterolemia leading to obstruction of blood flow, hypolipidemics, along with lifestyle changes are used for long-term therapy.

Anticoagulants are used to treat deep venous thrombosis by disrupting the coagulation process and formation of fibrin. Antiplatelet medications, such as frequently used aspirin, inhibit aggregation of platelets to prevent arterial thrombi formation.

Hematopoietic and erythropoietic agents are used to increase circulating blood cells when disease processes or disease treatment cause a drop in white or red blood cells. Treatment reduces the need for blood transfusions in persons undergoing chemotherapy, hemodialysis, or with infections such as human immunodeficiency virus.

Many medications affect the cardiovascular system and thrombus-forming blood disorders—major areas in medical treatment today. Cardiac glycosides and nitrates are medicines that have been in use for many years. Antihyperlipidemics are more recent additions for cardiac disease prophylaxis. Nitrates, particularly nitroglycerin, now come in various forms. Some are used as needed, whereas other forms are used on a daily basis, but the patient must be nitrate free at some point during the day to prevent development of tolerance to the medication.

As more information is gathered about the leading cause of sickness and death—cardiovascular disease—medications are changing rapidly. The lifelong need for treating hypertension continues. Vessel disease is still present, but prevention through lifestyle changes and medication will continue to improve quality of life for those prone to cardiovascular disease.

CRITICAL THINKING EXERCISES

Scenario

Mr. Jones has been diagnosed with essential hypertension. He asks how long he will need to take medications.

1. What do you tell him?
2. He also wants to know if there are any lifestyle changes that will help. Name several of these for Mr. Jones.
3. Given diuretics as his first medication, Mr. Jones needs to eat what foods to help keep potassium at acceptable levels?
4. How often does Mr. Jones need to check his blood pressure?
5. Can other medications be added to help bring his blood pressure to within an acceptable range if diuretics alone do not accomplish this? Explain your answer.

DRUG CALCULATIONS

1. Order: captopril 50 mg PO qam
   Available medication:

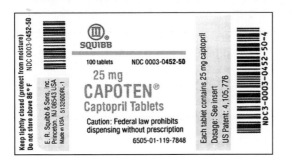

Dose to be administered: _____

2. Order: Lanoxin 375 mcg PO qam if P ↑60
   Available medication:

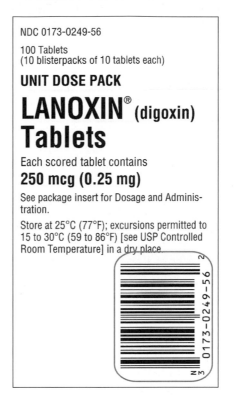

NDC 0173-0249-56

100 Tablets
(10 blisterpacks of 10 tablets each)

UNIT DOSE PACK

LANOXIN® (digoxin) Tablets

Each scored tablet contains
250 mcg (0.25 mg)

See package insert for Dosage and Administration.

Store at 25°C (77°F); excursions permitted to 15 to 30°C (59 to 86°F) [see USP Controlled Room Temperature] in a dry place.

Dose to be administered: _____

REVIEW QUESTIONS

1. How do cardiac glycosides work on heart tissue? _____

2. What chemical classification of medicines is used for anginal pain? _____

3. How do the cardiac glycosides work on the heart muscle in congestive heart failure? _____

4. What are the side effects of antidysrhythmics? _____

5. What are the five categories of medications used to treat hypertension? _____

6. What two categories of medications are used for the initial treatment of hypertension? _____
   _____
   _____

7. What is hyperlipidemia? What are the classifications of lipoproteins? _____
   _____
   _____

8. How do the statins decrease lipoprotein levels? _____
   _____
   _____

9. How do anticoagulants act? Thrombolytics? _____
   _____
   _____

10. How do antiplatelet medications stop thrombi? _____
    _____
    _____

CHAPTER 27

Urinary System Disorders

After studying this chapter, you should be capable of doing the following:

- Discussing specific electrolytes needed to achieve homeostasis and to balance extracellular and intracellular fluids.
- Describing how and what antiinfectives and antiseptics are used for urinary tract infections.
- Explaining the role of urinary tract analgesics and antispasmodics in treatment of urinary tract conditions.

- Discussing enuresis and medications used for treatment.
- Discussing medications used for treating an overactive bladder (OAB).
- Providing patient education for compliance with medications used to treat diseases and conditions of the urinary system.

Mrs. Smith calls to tell you that her 7-year-old son, James, is having a problem with bedwetting and she has tried withholding liquids at bedtime. This action does not seem to help James, and Dr. Merry orders DDAVP.

What is the form of this medication?
What side effects would be expected with this medication?
What is the youngest age the Food and Drug Administration considers to be safe for taking this medication?
What other suggestions may be made to assist with the control of enuresis?

KEY TERMS

Anorexia	Enuresis	Malaise	Solute
Ascites	Hematuria	Nocturia	Solvent
Diuresis	Incontinence	Oliguria	Urgency
Dysuria	Ion	Pyuria	Urinary frequency
Electrolyte	Lethargy	Replacement therapy	

EASY WORKING KNOWLEDGE OF INDICATIONS AND SIDE EFFECTS

Common Symptoms of Urinary System Disorders

Anorexia, nausea, vomiting

Malaise, fatigue, lethargy

Nocturia, hematuria, pyuria, proteinuria

Dysuria, urgency, frequency, incontinence

Pain in lumbar region or flank radiating into medial thighs, ranging from slight tenderness to intense pain

Fever

Edema and ascites

Symptoms of respiratory and cardiovascular disease including hypertension and shortness of breath

Common Side Effects of Medications for Urinary System Disorders

Drying of secretions

Drowsiness and dizziness

Rash and urticaria

Gastrointestinal symptoms (nausea, vomiting, diarrhea)

Headaches

Bradycardia, tachycardia

Discolored urine

EASY WORKING KNOWLEDGE OF DRUGS FOR URINARY SYSTEM DISORDERS

DRUG CLASS	PRESCRIPTION	OTC	PREGNANCY CATEGORY	MAJOR INDICATIONS
Diuretics (also see Chapter 26)	Yes	Yes	B, C	Hypertension and edema
Antiinfectives (also see Chapter 17)	Yes	No	B, C, D (sulfamethoxizole at term)	Urinary tract infections including pyelonephritis, cystitis, urethritis
Urinary tract antiseptics	Yes	Yes	B	Urinary tract irritation
Urinary tract antispasmodics	Yes	No	B	Genitourinary muscle relaxant
Medications for overactive bladder (OAB)	Yes	No	C	Treatment of OAB symptoms
Medications for enuresis	Yes	No	B	Enuresis in children older than 6

Urine is formed in kidney nephrons and then passes through two ureters into the urinary bladder for storage before excretion (Figures 27-1 and 27-2). The kidneys regulate homeostasis, maintain fluid and electrolyte balance, and eliminate body fluid wastes through urine. When the bladder is sufficiently filled (approximately 250 mL of urine), the person feels the urge to void, and urine voluntarily passes through the urethra from the body. When urine is retained for prolonged periods of time, urinary tract infections (UTIs) are more prevalent.

In males the urethra is surrounded by the prostate gland. If the prostate becomes enlarged, urine may be retained in the bladder because of urethral constriction. However, UTIs are more prevalent in women owing to proximity of the urethra, vagina, and anus, and the short length of the urethra. When medications have been ordered, patients should be aware that urine can change color with ingestion of certain drugs, an important element in patient education in the use of urinary tract medications (Table 27-1).

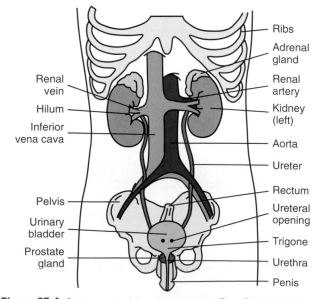

Figure 27-1 Components of the urinary system. (From Frazier MS, Drzymkowski JW: *Essentials of human diseases and conditions*, ed 4, St Louis, 2008, Saunders.)

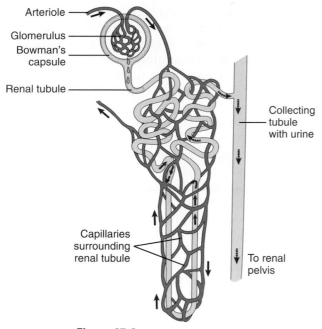

Arteriole
Glomerulus
Bowman's capsule
Renal tubule
Collecting tubule with urine
Capillaries surrounding renal tubule
To renal pelvis

Figure 27-2 Anatomy of a nephron.

TABLE 27-1 MEDICATIONS THAT MAY ALTER URINE COLOR

DRUG	POSSIBLE COLOR CHANGES
amitriptyline (Elavil)	Blue-green
Anticoagulants containing warfarin	Pink, red, or dark brown (indicative of systemic bleeding)
cascara sagrada	In acidic urine, brown
	In alkaline urine, yellow to pink
	In standing urine, black
iron salts	Brown to black
Laxatives containing senna	Pink to red to brown
Laxatives containing phenolphthalein	Pink to red
levodopa	Darkens urine and sweat
methyldopa	Pink or amber to dark urine
metronidazole	Dark urine
nitrofurantoin	Yellow to rusty brown
phenazopyridine	Orange-red urine that may stain clothing
phenytoin	Red-brown or darkened urine
phenothiazine	Pink, red, or orange urine
rifampin	Red, orange, or brown urine, saliva, sweat, or tears

FLUID AND ELECTROLYTE BALANCE

Diuretics (see Chapter 26 for use with cardiovascular diseases) modify kidney function to increase **diuresis.** Diuretics are also used to treat edema from cirrhosis, nephrotic disease, renal failure, hypertension, and cardiovascular disease. When body fluids are excreted, excessive sodium, potassium, and chlorides are also excreted, which results in possible electrolyte imbalances.

The amount of water excreted in urine is under the direct influence of antidiuretic hormone (ADH) and the concentration of waste products found in urine. Approximately 60% of body weight is water, in the form of intracellular and extracellular fluids. Three fourths of body fluid is intracellular fluid, which is absolutely essential for metabolic reactions. The largest portion of extracellular fluid is interstitial fluid. Intracellular fluid maintains the proper environment for homeostasis by supplying nutrients, oxygen, vitamins, and electrolytes and carrying off waste products.

Water is the **solvent** in which body substances are dissolved. In infants, up to 75% of body weight may be water; this percentage decreases with age. Infants and very young children are at greater risk for dehydration than older children and adults because of the high ratio of body surface area to body weight and immaturity of kidneys. Obese persons also have less fluid because fat contains little water. Elderly and obese individuals are at risk for dehydration in situations in which fluid loss occurs.

Electrolytes are substances dissolved in body fluids, called **solutes,** and are particles that develop an electrical charge when dissolved in water; examples are sodium, potassium, and chloride. Electrolytes, or **ions,** are found inside and outside of cells. Fluids and electrolytes are acquired through food and water. Normally fluid gain is approximately equal to fluid loss. Abnormal physical conditions can result in loss of fluids or electrolytes or both. When electrolytes or fluids are not present in normal amounts, **replacement therapy** is used to return the body to homeostasis.

Replacement Therapy

Fluids and electrolytes are interdependent because as the amount of water in a body increases, the concentration of electrolytes decreases, and vice versa. Replacement therapy may also be accomplished by oral or intravenous administration, but the oral route takes longer and is less efficient. Oral replacement is used in milder, chronic cases of imbalances such as diarrhea or excessive perspiration not requiring urgent and immediate treatment in

TABLE 27-2 SIGNS OF ELECTROLYTE IMBALANCES

ELECTROLYTE	SIGNS
SODIUM	
Depletion	Lethargy, hypotension, stomach cramping, vomiting, diarrhea
Excess	Edema, hypertonicity, red flushed skin, dry mucous membranes, thirst, elevated temperature
POTASSIUM	
Depletion	Impaired skeletal muscle function, weakness, paralysis
Excess	Abdominal distention, weakness, diarrhea, paralysis
CALCIUM	
Depletion	Muscle cramping and twitching; numbness and tingling of fingers, toes, and lips
Excess	Anorexia, nausea, weakness, vomiting, coma, constipation, apathy, depression, stupor, cardiac contractility
MAGNESIUM	
Depletion	Cardiac dysrhythmias, neurotoxicity
Excess	Flushing, sweating, hypothermia, paralysis, muscle excitability, cardiac depression

adults. Fluid and electrolyte imbalances usually occur at the same time and are corrected by giving fluids with proper electrolytes and nutrients such as glucose, potassium, sodium, and chlorides. When oral rehydration is not practical or not efficient for the needs, intravenous fluids may be used to replace lost electrolytes and glucose because glucose aids in absorption of electrolytes (see Chapter 19 for a discussion of vitamins and minerals and their replacement for homeostasis).

Electrolyte loss usually is a result of nausea, vomiting, renal disease, diarrhea, excessive sweating, burns, trauma, and overuse of diuretics. Each electrolyte has some specific signs of imbalance (Table 27-2). Various fluid bases, such as water and saline, may be used for the addition of fluids, nutrients, or electrolytes.

When electrolytes are lost during diuresis or disease conditions, fluid balance will also be affected. Sodium is the primary cation in interstitial fluids; thus when its concentration is reduced, fluid transfers from extracellular sources to maintain intracellular fluids.

Sodium loss will cause a patient to experience nausea, malaise, weakness, headaches, and drowsiness. The usual replacement is oral administration of sodium or sodium chloride compounds. An increase in pulse rate and blood pressure are good indications of the appropriate response. In patients with nephrotic disease, heart failure, or cirrhosis, and in patients using drugs such as corticosteroids and oral contraceptives, the plasma levels of sodium may be excessive, causing edema and disease conditions such as congestive heart failure. Restricting intake of salt and water is required with these diseases, and diuretics are given to increase excretion of excessive sodium and fluids.

Potassium may be lost in urine when diuretics are used, but more commonly loss results from disorders of the gastrointestinal (GI) tract such as vomiting, diarrhea, or excessive use of laxatives. Respiratory or metabolic acidosis, corticosteroid therapy, and renal diseases may also lead to potassium depletion. When potassium is lost, cardiac muscle conduction and nerve impulse conduction are interrupted. As a regulator in many metabolic activities, potassium replacement is necessary to maintain homeostasis. Signs of potassium loss include apathy, weakness, mental disturbances, cardiac arrhythmias, and thirst. Potassium may be given through intravenous replacement therapy, but oral replacement is preferred. Preparations come in slow-release tablets, effervescent tablets, and liquid preparations. Perhaps the easiest way to replace small potassium losses is through dietary intake.

Calcium deficits are associated with excessive losses from the GI tract, pancreatic diseases, and other diseases such as parathyroid diseases. Deficit signs are tingling of extremities, muscle cramps, tetany, and possibly convulsions. Dietary calcium is increased during replacement, and oral calcium supplements may be added. Vitamin D therapy is frequently added to enhance GI tract absorption of calcium. A good source of calcium for elderly women is Tums or other calcium antacids. Excessive amounts of calcium cause lethargy, decreased muscle tone, and deep bone pain. Cancer and trauma patients with multiple fractures may also have an increase in calcium absorption with the same effects. Nausea, vomiting, anorexia, constipation, and kidney stones may result from excess calcium intake. A sign of calcium depletion is muscle cramping for what seems to be an unknown reason.

Magnesium deficits are usually dietary in nature but may be caused by severe malnutrition, alcoholism, prolonged diarrhea, or intestinal malabsorption. People with magnesium deficits have neuromuscular excitability. Mild deficits are treated with the addition of magnesium-rich foods plus magnesium-based antacids. Excessive magnesium absorption is usually found with renal insufficiency. Signs of excessive magnesium are an increased sense of warmth, decreased deep tendon reflexes, low blood pressure, drowsiness, and lethargy. An electrocardiogram may show arrhythmias. Treatment is aimed at the cause of excess absorption, but renal dialysis may be required.

TREATING URINARY TRACT INFECTIONS

UTIs are the most common bacterial infections reported in the United States. Ten percent to 20% of women experience a UTI during their lifetime. An upper UTI (kidneys and ureters) may cause lower back, flank, or stomach pain with fever, sweating, headache, weakness, and nausea and vomiting. Lower UTIs, in the bladder and urethra, are associated with **urinary frequency, urgency, dysuria, incontinence, hematuria,** and **oliguria.** These infections may be from cross-contamination from the GI tract with *Escherichia coli,* which causes about 90% of all UTIs. Drug therapy for lower UTIs may be started before culture and sensitivity results are available because of the strong likelihood of GI contamination. When symptoms of lower UTI are related to dietary factors, strict adherence to a diet eliminating irritating foods should bring significant relief in a week to 10 days (Box 27-1 lists common foods that irritate the bladder). As symptoms subside, suspicious foods may be added back to the diet, one at a time. If the symptoms return, identification of the irritating food can be made and that food avoided. As foods are returned to the diet, significant amounts of water should be consumed to flush kidneys of irritants.

BOX 27-1 FOODS THAT IRRITATE THE BLADDER

The following foods are acidic and are considered irritants to the bladder that should be avoided by persons who are prone to lower urinary tract infections:

Alcoholic beverages
Guava
Apples and apple juice
Peaches
Cantaloupe
Pineapple
Carbonated beverages
Plums
Chili and other spicy foods
Strawberries
Chocolate
Citrus fruits
Tea
Coffee (including decaffeinated)
Tomatoes
Cranberries and cranberry juice
Vinegar
Grapes
Vitamin B complex

Drugs to Treat Urinary Tract Infections

Fosfomycin (Monaural) is a unique antibiotic approved for use with uncomplicated UTIs in women and complicated infections in men caused by *E. coli* or *Enterococcus faecalis.* The dose is in a water-soluble powder packet at 3 g/dose. Women receive one dose of the medication only, as further administration will not improve symptoms. Men receive two or three doses of the medication. Side effects are diarrhea, vaginitis, headache, and nausea (Table 27-3).

Other drugs used to treat UTIs and **pyuria** include antibacterials, antiseptics, and analgesics. Sulfonamides (see Chapter 17), the most commonly prescribed antibacterial agents for UTIs, work by suppressing the synthesis of folic acid. They have a high solubility in urine, achieve effective concentrations in the urinary tract, and are less expensive than the other antiinfectives. However, with recurrent infections, sulfonamides alone may not be adequate.

Short- and intermediate-acting sulfonamides including TMP-SMZ (trimethoprim-sulfamethoxazole) may be used to treat acute cystitis, acute urethral disease, acute pyelonephritis, and acute bacterial prostatitis, as well as for long-term prophylaxis for recurrent UTIs. Sulfonamides are used as first-line drugs in treatment of UTIs because of lower cost. Short-acting sulfonamides (sulfa medications), including **sulfisoxazole** (Gantrisin) and **sulfadiazine** (Microsulfon), are also included in the short-acting sulfa medications. Intermediate-acting sulfonamides may also be used as needed, depending on the extent of infection. The only intermediate-acting sulfonamide is **sulfamethoxazole** (Gantanol), which has the same urinary indications for use as short-acting medications. Because of its prolonged duration of action, it can be administered less frequently (see Table 17-8).

Trimethoprim (TMP) and **sulfamethoxazole** (SMZ) are marketed together as a fixed-dose combination known as TMP-SMZ (co-trimoxazole, Septra, Bactrim). This combination is a powerful antimicrobial and is used for uncomplicated UTIs. It is particularly useful for prophylaxis and for chronic or recurrent UTIs (see Table 27-3).

Antiinfectives

Penicillin, cephalosporins, tetracyclines, and fluoroquinolones may be added or used in conjunction with sulfonamides for bacterial infections (see Chapter 17 for specific discussion of antimicrobials). Penicillins are also used against enteric-caused bacterial infections, but their usefulness is decreasing as *E. coli* strains become resistant to penicillin. Cephalosporins are used for UTIs resistant to penicillin and TMP-SMZ. Tetracycline may be used to treat initial infections and chlamydial infections, but resistance to tetracyclines develops rapidly.

TABLE 27-3 DRUGS USED TO TREAT URINARY TRACT DISORDERS

GENERIC NAME/ TRADE NAME	USUAL DOSE, ROUTE, AND FREQUENCY	INDICATIONS FOR USE	DRUG INTERACTIONS
ANTIINFECTIVES*			
fosfomycin (Monural)	3 g powder packet PO single dose	Cystitis	Usually none
SHORT-ACTING SULFONAMIDES*		Urinary tract infections	
sulfadiazine	250-500 mg PO 4-6× qd		Usually none
Major Side Effects of Short- and Intermediate-Acting Sulfonamides: Nausea, vomiting, rashes			
SULFONAMIDE COMBINATIONS*		Urinary tract infections	
trimethoprim-sulfamethoxazole (TMP-SMZ) (Septra, Bactrim, Septra DS, Bactrim DS)	80/400 mg PO bid 160/800 mg PO bid		Usually none
Major Side Effects of Sulfonamide Combinations: Nausea, vomiting, rashes			
URINARY TRACT ANTIINFECTIONS*			
nitrofurantoin (Furadantin, Macrodantin, Macrobid)	50-100 mg PO bid therapeutically and prophylactically qhs 50-100 mg PO qid prophylactically qhs	Urinary tract infections	No significant
Major Side Effects of Urinary Tract Antiinfectives: *nitrofurantoin*—GI disturbances, headaches, vertigo, drowsiness			
URINARY TRACT ANALGESICS			
phenazopyridine (Pyridium*) (Azo†)	100-200 mg PO tid 100 mg PO tid	Urinary tract irritation	Usually none
pentosan polysulfate (Elmiron)*	100 mg PO tid	Interstitial cystitis	heparin, other anticoagulants
Major Side Effects of Drugs for Urinary Tract Analgesics: *pentosan polysulfate*—GI discomfort, hair loss, insomnia, headache			
DRUGS FOR OVERACTIVE BLADDER*			
tolterodine (Detrol,* Detrol LA)	1-2 mg PO bid 2-4 mg PO qd	Overactive bladder	None
trospium (Sanctura, Sanctura XR)	20 mg PO bid 60 mg PO qd		alcohol
solifenacin (VESIcare)	5-10 mg PO qd		
darifenacin (Enablex)	7.5-15 mg PO qd		
fesoterodine (Toviaz)	4-8 mg PO qd		

IM, Intramuscular; *IV,* intravenously; *PO,* orally; *SC,* subcutaneously, *XR,* extended release.
*Prescription medication.
†OTC medication.

TABLE 27-3 DRUGS USED TO TREAT URINARY TRACT DISORDERS—cont'd

GENERIC NAME/ TRADE NAME	USUAL DOSE, ROUTE, AND FREQUENCY	INDICATIONS FOR USE	DRUG INTERACTIONS
Major Side Effects of Drugs for Overactive Bladder: Dry mouth, constipation, blurred vision, dyspepsia			
URINARY TRACT ANTISPASMODICS*			
flavoxate (Urispas)	100-200 mg PO tid-qid	Genitourinary muscle relaxant	None
oxybutynin	5 mg PO bid-qid	Urinary antispasmodic, overactive bladder	Antihistamines
(Ditropan XL,	5-15 mg PO qd		
Oxytrol)	3.9 mg/day patch 2×/wk		
Oxytrol Transdermal	Transdermal gel 10%		
Gelnique	apply 1 pkg topically qd		
Major Side Effects of Urinary Tract Antispasmodics: *oxybutynin*—dry mouth, constipation			
DRUGS TO TREAT ENURESIS*			
imipramine (Tofranil)	6-12 yr: 25 mg PO >12 yr: 75 mg PO at bedtime	Enuresis in persons older than 6 yr	alcohol, phenothiazine, cimetidine, clonidine, phenytoin
desmopressin (DDAVP, Stimate)	1-4 sprays qd in divided dose		carbamazepine, chlorpropamide demeclocycline
Major Side Effects of Drugs to Treat Enuresis: *imipramine*—drowsiness, fatigue, dry mouth, blurred vision, constipation, impaired concentration; *desmopressin*—headaches, nosebleeds, increased blood pressure, sore throat			

Candidal overgrowth occurs most frequently with tetracyclines. Fluoroquinolones are broad-spectrum agents and are active against most organisms causing UTIs, but the cost of most agents is prohibitively high for some patients.

Patient Education for Compliance

1. Sulfonamides should be taken on empty stomach with full glass of water.
2. Entire course of treatment for urinary tract infection should be completed, even though symptoms may have improved.
3. Care should be taken to avoid prolonged exposure to sunlight when taking sulfonamides. If it is necessary to be in sun, sunscreens should be worn.
4. Drink eight to ten 8-oz glasses of water a day while taking sulfonamides.

Important Facts about Medications to Treat Urinary Tract Infections (UTIs)

- *Escherichia coli* is the most common cause of uncomplicated UTIs.
- Most UTIs can be treated on outpatient basis with oral medications.
- Sulfonamides are drugs of choice with UTIs, with TMP-SMZ being preferred medication.
- Sulfonamides should be discontinued at first sign of hypersensitivity reaction.
- Sulfonamides may increase effects of warfarin and oral hypoglycemics, and reduction in their dosage may be necessary.
- Prophylaxis for UTI may be achieved with low doses of trimethoprim, TMP-SMZ, or urinary antiseptics.

Urinary Tract Antiseptics

The most commonly used urinary tract antiseptic is **nitrofurantoin** (Furadantin, Macrobid, and Macrodantin). This agent may be used for prophylaxis and for treatment of upper UTIs but is primarily used in the lower urinary tract. Urinary tract antiseptics exert antibacterial activity in urine but have little or no systemic antibacterial effects (see Table 27-3).

MISCELLANEOUS URINARY TRACT MEDICATIONS

Urinary Tract Analgesics

Urinary tract analgesia may be accomplished through topical analgesia or local anesthesia on urinary tract mucosa. **Phenazopyridine** (Pyridium), an oral agent, is a dye that exerts topical anesthetic effect on the urinary tract lining. It has no antiinfective effect but relieves pain and burning on urination and urinary frequency found with UTIs. With the possibility of masking infection symptoms, phenazopyridine has minimal side effects and is for short-term use. **Pentosan polysulfate** (Elmiron) is a drug specific for prevention of irritation of the bladder wall found with interstitial cystitis. The drug has a blood thinning effect and may cause increased bleeding.

Patient Education for Compliance

1. Pyridium may change urine to orange-red color and may permanently stain clothing.
2. For urinary antiseptics to be most effective, urine should be acidic. Large doses of vitamin C, cranberries, and prunes will promote acidic urine.
3. Carbonated beverages and citrus fruits should be avoided with urinary antiseptics because they tend to make urine alkaline.
4. When taking pentosan polysulfate, the physician or dentist performing procedures needs to be informed of the administering of the medication.

Important Facts about Urinary Tract Antiseptics and Analgesics

- Urinary tract antiseptics are second-line drug choices for urinary tract infections.
- Pyridium is a dye used as an analgesic or local anesthetic on urinary tract mucosa and for symptomatic relief of burning, pain, discomfort, or urgency.

Urinary Tract Antispasmodics and Drugs for Overactive Bladder

Overactive bladder (OAB) syndrome is a form of urinary incontinence found in patients of all ages, but symptoms increase with age. Classic symptoms are urgency, frequency, and **nocturia.** Medications for treatment are aimed at increasing the volume of urine in the bladder, reducing the frequency of urination, and decreasing pressure and urgency, which cause the need to urinate, by relaxing bladder smooth muscles (see Table 27-3). **Flavoxate** (Urispas), a urinary antispasmodic and genitourinary muscle relaxant, is used to treat dysuria, urgency, nocturia, and the incontinence of cystitis and prostatitis. It may also be used for nocturnal **enuresis** in children older than 6 years of age. Patients with glaucoma must be closely monitored because of the possibility of increased intraocular pressure. **Oxybutynin** (Ditropan) relieves urinary symptoms associated with neurogenic bladder conditions. Oxybutynin is not a cure for neurogenic bladder or OAB but is a means for patients to live a relatively symptom-free life. **Tolterodine** (Detrol LA), **trospium** (Sanctura), and **darifenacin** (Enablex) are used to relieve urinary frequency and urgency, providing relief of OAB symptoms. The medications relax smooth muscles of the bladder. **Fesoterodine** (Toviaz) inhibits urinary bladder contractions to relieve symptoms of urgency and frequency.

Patient Education for Compliance

Urinary antispasmodics may cause drowsiness. Operating machinery may pose a danger.

Important Fact about Urinary Antispasmodics

Urinary antispasmodics reduce the strength and frequency of urinary bladder contractions.

Drugs for Enuresis

Bedwetting, or enuresis, is fairly common in children, with the percentage of bedwetters gradually decreasing by age 21. Some behavioral techniques may be used to achieve temporary improvement for those with a small or spastic-like bladder that seems to empty automatically when it contains a certain volume of urine. **Imipramine** (Tofranil), an antidepressant, improves symptoms of enuresis in some children. **Desmopressin** (DDAVP), an antidiuretic hormone (ADH), increases reabsorption of water. This nasal spray may be used in children 6 years of age or older and in elderly individuals who have enuresis (see Table 27-3).

Patient Education for Compliance

Withholding fluids at bedtime is not effective in treating enuresis except in cases of a small bladder.

Important Fact about Drugs for Enuresis

Drugs may be used to reduce incontinence, frequency, and urgency by reducing spasms of bladder smooth muscles.

SUMMARY

Urinary organs excrete fluid body wastes. The urinary tract is also a major component of maintaining homeostasis and in fluid and electrolyte balance. Edema may be caused by several medical conditions but is most frequently associated with cardiovascular diseases (see Chapter 26). Diuretics are grouped by sites of action to increase excretion of fluids, thereby reducing swelling. However, diuretics may cause excretion of electrolytes, and their loss may result in specific signs and symptoms, with replacement necessary. Chronic electrolyte imbalances may be treated as an ambulatory condition as well as in an inpatient setting.

UTIs are treated with sulfonamides and their derivatives as first choice. TMP-SMZ is the best medication to use with UTIs caused by enteric bacteria. UTI symptoms—urgency, frequency, dysuria, oliguria, and burning on urination—are relieved by both sulfonamides and TMP-SMZ. Some foods (cranberries and cranberry juice) are indicated to treat infections, to keep urine more acidic for better effectiveness of urinary antiseptics, but they should be avoided for routine ingestion by those prone to frequent UTIs because they tend to irritate the bladder. Fosfomycin, in a single dose for uncomplicated infections in women and two or three doses for complicated infections in men, is specific for infections caused by enteric cross-infection.

Urinary tract antiseptics are the second-choice medications for prevention and treatment of UTIs. These medications have little or no systemic effect, as they are urinary tract specific, and may be used for prophylaxis or long-term therapy.

Phenazopyridine is a local analgesic for UTIs, with no antiinflammatory properties. This agent relieves pain and burning associated with UTIs.

Urinary tract antispasmodics are used to relax genitourinary muscles to relieve incontinence, nocturia, and dysuria. Some newer medications are indicated to relieve the frequency and urgency of an OAB.

Enuresis is treated with medications in children older than age 7. Behavioral therapies may not be indicated, and withholding fluids at bedtime in children is not an effective treatment for small bladder or OAB in some children.

CRITICAL THINKING EXERCISES

Scenario

Mary comes to see Dr. Merry complaining of urinary frequency, burning, and dysuria.

1. Should you expect to get a urine sample from Mary? Why or why not?
2. If the sample shows bacteria and Dr. Merry orders sulfonamides for Mary, what side effects should she be aware of?
3. How long should she take sulfonamide medications?
4. What food should Mary avoid to prevent irritation of the bladder?
5. Could Mary expect to take sulfonamides on a daily basis for chronic UTIs? Why or why not?

DRUG CALCULATIONS

1. Order: Detrol LA 4 mg PO qam
   Available medication:

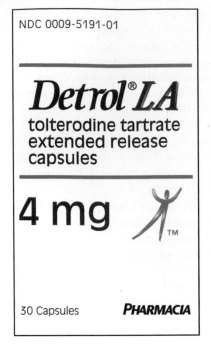

Dose to be administered: _____
_____

2. Order: trimethoprim-sulfamethoxazole 160/800 mg
   tab i qd × 14 days
   Available medication:

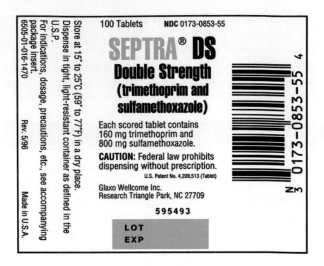

Dose to be administered: _____
_____

REVIEW QUESTIONS

1. What is an electrolyte? What are the four chief electrolytes? _____
_____
_____

2. What is replacement therapy? _____
_____
_____

3. What are the most commonly ordered medications for UTIs? _____
_____
_____

4. What is TMP-SMZ? What are the indications for this combination of medications? _____
_____
_____

5. How are the four urinary tract antiseptics effective in UTIs? _____
_____
_____

CHAPTER 28

Reproductive System Disorders

OBJECTIVES

After studying this chapter, you should be capable of doing the following:

- Discussing sex hormones and their function in human reproduction.
- Describing medications used in treating diseases specific to the male and female reproductive systems.
- Describing pros and cons of different forms of contraceptive medications.
- Discussing medications used to treat infertility and their effectiveness.
- Providing information on medications for premenstrual syndrome and dysmenorrhea.

- Identifying medications for endometriosis.
- Discussing medications for erectile dysfunction and the dangers when used with nitrate medications.
- Discussing categories of medications that impair sexual function as a side effect.
- Providing patient education for compliance with medications used to treat diseases and conditions of the reproductive system.

Mr. Husain, age 65, comes to Dr. Merry worried about an inability to void that has become progressively worse. At this time, he has not voided for about 8 hours. Dr. Merry examines Mr. Husain and prescribes Proscar.

For what disease process is Proscar indicated?
What medications for hypertension should not be used with Proscar?
If Mr. Husain were a younger man, would an enlarged prostate be as likely as it is after age 60?
Mr. Husain tells you that his libido has diminished since he started taking diphenhydramine for allergies. He wants to know if there is any connection between his diminished libido and the allergy medication. What is your response?

KEY TERMS

Anabolic steroids	Cryptorchidism	Galactorrhea	Ovum
Anabolism	Depot form of	Hirsutism	Priapism
Androgen	medication	Hypogonadism	Progesterone
Chloasma	Dyspareunia	Negative feedback	Progestin
Coitus	Estrogen	Oogenesis	Spermatogenesis
Contraception	Exogenous	Ovulation	Testosterone

EASY WORKING KNOWLEDGE OF DRUGS USED FOR REPRODUCTIVE SYSTEM DISORDERS

DRUG CLASS	PRESCRIPTION	OTC	PREGNANCY CATEGORY	MAJOR INDICATIONS
Androgens	Yes (anabolic androgens— Schedule III)	No	C, X	Hormone replacement
Benign prostatic hypertrophy agents	Yes	No	B, D, X (finasteride)	Reduce symptoms of benign prostatic hypertrophy
Estrogens, progestins	Yes	No	C, D, X	Menopause, replacement therapy, cancers in males and females
Oral and long-acting parenteral contraceptives	Yes	No	X	Prevention of pregnancy
Other contraceptives	Yes (diaphragm)	Yes	Nonapplicable	Prevention of pregnancy
Postcoital contraceptives	Yes	No	X	Prevention of pregnancy after unprotected sexual intercourse
Medications for PMS and dysmenorrhea	Yes	Yes	B, D	Relief of symptoms of PMS and menstrual cramping
Medications for infertility	Yes	No	X	Treatment of male and female infertility
Medications for erectile dysfunction	Yes	No	N/A	Treatment of erectile dysfunction

PMS, Premenstrual syndrome.

EASY WORKING KNOWLEDGE OF INDICATIONS AND SIDE EFFECTS

Common Symptoms of Reproductive System Disorders
Sexually Transmitted Diseases (STDs)
Pelvic or genital pain
Dysuria, hematuria, purulent discharge
Burning or itching on urination
Urinary frequency or incontinence
Dyspareunia
Fever, malaise
Lesions in genital area

Infertility
Abnormal pregnancies
Endometriosis or other reproductive tract disorders, including blocked fallopian tubes or tumors
Congenital malformations
Decreased sperm count

Specific to Female Reproductive System
Fever
Abnormal vaginal discharge or itching
Pain in lower abdomen or pelvic region
Dyspareunia or sexual dysfunction
Dysmenorrhea, amenorrhea, metrorrhagia, menorrhagia, or oligomenorrhea

Found with Reproductive Tract in Both Genders
Genital lesions
Breast changes (growths [benign and malignant], mastitis, discharge)
Psychologic response to hormone changes

Specific to Male Reproductive System
Frequency, urgency, pain, or burning on urination; oliguria
Sexual dysfunction, including impotence or erectile dysfunction
Pain, swelling, or lesions of any reproductive organ

Common Side Effects of Medications for the Reproductive System
Edema and weight gain
Acne and skin discoloration, especially of face (e.g., **chloasma**)
Increased or decreased sexual stimulation or libido
Enlarged breast tissue in both sexes
Hirsutism, deepening of voice, and amenorrhea in women
Nausea and vomiting
Anxiety, depression
Headaches
Increased risk of thromboembolic disorders
Hypertension, myocardial infarction, stroke
Increased risk of cervicitis
Increased risk of gallbladder disease
Menstrual irregularities
Visual disturbances

Because the reproductive system has been cloaked in secrecy and cultural inhibitions for centuries, many patients are uncomfortable discussing sexual matters, especially when the patient is of one gender and the physician is of the other. Because of social perceptions about reproductive organs and their functions, health care professionals face challenges obtaining information concerning reproductive system dysfunctions, making an open, trusting patient-professional relationship necessary. Medications used require teaching and counseling in personal and sensitive areas; therefore patient information must be presented and discussed with an understanding but positive approach.

In review, the major structures of the female reproductive system are the ovaries, fallopian tubes, uterus, and vagina (Figure 28-1). In the male, the urinary and reproductive systems are interrelated consisting of the testes, vas deferens, prostate gland, urethra, seminal vesicles, epididymis, ejaculatory duct, and penis (Figure 28-2). The male and female sex hormones are necessary for development and maintenance of secondary sex characteristics and for reproduction. The reproductive process begins with secretion of gonadotropic hormones from the anterior pituitary gland, stimulating development of sex organs. Follicle-stimulating hormone (FSH) stimulates oogenesis in ovaries and spermatogenesis in testes. Luteinizing hormone (LH) stimulates release of an egg and formation of corpus luteum. In the testes, spermatogenesis and secretion of androgens occur. The male sex hormones are called androgens; the female sex hormones are estrogen and progesterone (see Figure 28-1). See Chapter 20 for more information on these hormones.

INFLUENCE OF HORMONES ON THE REPRODUCTIVE SYSTEM

FSH and interstitial cell-stimulating hormone (ICSH) in males stimulate production of testosterone. Testosterone promotes adult male sexual characteristics, essential for regulating metabolism and growth of bone and skeletal muscles.

In females, FSH stimulates growth of a graafian follicle and production of estrogen. During the proliferative menstrual cycle phase, as estrogen increases, FSH decreases, preparing the uterus to receive and nourish a fertilized ovum. During the proliferative phase, the endometrium grows and endocervical glands secrete viscous mucus to nourish sperm before fertilization (Figure 28-3).

With ovulation at midcycle, LH influences formation of the corpus luteum, releasing estrogen and progesterone during the menstrual cycle secretory phase. If the ovum is fertilized, the increased endometrial lining will support growth and nourishment of the ovum. If fertilization does not occur, increased estrogen and progesterone decrease the release of FSH and LH by a negative feedback mechanism.

The chief agents affecting the reproductive system are hormones, with some agents stimulating secretions and others blocking these same secretions. Medication therapy for conditions of the reproductive system can be complicated, even with drugs with familiar names. Although hormones are naturally produced, some disorders are indications for use of exogenous male or female hormones. Such symptoms and diseases as deficiencies in hormone secretions, hypogonadism, and

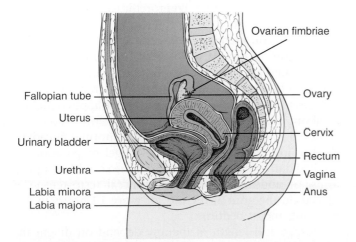

Figure 28-1 The female reproductive system. (From Frazier MS, Drzymkowski JW: *Essentials of human diseases and conditions*, ed 4, St Louis, 2008, Saunders.)

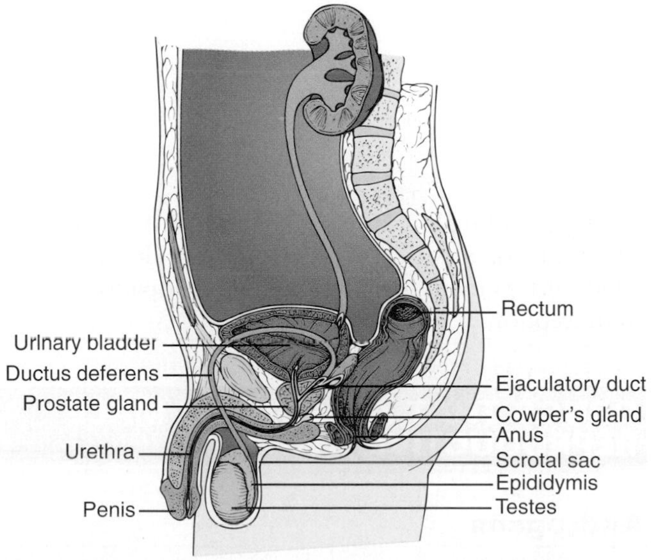

Figure 28-2 The male reproductive system. (From Frazier MS, Drzymkowski JW: *Essentials of human diseases and conditions*, ed 4, St Louis, 2008, Saunders.)

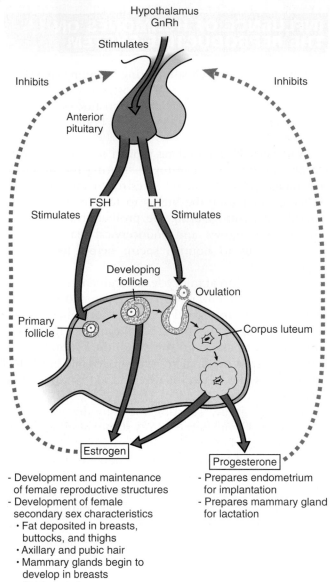

Figure 28-3 Hormone regulation of the menstrual cycle and ovarian function. (From Applegate EJ: *Anatomy and physiology learning system,* ed 4, St Louis, 2010, Saunders.)

carcinomas of male and female reproductive organs may be reason for this treatment. Hormones are also indicated for treatment of symptoms of menopause and for contraception.

DRUGS THAT AFFECT THE MALE REPRODUCTIVE SYSTEM

Androgens

The male sex hormones are called *androgens;* the major hormone is **testosterone.** Androgens are given therapeutically to men for various conditions, such as to supplement low levels of testosterone to correct **hypogonadism** or **cryptorchidism;** to increase sperm production in cases of infertility; and to stimulate production of red blood cells. An increase in red blood cells and in protein synthesis causes muscle mass to increase, so athletes may use androgens to improve athletic performance.

Testosterone

Testosterone brings about a sense of well-being, restores mental equilibrium and energy, and increases the resistance of the central nervous system to fatigue. Two types of testosterone are available for replacement therapy: natural testosterone from testes of bulls, and synthetic androgens. **Anabolism,** the constructive metabolic process for converting substances into other chemical compounds that are required for cell repair and growth, is stimulated by testosterone. Testosterone functions to build new body tissue and to increase muscle strength and endurance. Natural types are preferred, to achieve adequate blood drug levels. Administration by intramuscular injection is necessary because oral testosterone is highly metabolized in the intestines and the liver before reaching the bloodstream, which lowers its effectiveness. Medication is available in aqueous bases for short action, in oil bases, or in the **depot form of medication** for action up to 4 weeks. Testosterone pellets are available for subcutaneous implantation, with extended duration of action of 2 to 6 months. Methyltestosterone may be administered by the buccal route, whereas synthetic androgens may be effectively administered orally (Table 28-1).

Transdermal testosterone preparations are applied in different ways. The testosterone patch, Testoderm, is applied to scrotal skin for absorption at a high rate five times greater than at other dermal sites. The patch is left on the scrotal area for 24 hours and is changed daily. When used for treating cryptorchidism to encourage descent of testes into the scrotal sac an 8 week course of therapy s recommended. The second testosterone patch, Androderm, is applied to the back, abdomen, arms, or thighs daily, with the application site changed every 24 hours so that no site is used more frequently than once in 7 days. Both of these patches should be applied nightly at about 10:00 PM so that maximum serum levels are achieved in the morning, to stimulate normal circadian rhythm in young boys. AndroGel, a gel preparation, is applied daily to a clean, dry area on the shoulders, upper arms, or abdomen at bedtime. Buccal testosterone is placed on the gum at the incisor every 12 hours in the morning and at bedtime.

Dosage and length of therapy depend on diagnosis, patient's age and gender, and side effects or adverse reactions that occur. In males with delayed puberty, the dose may be low initially then gradually increased according

TABLE 28-1 ANDROGENS

GENERIC NAME/ TRADE NAME	USUAL ADULT DOSE, ROUTE, AND FREQUENCY	INDICATIONS FOR USE	DRUG INTERACTIONS
testosterone (Testopel)	2-6 pellets SC q3-6mo	Palliation of metastatic breast cancer Replacement therapy Postpartal breast pain	Oral anticoagulants
(Delatestryl, Depo-Testosterone, Depotest, Duratest) (long-acting injectable)	50-400 mg IM q2-4wks		
(Androderm) (transdermal)	1 patch q24h		
(AndroGel 1%, Testim)	5 mg topically qd		
(Striant)	1 buccal application bid		
fluoxymesterone (Androxy)	5-20 mg PO*‡ qd		
methyltestosterone (Adroid, Methitest, Testred, Virilon)	10-50 mg PO* qd		
danazol	200-400 mg PO daily in divided doses	Endometriosis	lovastatin, oral anticoagulants
Androgen inhibitor	1000 mg PO qd	Advanced metastatic	CYP2D6
abiraterone (Zytiga)	E Prednisone 5 mg	Prostate cancer	

Major Side Effects: *Females*—oily skin, acne, increased hair growth, increased libido, irregular menses, deepening voice; *males*—urinary urgency, swelling or tenderness of breasts, frequent erections, priapism; *both genders*—change of skin color, abdominal pain, insomnia, mouth soreness, diarrhea, constipation, dizziness, headaches, confusion, depression, edema of legs

IM, Intramuscular; *PO*, orally; *SC*, subcutaneous.
*Used as replacement therapy.
†Used for postpartum breast pain.
‡Used to palliate metastatic breast cancer.

to need and response. Treatment may last for several months or may continue throughout puberty. These drugs are also used for antineoplastic therapy in men and women; a 3-month period is necessary to evaluate treatment effectiveness. Women should receive a short-acting androgen because they may occasionally increase the extent of breast cancer. Because of drug interactions with anticoagulants, an increase in bleeding episodes may occur and an unusual increase or decrease in libido may occur.

Anabolic Steroids

Anabolic steroids, which are used to bring about a feeling of well-being, are actually natural or synthetically produced androgens. In the male, androgens function to build new body tissue and to greatly increase muscle strength and endurance (the abuse of anabolic steroids is discussed in Chapters 20 and 31). Anabolic steroids, or 17-alpha-alkylated androgens, are classified as Schedule III medications because of the potential for abuse or misuse and their serious side effects. Men who think the anabolic action will maintain strength, especially in sports, and virility into the older adult years, are those who usually use these drugs. Mood, libido, and cholesterol levels may be improved, and muscle mass may increase, but the dangers far outweigh the benefits. Therapeutically these drugs administered orally, intramuscularly, and topically, may be used to treat anemias from renal disease in both genders. For conditions characterized by a breakdown in protein metabolism, anabolic steroids may be used to promote weight gain. These medications are hepatotoxic, and irreversible liver damage can occur (Table 28-2).

TABLE 28-2 ANABOLIC STEROIDS

GENERIC NAME/ TRADE NAME	USUAL ADULT DOSE AND ROUTE	INDICATIONS FOR USE	DRUG INTERACTIONS
nandrolone (Deca-Durabolin)	50-100 mg IM	Breast cancer and anemias caused by renal disease	Anticoagulants, antidiabetics, immunosuppressants

Major Side Effects: Rash, hematuria, elevated blood pressure, amenorrhea, nausea, vomiting, changes in libido, headaches, insomnia, increased aggression and irritability

IM, Intramuscularly; *PO*, orally

Patient Education for Compliance

1. Patients using Testoderm should shave scrotum before applying patch.
2. Sodium and water retention may occur with use of testosterone, with resultant weight gain and extremity edema.
3. Buccal testosterone should be placed with rounded surface against gum at incisor site and held in place for 30 seconds with finger over lip. Do not chew or swallow buccal application of testosterone. Rotate placement with each administration.
4. Signs of hepatic toxicity such as jaundice, chalky stools, and pain in right shoulder should be reported immediately when using androgens.
5. Oral androgens should be taken with food to avoid gastrointestinal upset.

Important Facts about Androgen Preparations

- Testosterone is principal androgen.
- Androgens stimulate production of red blood cells and increase muscle mass. Androgens are used therapeutically as replacement therapy for anemias from renal disease, to treat female breast engorgement, and palliatively in metastatic breast cancer.
- Testosterone taken orally is metabolized by the liver before absorption, so testosterone is usually given by injection or transdermally. Testosterone gel and buccal tablets are also available for ease of administration.
- Two transdermal forms of testosterone are available. One is applied to scrotum; other is applied to extremities or back, and sites should be rotated.
- Anabolic steroids have toxic effects on liver and are Schedule III drugs because of potential for abuse.

Medications for Benign Prostatic Hypertrophy

Benign prostatic hypertrophy (BPH) is an increase in glandular and connective tissue mass of the prostate surrounding the male urethra. Development of BPH is considered a normal age-related change in men after age of 40, with 73% of men by age 70 having symptoms of BPH requiring medical intervention. BPH obstructs the bladder neck and compresses the urethra, resulting in urinary retention and an increased risk of urinary tract infections. Symptoms of BPH are hesitancy on urination, decrease in stream and force of urine, postvoiding dribbling, and sensation of incomplete bladder emptying, resulting in frequency and nocturia.

The goal of treatment of BPH is to relieve bothersome symptoms. Alpha-adrenergic blockers such as ***tamsulosin*** (Flomax), ***terazosin*** (Hytrin), and ***doxazosin*** (Cardura) are preferred for BPH treatment in patients with relatively small prostates. These medications relax the smooth muscles of the bladder neck and prostate for ease of voiding while acting as hypotensives; thus these medications are useful for both prostate disease and hypertension.

Finasteride (Proscar) and ***dutasteride*** (Avodart), 5-alpha-reductase inhibitors, are appropriate for patients with large prostate glands to promote prostate shrinkage. Benefits develop slowly, taking up to 12 months to appear. This medication prevents testosterone conversion to dihydrotestosterone (DHT), the androgen found in prostate gland. The powdered DHT decreases prostate growth to relieve BPH symptoms. Women of childbearing age should not handle this medication, because any amount absorbed through the skin may cause birth defects. Women of childbearing age with partners undergoing finasteride therapy should use contraception (Table 28-3). A new group of androgen inhibitors used for advanced metastatic prostate cancer had been introduced. ***Abiraterone*** (Zytiga) is a pregnancy category X drug that is taken concurrently with prednisone.

LEARNING TOP

Adrenergic antagonists used for BPH usually end in "sin" and 5-alpha reduction inhibitors used for BPH usually end in "ride."

Did You Know?

Finasteride is marketed as Proscar 5 mg tablets for BPH and as Propecia 1 mg tablets for alopecia.

TABLE 28-3 DRUGS USED TO TREAT BENIGN PROSTATIC HYPERTROPHY

GENERIC NAME/ TRADE NAME	USUAL ADULT DOSE, ROUTE, AND FREQUENCY	INDICATIONS FOR USE	DRUG INTERACTIONS
ADRENERGIC ANTAGONISTS (BLOCKERS)		Benign prostatic hypertrophy	
silodosin (Rapaflo)	8 mg PO qd		itraconazole or ritonavir, CYP3A4 inhibitor, ketoconazole
terazosin	1-10 mg PO qd		ACE inhibitors, NSAIDs, propranolol
tamsulosin (Flomax)	0.4 mg PO qd		Beta blockers, other adrenergic antagonists
doxazosin (Cardura)	1-8 mg PO qd	Hypertension	ACE inhibitors, indomethacin, verapamil, nifedipine
alfuzosin (Uroxatral)	10 mg PO qd		alcohol
5-ALPHA REDUCTASE INHIBITORS			
dutasteride (Avodart)	0.5 mg PO qd		None
finasteride (Proscar)	5 mg PO qd		No significant interactions but should not be handled by women of childbearing age

ACE, Angiotensin-converting enzyme; *NSAIDs*, nonsteroidal antiinflammatory drugs; *PO*, orally.

Patient Education for Compliance

1. Patients taking alpha-adrenergic blockers should take medications at bedtime because of "first-dose" orthostatic hypotension and dizziness.
2. Treatment for benign prostatic hypertrophy is suppressive rather than curative, and symptoms may return if medication is withdrawn.
3. 5-alpha reductase inhibitors may be teratogenic to male fetuses, so all women of childbearing age should not handle drug. Sexual partner should not become pregnant while partner is taking drug.

Important Facts about Drugs to Treat Benign Prostatic Hypertrophy

- Benign prostatic hypertrophy (BPH) occurs in 73% of men by age 70, causing sufficient symptoms to require medical intervention with drugs.
- Symptoms of BPH result from mechanical obstruction of urethra from overgrowth of epithelial or smooth muscle cells.
- Alpha-adrenergic blockers, which are also used as antihypertensives, relax the smooth muscles of the bladder and prostate to relieve BPH symptoms.
- 5-alpha reductase inhibitors promote regression of prostate epithelial tissue and reduce mechanical obstruction, being more effective in men whose prostate is significantly enlarged.

DRUGS THAT AFFECT THE FEMALE REPRODUCTIVE SYSTEM

Medications used to treat conditions of the female reproductive system are similar to the hormones naturally produced by females but also includes use of androgens in some cases. The medications—provided as the female hormones estrogen and progesterone (or progestin, the synthetic equivalent)—are prescribed to supplement low levels of natural hormones, to correct hormone imbalances that cause abnormal uterine bleeding, to reverse abnormal ovulation, to enhance fertility, and to be used for oral contraception.

Occasionally women are treated with androgens palliatively for metastatic breast cancer and as therapy for postpartum breast engorgement, endometriosis, and fibrocystic breast disease. Women receiving androgen preparations may have irreversible voice deepening.

Estrogens

Estrogens support development and maintenance of reproductive organs and secondary sex characteristics in females. These hormones also have profound influences on reproductive physiology, from their actions during the menstrual cycle to stimulation of uterine growth and blood flow during pregnancy. In premenopausal women, the ovary is the principal organ of estrogen production in estradiol form.

Estrogens have a positive effect for blocking bone mass resorption and promoting mineral deposits. During puberty, estrogens promote growth of long bones. In postmenopausal women, estrogen replacement helps to maintain bone mass.

Estrogens are the dominant form of medicinal therapy for female reproductive system conditions as well as having a direct effect on bone and cardiovascular function and insulin sensitivity. Estrogens reduce levels of low-density lipoproteins (LDLs) and increase levels of high-density lipoproteins (HDLs), thought to reduce risk of heart attacks in premenopausal women. As estrogen levels begin to fall during menopause, the incidence of heart attacks in females rises. Estrogens also increase bile's cholesterol content, explaining why women taking estrogens may develop gallstones.

Estrogens have several uses in both genders, including adjuvant therapy for certain cancers—male prostate cancer and non–estrogen-dependent breast cancers in both genders. Hormone replacement therapy (HRT) using estrogen preparations is prescribed for women who had their ovaries removed during the reproductive years and in older women for prevention and treatment of osteoporosis. A family or personal history of breast cancer may be a contraindication for use of HRT.

Use of estrogen without added **progestins** in postmenopausal women increases risk of endometrial hyperplasia and of endometrial and breast cancer; estrogens alone cause endometrial lining proliferation. A woman with an intact uterus who receives replacement therapy should be followed closely with physical examinations and Pap smears to ensure early detection of disease. Addition of progestins reduces endometrial cancer risk by down-regulating estrogen receptors.

Recent studies have shown that with HRT therapy in postmenopausal women who took conjugated estrogens for 10 years, the risk of death from any cause was decreased by 37%. Risk of death from heart disease was decreased by 53% and from stroke was decreased by 32%. However some scientists are of the opinion that HRT may be more harmful than helpful because of the increased risk of reproductive tract cancer. Some women who are given prescriptions for estrogen replacement therapy never fill the prescription out of fear of developing endometrial or breast cancer. Women who had an early menarche and a late menopause and who take HRT appear to have a greater incidence of breast cancer. Whether incidence is higher because of an actual disease increase or because of earlier detection of breast cancer in women who have regular, frequent examinations is unknown.

Estrogens are available in conjugated doses from natural sources, including the urine of pregnant mares, and are also synthetically formulated. Estriol and estrone are naturally occurring estrogens that occur when estradiol secreted by the ovaries is converted. *Conjugated estrogens* (Premarin) are available in mixtures of estrogenic medications in oral, parenteral, transdermal, and percutaneous forms. Transdermal patches, vaginal rings, percutaneous creams, and emulsions of estrogen preparations are most often used for urogenital atrophy. Estradiol used by women with estrogen deficiency may be delivered transdermally to provide its continuous release. The lowest estrogen dose needed to produce the desired effect should be administered over the shortest period of time to reduce the potential for serious side effects.

Estrogens should be used with caution in patients with endometriosis, gallbladder and liver disease, pancreatitis, and elevated lipoprotein levels. Women with a history of estrogen hypersensitivity, hypercalcemia, and thrombophlebitis or thromboembolic disease should avoid estrogens unless the benefit outweighs the risk. Glucose tolerance is decreased with estrogen therapy, occasionally leading to symptoms of diabetes mellitus. Estrogens tend to cause retention of sodium and water and therefore may aggravate asthma, epilepsy, migraine headaches, heart disease, and kidney disease. People who wear contact lenses may note intolerance for lens wear because edema changes the corneal shape and results in improper lens fit.

Forms of Estrogen Preparations

Estrogens are available in several forms with unique means of administration. Estrogen and progesterone products are available orally, parenterally (intramuscularly), vaginally, topically, and as intradermal implants. To lengthen the onset and duration of action, hormones may be administered parenterally in an oil base—the "depot" form—for slower absorption from muscle tissue. Transdermal estrogen patches, applied to a dry surface on the abdomen or buttocks, bypass hepatic metabolism. Administration of transdermal medication is 1 or 2 times a week, rather than daily. An innovative form of estrogen therapy for menopausal hot flashes is an estradiol emulsion to be rubbed on each leg daily in morning, much like a lotion. The lower dose of estradiol is absorbed through the skin into the bloodstream. Another unique delivery system is a drug-laden vaginal ring pressed into the vaginal canal for continuous release of medication into local tissues. Vaginal inserts and creams are formulated to release hormones into the vagina on contact.

New oral forms are most commonly used, with the trend toward long-acting products that are taken daily for up to 3 months before stoppage to allow for a menstrual period. The U.S. Food and Drug Administration (FDA) now allows indefinite use of some medications for prevention of menses, as well as for oral contraception.

Implants containing contraceptives are surgically placed under upper arm skin to prevent pregnancy. Older implant forms contained multiple rods that were changed every 5 years. The newest implant, consisting of one rod for a 3-year duration, is expected to stop menstruation in most women.

Oral estrogen may be prescribed in cyclic doses, in which 3 weeks of estrogen are followed by a week off, or by progestin addition for the last 10 to 13 days of the cycle. Newer low-dose oral contraceptives rarely include more than 50 mcg of estrogen; in most cases, the use of 20 to 30 mcg of estrogen is adequate for birth control. Lower doses with effective coverage improve oral contraceptive safety (Table 28-4).

Progesterone

Progesterone, stimulated by LH and produced by the ovaries, is a naturally occurring but also may be synthetic progestin with similar pharmacologic effects. Advantages of progestin over progesterone are that a lower dose of progestin is necessary to produce the desired response, progestin has a longer duration of action than progesterone, and progestin is available in oral and sublingual forms for easier administration. Progestin is used for treating amenorrhea and abnormal uterine bleeding from hormone imbalances, for contraception or in combination with estrogen for postmenopausal HRT, and as adjuvant or palliative therapy for renal or endometrial cancer. When in combination with progesterone, the estrogen component is most often stated in micrograms with the progestin component stated in milligrams. A combined-continuous regimen for HRT is estrogen and progestin combined in a single tablet for daily administration see Table 28-4).

Patients with a history of migraines, diabetes mellitus, hyperlipidemia, thrombophlebitis, and undiagnosed bleeding from the reproductive tract should be watched closely when taking progestin.

TABLE 28-4 SELECT ESTROGENS AND PROGESTINS

GENERIC NAME/ TRADE NAME	USUAL ADULT DOSE, ROUTE, AND FREQUENCY	INDICATIONS FOR USE	DRUG INTERACTIONS
ESTROGENS			
estradiol (Estrace)	0.5-2 mg PO daily in cycles	Menopausal symptoms, hypogonadism	bromocriptine, hepatotoxic drugs
(Estraderm, Vivelle, Climara)	0.025-0.1 mg patch		
(Estring)	2 mg vaginal ring every 3 mo		
(Estrasorb)	2.5 mg applied onto each leg qd (emulsion)		
(Evamist)	1.53 mg spray on inner surface of forearm qd		
(Vagifem) (vaginal tablet)	10 mg topically in vagina		
(Elestrin) (gel)	0.87 g topically to upper arm qd		
estradiol cypionate (Depo-Estradiol, Dura-Estrin)	1-5 mg IM every 3-4 wks		
estradiol valerate (Delestrogen)	10-20 mg IM every 3-4 wks	Menopausal symptoms Hypogonadism, and prostatic cancer	tobacco
estradiol, ethinyl	1-2 mg PO bid-tid	Prostatic cancer	
esterified estrogen (Menest)	0.3-1.25 mg PO qd		
estropipate	0.75-3 mg PO qd	Same as other estrogens and osteoporosis	None noted

IM, Intramuscularly; *PO,* orally.

Continued

TABLE 28-4 SELECT ESTROGENS AND PROGESTINS—cont'd

GENERIC NAME/ TRADE NAME	USUAL ADULT DOSE, ROUTE, AND FREQUENCY	INDICATIONS FOR USE	DRUG INTERACTIONS
PROGESTINS			
progesterone (Crinone) (Prometrium)	5-10 mg IM Vaginal gel/suppository topically 200 mg PO qd ×12/day	Amenorrhea, abnormal uterine bleeding, infertility	None noted
medroxyprogesterone (Provera)	2-10 mg PO qd	Endometrial hyperplasia, secondary amenorrhea, abnormal uterine bleeding	None noted
(Depo-Provera)	150 mg IM q 3 months 400-1000 mg IM wkly 1-7 g/wk	Contraception Endometrial carcinoma Endometrial cancer	
megestrol (Megace)	40 mg PO qid 40-320 mg PO qd 800 mg PO qd	Breast cancer Endometrial cancer Anorexia, cachexia	None noted
norethindrone	0.5-2.0 mg PO qd	Amenorrhea, abnormal uterine bleeding	None noted
(Camila, Errin, NorQD, Jolivette)	0.35 mg PO qd 5 mg PO qd	Contraception Prevention of endometrial hyperplasia with estrogen therapy	
norethindrone acetate (Aygestin)	2.5 mg PO qd	HRT replacement, abnormal bleeding, endometriosis	
COMBINATION ESTROGEN AND PROGESTERONE MEDICATIONS			
esterified estrogen with methyltestosterone (Covaryx, EEMT)	1.25 mg/2.5 mg PO qd	Menopausal symptoms, hypogonadism, and breast cancer	None noted
esterified estrogen with medroxyprogesterone (PREMPRO, Premphase)	0.625 mg/2.5 mg PO qd 0.625 mg/5 mg PO qd	Same as other estrogens	None noted
estradiol, norethindrone (Combipatch, Activella) (Mimvey)	dose varies with drug	HRT replacement	None noted
estradiol, norgestimate (Prefest)	1 tab qd in cycles 1 mg/0.09 mg PO qd	HRT replacement	
estradiol, norethindrone (Femhrt)	5 mcg/1 mg PO qd	HRT replacement	
estradiol, drospirenone (Angeliq)	5 mcg/1 mg PO qd	HRT replacement	
conjugated estrogens (Premarin) (Premarin vaginal cream)	0.3-2.5 mg PO qd 2-4 g topically qd	Menopausal symptoms, osteoporosis prevention, prostate cancer, breast cancer, hypogonadism, and atrophic vaginitis	None noted
conjugated estrogen, synthetic A (Cenestin)	0.3-1.25 mg PO qd in cycles		
conjugated estrogen, synthetic B (Enjuvia)	0.3-1.25 mg PO qd in cycles		

Patient Education for Compliance

1. Before starting any estrogen therapy, a female patient should undergo full physical examination including breast and pelvic examinations, Pap smear, blood pressure, and lipid profile, followed by yearly reexaminations and monthly breast self-examinations. For women older than age 40, a mammogram may be indicated.
2. Estrogens can cause genital abnormalities in male fetus and vaginal cancer in female fetus. Estrogens should be discontinued as soon as pregnancy is suspected.
3. To reduce side effects of estrogen and progesterone, take medication with food.
4. If persistent vaginal bleeding develops in menopausal women, the physician should be notified.
5. Estrogen and progestin may cause a sunburn-like reaction on exposure to sunlight or ultraviolet light.
6. Blood glucose levels should be checked more frequently in people with diabetes mellitus taking estrogens.
7. Estradiol transdermal patches should be applied to a clean, dry area of intact skin on the abdomen or trunk, pressing it firmly in place with palm of hand for 10 seconds. If patch falls off, reapply same patch. Application site should be changed with each new patch. Avoid applying estradiol transdermal patches at waist or breasts, or in places where clothing will loosen edges of patch.
8. Intravaginal estrogen preparations should be positioned high in vagina. A recumbent position for 30 minutes is necessary after application to allow medications to remain in place for effectiveness. If patient is in upright position, medications will be expelled by gravity.
9. Patient should avoid sunscreens when using estrogen emulsion.

Important Facts about Estrogen-Progesterone Preparations

- Estradiol is the principal endogenous estrogen with a role in the menstrual cycle and is required for growth and maturation of reproductive organs.
- Estrogens raise levels of high-density lipoproteins (HDL) and reduce levels of low-density lipoprotein (LDL), which may explain why premenopausal women may not be as susceptible to coronary heart disease.
- Nausea is the most common side effect of estrogen preparations.
- Prolonged use of estrogens alone is associated with an increased risk of endometrial carcinoma; when used with progesterone, there is little or no risk of uterine cancer.
- Estrogens taken for less than 5 years pose a smaller risk for breast cancer.
- Progestins may cause breakthrough bleeding, spotting, and amenorrhea.

Important Facts about Estrogen-Progesterone Preparations—cont'd

- Natural estrogen losses in menopause may cause hot flashes, loss of bone mass, and an increased risk of coronary heart disease.
- Hormone replacement therapy in postmenopausal women usually consists of estrogen combined with progestin. Estrogens and progestins are contraindicated during pregnancy and in women with estrogen-dependent carcinomas, undiagnosed abnormal vaginal bleeding, and thromboembolic disorders.

FORMS OF CONTRACEPTION

Chief factors to consider when choosing a method of *birth control* are effectiveness, safety, and personal preference. **Contraception** denotes prevention of ovum fertilization and subsequent onset of pregnancy. Birth control may be accomplished using pharmacologic methods such as oral contraceptives, medication-laden implants, injectable hormones, and intrauterine devices (IUDs). Nonpharmacologic methods include surgical sterilization, mechanical devices, and the rhythm method. The best form of contraception will be ineffective if improperly practiced.

Safety of birth control measures is a complex area. Of contraceptive methods available, oral contraceptives have the largest spectrum of adverse effects—from nausea to menstrual abnormalities to rare thromboembolytic disorders. The lowest mortality rate is seen with barrier methods, but oral contraceptives are relatively safe in nonsmoking women with normal cardiovascular function.

Oral Contraceptives

Oral contraceptives are the most effective form of easily reversible birth control presently available. First made available in the late 1950s, these medications have had a large impact on socioeconomic conditions in the United States because their use has reduced family size. Early dosages of contraceptives were much stronger with greater side effects than those found today. Millions of women have used these medications; through this experience, risk factors, dosages, and effectiveness have been evaluated and modified. Newer low-dose oral contraceptives are associated with lower risk of adverse effects.

Did You Know?

The first oral contraceptives contained from 10 to 20 mg of estrogen per tablet compared to 0.5 to 1 mcg per tablet currently.

Combination oral contraceptives, which consist of some estrogen and progestin formulation, inhibit ovulation by increasing hormone levels and increasing the cervical mucus viscosity, thus creating a barrier to sperm. Two main categories of oral contraceptives that are nearly 100% effective are (1) those containing estrogen and progestin, known as *combination oral contraceptives*, and (2) those containing only progestins, or "minipills." Combination oral contraceptives are manufactured in monophasic, biphasic, triphasic, and estrophasic formulations. In monophasic regimens, daily doses of estrogen and progestin remain constant throughout the menstrual cycle. In biphasic regimens, the estrogen dose remains constant but the progestin dose is increased during the second half of the cycle. Triphasic regimens divide the menstrual cycle into three phases, with the progestin amount changing in each phase of cycle. In estrophasic regimens, the amount of progestin remains constant and the estrogen dose is gradually increased throughout the cycle.

Estrogen components have been associated with venous and arterial thromboembolism, causing myocardial infarctions and strokes. Associated risk of hypertension increases with prolonged oral contraceptive use and increasing age. Risk of adverse cardiovascular reactions and breast cancer is greatly increased in women who smoke while taking oral contraceptives. Cancer risk is low, especially when compared with the endometrial cancer risk found with postmenopausal estrogen therapy. Oral contraceptives containing progestins can elevate blood sugar levels and cause gallbladder disease.

The efficacy of oral contraceptives can be affected by medications, and oral contraceptives in turn can affect the dosage of some medications (Box 28-1).

BOX 28-1 MEDICATIONS THAT CHANGE THE EFFECTIVENESS OF ORAL CONTRACEPTIVES

Drugs that Reduce Effects of Oral Contraceptives
rifampin (tuberculosis)
phenobarbital, phenytoin, and primidone (antiseizure)
tetracycline and penicillin derivatives (antiinfective)
St John's Wort (herbal)
ritonavir (antiviral)

Drugs Whose Effects are Reduced by Oral Contraceptives
warfarin (anticoagulant)
insulin and other hypoglycemic agents (for diabetes mellitus)

Drugs Whose Effects are Increased by Oral Contraceptives
theophylline (for asthma)
tricyclic antidepressants (for depression)
diazepam (anti-anxiety)
chlordiazepoxide (anti-anxiety)

Taking Oral Contraceptives Effectively

Most oral contraceptives are taken in a sequence of 21 days, followed by 7 days of no pill, an inert pill, or an iron-containing pill. Some oral contraceptives are started on the fifth day of the menstrual cycle to be taken at the same time daily. Successive cycles begin every 28 days. Other oral contraceptives are started on the first day of the menstrual cycle and are continued daily throughout the cycle. These medications may contain iron supplements or placebos during the last 7 days. During the first cycle of use, other birth control forms should be used. If a single dose of oral contraceptive is missed, the chance of ovulation is small. However, risk of ovulation becomes greater with each consecutive pill omitted. If one dose is missed, it should be taken the next day. If two doses are missed, two tablets should be taken on the next 2 days. If three doses are missed, a new medication cycle should be started 7 days after the last pill was taken. Additional birth control should be used during the first 2 weeks of the new cycle. If this routine is not followed, pregnancy due to ovulation may occur (Table 28-5).

Patient Education for Compliance

1. Breakthrough bleeding, spotting, amenorrhea, and breast tenderness are possible with estrogen and progestin preparations.
2. Oral contraceptives should be taken at same time daily, beginning at the appropriate time during menstrual cycle. Monophasic medications are taken for 21 days, followed by no drug for 7 days. Other formulations may provide tablets containing iron or placebos so tablets are taken on daily basis.
3. Shortness of breath, leg tenderness, chest pain, headaches, or visual disturbances while taking oral contraceptives should be reported to physician immediately. Yearly physical examinations are necessary.
4. If two consecutive menstrual periods are missed, the possibility of pregnancy must be evaluated.
5. Menses may be irregular for several months after discontinuation of oral contraceptives.
6. Oral contraceptives cannot be used during breastfeeding because hormones will enter breast milk and pass to infant.
7. Persons with diabetes mellitus taking oral contraceptives should monitor blood glucose levels closely.
8. Incidence of multiple births is increased if conception occurs shortly after oral contraceptives are stopped. To reduce this chance, other forms of birth control should be used for 3 months after termination of oral contraceptive use.
9. Additional forms of contraception should be used during initial cycle of oral contraceptive use.

TABLE 28-5 SELECT CONTRACEPTIVES*

GENERIC NAME/TRADE NAME	USUAL ADULT DOSE, ROUTE, AND FREQUENCY	INDICATIONS FOR USE	DRUG INTERACTIONS
MONOPHASIC COMBINATION MEDICATIONS		Prevention of pregnancy	See Box 28-1 for drug interactions with this group of drugs
ethinyl estradiol/norethindrone (in various strengths) (Loestrin, Loestrin 24 FE, Ovcon 35, Brevicon, Modicon, Norinyl, Ortho-Novum, Junel, Microgestin)	1 tab PO qd (the estrogen component is in micrograms; the progestin component is in milligrams)		
ethinyl estradiol/drospirenone (Yasmin, Yaz)	1 tab PO qd in cycles		
ethinyl estradiol/norelgestromin (Ortho Evra)	Apply patch topically once wkly		
ethinyl estradiol/levonorgestrel (Alesse, Nordette, Altavera)	1 tab PO qd in cycles		
ethinyl estradiol/norgestrel (Lo/Ovral, Ovral)	1 tab PO qd in cycles		
ethinyl estradiol/desogestrel (Desogen, Ortho-Cept)	1 tab PO qd in cycles		
ethinyl estradiol/norgestimate (Previfem, Ortho-Cyclen)	1 tab PO qd in cycles		
ethinyl estradiol/ethynodiol diacetate (Zovia)	1 tab PO qd in cycles		
mestranol/norethindrone (Norinyl, Ortho-Novum 1/50, Necon 1/50)	1 tab PO qd in cycles		
estrogen/progestin (Necon 1/35, Alesse-28, Ortho-Novum 1/35)	1 tab PO qd in cycles		
BIPHASIC COMBINATION MEDICATIONS			
ethinyl estradiol/norethindrone (Ortho-Novum 10/11, Necon 10/11)	1 tab PO qd in cycles		
ethinyl estadiol/desogestrel (Mircette)	1 tab PO qd in cycles		
TRIPHASIC COMBINATION MEDICATIONS			
ethinyl estradiol/norethindrone (Tri-Norinyl, Ortho-Novum 7/7/7)	1 tab PO qd in cycles		
ethinyl estradiol/levonorgestrel (Triphasil, Trivora)	1 tab PO qd in cycles		
ethinyl estradiol/norgestimate (Ortho Tri-Cyclen†)	1 tab PO qd in cycles		
ESTROPHASIC COMBINATION MEDICATIONS			
ethinyl estradiol/norethindrone (Estrostep)	1 tab PO qd in cycles		

FE, Iron; *IM*, intramuscularly; *IUD*, intrauterine device; *PO*, orally.

*For drugs separated by a slash, the first drug listed is an estrogen component and the second drug is a progestin component.

†Food and Drug Administration approved for use with acne.

Continued

TABLE 28-5 SELECT CONTRACEPTIVES—cont'd

GENERIC NAME/TRADE NAME	USUAL ADULT DOSE, ROUTE, AND FREQUENCY	INDICATIONS FOR USE	DRUG INTERACTIONS
PROGESTIN-ONLY MEDICATIONS			
norethindrone (Ortho-Micronor)	1 tab PO qd in cycles		
LONG-ACTING CONTRACEPTIVES			
ethyl estradiol/levonorgestrel (Seasonale, Seasonique, LoSeasonique)	1 tab PO for 91 days		
	1 tablet PO for 84 days		
(Lybrel)	1 tab PO indefinitely		
medroxyprogesterone (Depo-Provera, Depo-subQ)	150 mg q3mo IM		
	104 mg q 3 mo SC		
levonorgestrel (Implanon)	1 rod subdermal q3yr		
INTRAUTERINE PROGESTERONE CONTRACEPTIVE SYSTEM			
levonorgestrel (Mirena)	IUD q5yr	None noted	

Important Facts about Oral Contraceptives

- Two main categories of oral contraceptives are combinations of estrogen plus progestin and progestin-only medications (minipills).
- Combination oral contraceptives primarily inhibit ovulation.
- Serious adverse reactions from oral contraceptive use are rare, although side effects and some complications occur. Adjusting estrogen and progestin content may minimize problems.
- Low-estrogen combination oral contraceptives pose only minimal thromboembolism risk except in women with past history of thromboembolic disease or in those who smoke.
- Oral contraceptives are teratogenic and may cause cancer in female offspring; therefore they are contraindicated during pregnancy.
- Progestins are slightly safer than combination oral contraceptives but are less effective and cause more menstrual irregularity.
- Progestin-only oral contraceptives increase viscosity of cervical mucus, creating a barrier to sperm and suppressing growth of endometrium to prevent fertilized ovum implantation.
- Combination oral contraceptions protect against ovarian and endometrial cancer. They do not cause breast cancer.

Other Forms of Contraception

Implants and Transdermal Patches

Other medications are used for long-acting contraception. A subdermal system, Implanon, provides synthetic progestin, **levonorgestrel,** as the most effective long-term, reversible method of contraception. The six tiny capsules containing synthetic progestin are surgically implanted inside the upper arm. Levonorgestrel diffuses slowly and continuously at a rate of about 80 mcg/day to provide contraception for up to 5 years. The implant must be surgically removed when no longer desired or effective.

A monophasic transdermal patch holds a combination of **ethinyl estradiol** and **norelgestromin** (Ortho-Evra) to provide contraception much like oral preparations with the same indications and contraindications. Patches are applied to the upper arms, back, abdomen, or buttocks and are worn in either weekly or biweekly cycles. The patch is applied on the same day of the week for 3 weeks, with the fourth week being patch free. With correct use, effectiveness of contraception is equal to that of oral medications without the need to remember to take daily medication doses. This medication has proven less effective in women weighing 198 lb or more, indicating the need for other means of contraception in obese women. Women using this medication should not be without a patch for longer than 7 days in a row, or pregnancy is possible. If a patch becomes loose or falls off for less than 1 day, either the patch should be reapplied or a new patch should be applied, and the regular day for changing should remain the same. If the patch is off for more than 1 day or if the time off is unknown, a new 4-week cycle should begin immediately and a backup method of contraception should be used the first week of the cycle (see Table 28-5).

Contraception by Injection

A single injection of **medroxyprogesterone** (Depo-Provera, 150 mg indepot form or Depo-subQ 104 mg in subcantaneous form) provides contraception safely and effectively for 3 months or more. Injections prevent pregnancy in three ways: (1) by suppressing ovulation, (2) by thickening the cervical mucus, and (3) by altering the endometrium to discourage fertilized ovum implantation. When injections are discontinued, an average of 12 months is required for fertility to return, with some women remaining infertile for 2 or more years (see Table 28-5).

Intrauterine Devices

IUDs, another relatively long-term effective reversible form of birth control, are inserted using minor surgical procedures. The principal problem with IUD use is pelvic inflammatory disease. The major side effect is cramping. The IUD should be used by women at low risk for sexually transmitted diseases (STDs). Three IUDs are available: the Copper T 380A (ParaGard) IUD and the intrauterine progesterone contraceptive system (Progestasert) and levonorgestrel (Mirena). IUD ParaGard may remain in place for 8 years and is more widely used. The Progestasert must be replaced annually, and Mirena is effective for 5 years (see Table 28-5).

Spermicides

With minimal adverse reactions, spermicides come in foams, gels, creams, and suppositories that may be purchased without a prescription. Spermicides, **nonoxynol-9** (Delfen, Ensure) and **octoxynol-9** (Ortho-Gynol, Koromex cream), provide effective contraception when used as directed, with increased effectiveness when used with a diaphragm or condom. The active ingredient, a chemical surfactant, kills sperm by destroying their cell membranes. The adverse reactions are minimal. A spermicide must be applied before coitus but no more than 1 hour in advance if used alone. Spermicides must be reapplied each time intercourse is anticipated. Foams must be thoroughly shaken before each use to ensure dispersal of active ingredients. Suppositories or tablets should be inserted into the vagina a minimum of 10 to 15 minutes before intercourse to allow time for these forms of contraception to dissolve. Douching should be postponed for at least 6 hours after coitus with any spermicidal use. Recent data indicate that use of nonoxynol-9, the ingredient in most spermicides, can increase the risk of HIV transmission (Table 28-6).

TABLE 28-6 COMMON SPERMICIDALS		
MEDICATION TYPE	**ACTIVE INGREDIENT***	**TRADE NAME**
Foam	nonoxynol-9	Delfen, Koromex
Jelly	nonoxynol-9	Gynol II
Gel	nonoxynol-9	Conceptrol, Advantage 24,[†] Advantage-S, Aqua Lube Plus, K-Y Plus,[†] Gynol II,[†] Koromex[†]
	octoxynol-9	Ortho-Gynol[†]
Suppository	nonoxynol-9	Encare, Semicid
Vaginal film	nonoxynol-9	VCF, Ortho Options

Major Side Effects: Nausea, vomiting, infertility, breast tenderness, ectopic pregnancy, blood clot formation

*Side effects minimal.
[†]To be used only in combination with a diaphragm.

Barrier Devices

Barrier devices, nonpharmacologic methods of birth control, include male and female condoms, diaphragms, and cervical caps. The most commonly used barrier contraceptive device is the male condom.

Condoms are made from three materials—latex, polyurethane, and lamb intestine. Most condoms in the United States are made from latex, which is impenetrable by bacteria and viruses. In addition to use for contraception, the latex condom protects against STDs. Lubricants containing mineral oil can decrease the barrier strength of latex by as much as 90% and should therefore be avoided. Polyurethane condoms are thinner, are possibly stronger, and do not cause allergies (a possibility with latex), while still providing protection against STDs. Lamb intestine condoms allow viral transmission and so do not protect against viral STDs. Male condoms have a 12% failure rate in preventing pregnancy.

The female condom, Reality, is a loose-fitting tubular polyurethane pouch with flexible rings at both ends. The ring at the closed end anchors the pouch on the cervix. On the open end, the pouch has a larger ring to be placed over the labia as an external anchor. This mechanism provides some protection against STDs. The Reality condom is prelubricated, available over the counter

(OTC), and cannot be combined with a male condom. Failure rate for pregnancy is about 21%.

The diaphragm is a soft rubber cap with a metal spring to reinforce the rim. For proper sizing the device must be fitted by a health care provider and is bought with a prescription. Before insertion, the diaphragm should be filled with spermicide to completely block the cervix. A diaphragm may be inserted up to 6 hours before intercourse but must remain in place for at least 6 hours after. Failure rate for pregnancy is about 18%.

The cervical cap is a small, pliant, cup-shaped device that fits directly over the cervix, where it is held in place by suction. Like the diaphragm, the cap is not available OTC but must be fitted by a health care professional, and spermicides must be used as a barrier. The failure rate for women who have previously given birth is around 40%, whereas the failure rate is about 20% for women who have not given birth.

Postcoital Contraception

Medications used as postcoital contraceptives may be either "morning-after" pills or "abortion" pills to prevent pregnancy after intercourse. These drugs are not to be used routinely because of the dangers from potential side effects; rather, emergency contraception pills (ECPs) are meant to provide one-time emergency protection from unplanned and unwanted pregnancies occurring from unprotected sexual intercourse resulting from sexual attack, contraception failure, and the like.

The morning-after pill has three possible modes of action: (1) inhibiting ovulation, (2) altering the menstrual cycle to prevent ovulation, and (3) irritating the uterine lining so rejection of a possible fertilized egg occurs. A high-dose oral contraceptive, the pill is formulated of either progestin alone, estrogen alone, or both of these artificial steroids together. Medications with combined hormones are called *combined ECPs*. A specially packaged combination of high doses of estrogen and progestin, Preven, has a dose of two pills. The only drug packaged for ECP is Plan B, the remainder of the medications are contraceptions that are used as ECP. Combined ECPs are 75% effective in women who would otherwise become pregnant from unprotected sex. The other type of ECP, or progestin-only (Plan B) ECP, with a dose of one tablet, is even more effective, at an 85% rate.

The pill may be taken immediately after the unprotected intercourse, but the first pill must be taken within the first 72-hour period. A second pill must be taken 12 hours after the first dose.

Danger signals for a few weeks after use of morning-after pills are severe pain in the legs, severe abdominal pain, chest pain, shortness of breath, blurred vision, trouble speaking, loss of vision, or jaundice. The next menstrual period may be earlier or later than usual. If the menstrual period does not begin for 3 weeks, a pregnancy test and a pelvic examination should be done. If pregnancy occurs, an abortion should be considered because of the teratogenicity of estrogen to the fetus. See Table 28-7 for a list of oral contraceptives that can be used as ECPs.

Important Facts about Methods of Contraception

- Long-lasting methods of birth control, such as Implanon implants, intrauterine devices (IUDs), and sterilization, should be used when compliance may be a problem. Oral contraceptives are a close second for effectiveness of birth control.
- Norplant, which acts similarly to progestin, is effective for 5 years and is the most effective method of contraception.
- Medroxyprogesterone (Depo-Provera) is given intramuscularly, works for 3 months, and is highly effective.
- Morning-after pills are not to be used as routine means of contraception. These drugs are for emergency situations only. These medications may be a combination of estrogen and progestin or a progestin-only medication.

TABLE 28-7 SELECT MEDICATIONS THAT MAY BE USED AS EMERGENCY CONTRACEPTIVES

TYPE OF MEDICATION	TRADE NAME	USUAL DOSE, ROUTE, AND FREQUENCY
progestin-only ECP[†]	Plan B*	1 pill within 72 hr and another 12 hr later
Combined ECP	Preven	2 pills within 72 hr and 2 more pills 12 hr later
Combined oral contraceptive	Ovral	2 pills within 72 hr and 2 pills 12 hr later
	Nordette, Levlen, Levora Lo/Ovral, Low-Ogestrel	4 pills within 72 hr and 4 pills 12 hr later
	Alesse, Levlite	5 pills within 72 hr and 5 pills 12 hr later
mifepristone (RU-486)	Mifeprex	3 pills (600 mg) within 63 days of LMP, 2 tab misoprostol 2 days later

Major Side Effects: Excessive bleeding, cramping, nausea, vomiting, fatigue, weakness, headache, diarrhea

ECP, Emergency contraception pill; *LMP*, Last menstrual period.
*As of February 2007, Plan B is available OTC in some states.
[†]Only medication specific as ECP.

RU-486 (Abortion Pill)

Mifepristone (RU-486) is approved by the FDA as a post-coital contraceptive agent to stop gestation. Similar in structure to progesterone, **mifepristone** (Mifeprex) is the first of a new generation of birth control pills called *antiprogestins*. It works only in the first 9 weeks of pregnancy, or up to 63 days from the start of the last menstrual period, to produce a medical-chemical abortion by stimulating uterine contractions and preventing the fertilized egg from attaching to the uterus. After the first 7 weeks of pregnancy, the natural progesterone found in the pregnant woman is too great to allow medication to be effective. Bleeding and cramping that typically occur after administration are similar to or greater than a heavy menstrual period and last for 9 to 16 days. Efficacy is 92% to 95%.

Women using this medication must be carefully screened, and medicine must be administered by specially trained health care providers who have the capability of surgical intervention if needed for an incomplete abortion or for excessive bleeding. Mifepristone should not be used with the following conditions: confirmed or suspected tubal pregnancies; IUD in place; chronic adrenal gland disease; current long-term therapy with corticosteroids; history of allergy to mifepristone, misoprostol, or other prostaglandins; and bleeding disorders or current anticoagulant therapy.

Eligible women will need to see the health care provider three times for completion of entire procedure: (1) initially, to receive a three-pill dose by mouth; (2) to take a dose of misoprostol, a prostaglandin, 2 days later to complete the abortion; and (3) finally, a return visit approximately 2 weeks later to be certain the abortion was complete. If abortion is not complete, a surgical procedure may be necessary to terminate the pregnancy. However, methotrexate (an antimetabolite) and an intravaginal insertion of misoprostol is a safe and effective alternative to surgical intervention.

Did You Know?

The medical community has identified RU-486 as having promising effects in treatment of some breast cancers, endometrial cancer, brain tumors, endometriosis, uterine fibroid tumors, adrenal cancer, glaucoma, and in inducing labor.

Forms of Contraception on the Horizon

Researchers are pursuing new vaccines for both men and women. A male vaccine has been shown to be 99% effective in suppressing sperm production. This vaccine requires weekly injections of testosterone at present, but scientists are looking at implants or longer-acting injections.

Patient Education for Compliance

1. Barrier contraceptives used by women should remain in place for prescribed time after sexual intercourse and should be used with spermicide as suggested by manufacturers.
2. Lubricants containing mineral oil should not be used with latex condoms because strength of latex may be decreased by as much as 90%.
3. Barrier contraception devices such as diaphragms and cervical caps must be fitted professionally.
4. "Morning-after" contraception must be accomplished within 72 hours of unprotected sex and should be used only as emergency means of contraception, not as routine means of contraception.
5. "Abortion pill" must be administered by health care professional within 7 weeks of the last menstrual period. Pregnancy should be confirmed before use of RU-486.

DRUGS FOR PREMENSTRUAL SYNDROME AND DYSMENORRHEA

Premenstrual syndrome (PMS) is a group of physical and psychologic symptoms that occur just before menstruation and resolve a few days after onset of menses. See Box 28-2 for common PMS symptoms. For PMS to be diagnosed, symptoms must be intense and related to a woman's menstrual cycle. For mild symptoms, lifestyle changes including dietary supplements, exercise, eating carbohydrate-rich foods, and reducing salt intake are the

BOX 28-2 COMMON SYMPTOMS OF PREMENSTRUAL SYNDROME

Psychologic and Behavioral Symptoms
Irritability and crying
Depression, sadness, feeling of helplessness
Alternating sadness and anger
Hypersensitivity to trivial events
Social withdrawal
Anxiety and tension
Difficulty concentrating
Reduced efficiency in work performance
Restlessness and agitation

Physical Symptoms
Acne
Breast tenderness
Abdominal bloating, ankle edema
Weight gain from water retention
Food cravings
Fatigue
Headache
Backache, joint and muscle pain
Nausea, vomiting, constipation, or diarrhea

first line of treatment. For more severe symptoms, two types of drug therapy using different agents are indicated. The most prescribed medications are mood-altering drugs and those used to suppress ovulation, although other medications may be used to relieve specific symptoms.

Mood-altering drugs (discussed in Chapter 30) that are often used are (1) selective serotonin reuptake inhibitors (SSRIs) such as *fluoxetine* (Prozac) and *sertraline* (Zoloft), the first drugs of choice to relieve psychologic PMS symptoms; (2) *alprazolam* (Xanax), a member of the benzodiazepine family, used to reduce irritability, anxiety, and tension of PMS; (3) ovulation suppressants, including two classes of drugs—oral contraceptives and gonadotropin-releasing hormone (GnRH) agents—helpful with primarily physical symptoms; and (4) *leuprolide* (Lupron), used to reduce breast tenderness, bloating, anxiety, and nervous tension.

Some other medications for specific symptoms include *spironolactone* (Aldactone), a potassium-sparing diuretic, used to treat bloating and urine retention; calcium to decrease mood swings and depression, aches, pains, food cravings, and water retention; and analgesics such as *aspirin, acetaminophen, naproxen* (Naprosyn), and *ibuprofen,* which may relieve cramps, headaches, dysmenorrhea, and muscle and joint pain. Ibuprofen is considered superior medication for relief of primary dysmenorrhea. Aspirin and naproxen relieve primary dysmenorrhea because they suppress prostaglandins that cause smooth muscle cramping. Drugs known not to work for dysmenorrhea are progesterone, pyridoxine, tamoxifen, lithium, and magnesium.

MEDICATIONS FOR INFERTILITY

Infertility is the decreased ability to reproduce; *sterility* is the absence of reproductive ability. Infertility is experienced by 15% of couples trying to conceive children, and it may be the result of reproductive dysfunction in either partner or both. With medical care, approximately half of the couples are able to achieve fertility when medication is matched to the cause.

Fertility depends on secreting proper amounts of hormones by the endocrine system. Deficiencies in hormones responsible for production of ova or sperm may lead to infertility. Cysts, tumors, or infections of reproductive organs or obstruction of tubal structures that transport ova or sperm may cause difficulty in conception. Some conditions can be treated medicinally; others require surgical intervention.

Treatment by Follicular Stimulation

Anovulation, a cause of infertility, frequently can be corrected by pharmaceutical means to promote follicle maturation and produce ovulation. *Clomiphene*

(Clomid) and *gonadorelin* (Fractal, Lutrepulse) have antiestrogenic effects to cause ovarian stimulation, maturation of ovarian follicles, and development of corpus luteum. *Menotropin* (Pergonal, Humegon), a hormonal preparation with LH and FSH activity in equal amounts, is used to provide adequate ovarian stimulation when pituitary hormones are insufficient. The cost for a single medication treatment can be as high as $1500, but the rate of ovulation approaches 100%. *Human chorionic gonadotropin* (hCG) is also given after 4 days of menotropin to stimulate ovulation. Of interest, these medications are also used to treat infertility in males. *Urofollitropin* (Metrodin), similar to menotropin, obtained from the urine of postmenopausal women, contains FSH. hCG is administered after urofollitropin to stimulate natural ovulation.

Treatment of Amenorrhea

Bromocriptine (Parlodel) is used to correct amenorrhea and infertility associated with excessive prolactin secretion. In some persons, a common first-dose side effect is the phenomenon of dizziness or syncope on change of position. Some conditions of the female reproductive tract such as polycystic ovaries, endometriosis, and uterine fibroid tumors may be exacerbated; medication is then contraindicated (Table 28-8).

Male Infertility

Male reproductive system dysfunction is the cause of 30% of cases of infertility, which frequently are unresponsive to medications. This failure may be caused by decreased density or motility of sperm or to abnormal quality or volume of semen. In men who do not produce sperm because of insufficient secretion of hormones, drug therapy may be helpful. Sperm counts may be increased with the use of hCG alone or in combination with menotropin. Combination therapy is expensive and may require prolonged treatment for 3 to 4 years. If hormone deficiency is severe, androgens may be used for drug therapy.

Important Facts about Medications for Infertility

- Infertility is decreased ability to reproduce; sterility is absence of ability to reproduce.
- Infertility may occur in either partner or both.
- Clomiphene promotes follicular maturation and ovulation.
- Menotropin is a 50:50 mixture of luteinizing hormone and follicle-stimulating hormone that promotes follicular maturation and ovulation.

TABLE 28-8 DRUGS USED TO TREAT INFERTILITY

GENERIC NAME/ TRADE NAME	USUAL ADULT DOSE, ROUTE, AND FREQUENCY	INDICATIONS FOR USE	DRUG INTERACTIONS
clomiphene (Clomid, Serophene)	50 mg PO qd × 5 days, starting on the fifth day of menstrual cycle; may be used for 3 or 4 cycles and then increased to 75-100 mg/day	Female infertility	None noted
menotropin (Repronex)	75 units each of FSH and LH IM, SQ	Stimulates follicles to mature by acting on FSH and LH	None noted
(Menopur)	75 units each of FSH and LH IM, SC		
urofollitropin (Bravelle)	75 mg/day × 1 week IM/SQ or more, followed by 5000 to 10,000 units of hCG on day after last dose of urofollitropin	Stimulates follicle maturity in males and females	None noted
bromocriptine (Parlodel)	2.5-7.5 mg PO qd		None noted
human chorionic gonadotropin, hCG (A.P.L., Pregnyl, Novarel)	5000-10,000 units IM on day 1 after last dose of tropins	Stimulates production of progesterone from the corpus luteum	None noted

FSH, Follicle-stimulating hormone; *hCG*, human chorionic gonadotropin; *IM*, intramuscularly; *LH*, luteinizing hormone; *PO*, orally; *SC*, subcutaneously.

MEDICATIONS FOR MISCELLANEOUS REPRODUCTIVE CONDITIONS

Danazol (Danocrine), used to treat endometriosis and associated infertility, may temporarily impair the ability of the endometrium to support a pregnancy, so attempts at conception should be postponed for 3 months after completion of treatment. The medication causes atrophy of endometrial tissue and is weakly androgenic (see Table 28-1).

Goserelin (Zoladex), an injectable implant administered into the abdominal wall every 4 weeks for 6 months to treat endometriosis, is pregnancy category X. Goserelin is also used as an antineoplastic agent in breast and prostate cancer.

Two GnRH agents are used for endometriosis—**leuprolide** (Lupron) and **nafarelin** (Synarel). Nafarelin, the drug of choice for treating endometriosis if future fertility is an issue, is a gonadotropin used to treat endometriosis in females and precocious puberty in both sexes. Because the route of administration is nasal, rhinitis may occur. (This drug may also be used to treat prostate cancer.) Leuprolide, similar to goserelin in action and side effects, is also used for uterine fibroids (Table 28-9).

Patient Education for Compliance

Women taking danazol for endometriosis should refrain from becoming pregnant for 3 months after treatment because of possible masculinization of fetus.

MEDICATIONS FOR ERECTILE DYSFUNCTION

Sildenafil (Viagra), the first medication for treatment of impotency, was first released as a cardiovascular agent to lower blood pressure; today it is used for erectile dysfunction in men. Newer drugs such as **tadalafil** (Cialis) and **vardenafil** (Levitra) have rapidly joined this group for use with erectile dysfunction. These medications act to increase blood flow to produce penile rigidity when associated with sexual stimulation. Sildenafil and vardenafil should be taken one hour before sexual activity and not more than once a day. However, tadalafil has a more rapid onset and prolonged effects, providing effectiveness for up to thirty-six hours with a new lower dose that may be taken daily. Investigations are being conducted to evaluate potential effectiveness for use in women.

TABLE 28-9 MISCELLANEOUS MEDICATIONS USED FOR REPRODUCTIVE TRACT CONDITIONS

GENERIC NAME/ TRADE NAME	USUAL ADULT DOSE, ROUTE, AND FREQUENCY	INDICATIONS FOR USE	DRUG INTERACTIONS
DRUGS FOR ENDOMETRIOSIS			
danazol	200-800 mg PO daily in divided doses	Endometriosis	None noted
goserelin (Zoladex)	3.6 mg SC monthly		
GnRH Agonists			
leuprolide (Lupron)	3.75 mg/dose IM monthly	Endometriosis and uterine fibroids	None noted
nafarelin (Synarel)	200-400 mcg as nasal spray bid	Endometriosis and precocious puberty	Nasal topical decongestants
Major Side Effects of Drugs for Endometriosis: Anxiety, headaches, CVA, hot flashes, breakthrough bleeding, breast tenderness			
DRUGS FOR ERECTILE DYSFUNCTION			
sildenafil (Viagra)	50 mg PO 1 hr before sexual activity	Erectile dysfunction in male	nitrate preparations
tadalafil (Cialis)	5-20 mg PO before sexual activity or 5 mg PO qd		nitrates, some antivirals
vardenafil (Levitra) (Staxyn)	5-20 mg PO before sexual activity oral disintegrating tab before sexual activity		nitrates, alpha blockers
Major Side Effects of Drugs for Erectile Dysfunction: Headache, flushing, GI upset, nasal congestion, diarrhea, rash, visual disturbances			

CVA, Cerebrovascular accident; *GI,* gastrointestinal; *IM,* intramuscularly; *PO,* orally; *SC,* subcutaneously.

These medications have not been associated with **priapism,** but these drugs should be used with care in the patient who is predisposed to the condition. An erection lasting longer than 4 hours should be immediately reported to the physician (see Table 28-9).

CLINICAL TIP

Drugs for erectile dysfunction should not be given with nitrates because of severe hypotension and danger of myocardial infarction.

LEARNING TIP

The generic names for medications for erectile dysfunction end in "afil."

MEDICATIONS THAT IMPAIR OR ENHANCE LIBIDO AS A SIDE EFFECT

Some medications can have side effects or adverse reactions that decrease libido in both genders. A decreased level of testosterone in either gender lowers the sex drive. Centrally acting alpha₂ agonists (**methyldopa** [Aldomet], **clonidine** [Catapres], and **guanfacine** [Tenex]) for hypertension have been associated with impotency and sexual dysfunction. **Guanethidine** (Ismelin) and **reserpine** have been reported to cause difficulty with male ejaculation. Anticholinergic agents used for hypertension may also cause impotence. Thiazide diuretics may induce sexual dysfunction and decrease libido, with impotency and breast changes. **Spironolactone** (Aldactone) seems to be the chief agent of this group to cause sexual dysfunction.

Continuous use of antihistamines will also interfere with sexual activity. Some well-known medications, such as **diphenhydramine** (Benadryl), **promethazine** (Phenergan), and **chlorpheniramine** (Chlor-Trimeton), are used as antiemetics and sedatives and to control allergy symptoms; however, these drugs also block parasympathetic nerve impulses to sex glands and organs.

Many of the centrally acting antianxiety and psychotropic medications, including benzodiazepines such as **diazepam** (Valium), affect sexual interest and capability. While a patient is undergoing therapy, phenothiazines decrease sexual interest by inhibiting sexual function, causing decreased libido and the inability to ejaculate. Impotence and prolonged amenorrhea are also possible. **Ethyl alcohol** is a sexual depressant, although moderate amounts may enhance sexual activity by decreasing inhibitions.

Histamine$_2$ (H$_2$)-receptor antagonists **cimetidine** (Tagamet) and **ranitidine** (Zantac) lead to impotency when used for long periods of time. Some calcium channel blockers cause erectile dysfunction, and beta blockers, especially **propranolol** (Inderal), have been associated with decreased libido and erectile dysfunction. The tricyclic antidepressant **clomipramine** (Anafranil) may induce a spontaneous orgasm as a side effect.

Opioids and psychotic agents such as LSD, cocaine, marijuana, and amphetamines are considered aphrodisiacs in contemporary society. More commonly, sexual behavior is decreased. The user's state of mind and the amount of medication consumed contribute to sexual effects of medication.

Some elderly patients taking **levodopa** (Dopar) have observed a sexual rejuvenation. **Amyl nitrate,** a vasodilator used for angina pectoris, has been alleged to enhance sexual activity and to intensify orgasmic experiences for men; however, loss of erection and delayed ejaculation may also result.

Many medications, both legal and illegal, may affect sexuality and sexual behavior. For patients taking therapeutic doses of medications interfering with sexual behavior, allied health care professionals should take an accurate history to develop awareness of the patient's needs and provide this information to the physician so treatment may be altered as needed to ensure medication compliance. Listening to patients' concerns about medications and sexual function is an important role of the allied health professional.

Patient Education for Compliance

Some drugs cause impairment of sexual function. These concerns should be discussed with the health care professional to allow changes in medications if possible.

SUMMARY

Androgens, necessary for normal development of male sex characteristics and for spermatogenesis, may be used therapeutically as hormonal replacement therapy in males or for breast cancer treatment.

Finasteride is a drug specific for BPH, a common reproductive system disorder in older males.

Testosterone, the primary male hormone or androgen, comes in several forms for treatment of certain types of cancer. Patches must be applied to the proper sites, whereas injectable forms may be short or long acting. Anabolic steroids are synthetic androgens often used by athletes to enhance performance. Although steroids have potential, the risks that accompany their use are substantial, making these medications Schedule III drugs because of the danger of abuse.

Estrogens and progestins are necessary for development of female sex characteristics and reproduction. Estrogens and progestins are used for contraception and for noncontraceptive applications such as HRT and treatment of breast and prostate cancer. Estrogens reduce the incidence of osteoporosis and coronary artery disease; therefore postmenopausal women should be evaluated for prophylactic use. Progestins are indicated for HRT and also for treatment of endometriosis and carcinomas, as well as to prevent pregnancy. Estrogens, progestins, and androgens are teratogenic. All oral contraceptives containing combinations of estrogens and progestins are an effective form of birth control. These medications are widely used because of ease of administration. Thromboembolytic disease is a dangerous adverse reaction.

Medications are available for treatment of infertility and sexual dysfunction and should be used with care because of their possible side effects. Drugs for female infertility must be taken exactly as ordered, with coitus occurring at a specific time in relation to drug administration to encourage pregnancy. Products available for erectile dysfunction should not be used with nitrates.

The morning-after pill for postcoital contraception must be taken within 72 hours after unprotected intercourse and should not be used as a means of routine contraception. The "abortion pill" must be administered by a specially trained health care professional requiring a specific regimen of three office visits.

The use of medications for any reproductive condition is a sensitive area for most patients. Allied health professionals should be empathic and discreet when discussing reproductive tract conditions and their treatments with clients.

CRITICAL THINKING EXERCISES

Scenario

Erin is taking an oral contraceptive but states that when she had the flu, she forgot to take her pills for 3 days. Also, the physician gave her a prescription for ampicillin for a bacterial infection.

1. Does the ampicillin have any bearing on the efficacy of the oral contraceptive? If so, what?
2. What should Erin do to resume her schedule of oral contraceptive use?
3. Should she use additional means of contraception at any point? Explain your answer.
4. Erin wants to know why 21 tablets in the prescription for the contraceptive look alike and seven look different. What is your response?

DRUG CALCULATIONS

1. Order: medroxyprogesterone acetate 0.2 g stat
   Available medication:

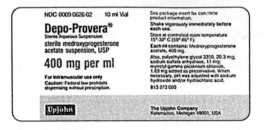

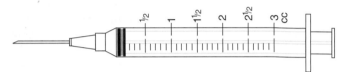

Show the volume of medication on the syringe shown.

Volume to be administered: _____

2. Order: Premarin 1.25 mg PO qd
   Available medication: Premarin 0.625 mg per tablet
   Amount to be administered with each dose: _____
   _____

REVIEW QUESTIONS

1. What is the collective name for male sex hormones? _____
   _____

2. What hormone is primarily responsible for the development of secondary sex characteristics in the male?
   _____
   _____

3. What is the goal of pharmaceutical treatment for benign prostatic hypertrophy? _____
   _____

4. What are some of the risks associated with female hormone replacement therapy? _____
   _____

5. What does *conjugated estrogen* mean? _____
   _____

6. What are some of the side effects of estrogen therapy? _____
   _____

7. Why are combination oral contraceptives so effective? _____
   _____

8. What is the main component of the minipill? _____
_____

9. Explain the differences among monophasic, biphasic, triphasic, and estrophasic oral contraceptives.
_____
_____
_____
_____

10. What medications reduce the effectiveness of oral contraceptives? _____
_____
_____
_____

11. What medication category is most effective for dysmenorrhea? _____
_____

12. What medications are considered dangerous for use with sildenafil? _____
_____

CHAPTER 29

Drugs for Neurologic System Disorders

After studying this chapter, you should be capable of doing the following:

- Briefly describing how analgesics and general anesthetics work.
- Explaining actions of local anesthetics.
- Discussing how hypnotics and sedatives affect the body.
- Describing antiseizure medications and their actions.
- Explaining how medications can be used to relieve Parkinson's disease symptoms.
- Describing how medications are used for headaches and migraines.
- Discussing how drugs are used to relieve spasticity.
- Identifying central nervous system stimulants and their actions.
- Explaining action of medications on autonomic and peripheral nervous system.
- Providing patient education for compliance with medications used to treat diseases and conditions of the neurologic system.

Katherine, age 32, has a family history of migraine headaches with auras. In the past few months, Katherine has had two migraine headaches related to menstruation. She thinks these may have been caused by tension and fatigue from her new job.

What nondrug measures might Katherine try for early relief of headaches?
What are causes of nonmigraine headaches?
What group of medications specific is for migraine headaches?

KEY TERMS

Absence or petit mal seizures	Blood-brain barrier	Hypnotic	Seizure
Acetylcholine (ACh)	Cataplexy	Narcolepsy	Spasticity
Adrenergic (sympathomimetic) agonists	Catecholamines	Neurohormones	Sympathetic nervous system
	Central nervous system	Neuron	
	Cholinesterase	Parasympathetic nervous system	Sympatholytic (or adrenergic blocking) agent
Amyloid blockers	Clonic		
Analeptics	Convulsion	Parasympatholytic (cholinergic) agent	Sympathomimetic (adrenergic or adrenergic-acting agents)
Analgesic	Diaphoresis		
Anesthesia	Dyskinesia	Peripheral nervous system	
Anorexiant	Dystonia		
Aura	Euphoria	Physical dependence	Tolerance
Autonomic nervous system (ANS)	Focal (partial) seizure	Restless legs syndrome	Tonic
	Generalized seizure		Xerostomia
	Grand mal seizure	Sedative	

EASY WORKING KNOWLEDGE OF DRUGS USED IN NEUROLOGIC SYSTEM DISORDERS

DRUG CLASS	PRESCRIPTION	OTC	PREGNANCY CATEGORY	MAJOR INDICATIONS
Analgesics	Yes	Yes	B, C, D	Relief of pain, RLS
Anesthetics	Yes	Yes	C, D	Blocking nerve endings causing pain
Sedatives, hypnotics	Yes	Yes (alcohol)	D (many not categorized)	Sedation and treatment of insomnia, RLS
Antiseizure medications	Yes	No	C, D	Epilepsy and associated seizure disorders, RLS
Antiparkinsonism medications	Yes	No	B, C	Parkinson's disease and Parkinson's syndrome, RLS
Medications for headaches	Yes	Yes	B, C, X (ergot preparations and sumatriptan)	Headaches, especially migraine headaches
Medications for spasticity	Yes	Yes	C	Muscle spasticity
CNS stimulants	Yes	Yes	B, C	ADD, ADHD, anorexiants, fatigue
Cholinergics (amyloid blockers)	Yes	No	C, X (isoflurophates)	Glaucoma, myasthenia gravis, Alzheimer disease
Anticholinergics	Yes	No	B, C	Gastric antispasmodic and antiulcer treatment, mydriatic, Parkinsonism
Adrenergics	Yes	Yes	B, C, D	Cardiovascular and respiratory conditions, shock
Adrenergic blockers	Yes	Yes	B, C	Hypertension, angina, glaucoma

ADD, Attention-deficit disorder; *ADHD,* attention-deficit/hyperactivity disorder; *CNS,* central nervous system; *RLS,* restless legs syndrome.

EASY WORKING KNOWLEDGE OF INDICATIONS AND SYMPTOMS

Common Signs and Symptoms of Neurologic Disorders
Headaches and fever
Nausea and vomiting
Weakness and motor disturbances
Mood swings and memory impairment
Drowsiness, stupor, coma
Seizures, paralysis, convulsions, numbness
Muscle rigidity or flaccidity
Disturbances in speech, vision, hearing, taste
Tremors
Radiating pain

Common Side Effects of Medications for Neurologic Disorders
Visual disturbances
Lack of muscular coordination
Skin rashes
Drowsiness
Anorexia
Irritability
Headaches
Impotence
Dry mouth
Nightmares

The nervous system is composed of the brain and spinal cord (the **central nervous system [CNS]**) and the nerves (**peripheral nervous system [PNS]**) (Figure 29-1). **Neurons,** the basic cells of the nervous system, carry nerve impulses from one part of the body to another. Axons carry nerve information away from the nerve cell body, and dendrites carry information to the nerve cell body (Figure 29-2). At the junction of neurons, the continuation of the messages is performed by neurotransmitters such as **acetylcholine (ACh),** which stimulates the nerve ending, and **cholinesterase,** which enzymatically breaks down ACh to inhibit its actions (Figure 29-3). Other neurotransmitters, or **neurohormones,** include the **catecholamines,** serotonin, and peptides such as endorphins.

Incoming messages are received and passed through dendrites, processed in the cell body, and transported to the axon. Messages exit by an axon terminal and

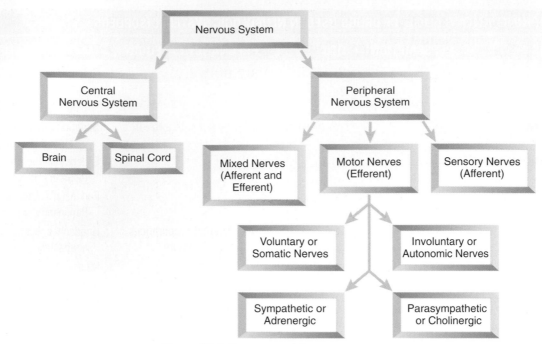

Figure 29-1 Components of the nervous system.

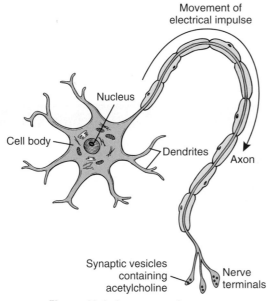

Figure 29-2 Components of a neuron.

continue by either electrical or chemical transport across the synapse to form electrical impulses for moving the impulse through the nerve tract, allowing nerves to react. Drugs can act directly on impulses and their receptors to induce or reduce nerve transmission.

As a neurotransmitter, ACh has various parasympathetic effects such as peristalsis, vasodilation, and cardiac inhibition. Voluntary muscles are contracted by release of ACh at the neuromuscular junction, causing muscle fibers to contract simultaneously for body movement.

Variations in ACh transmission and inhibition by cholinesterase cause diseases related to body movement.

Catecholamines, stored in the brain, are attached to sympathetic effector cells of the **autonomic nervous system (ANS)** to depress brain stimulation. An increase in catecholamines and serotonin causes cerebral stimulation, allowing drugs to have a depressing effect in the brain.

Neuroactive peptides such as endorphins or enkephalins affect neuron activity by either increasing or decreasing synthesis, release, or breakdown of neurotransmitters at the synapse. Endorphins are peptides that suppress pain and are the basis for acupuncture and transcutaneous electrical nerve stimulation (TENS) for pain relief. Enkephalins decrease perception and emotional aspects of pain by blocking spinal cord receptors. (Research the nervous system and its anatomy and physiology for more in-depth information about nerve transmissions.)

The brain is covered by nerve cells that encircle its capillary walls to form the **blood-brain barrier.** This barrier prevents passage of many drugs and large molecules into the brain but allows substances with small molecules (such as water, alcohol, oxygen, and carbon dioxide, as well as glucose and lipid-soluble materials) to pass for absorption and is a type of security system against toxic effects of some drugs on the CNS. Today's pharmaceutical research involves ways to increase blood-brain barrier permeability so specific medications needed for treatment of brain diseases can be absorbed directly. Drug actions requiring brain use are directly related to the section of the brain affected by medications. Figure 29-4 shows brain areas and the specific function of each.

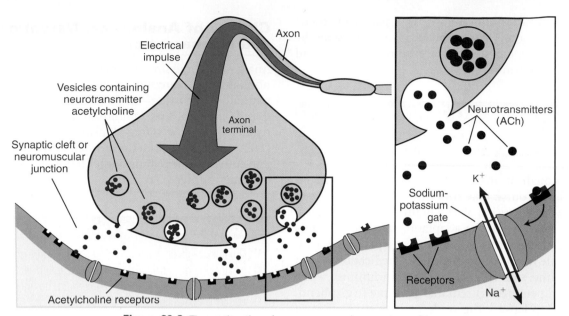

Figure 29-3 The continuation of nerve messages by neurotransmitters.

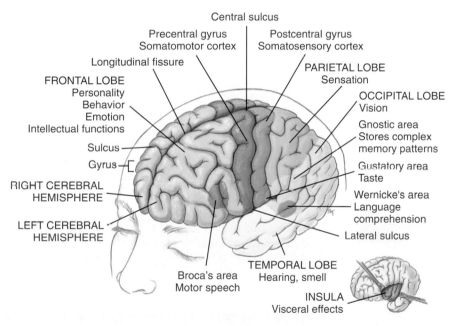

Figure 29-4 The areas of the brain and their function in homeostasis. (From Applegate EJ: *The anatomy and physiology learning system,* ed 4, St Louis, 2011, Saunders.)

When neurons are over active or hyperexcited, too many messages are transmitted at a rapid, irregular rate, leading to distortion and incorrect interpretations of stimuli, which result in seizures. If neurons are not receiving sufficient stimulation, neurons cannot detect nerve transmissions, causing a decrease in body function. Thus nervous system medications are dependent on neuron stimulation, as well as the ability to cross the brain-blood barrier and neuromuscular junctions.

The ANS is also dependent on neuronal actions. The *sympathetic* nerves, also called *adrenergic* nerves, are responsible for body safety through the "fight-or-flight" mechanism by stimulating two neurohormones—epinephrine or adrenaline, and norepinephrine or noradrenaline. This mechanism supplies functions vital to body survival when the person must either react (fight) or run away (flight). When the ANS responds to stimuli, blood and nerve stimulation bypasses body parts and organs not vital for survival, causing extra blood and nerve supply to be sent to areas of stress.

The **parasympathetic nervous system** or *cholinergic system* conserves energy through the neurohormone ACh and the enzyme cholinesterase. The parasympathetic system controls the "feed-or-breed" body functions by slowing the heart, digesting food, eliminating waste, and producing sex hormones.

EFFECTS OF LONG-TERM DRUG USE ON THE CENTRAL NERVOUS SYSTEM

When CNS medications are taken chronically, the effects from the long course may differ from those seen when the agent was first used, as the brain adapts to medications over time. When the adaptation is beneficial, it is considered therapeutic; detrimental adaptation is considered a side effect. With some CNS medications taken for a long time, side effect intensity may diminish while desired therapeutic effect remains the same (e.g., phenobarbital for epilepsy). The undesired sedative effect of phenobarbital is decreased over time while the desired anticonvulsant therapy is retained.

Certain drugs, typically antipsychotics and antidepressants, must be taken for several weeks before full therapeutic effects appear or until the CNS responds and modifies its response to drug exposure, although side effects may occur immediately. In the meantime, these drugs have an increased therapeutic effect that is not readily detected. **Tolerance,** an adaptation of the brain to a medication, and **physical dependence,** in which the drug-adapted brain requires the medication or withdrawal symptoms occur when the medication is stopped, are also manifestations of the CNS and its adaptive abilities. These responses are seen with medications used over prolonged periods (see Chapters 2 and 31).

ANALGESICS

Analgesics are used to relieve pain—a unique and subjective symptom that is a highly individualized response. Types, signs, and symptoms of pain and interventions for controlling or preventing pain are different for each person. A feared symptom, pain is important because it warns that the body is malfunctioning or is out of homeostasis. Only the person experiencing pain can describe the symptoms, intensity, and site.

Analgesics are the subject of Chapter 15, but a short review is included here because of their interactions with the nervous system. The physical discomfort of pain may cause ANS responses such as hypertension, **diaphoresis,** pallor, restlessness, anxiety, tensed muscles, and inability to concentrate. Pain impulses are transmitted on afferent, or sensory, nerve fibers to the CNS for interpretation. The brain releases the natural pain relievers enkephalins and endorphins to control pain. When these are not fully effective, analgesics are ordered for pain relief.

Classes of Analgesics: Narcotics and Nonnarcotics

Analgesics come in two main groups—narcotics and nonnarcotics. Narcotic analgesics are either opioids—naturally occurring—or opiates—synthetically produced—medications. Opioids and some nonopioids are regulated by the Drug Enforcement Administration (DEA), others are prescription items without regulation, and some with less abuse potential may even be bought over the counter (OTC).

Patient Education for Compliance

1. Opioids are given in specific doses that should not be adjusted or abruptly discontinued without medical direction.
2. Dietary fiber and fluid intake should be increased when taking analgesics, especially with opioids. If constipation occurs, a laxative may be indicated.
3. Initial doses of opioids may cause nausea and vomiting, which can be minimized with an antiemetic and by remaining calm. Side effects usually subside with each administered dose.
4. Analgesics may cause drowsiness, decreased mental alertness, and decreased physical coordination; hazardous activities should be stopped while evaluating drowsiness.
5. Orthostatic hypotension may occur with analgesics, especially opioids. Care should be taken with position changes. Opioid medications may increase effects of antihypertensives, especially causing orthostatic hypotension.
6. Severe or recurrent pain for more than 10 days or high continuous fever for more than 3 days should be reported to health care provider.
7. Potential for physical and psychologic dependence and tolerance with opioids, sedatives, analgesics, and hypnotics exists. These drugs should be taken on a limited basis for short periods of time *except* by terminally ill patients. Terminally ill patients should be kept as pain-free as possible.

Important Facts about Analgesics

- Analgesics are used to relieve pain without loss of consciousness. Some types of pain such as neuropathic pain and pain from inflammatory processes may not respond to opioid medications.
- Opioids are the most effective analgesics, with morphine being the prototype for analgesic relief.
- Respiratory depression is a serious adverse reaction to opioids, as are constipation, urinary retention, orthostatic hypotension, and vomiting.
- Because prolonged opioid use leads to physical dependence and abrupt stoppage will lead to withdrawal symptoms, these drugs should be gradually withdrawn.

ANESTHETICS

Two types of anesthesia are general and local. Anesthesia by definition is used to produce a loss of sensation. Patients are often fearful when anticipating surgery because of surgery itself or fear of feeling pain during the procedure. The allied health professional should attempt to dispel fear by assuring the patient that anesthesia provides sleep throughout with amnesia about the experience. This educational step is important because excessive fear may disrupt surgical procedures. Therefore this section on anesthesia is presented to assist with patient education.

General Anesthetics

General anesthetics produce their desired effects by blocking all sensory impulses to the brain, causing unconsciousness. Stages of anesthesia are controlled and passed through during induction and are reversed during recovery. Patients undergoing surgery are usually taken to stage 3 to allow muscular relaxation.

Stage 1: Analgesia starts with administration of anesthetic and lasts to loss of consciousness. Characteristics are euphoria, distortions of perceptions, and amnesia. Some surgery can be performed at this level.

Stage 2: Delirium begins with loss of consciousness and extends to the beginning of surgical anesthesia. During this stage, through which induction is rapid, involuntary muscles are active, breathing is irregular, and hypertension and tachycardia may occur because of muscle excitability.

Stage 3: Surgical anesthesia occurs, with muscle relaxation and respiratory depression, lasting until spontaneous respirations cease.

Stage 4: Medullary depression is usually caused by anesthesia overdose, beginning with cessation of respirations and ending with circulatory collapse causing death.

The most common route of administration for general anesthesia is inhalation, although some general anesthetics are given intravenously (IV). The main intravenous drugs are thiopental (Pentothal), ketamine (Ketalar), and midazolam (Versed). Diazepam (Valium) may be used to aid induction of anesthesia or as a preoperative medication.

Preanesthetic Medications

Preanesthetic medications are given to reduce anxiety, to produce preoperative amnesia, and to relieve preoperative and postoperative pain. Medications are also often used prophylactically to reduce adverse reactions such as excessive salivation, coughing, vomiting, and increased bronchial secretions. Benzodiazepines such as diazepam and barbiturates such as secobarbital or pentobarbital are given to reduce anxiety and produce amnesia by producing mild sedation. Anticholinergic medications such as atropine decrease the bradycardia risk during surgery while also drying secretions.

Midazolam for Conscious Sedation

Intravenous midazolam may be used for induction of anesthesia or for conscious sedation. The patient is unperturbed and passive but is capable of responding to commands needed for minor surgery or endoscopic procedures. Versed does cause respiratory and cardiac depression.

Local Anesthetics

Pain perception is the first sensation lost, followed by cold, warmth, touch, and deep pressure, in that order. Local anesthetics work by interfering with nerve conduction and pain perception from the body to CNS. The great advantage over general anesthesia is that pain is suppressed without loss of consciousness and nervous system depression, allowing medical and surgical procedures to be performed with less risk and pain.

The duration of action of local anesthetics with rapid onset in most cases is longer than necessary, whereas prolonged procedures may necessitate repeated administration. Vasoconstrictors—usually epinephrine—are often added to local anesthetics to prolong anesthesia and reduce risk of toxicity. Systemic reactions such as palpitations, tachycardia, nervousness, and hypertension may occur with vasoconstrictor use.

In the anesthetized area, blood flow is important in determining how long anesthesia will last. In areas with many blood vessels, the anesthetic effect is quickly carried away; in areas where few blood vessels are found or blood flow is restricted, a prolonged duration will occur. If local anesthetics are absorbed into the bloodstream, adverse reactions such as bradycardia and symptoms related to the heart conduction impulses may occur. CNS excitability followed by depression and drowsiness may occur if large doses are given; allergic reactions are not common but may occur.

Local anesthetics may be administered either topically as surface anesthetics applied to the skin or a mucous membrane or by infiltration as injections. Therapeutic uses for topically applied anesthetics are to relieve pain, itching, and soreness from infections, burns, sunburns, diaper rash, wounds, bruises, abrasions, plant poisoning, and insect bites and neuropathic-type pain. Applications to mucous membranes include those in the nose, mouth, pharynx, larynx, trachea, vagina, and urethra. Local anesthetics may also be used for hemorrhoids, anal fissures, and anal pruritus. Infiltration anesthesia stops conduction of nerve impulses and blocks motor neurons by injecting local anesthetics, such as procaine and lidocaine, into specific areas for surgery or orthopedic manipulation.

Procaine

Procaine (Novocain), a local anesthetic agent first made in 1905, is not effective topically and so must be administered by injection, often given in combination with epinephrine to slow the absorption. Procaine is available in 1%, 2%, and 10% solutions for injection and with epinephrine added in ratios of 1:1000, 1:10,000, and 1:50,000. The allied health professional should carefully read labels to ensure selection of the correct medication as ordered by percentage of procaine and correct ratio of epinephrine.

Lidocaine

Lidocaine (Xylocaine), introduced in 1948, is one of the most widely used local anesthetics because it may be administered topically or by injection with rare allergic reactions. This agent produces anesthesia more rapidly, more intensely, and with a more prolonged effect than procaine. The effects may be prolonged further by adding epinephrine. Injectable lidocaine comes in concentrations ranging from 0.5% to 20%. Forms of lidocaine include creams, ointments, gels, aerosols, and solutions.

Did You Know?

Because lidocaine suppresses cardiac muscle excitability by blocking sodium channels, it is also used to treat cardiac arrhythmias.

Cocaine

Cocaine, an excellent topical anesthetic that acts rapidly and has a duration of effect of about an hour, is used primarily for anesthesia of the ear, nose, and throat. A

TABLE 29-1 TOPICAL LOCAL ANESTHETICS

GENERIC NAME/ TRADE NAME	SITES OF APPLICATION	TIME TO PEAK EFFECT (MIN)	DURATION OF ACTION (MIN)
dibucaine (Nupercainal)	Skin	<5	15-45
lidocaine (Xylocaine)	Skin, mucous membranes	2-5	15-45
benzocaine (many trade names)	Skin, mucous membranes	<5	30-60
cocaine	Mucous membranes	3-8	30-60
tetracaine (Pontocaine)	Skin, mucous membranes	3-8	30-60

TABLE 29-2 INJECTABLE LOCAL ANESTHETICS

GENERIC/TRADE NAME	ONSET OF ACTION (MIN)	DURATION OF ACTION (MIN)*
procaine (Novocain)	2-5	15-60
tetracaine (Pontocaine)	≤15	120-180
lidocaine (Xylocaine and others)	<2	30-60
mepivacaine (Carbocaine, Polocaine)	3-5	45-90
bupivacaine (Marcaine, Sensorcaine)	5	120-240

*Epinephrine may increase anesthesia duration by two to three times.

Schedule II controlled medication, cocaine causes vasoconstriction and so should not be given with epinephrine because of an increased risk of cardiovascular toxicity. The medication is available as soluble tablets, powder, and 4% solution, the usual form used (Tables 29-1 and 29-2).

Patient Education for Compliance

Patients who have received local anesthetics should take care to avoid activities that might injure anesthetized areas that cannot respond to pain signals.

TABLE 29-3 EFFECTS OF SEDATIVES AND HYPNOTICS ON THE CENTRAL NERVOUS SYSTEM (CNS)

INCREASED DOSE OF MEDICATION	EFFECTS OF DRUG	PSYCHOLOGIC AND PHYSICAL RESPONSE	CNS STIMULATION
Low dose	No drug ↓	Stress, tension	CNS stimulated
↓	Tranquilizing ↓	Calm	Gradual depression of CNS
↓	Hypnotic ↓		
High dose	Relaxed, drowsy	Sleep	CNS depressed

Important Facts about Anesthetics

- General anesthetics produce unconsciousness and insensitivity to painful stimuli.
- Local analgesics reduce sensitivity to pain without loss of consciousness. Some local anesthetics may be mixed with epinephrine to cause vasoconstriction and prolong anesthetic effects.

SEDATIVES AND HYPNOTICS

All body activities are influenced by the CNS. Depression of the CNS reduces physical and mental activity and is often related to use of barbiturates and alcohol (see Chapter 30). **Sedatives** and **hypnotics** such as **pentobarbital** (Nembutal) and **phenobarbital** (Luminal) are used therapeutically to decrease CNS activity. The major difference between drugs being used as hypnotics and sedatives is the amount of depression and sedation induced. Small doses of medication may be used for daytime sedation, whereas larger doses of the same drug may be used to produce hypnotic effects and produce sleep induction (Tables 29-3 and 29-4).

Sedatives, used to reduce nervousness, excitability, and irritability, produce calming effects. When various emotional or medical conditions cause anxiety or tension, sleep may be interrupted and sedation may be indicated. Benzodiazepines such as **diazepam** (Valium) and **lorazepam** (Ativan) are used for their sedative effects as well as for controlling stress related to hypertension (Table 29-5).

Hypnotics, used to induce and maintain sleep, should be used intermittently only when needed for transient insomnia. Some drugs more frequently used as hypnotics are **chloral hydrate** (Noctec) and **temazepam** (Restoril). Because tolerance to hypnotics develops and effectiveness decreases after several weeks of continuous

TABLE 29-4 ACTION TIMES OF BARBITURATES

CLASSIFICATION	DURATION OF ACTION	TYPICAL MEDICATIONS
Ultra-short-acting agent	20 minutes or less	thiopental (Pentothal)
Short-acting agents	3-4 hr	secobarbital (Seconal)
		pentobarbital (Nembutal)
Intermediate-acting agents	6-8 hr	amobarbital (Amytal)
		aprobarbital (Alurate)
		butabarbital (Butisol)
Long-acting agents	10-16 hr	phenobarbital (Luminal)
		mephobarbital (Mebaral)

BOX 29-1 GENERAL GUIDELINES FOR DRUG THERAPY FOR TRANSIENT INSOMNIA

Use short-term therapy with lowest effective dose for shortest time period.
Assess patient regularly to ensure need for continued therapy and that underlying pathology is not a cause.
Interrupt therapy to allow tolerance to decline.
Use hypnotics cautiously with those who snore heavily, are in respiratory distress, or are pregnant or suicidal.

use, hypnotic use should be limited to 2 to 4 weeks. Benzodiazepines are frequently used over barbiturates as sedatives or hypnotics because of their safety. Other CNS depressants such as alcohol should not be used with antianxiety drugs and hypnotics and sedatives. Box 29-1 lists general rules for treatment of transient insomnia.

TABLE 29-5 SELECT SEDATIVES AND HYPNOTICS

GENERIC NAME/TRADE NAME (SCHEDULE)	USUAL ADULT DOSE, ROUTE, AND FREQUENCY	INDICATIONS FOR USE	DRUG INTERACTIONS
BARBITURATES		Hypnotic, sedative	alcohol, analgesics, MAOIs, other sedatives, theophylline, corticosteroids, oral contraceptives, oral anticoagulants
amobarbital (II)* (Amytal)	Hypnotic: 65-200 mg IM 1-2 hr before surgery		
mephobarbital (IV)† (Mebaral)	Sedative: 32-100 mg PO tid-qid Epilepsy: 400-600 mg PO qd or divided	Also used with epilepsy	
pentobarbital (II)* (Nembutal)	Sedative: 30-120 mg PO qd, IM, IV Hypnotic: 100-200 mg PO hs Preoperative use: 100-200 mg IM		
secobarbital (II)‡ (Seconal)	Hypnotic: 100-200 mg PO qd, IM		
phenobarbital (IV)† (Luminal)	Hypnotic: 100-320 mg IM, IV, PO hs		
BENZODIAZEPINES			
alprazolam*‡ (III) (Xanax)	0.25-1 mg PO tid	Sedative, anxiety, alcohol withdrawal	cimetidine, digoxin, macrolides, ethanol, grapefruit juice, phenytoin, carbamazepine
chlordiazepoxide† (IV) (Librium)	5-25 mg PO tid-qid 50-100 mg IM, IV		ethanol, cimetidine, fluconazole, levodopa
clonazepam*‡ (IV) (Klonopin)	0.5-2 mg PO tid	Also used for seizures	valproic acid, disulfiram
clorazepate† (III) (Tranxene)	30 mg/day PO bid-tid	Also used for seizures	cimetidine, ethanol, rifampin, disulfiram
diazepam† (III) (Valium)	2-10 mg PO tid-qid, IM, IV	Also used with skeletal muscle relaxants and for seizures	See alprazolam
estazolam*‡ (IV) (ProSom)	1-2 mg PO hs	Insomnia	ethanol, cimetidine, disulfiram, macrolides, rifampin
flurazepam†§ (IV)	15-30 mg PO hs	Insomnia	beta blockers, isoniazid (INH), cimetidine, clozapine, disulfiram, loxapine, macrolides, rifampin, omeprazole
lorazepam† (III) (Ativan)	1-10 mg PO bid-tid in divided doses	Anxiety, insomnia, alcohol withdrawal	ethanol, fluconazole, itraconazole
midazolam‡ (II) (Versed)	IM, IV, varies with level of sedation	Sedation	calcium channel blockers, macrolides, lorazepam, and ethanol

CNS, Central nervous system; *IM*, intramuscularly; *IV*, intravenously; *MAOI*, monoamine oxidase inhibitor; *OTC*, over the counter; *PO*, orally.
*Intermediate acting.
†Long acting.
‡Short acting.
§Dangerous in older adults.
Note: The Roman numerals in parenthesis behind the generic name is the indication of the DEA schedule that applies to that medication.

TABLE 29-5 SELECT SEDATIVES AND HYPNOTICS—cont'd

GENERIC NAME/TRADE NAME (SCHEDULE)	USUAL ADULT DOSE, ROUTE, AND FREQUENCY	INDICATIONS FOR USE	DRUG INTERACTIONS
oxazepam*‡ (III)	10-15 mg PO tid-qid	Anxiety, alcohol withdrawal	
prazepam† (IV) (Centrax)	20-40 mg PO qd	Anxiety, alcohol withdrawal	See estazolam
temazepam*‡ (IV) (Restoril)	15-30 mg PO hs	Sedative, hypnotic	alcohol, CNS depressants
triazolam*‡ (IV) (Halcion)	0.125-0.5 mg PO hs	Hypnotic, insomnia	alcohol, CNS depressants
zaleplon (IV) (Sonata)	5-10 mg PO hs	Insomnia	alcohol
eszopiclone (IV) (Lunesta)	1-3 mg PO hs	Insomnia	alcohol
ramelteon (Rozerem)	8 mg PO hs	Insomnia	rifampin
chloral hydrate (IV)	250 mg-1 g PO hs	Sedative, hypnotic	alcohol, anticoagulants
zolpidem (IV) (Ambien)	5-10 mg PO hs	Hypnotic	CNS depressants, alcohol
buspirone¶ (BuSpar)	15-30 mg PO bid-tid	Hypnotic, sedative	MAOIs
hydroxyzine¶ (Atarax)	5-100 mg PO qid, IM	Antianxiety, antiemetic	alcohol
(Vistaril)	25-100 mg PO qid, IM	Sedative, hypnotic	
INSOMNIA MEDICATIONS			
diphenhydramine (OTC) (Nytol, Sominex, Sleep-Eze, Benadryl)	According to package instructions		alcohol
doxylamine (OTC) (Unisom)	According to package instructions		

¶Not included in Controlled Substances Act—no evidence for abuse.

Treatment of Sleep Disorders

Some medication classes, such as barbiturates and benzodiazepines as well as some OTC medications, are used for treating sleep disorders.

Barbiturates

Barbiturates, some of the oldest drugs, produce dose-dependent depression of CNS. Most of these medications are classified as either Schedule II or III medications, although phenobarbital is a Schedule IV drug in most states (see Table 29-5). Depending on the amount given, these medications produce CNS depression and mood alteration from reduced excitation to sedation followed by hypnosis and deep coma. After 2 weeks of continuous use, the desired effects at the same dose are not produced. The tendency is then to increase the dose to produce desired effects, leading to physical and psychologic dependence. After prolonged use of barbiturates,

withdrawal symptoms may occur when medication is stopped. These medications must be used with care in the elderly, in debilitated persons, in those with severe renal and liver disease, and in those who have suicidal tendencies. Barbiturates should be avoided in geriatric patients because CNS depression, confusion, and ataxia are often reported (Box 29-2). The short-acting benzodiazepines are safer agents than barbiturates and so are used more often.

Elderly individuals consume one third to one half of the sedatives and hypnotics prescribed because most, especially women, have changes in sleep patterns that come with age. The most common reasons the elderly give for being unable to sleep include respiratory problems, pain, and cramping of leg muscles. Of concern is the susceptibility to many side effects occurring with sedatives and hypnotics. Elderly patients need to be watched for increased excitability, hostility, confusion, and hallucinations.

BOX 29-2 IMPLICATIONS OF SEDATIVE AND HYPNOTIC USE IN THE ELDERLY

Sleep disturbances are common in elderly because preexisting conditions, such as arthritis, dyspnea, and cardiac arrhythmias, interrupt sleep.

Hypnotics should be used for short duration to treat acute insomnia and should not be given long enough for tolerance or dependency to develop.

Daytime sedation may occur when long-acting hypnotics are prescribed.

Use of relaxation techniques, establishment of regular bedtimes, and avoidance of caffeine should be attempted before use of hypnotic medications.

OTC sleeping aids often contain antihistamines, which may cause dizziness, tinnitus, blurred vision, gastrointestinal disturbances, and dry mouth.

 LEARNING TIP

Most generic names for barbiturates end in "barbital," and the trade names end in "al."

TABLE 29-6 SAFETY OF BENZODIAZEPINES VERSUS BARBITURATES

FACTORS RELATED TO SAFETY	BENZODIAZEPINES	BARBITURATES
Relative safety	High	Low
Depression of central nervous system function	Low	High
Respiratory depression	Low	High
Potential for suicide	Low	High
Chance of causing physical dependency	Low	High
Potential for abuse	Low	High
Tolerance potential	Low	High

Benzodiazepines

Benzodiazepines, or anxiolytics, are among the most widely prescribed medications because of many advantages over older medicines such as barbiturates, *meprobamate,* and alcohol. *Diazepam* (Valium), the prototype of this class of medications, is indicated for anxiety disorders, alcohol withdrawal, preoperative medications, insomnia, seizures, and neuromuscular diseases such as skeletal muscle spasms or neuron dysfunction. Like barbiturates, benzodiazepines are Schedules III and IV medications with short- to long-acting effects. These drugs have fewer deaths from toxicity and overdose, a lower potential for abuse and side effects, and fewer drug interactions. These drugs have muscle relaxant, antianxiety, anticonvulsant, and sedating and hypnotic effects (see Table 29-5). See Chapter 30 for more information on benzodiazepines as anxiolytics.

LEARNING TIP

Many of the generic names for benzodiazepines end in "pam" or "lam."

When comparing barbiturates and benzodiazepines for uses or abuses, these medications are at opposite poles. Whereas barbiturates are dangerous, benzodiazepines are much safer (Table 29-6).

Other Medications Used as Sedatives and Hypnotics

A number of antianxiety drugs and sedatives and hypnotics do not fall into the categories previously listed. Their actions are similar, causing sedation and hypnosis; agents such as *zolpidem* (Ambien) are therefore Schedules III and IV medications, with a potential for misuse and abuse especially by the elderly. *Buspirone* (BuSpar) does not cause sedation, has no abuse potential, and does not intensify CNS depressants and its antianxiety effects take an extended time to develop; it is the drug of choice because of these properties (see Table 29-5).

Other Products Available OTC for Insomnia

Antihistamines may cause excessive drowsiness when given with sedatives and hypnotics and may even produce a "hangover," or sedative effect, the next day. The Food and Drug Administration (FDA) has approved two antihistamines for use with insomnia—*diphenhydramine* (Nytol, Sominex, Benadryl) and *doxylamine* (Unisom). These medications are not as effective as benzodiazepines, and tolerance to the hypnotic effect develops quickly, often in less than 2 weeks (see Table 29-5).

Alternative products that do not require a prescription such as valerian root (an herbal supplement) and melatonin (a dietary supplement) have been employed to promote sleep. Valerian root can assist with falling asleep but does not help maintain sleep and must be taken for a week or more to be effective. Melatonin is secreted by the pineal gland with an action that is stimulated with darkness. Trials have indicated that melatonin supplements can promote sleep. Large doses have side effects such as headaches, hangover, nightmares, hypothermia, and transient depression.

Patient Education for Compliance

1. Potential for overdose with elderly using sedatives is always present, and signs of confusion, agitation, hallucinations, and hyperexcitability may show that this reaction is occurring.
2. Withdrawal from analgesics, hypnotics, and sedatives after prolonged use may lead to nightmares, hallucinations, insomnia, or a combination of these.
3. With sedatives and hypnotics, daytime sedation is possible, and individuals taking these drugs should avoid hazardous activities.
4. Medications for sedation and sleep should be taken at lowest dose possible for shortest period of time.
5. Alcohol and all other CNS depressants such as antihistamines (e.g., OTC cold, cough, or allergy medications) should be avoided when sedatives are being taken. Some medications contain antihistamines and accentuate drowsiness, whereas others contain CNS stimulants and defeat the purpose of sedatives.
6. Patients having difficulty sleeping should try to identify the cause. Ideally, the cause rather than sleep disturbance should be treated.

Important Facts about Sedatives and Hypnotics

- Drugs that promote sleep are called *hypnotics,* with daytime sedation and amnesia being chief side effect.
- Barbiturates, regulated by Drug Enforcement Administration (DEA), have high potential for abuse and cause significant tolerance and physical dependence.
- Benzodiazepines are safer with low abuse potential and cause less tolerance and dependence; therefore these medications are preferred to barbiturates and other general CNS depressants.
- Principal indications for benzodiazepines are insomnia, anxiety, and seizure disorders. Benzodiazepines are drugs of choice for transient insomnia. Administration should be intermittent and the drugs should be given for only 2 to 3 weeks because of physical dependence, but withdrawal syndrome is usually mild. With longer use, drugs should be decreased over several weeks to months to prevent seizures.

ANTISEIZURE MEDICATIONS

Epilepsy, a group of disorders characterized by hyperexcitability within the CNS, is present in approximately 2.5 million Americans. Abnormal stimuli can produce many symptoms from short periods of unconsciousness to violent **convulsions.** *Seizure* is a term for all epileptic events, whereas *convulsion* relates to abnormal motor movements such as the jerking movements of **grand mal seizures.** Seizures are of two broad types: **focal (partial) seizures** and **generalized seizures.** Box 29-3 compares different types of seizures.

Epilepsy may be controlled but cannot be cured. Early epilepsy control began in the mid-nineteenth century, when bromides were used to reduce seizures. In 1912 phenobarbital was found to produce depression of the brain's motor cortex to reduce the number of seizures; however, the drug had the unpleasant side effect of depressing sensory and motor areas.

BOX 29-3 TYPES OF SEIZURES

I. Focal or partial seizures (limited spread)
   A. Simple seizures: Convulsion of single limb or muscle group with no loss of consciousness
   B. Complex partial seizures: Confused, bizarre behavior with impaired consciousness
II. Generalized seizures (generally produce loss of consciousness)
   A. Nonconvulsive
      1. Absence or petit mal seizures: Loss of consciousness for a short time (10 to 30 seconds) with mild symmetric motor activity to no motor activity at all—may be as mild as only eye blinking
   B. Convulsive
      1. Tonic-clonic or grand mal seizures: Major convulsions with muscle rigidity and synchronous muscle jerks; marked impairment of consciousness
      2. Tonic-psychomotor seizures: Tonic muscle contractions
         a. Uncontrolled seizures: Usually children; multiple seizures per day (up to 100)
         b. Atonic or akinetic seizures: Sudden loss of muscle tone causing collapse of the body or body part without muscular contractions
         c. Myoclonic seizures: Sudden, rapid muscle contractions
         d. Febrile seizures: Tonic-clonic seizures of short duration, usually seen in children with moderate to high temperature levels (children more likely to develop epilepsy later)
      3. Status epilepticus: Uncontrolled seizures lasting 30 minutes or more; may be life threatening

Antiseizure medications allow individuals to have greater self-control by suppressing neuronal malfunction at the seizure focus. Reduction in brain cell excitability reduces the incidence and severity of seizures. Medications control 40% of **absence or petit mal seizures** and reduce the frequency of another 35%. **Tonic-clonic** (grand mal) seizures are better controlled, with complete control achieved in 50% of the patients and greatly reduced frequency in another 35%. **Tonic** (psychomotor) seizures, characterized by tense movements, are controlled in only 35% of patients, but frequency is reduced in another 50% of patients. Antiseizure medicines require dosage adjustments during times of stress or severe illness or with the addition of medications taken for other medical conditions.

Medications for seizures include barbiturates (discussed earlier), with phenobarbital being most frequently used for its antiepileptic properties. Sedative and hypnotic effects are undesired side effects; however, tolerance to sedation develops as a positive effect when barbiturates are used chronically. Sudden withdrawal of barbiturates in seizure-prone patients can produce seizures. Therefore if withdrawal of barbiturates is desired, the dose should be gradually reduced (see Table 29-5).

The benzodiazepines **diazepam** (Valium), **clonazepam** (Klonopin), and **lorazepam** (Ativan) are also used as antiseizure drugs. Diazepam and lorazepam are used to halt seizures in progress. Clonazepam is used for myoclonic, akinetic-atonic, and absence seizures (Table 29-5).

Hydantoins include **phenytoin** (Dilantin), a potent broad-spectrum antiseizure medication for partial and tonic-clonic seizures. These drugs change the nerve cell excitability by decreasing the sodium effect in the brain. Because hyperexcitability is decreased, seizure reduction occurs in most patients. Good dental hygiene and gum care are important with patients taking hydantoins because of gum hyperplasia (Table 29-7).

Fosphenytoin (Cerebyx), used parenterally, is used for status epilepticus and when substitution for oral antiseizure medications is necessary, such as with surgical procedures (see Table 29-7).

✎ LEARNING TIP

Most hydantoins have names that end in "nytoin."

Succinimides, used exclusively for the treatment of absence or petit mal seizures, decrease calcium currents in the brain to play an important role in treating these seizures. The most commonly used succinimide is **ethosuximide** (Zarontin), with **methsuximide** (Celontin) and **phensuximide** (Milontin) being two other medications in the group (see Table 29-7).

TABLE 29-7 ANTISEIZURE MEDICATIONS

GENERIC NAME/ TRADE NAME	USUAL ADULT DOSE, ROUTE, AND FREQUENCY	INDICATIONS FOR USE	DRUG INTERACTIONS
BARBITURATES phenobarbital, mephobarbital, and so on (see Table 29-5)		Epilepsy—partial tonic-clonic seizures	See Table 29-5
BENZODIAZEPINES diazepam, clonazepam, lorazepam, clorazepate (see Table 29-5)		Myoclonic, absence, and akinetic seizures and status epilepticus	See Table 29-5
HYDANTOINS	All are highly individualized	Partial and tonic-clonic seizures	Oral contraceptives for all
phenytoin (Dilantin)	50-200 mg PO bid-tid		glucocorticoids, isoniazid (INH), diazepam, amantadine, phenobarbital, alcohol
fosphenytoin (Cerebyx)	Individualized, IM, IV	For use when oral medications cannot be used	

GI, Gastrointestinal; *IM,* intramuscularly; *IV,* intravenously; *PO,* orally; *TB,* tuberculosis.

TABLE 29-7 ANTISEIZURE MEDICATIONS—cont'd

GENERIC NAME/ TRADE NAME	USUAL ADULT DOSE, ROUTE, AND FREQUENCY	INDICATIONS FOR USE	DRUG INTERACTIONS
Major Side Effects of Hydantoins:			
Skin rashes, hirsutism, overgrowth of mouth gums, gingivitis, dizziness, visual disturbances, postural imbalance			
SUCCINIMIDES		Absence seizures	None indicated
ethosuximide (Zarontin)	500 mg/day PO qd-tid		
phensuximide (Milontin)	1-3 g PO tid-qid		
methsuximide (Celontin)	300-1200 mg PO tid-qid		
Major Side Effects of Succinimides:			
GI symptoms, drowsiness, diarrhea, dizziness, blood dyscrasias			
MISCELLANEOUS ANTISEIZURE AGENTS		Partial and generalized tonic-clonic seizures and mixed seizures	steroids, cimetidine, anticoagulants, lithium
carbamazepine (Tegretol)	Varies		acetaminophen, antidepressants, oral contraceptives, calcium channel blockers
valproic acid (Depakene)	100-200 mg PO varies	All generalized seizures and partial seizures	Other antiseizure drugs, medications for TB, salicylates, macrolides
valproate (Depakote)	125-250 mg PO (as sprinkle or tablet)	As with valproic acid	Same as valproic acid
primidone (Mysoline)	250 mg-500 PO tid-qid	Psychomotor seizures	digoxin, alcohol, oral anticoagulants, valproic acid, carbamazepine
gabapentin (Neurontin)	100-800 mg PO tid	Partial seizures	antacids
lamotrigine (Lamictal)	Varies	Partial seizures	carbimazole, valproic acid, phenytoin, phenobarbital
levetiracetam (Keppra) (Keppra XR)	500-1000 mg PO, IV bid 500-1000 mg bid PO	Partial seizers	Basically none
oxcarbazepine (Trileptal)	300-1200 mg PO bid	Partial seizures	Same
topiramate (Topamax)	25-400 mg PO in divided doses	Partial seizures	Same
tiagabine (Gabitril)	4 qd-56 mg PO in divided doses	Partial tonic-clonic seizures, migraine headaches, alcohol treatment	Same, oral contraceptives
zonisamide (Zonegran)	100-500 mg PO qd	Partial seizures and others as needed	Antifungals

Major Side Effects of Miscellaneous Antiseizure Agents:

carbamazepine—sedation, GI symptoms; *valproic acid and valproate*—nausea, vomiting, diarrhea, tremors; *primidone*—GI symptoms, anorexia, drowsiness; *gabapentin*—sleepiness, ataxia, fatigue, nausea, severe dizziness; *lamotrigine*—dizziness, serious rash, diplopia, headache, ataxia, somnolence; *levetiracetam*—drowsiness, asthenia; *oxcarbazepine*—dizziness, nausea, headache, diarrhea, ataxia, nervousness; *topiramate*—dizziness, asthenia, somnolence, confusion, headache, tremors; *tiagabine*—somnolence, dizziness, ataxia, diplopia, nystagmus, nervousness, nausea, tremor; *zonisamide*—drowsiness, dizziness, headaches, nausea, impaired speech

Other antiseizure medications include new drugs, as well as drugs that have been around for a long time:

- **Carbamazepine** (Tegretol), similar to tricyclic antidepressants, blocks sodium ion channels, much like phenytoin. This medication also possesses analgesic properties for neuralgia and is used to treat bipolar disorders.
- **Oxcarbazepine** (Trileptal), a derivative of carbamazepine, is better tolerated and may be used for partial seizures in adults and children.
- **Valproic acid** (Depakene) and **valproate** (Depakote) can be used with all types of seizures, as well as for migraine headache prophylaxis, by inhibiting neurotransmitters to the CNS. These medications have the potential to cause fatal liver toxicity.
- **Primidone** (Mysoline), related chemically to barbiturates, is metabolized and converted into phenobarbital.
- **Gabapentin** (Neurontin) suppresses neuron excitability, which initiates epileptic seizures much like brain neurons excitability.
- Several new drugs such as **lamotrigine** (Lamictal), **tiagabine** (Gabitril), and **zonisamide** (Zonegran) for control of partial seizures have been introduced.
- **Topiramate** (Topamax) has been introduced for partial seizures and tonic-clonic seizures, as well as treatment of alcoholism and prevention of migraine headaches.
- **Levetiracetam** (Keppra) is used in adults for adjunctive therapy in partial seizures, with the advantage of not interacting with other medications (see Table 29-7).

Did You Know?

Neurontin, first introduced as an antiseizure medication, is being used for severe neurogenic pain.

Patient Education for Compliance

1. Persons taking antiseizure medications should not omit, increase, or decrease medications without permission of the health care provider.
2. Antiseizure medications should not be discontinued abruptly.
3. Antiseizure medications may cause drowsiness or dizziness; therefore avoid hazardous tasks until side effects are evaluated.

Patient Education for Compliance—cont'd

4. OTC medications should not be used with antiseizure medications without physician's permission.
5. No alcohol should be consumed while taking antiseizure medications.
6. Use good dental hygiene after each meal, especially with hydantoins, because of gum tissue overgrowth.
7. Keep a record of all seizures—date, time, length, and so forth.

Important Facts about Antiseizure Medications

- The goal of antiseizure medication is to reduce seizures to the extent that the patient can live a normal life; however, complete seizure elimination may not be possible. Most antiseizure medications are selective for particular seizure types. Successful treatment depends on finding the most effective drug for each individual patient. Noncompliance is the main reason for treatment failure.
- Antiseizure medication must be tapered and not abruptly withdrawn.
- Most antiseizure medication causes central nervous system (CNS) depression; other CNS depressants such as alcohol, opioids, and antihistamines should not be used concurrently.
- Phenytoin, phenobarbital, and carbamazepine are active against partial and tonic-clonic seizures but not absence seizures.
- Phenytoin causes gingival hyperplasia.

DRUGS FOR PARKINSON'S DISEASE

Parkinson's disease is thought to be caused by dopamine deficiency and an ACh excess within the CNS. When regulating voluntary muscle movements, ACh is an excitatory neurotransmitter, with dopamine inhibiting, or stopping, the ACh neurotransmitters to decrease muscle movements. Normally ACh and dopamine are balanced, providing smooth, better-controlled muscle movement. A decrease in dopamine produces excesses in ACh, causing tremors and muscle rigidity typical of parkinsonism. Drug treatment is effective in reducing symptoms, but patients become progressively disabled and may become immobile in later stages. Depression or dementia may occur, causing memory impairment and alterations in thinking. Medications for parkinsonism involve increasing dopamine levels by administering levodopa—a precursor of dopamine—or administering medications that stimulate dopamine receptors. Reduction of ACh

BOX 29-4 NOMENCLATURE FOR DRUGS ACTIVE ON THE AUTONOMIC NERVOUS SYSTEM

Division of the Autonomic Nervous System	Important Neuroactive Substances	Drugs That Promote or Reproduce Effects of This System	Drugs That Reduce or Block Effects of This System
Parasympathetic (cholinergic)	acetylcholine cholinesterase	**Parasympathomimetic (cholinergic agents;** also called *cholinergic agonists*)	**Parasympatholytic (anticholinergic or cholinergic blocking agents;** also called *cholinergic antagonists*)
Sympathetic (adrenergic)	epinephrine norepinephrine dopamine	**Sympathomimetic (adrenergic or adrenergic-acting agents;** also called *adrenergic agonists*)	**Sympatholytic (antiadrenergic or adrenergic-blocking agents;** also called *adrenergic antagonists*)

Agonist (agonistic): Entity that activates; in pharmacology, a drug that stimulates the activity of cell receptors normally responsive to naturally occurring chemical substances. *Antagonist* (antagonistic): Entity that counteracts the action of another substance; in pharmacology, a drug that prevents stimulation of a receptor site.

activity may also be used for drug therapy with parkinsonism (Box 29-4).

- **Levodopa** (Dopar) converts into dopamine to lessen symptoms of parkinsonism and to provide significant improvement in physical activity, allowing many patients to resume normal activity. Levodopa can cross the blood-brain barrier (dopamine does not have this capability) to be metabolized into dopamine.
- **Carbidopa** (Lodosyn) is given with levodopa to prevent peripheral conversion of levodopa to dopamine, making more levodopa available to enter the brain. Carbidopa has no therapeutic effect and no side effects when given alone; however, the combination of **carbidopa and levodopa** (Sinemet) improves mobility by decreasing tremors.
- **Entacapone** (Comtan) and **tolcapone** (Tasmar) are used with levodopa-carbidopa to improve the ability of patients with parkinsonism to accomplish activities of daily living.
- **Amantadine** (Symmetrel) promotes dopamine release from brain storage sites. Effects were found by accident while the drug was being used primarily as an antiviral. Levodopa and amantadine are used to treat drug-induced **dyskinesia.** Some patients experience a skin discoloration that disappears on drug discontinuation.
- **Selegiline** (Eldepryl, Cortex), a monoamine oxidase inhibitor (MAOI), reduces the "wearing out" effect of levodopa and is neuroprotective to delay disease progression.
- **Bromocriptine** (Parlodel), a direct-acting dopamine agonist, is often used with levodopa to decrease dyskinesias.

- **Pergolide** (Permax), similar to bromocriptine, can prolong control of parkinsonism symptoms, reduce fluctuations in motor response, and reduce dyskinesia induced by levodopa.
- **Pramipexole** (Mirapex) and **ropinirole** (Requip) may be used alone in early Parkinson's disease or may be used with levodopa as the disease progresses and greater drug therapy is required (Table 29-8).

Patient Education for Compliance

1. Antiparkinsonism medications may cause dizziness, drowsiness, and blurred vision. No alcohol should be consumed with these drugs.
2. Medications for parkinsonism should be taken with food to prevent gastrointestinal disturbances that may occur.
3. Avoid vitamin B_6 with levodopa, as it accelerates breakdown of dopamine to decrease levodopa effects.

Important Facts about Antiparkinsonism Medications

- Parkinsonism is treated by activating dopamine receptors and use of acetylcholine (ACh) blocking drugs.
- Levodopa is the most effective treatment for Parkinson's disease.
- Levodopa and monoamine oxidase inhibitors (MAOIs) taken together can cause a hypertensive crisis.
- Amantadine relieves symptoms of early parkinsonism.

TABLE 29-8 MEDICATIONS USED FOR PARKINSONISM

GENERIC NAME/ TRADE NAME	USUAL ADULT DOSE, ROUTE, AND FREQUENCY	INDICATIONS FOR USE	DRUG INTERACTIONS
DRUGS TO INCREASE DOPAMINE		Parkinsonism	vitamin B_6, antipsychotics, carbidopa, anticholinergics, amantadine, pergolide, MAOIs
levodopa, (L-dopa Dopar, Larodopa)	0.5-1 g PO qd; increase to 4-8 g		
carbidopa-levodopa (Sinemet 10/100, Sinemet 25/100, Sinemet 25/250)	Individualized but usually 1 tab PO tid		
amantadine* (Symmetrel)	100-200 mg PO bid		alcohol
selegiline (Eldepryl, Zelapar)	5 mg PO bid Orally dissolving tablet 1.25-2.5 mg qd	Increases response to levodopa-carbidopa	meperidine, tricyclic antidepressants
rasagiline (Azilect)	0.5 mg-1 mg PO qd	Same as for selegiline	meperidine, MAOIs, antidepressants, dextromethorphan

Major Side Effects of Drugs to Increase Dopamine:

levodopa and carbidopa-levodopa—dystonia, nausea, vomiting, abdominal pain, dysphagia, dry mouth, mental changes, headache, dizziness, hand tremors, dyskinesia; *amantadine*—dry mouth, GI disturbances, CHF, visual disturbances, dizziness, confusion; *selegiline*—nausea, hallucinations, confusion, depression, loss of balance, dizziness; *rasagiline*—visual disturbances, headaches, seizures, nausea and vomiting

GENERIC NAME/ TRADE NAME	USUAL ADULT DOSE, ROUTE, AND FREQUENCY	INDICATIONS FOR USE	DRUG INTERACTIONS
DOPAMINE AGONISTS			
bromocriptine (Parlodel)	1.25 mg PO bid		neuroleptics, erythromycin
entacapone (Comtan)	200 mg with each dose of carbidopa-levodopa		methyldopa, dobutamine, isoproterenol
pramipexole (Mirapex)	1.5-4.5 mg PO qd	Early or late parkinsonism and restless legs syndrome	cimetidine, dopamine antagonists, levodopa, ciprofloxacin, estrogens
ropinirole (Requip)	0.25 mg PO tid (immediate release)		
tolcapone (Tasmar)	100-200 mg PO tid		levodopa, dopamine antagonists

Major Side Effects of Dopamine Agonists:

bromocriptine and pergolide—nausea, psychotic reactions, confusion, nightmares, agitation, hallucinations, paranoia; *entacapone*—nausea and vomiting, dyskinesias, orthostatic hypotension, hallucinations, sleep disturbances; *pramipexole, ropinirole, tolcapone, pramipexole*—nausea, dizziness, somnolence, hallucinations, orthostatic hypotension, agitation, confusion

GENERIC NAME/ TRADE NAME	USUAL ADULT DOSE, ROUTE, AND FREQUENCY	INDICATIONS FOR USE	DRUG INTERACTIONS
ANTICHOLINERGIC MEDICATIONS		Adjunctive treatment for parkinsonism	alcohol, amantadine, quinidine, procainamide
benztropine mesylate (Cogentin)	1-6 mg PO qd, IM, IV		
ANTIHISTAMINES			
diphenhydramine (Benadryl)	25-50 mg PO tid-qid, IM, IV	Reduce drug-induced extrapyramidal effects	alcohol

CHF, Congestive heart failure; *GI*, gastrointestinal; *IM*, intramuscularly; *IV*, intravenously; *MAOI*, monoamine oxidase inhibitor; *PO*, orally.
*Also used with influenza to relieve aching and muscle shaking.

DRUGS FOR RESTLESS LEGS SYNDROME

Restless legs syndrome (RLS), affecting two out of 10 Americans, is characterized by an uncontrollable urge to move the legs when sitting or lying down. The person simply cannot sit still. The cause is unknown, although the syndrome may be familial. Treatment includes using medications for parkinsonism, such as **pramipexole** (Mirapex) (see Table 29-8), opioids, muscle relaxants (see Table 24-3), and medications for epilepsy (see Table 29-7). The only FDA-approved drug for RLS is **ropinirole** (Requip), a dopamine agonist (see Table 29-8).

DRUGS FOR HEADACHES

Headaches are common symptoms caused by a variety of reasons including fatigue, illness, alcohol, and stress. Many headaches are relieved by OTC medications, but some patients have debilitating, severe, recurrent headaches requiring frequent medical attention (Figure 29-5). Severe headaches may be further subdivided into those with identifiable causes such as infections, hypertension, or tumors and those with no identifiable cause such as migraine or cluster headaches. When the cause of headaches is known, that cause is the center of treatment.

Migraine Headaches

Migraine headaches are characterized by unilateral, throbbing or nonthrobbing pain often accompanied by nausea, vomiting, and sensitivity to noise and light. Some migraines have an **aura** (formerly known as *classic migraines*), and some have no aura (formerly known as *common migraines*), the type most commonly found. Migraine attacks may be precipitated by hormones because the headaches seem to be worse during menstruation and women seem to cease having migraines

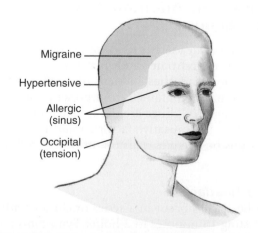

Migraine
Hypertensive
Allergic (sinus)
Occipital (tension)

Figure 29-5 Differentiation of headaches by location of pain.

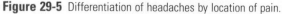

with menopause. Familial tendencies are another common cause of migraine headaches. Some medical professionals believe that migraine headaches are vascular in origin.

Treatment of Migraines

Drugs for migraines have two methods of action: to treat an ongoing headache and to prevent attacks. Medication individualization is necessary because some medications can cause dependency. Treatments for migraines include use of nonsteroidal antiinflammatory drugs (NSAIDs), opioid analgesics, and ergot alkaloids. Aspirin, acetaminophen, ibuprofen, and other aspirin-like NSAIDs can relieve mild to moderate migraine headaches and may be combined with **metoclopramide** (Reglan) for enhanced aspirin absorption. **Fiorinal** contains aspirin, caffeine, and butalbital; **Fioricet** is similar to Fiorinal but contains acetaminophen rather than aspirin. Another popular combination is **Midrin** (acetaminophen, a sedative, and a sympathomimetic) for pain relief. Midrin is contraindicated with glaucoma, severe renal disease, and severe liver and heart diseases caused by vasoconstriction.

Opioid analgesics are used with severe headaches that do not respond to nonopioids. The most frequently used are **meperidine** (Demerol) and **butorphanol nasal spray** (Stadol NS) (see analgesics in Chapter 15).

Medications specific for migraine headaches are in the triptan family, such as **eletriptan** (Relpax). By reducing the swelling of blood vessels surrounding the brain, it has a fairly rapid onset, with relief for most people in 2 hours. Persons with vascular or coronary diseases should not use this medication. **Sumatriptan** (Imitrex), related to serotonin and available for oral and subcutaneous administration, relieves both headaches and accompanying symptoms. Sumatriptan is teratogenic and should not be used in pregnancy. Other triptans include **zolmitriptan** (Zomig) and **rizatriptan** (Maxalt), which are similar to sumatriptan, with similar effects and side effects (Table 29-9).

Prevention of Migraine Headaches

Nondrug measures such as biofeedback and other relaxation techniques are helpful in controlling or eliminating causative factors of migraine headaches. Rest in a quiet, dark atmosphere is often indicated as early prophylaxis. Some medications are given prophylactically to reduce frequency and intensity of attacks, including beta blockers such as **amitriptyline** (Elavil), calcium channel blockers, **methysergide** (Sansert), and **valproic acid** (Depakene) among others. Prophylaxis is indicated for those who have frequent or severe migraines or for those who do not respond adequately to other therapy. **Propranolol** (Inderal), a beta blocker, is the drug of choice for prophylaxis. **Phenelzine** (Nardil), an MAOI-type antidepressant, is useful against migraines but is potentially dangerous, so it is not used routinely (see Chapter 30).

TABLE 29-9 MEDICATIONS SPECIFIC FOR USE WITH HEADACHES

GENERIC NAME/TRADE NAME (SCHEDULE)	USUAL ADULT DOSE, ROUTE, AND FREQUENCY	INDICATIONS FOR USE	DRUG INTERACTIONS
NONOPIOID ANALGESICS			
aspirin 325 mg + butalbital 50 mg + caffeine 40 mg (Fiorinal*) (III)	1 or 2 tabs PO q3-4h	Tension headache	Same as the ingredients included
acetaminophen 325 mg + caffeine 40 mg + butalbital 50 mg (Fioricet*) (III)	1 or 2 tabs PO q3-4h	Tension headache	Same as for Fiorinal
acetaminophen 325 mg + dichloralphenazone 100 mg + isometheptene 65 mg (Midrin) (IV)	1 or 2 caps PO up to 8 per day	Tension, vascular headache	bromocriptine
TRIPTANS			
naratriptan (Amerge)	1-2.5 mg PO prn q4h; max 5 mg/day	Migraine headaches	ergot preparations, other 5-HT₁ agonists, MAOIs
almotriptan (Axert)	6.25-12.5 mg PO qd; max 25 mg/day	Migraine headaches	Same as Amerge
rizatriptan (Maxalt)	5-10 mg PO; max 30 mg q24h	Migraine headaches	Same as Amerge
eletriptan (Relpax)	20-40 mg PO qd	Migraine headaches	ergotamine antifungals, nefazodone, macrolides, antivirals
frovatriptan (Frova)	2.5 mg PO; max 7.5 mg PO q24h	Migraine headaches	ergotamine, oral contraceptives, propranolol
sumatriptan (Imitrex)	25-100 mg PO; 6 mg SC; 5-20 mg intranasal q2h	Severe migraine or cluster headaches	ergotamine, dihydroergotamine
zolmitriptan (Zomig)	2.5-5 mg PO/nasal spray topically	Migraine headaches	MAOIs, SSRIs, oral contraceptives

Major Side Effects of Triptans:

eletriptan—dizziness, nausea, weakness, fatigue, pressure sensation in chest or throat; *frovatriptan*—hot or cold sensations, dizziness, fatigue, chest pain, skeletal pain, dry mouth, dyspepsia, flushing; *sumatriptan, zolmitriptan*—angina-like pain, pain in neck or throat, vertigo, malaise, fatigue

MAOI, Monoamine oxidase inhibitors; *PO,* orally; *SC,* subcutaneously.
*May have codeine added in gr ⅛; gr ¼, or gr ½.

Important Facts about Prevention of Migraine Headaches

- Drugs for migraine headaches are used for either treatment of existing headaches or prophylaxis.
- The goal of treatment for migraine headaches is to eliminate the pain, nausea, and vomiting associated with headaches.
- The goal of prophylactic therapy is to reduce the incidence of migraine attacks.
- Aspirin-like analgesics are effective for treating mild to moderate migraines.
- Opioids may be used for severe migraine headaches not responding to other medications.

Treatment of Additional Types of Headaches

More common headaches that cause pain and often inability to concentrate and perform needed tasks include cluster headaches and tension headaches. Relief of the pain may be obtained from prescription medications, or often OTC drugs are used. As with other types of headaches, the causative factor should be identified, whether this be allergies, tension, or other precipitating matters.

Cluster Headaches

Cluster headaches occur in a series or cluster, with each attack lasting 15 minutes to 2 hours. Symptoms include severe, nonthrobbing, unilateral pain usually located

TABLE 29-10 DRUGS FOR SPASTICITY

GENERIC NAME/ TRADE NAME	USUAL ADULT DOSE, ROUTE, AND FREQUENCY	INDICATIONS FOR USE	DRUG INTERACTIONS
baclofen	10-20 mg PO qid	Muscle spasticity of CNS origin	alcohol, insulin
dantrolene (Dantrium)	25 mg PO qd; up to 100 mg PO in divided doses		calcium channel blockers, alcohol, estrogens

CNS, Central nervous system; *PO,* orally.

around the eye that is not preceded by an aura, does not include nausea and vomiting, is not familial in nature, and occurs more often in males. These attacks consist of one headache or more every day for 4 to 12 weeks, with an interval of months to years of separation in each incident. **Verapamil** (Calan), a calcium channel blocker; lithium (see Chapter 30); and glucocorticoids (see Chapter 20) are used for cluster headaches.

Tension Headaches

Tension or muscle contraction headaches, the most common type of headaches, are characterized by moderate, nonthrobbing pain distributed in the head, neck, and scalp with tightness and pressure-like pain. Tension headache may occur with migraines. Precipitating factors are stress and eye strain. An acute attack is treated with combination medications such as **butalbital** (Fiorinal or Fiorrcet) and muscle relaxants such as **cyclobenzaprine** (Flexeril) (see Table 29-9). **Amitriptyline** (Elavil), a tricyclic antidepressant, is the drug of choice for prophylaxis.

Patient Education for Compliance

1. Possible causes of headaches such as eye diseases, sinusitis, or infections should be identified and treated. Patients may be able to find ways to avoid, control, or eliminate the factors that precipitate headaches.
2. Resting in a quiet, dark room for 2 to 3 hours after taking medications will usually ease headache pain.
3. Medications for headaches should be taken at the onset of symptoms unless prophylactic therapy is prescribed for patients with frequent migraine headaches.

DRUGS FOR SPASTICITY

Loss of dexterity, spasm, and increased muscle tone characterize **spasticity,** as found with multiple sclerosis or muscular dystrophy. Spasticity is a phenomenon in which uncoordinated movements are caused by CNS overstimulation. Trauma to the spinal cord or stroke may also cause muscle spasms. Drugs and physical therapy are treatments of choice. Muscle relaxants are not effective in treating spasticity. **Baclofen** (Lioresal) is used to reduce spasticity caused by multiple sclerosis, spinal cord

injury, and cerebral palsy but not by strokes. It decreases flexor and extensor muscle spasm, reducing spasticity discomfort. If medication is stopped, withdrawal should be accomplished slowly over 1 to 2 weeks. **Diazepam** (Valium) has similar actions but does not affect skeletal muscles directly. **Dantrolene** (Dantrium) is related to phenytoin and directly relaxes skeletal muscles by interfering with release of calcium, thus decreasing the skeletal muscles' ability to contract. This medicine is used with multiple sclerosis, cerebral palsy, and spinal cord injuries. The medication may take as long as 45 days to develop effectiveness. Unfortunately, Dantrium causes dose-related liver toxicity (Table 29-10).

CENTRAL NERVOUS SYSTEM STIMULANTS

The CNS processes information to and from the PNS and is the coordination control center for the entire body. Stimulants increase CNS neuron activity. Many medications stimulate the CNS, but their therapeutic usefulness is limited by side effects. Chronic use and misuse may occur, leading to drug tolerance, drug dependence, and drug misuse or abuse.

CNS stimulants, also called **analeptics,** are used to fight fatigue, alleviate mild pain, and counteract side effects of depressing medications to relieve respiratory distress (see Chapter 25). The most common analeptic is caffeine, found in many foods, drinks, and drugs such as Excedrin, Anacin, and OTC decongestants. Caffeine, a stimulant that gives a "quick picker-upper," may produce habituation and psychologic dependence causing withdrawal signs such as headaches, irritation, nervousness, anxiety, and dizziness on abrupt discontinuation. Caffeine should be used with care during pregnancy because it crosses the placenta to the fetus and is passed from mother to child in breast milk.

Did You Know?

Chocolate contains caffeine with theobromine that are CNS stimulates. Large amounts of chocolate ingestion may cause seizures and can be lethal. Chocolate truly is a quick picker-upper.

CNS stimulants, such as amphetamines, have been prescribed for exogenous obesity, but this use is considered obsolete and dangerous. These medications depress appetite by stimulating the cerebral cortex to produce euphoria and wakefulness, but tolerance usually occurs within 2 weeks—less time than required to achieve the weight reduction goal. Because of the high abuse potential and dangers of addiction, amphetamines are classified as DEA Schedule II drugs. Their many side effects cause these drugs to have little use. These medications should be avoided in patients with hyperthyroidism, hypertension, glaucoma, a history of drug abuse, and severe arteriosclerosis (Table 29-11).

Anorexiants, used for short-term treatment of obesity, suppress appetite by directly stimulating the satiety center of the hypothalamus. Some agents work on **sympathetic nervous system** pathways, whereas others work with adrenergic and dopamine pathways. These Schedule II through Schedule IV agents have a high potential for abuse. Caution must be used when anorexiants are prescribed for people with hypertension, cardiac disease, and a history of seizures (see Chapter 24 and Table 29-11 for further information on anorexiants).

Stimulants are also used for **narcolepsy, cataplexy,** sleep apnea, shift work sleep disorders, and auditory or visual hallucinations at sleep onset and to control daytime drowsiness and excessive sleep patterns. Stimulation results in an increase in motor function and mental alertness and a decrease in sense of fatigue and produce a euphoric state (see Table 29-11).

Psychomotor stimulants also have uses similar to those of CNS stimulants in inhibition of impulsive behaviors associated with attention-deficit disorder (ADD) and attention-deficit/hyperactivity disorder (ADHD). These medications are believed to activate portions of the CNS that inhibit impulsive behaviors (see Table 29-11 and Chapter 30).

AUTONOMIC NERVOUS SYSTEM DRUGS

The ANS can be thought of as a self-governing, an involuntary, or an automatic nervous system. Persons have no control over ANS, which is divided into sympathetic and parasympathetic divisions. These systems keep internal body organs in homeostasis or at their highest level of function to control smooth muscle, cardiac muscle, and glandular secretions (Figure 29-6).

Parasympathetic and sympathetic systems simultaneously innervate many of the same organs, opposing each other to balance innervations or provide negative feedback (Figure 29-7). The parasympathetic system has the primary function of conserving energy and restoring body resources for rest and digestion, or "feed-or-breed" responses. The sympathetic system mobilizes during emergency or stress situations, or "fight-or-flight" actions. These responses raise energy expenditures and increase body functions for response to energy requirements while decreasing digestive functions.

Medications affecting the ANS may mimic, intensify, or block effects of the sympathetic or parasympathetic divisions. Cholinergic medications mimic the parasympathetic system and so are called *parasympathomimetic drugs.* Anticholinergic or cholinergic blocking agents, also called *parasympatholytics,* block transmissions of the parasympathetic nervous system. Adrenergic drugs, or sympathomimetic agents, act to facilitate actions of

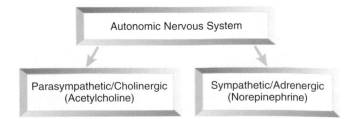
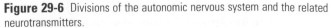

Figure 29-6 Divisions of the autonomic nervous system and the related neurotransmitters.

TABLE 29-11 CENTRAL NERVOUS SYSTEM STIMULANTS

GENERIC NAME/ TRADE NAME (SCHEDULE)	USUAL ADULT DOSE, ROUTE, AND FREQUENCY	INDICATIONS FOR USE	DRUG INTERACTIONS
caffeine (NoDoz [OTC], Vivarin [OTC], Caffedrine [OTC])	100-200 mg PO q3-4h	Promote mental alertness, decrease respiratory depression	fluoroquinolone antibiotics, fluconazole

Major Side Effects:
Insomnia, nervousness, tremors

AMPHETAMINES

amphetamine and dextroamphetamine (Adderall) (II)	5-30 mg PO bid	Narcolepsy, ADD, obesity	antacids, MAOIs, guanethidine, cardiac glycosides, beta blockers
dextroamphetamine (Dexedrine) (II)	5-20 mg PO qd-tid	Same as for amphetamine	MAOIs, antacids, antidepressants
methylphenidate (Ritalin) (II)	10-60 mg PO daily in 2-3 divided doses	ADD, narcolepsy	MAOIs, tricyclic, antidepressants, vasopressors
methamphetamine (Desoxyn) (II)	20-25 mg PO/day in 2 divided doses	ADHD and obesity	same as for amphetamine

Major Side Effects of Amphetamines:

amphetamine—insomnia, weight loss, restlessness, euphoria, irritability, visual disturbances, excessive sweating, dry mouth, nausea and vomiting, anorexia, tachycardia, chest pain, impotence; *dextroamphetamine*—increased irritability, nervousness, insomnia, headaches, nausea and vomiting, sweating, tachycardia

CENTRAL NERVOUS SYSTEM STIMULANTS USED AS ANOREXIANTS

		Exogenous obesity	
phentermine (Adipex-P) (IV)	15-37.5 mg PO qd		None
benzphetamine (Didrex) (IV)	25-50 mg PO tid		None
phendimetrazine (Bontril) (IV)	17.5-35 mg PO bid-tid; or 105 mg extended release qd		None

OTHER CNS STIMULANTS

modafinil (Provigil) (IV)	200 mg PO qd	Narcolepsy, sleep apnea	Oral contraceptives, cyclosporine
armodafinil (Nuvigil) (IV)	150-250 mg PO qd	Narcolepsy, sleep apnea	

Major Side Effects of CNS Stimulants:
Increased irritability, euphoria, nervousness, insomnia, headache, nausea and vomiting, sweating, tachycardia

ADD, Attention-deficit disorder; *ADHD,* attention-deficit/hyperactivity disorder; *CNS,* central nervous system; *MAOI,* monoamine oxidase inhibitor; *PO,* orally.

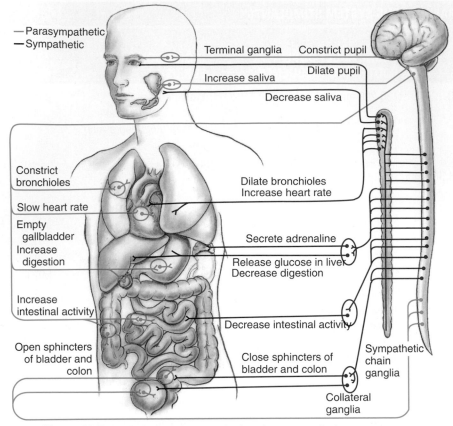

Figure 29-7 Comparison of the sympathetic and parasympathetic nervous systems.

the sympathetic nervous system. Adrenergic blockers, or sympatholytic drugs, block sympathetic responses. Terminology for substances active on the ANS is summarized in Box 29-4.

✏ LEARNING TIP

Mimetic means to imitate or mimic, so *parasympathomimetic* means to mimic parasympathetic nervous system, or acetylcholine (ACh) action. *Sympathomimetic* means to mimic sympathetic nervous system transmitters such as norepinephrine and epinephrine. *Lysis* means to relieve or reduce action of; *lytic* comes from the term *lysis*, so parasympatholytics act as cholinesterase to decrease ACh action. Sympatholytics are used to block the sympathetic nervous system; they are also called *adrenergic blockers*.

Cholinergic or Parasympathomimetic Medications

The parasympathetic nerve fibers liberate ACh as the facilitator to transmit nerve impulses in both phases of the ANS. Cholinergic or parasympathomimetic agents,

also called muscarinic agonists, are obtained from plant or synthetic sources because natural ACh's duration is too short to be pharmacologically effective. Synthetic medications are more stable, being subdivided into two groups: direct-acting and indirect-acting drugs. Direct-acting medications such as **bethanechol** (Urecholine) attach to receptors to mimic or increase ACh. Indirect-acting medications such as **neostigmine** (Prostigmin) inhibit the enzyme acetylcholinesterase or directly allow ACh to accumulate at receptor sites.

Cholinergic medications (parasympathomimetic agents) produce actions similar to those of ACh and are used in conditions that require (1) stimulating the intestines to increase peristalsis or the bladder to increase urination, (2) lowering intraocular pressure with glaucoma because of ophthalmic miotic response, (3) increasing salivation and sweating, and (4) reversing effects of curare-like medications used for relaxation during anesthesia. These medications are contraindicated in benign prostatic hypertrophy, gastric ulcers, intestinal obstructions, asthma, and cardiac disorders (Table 29-12).

Some physicians use cholinergic agents or **amyloid blockers** to increase the brain's ACh levels at nerve synapses for treating Alzheimer disease. Memory loss,

TABLE 29-12 CHOLINERGIC (PARASYMPATHOMIMETIC) AGENTS

GENERIC NAME/ TRADE NAME	USUAL ADULT DOSE, ROUTE, AND FREQUENCY	INDICATIONS FOR USE	DRUG INTERACTIONS
DIRECT-ACTING MEDICATIONS			
acetylcholine (see Chapter 21 for ophthalmic preparations)			
bethanechol (Urecholine, Duvoid)	10-50 mg PO tid-qid	Urinary retention	ambenonium, neostigmine, atropine, quinidine, procainamide, epinephrine
cevimeline (Evoxac)	30 mg PO tid	**Xerostomia**	Beta blockers, antihistamines, tricyclic antidepressants, phenothiazines

Major Side Effects of Direct-Acting Medications:
Nausea and vomiting, diarrhea, muscle cramps, muscle weakness, slowing of heart, hypotension, respiratory depression, bronchospasm, flushing, sweating, excessive saliva, tearing

INDIRECT-ACTING MEDICATIONS (see Chapter 21 for ophthalmic preparations)			
ambenonium (Mytelase)	5-75 mg PO tid-qid	Myasthenia gravis	tacrine
edrophonium (Enlon)	1-2 mg IM, IV, followed by anticholinesterase PO 1 hr later	Testing for myasthenia gravis	procainamide and tacrine
neostigmine (Prostigmin)	15-375 mg PO, IM in divided doses	Also used with treatment of myasthenia gravis	succinylcholine, same as for bethanechol

IM, Intramuscularly; *IV,* intravenously; *PO,* orally; *SC,* subcutaneously.

dementia, and deterioration of mental function are thought to occur because of lack of ACh in synapses. Use of these medications in Alzheimer disease is discussed in Chapter 30.

Did You Know?

Malathion, an insecticide, acts as a cholinergic agent on insects.

Anticholinergic or Parasympatholytic Medications

Cholinergic blocking agents such as **hyoscyamine** (Levsin) and **scopolamine** are referred to as *anticholinergics* or *parasympatholytic agents* or *muscarinic antagonists.*

These medications do not allow adequate ACh to bind to receptor sites, preventing ACh action—the opposite of the effect found with cholinergic agents. These drugs cause mydriasis (dilation) of the eye pupil; drying of the mouth, nose, throat, and bronchial secretions; decreased secretions and motility in the gastrointestinal tract; increased heart rate; and decreased sweating. Medications used are (1) antispasmodic and antisecretory agents in the gastrointestinal and genitourinary tracts, (2) neuromuscular blockers with spastic disorders, (3) antidotes for insecticide and mushroom poisoning, (4) for emergency care for bradycardia and atrioventricular heart block, (5) for dilation of pupils, and (6) for prevention and treatment of bronchospasm. Contraindications are chronic obstructive pulmonary disease (COPD), asthma, closed-angle glaucoma, gastrointestinal and genitourinary obstruction, cardiac arrhythmias, hypertension, hypothyroidism, and liver and renal disease (Table 29-13).

TABLE 29-13 ANTICHOLINERGIC (PARASYMPATHOLYTIC) AGENTS*

GENERIC NAME/ TRADE NAME	USUAL ADULT DOSE, ROUTE, AND FREQUENCY	INDICATIONS FOR USE	DRUG INTERACTIONS
atropine (Iso-Atropine, Sal-Tropine)	0.4-1 mg PO q4-6h	Bradycardia, GI and GU hypermotility, preoperatively to decrease secretions	amantadine, quinidine, disopyramide, levodopa, procainamide
hyoscyamine (Levsin, Cystospaz)	0.125-0.25 mg PO q4h, IM, SC, SL	Peptic ulcers, irritable bowel syndrome, vertigo, enuresis, parkinsonism, urinary tract spasms	None
scopolamine (Transderm-Scop)	1 patch transdermally q72h	Motion sickness	None
dicyclomine (Bentyl, Antispas)	20-40 mg PO tid-qid	Irritable bowel syndrome, infant colic, antispasmodic	amantadine, levodopa, tricyclic antidepressants, MAOIs, H₁ antihistamines, phenothiazines, ketoconazole

Major Side Effects: atropine—flushing, blurred vision, dry mouth, constipation, urinary retention, headaches, confusion, tachycardia

GI, Gastrointestinal; *GU,* genitourinary; *IM,* intramuscularly; *MAOI,* monoamine oxidase inhibitor; *PO,* orally; *SC,* subcutaneously; *SL,* sublingually.
*See Chapter 21 for ophthalmic uses and Chapter 27 for urinary tract uses.

Did You Know?

Belladonna alkaloids, often used as anticholinergic agents, are found in OTC preparations and in many common plants and inedible berries, causing danger for young children and pets. OTC preparations are used for infant colic, gastrointestinal spasms, and diarrhea.

Patient Education for Compliance

1. Patients taking cholinergic medications or those exposed to insecticides such as malathion should report such symptoms as decreased heart rate, decreased respirations, gastrointestinal distress, and excessive perspiration to a physician.
2. Cholinergic medications should not be combined with heart medications or antibiotics.
3. Medic-Alert tags should be worn when using cholinergic medications.
4. Persons taking cholinergic blockers should practice frequent mouth care and good dental hygiene.
5. Fluids such as water should be available when taking cholinergic blockers to combat dry mouth effects. Chewing gum and hard candy may be useful.
6. Report rapid heart rate or palpitations and blurred vision when taking anticholinergics.
7. Avoid oral anticholinergics with chronic obstructive pulmonary disease (COPD) or asthma and use only prescribed inhalants. No OTC products should be used.
8. Anticholinergics may cause photophobia, so sunglasses outside and reduced light indoors may be necessary.

Important Facts about Cholinergic and Anticholinergic Medications

- Cholinergic medications, or parasympathomimetics, mimic ACh effects and act either directly on cholinergic receptors or indirectly by inhibiting cholinesterase action.
- Cholinergic medications stimulate peristalsis and urination, lower intraocular pressure with glaucoma, and treat myasthenia gravis by innervating skeletal muscles, much as ACh does.
- Cholinergic blocking agents (parasympatholytics) do not allow binding of ACh at receptor sites. Consequently these medications produce mydriasis, drying of secretions, decreased motility of gastrointestinal tract, and increased heart rate.
- Cholinergic blocking agents, especially atropine, are used as antispasmodics and antisecretory agents and as antidotes for insecticide poisoning.

Adrenergic Agonists or Sympathomimetic Drugs

The sympathetic nervous system is considered the emergency system to mobilize the body for a quick response to frightening situations—"fight-or-flight" response. Blood pressure, pulse, and respirations increase; peripheral blood vessels constrict to allow flow of blood to vital organs; pupils dilate; and bronchioles dilate to supply more oxygen. Adrenergic agonists have a broad spectrum

- Sympathomimetics are used to restore cardiac rhythm and elevate blood pressure in shock and emergency situations.
- In the medical office, adrenergic agonists may be used to constrict capillaries to control bleeding from nosebleeds or to alleviate nasal congestion.
- Addition of these agents to local anesthetics to control bleeding is commonly found in medical and dental practice.
- Epinephrine-type medications are used to dilate bronchioles in asthma attacks, bronchospasm, or with anaphylactic reactions.
- When agents are used on lacerations found in peripheral tissues such as nose, fingers, or toes, tissue necrosis may occur.
- Because of side effects, adrenergics should be used with extreme caution in patients with angina, coronary insufficiencies, hypertension, cardiac arrhythmias, angle-closure glaucoma, organic brain damage, and hyperthyroidism.

of clinical applications in many specialty areas from obstetrics to cardiovascular medicine.

Medications found within the *adrenergic sympathomimetic agonist* or classification are catecholamines and noncatecholamines. The catecholamines such as *epinephrine* (adrenalin) and *dopamine* (levodopa), found naturally, are secreted at nerve terminals. Epinephrine is found in the adrenal medulla, whereas dopamine is from sites in the brain, kidneys, and gastrointestinal tract. These agents are available synthetically to produce the same effects as naturally secreted neurotransmitters (Box 29-5). Noncatecholamines including *ephedrine* and *phenylephrine* (Sudafed) have actions somewhat similar to those of catecholamines, being more selective of receptor sites and having a longer duration but slower actions (Table 29-14).

Adrenergic Blocking Agents or Sympatholytic Drugs

Adrenergic blockers are composed of two groups— alpha- and beta-adrenergic blocking agents—depending on the blocked receptors. These agents plug or block receptors, preventing other agents from stimulating the receptor sites. The alpha blockers such as *prazosin* (Minipress) and *terazosin* (Hytrin) prevent norepinephrine from producing a sympathetic response. The major effects of alpha blockade are lowering of blood pressure and vasodilation (antihypertensive effects of alpha blockers are discussed in Chapter 26). These agents are also used to treat peripheral vascular conditions such as Raynaud disease and to diagnose pheochromocytoma, a

tumor of the adrenal medulla (Table 29-15). See chapter tables related to use in specific body systems.

Beta-Adrenergic Receptor Blockers (Beta Blockers)

Beta blockers, such as *metoprolol* (Lopressor) and *nadolol* (Corgard), bind to beta-adrenergic receptors, especially in the heart. Clinical use of beta blockers is to decrease cardiac activity—heart rate, force of cardiac contractions, and impulse conduction. Reduction in heart work causes a decrease in oxygen need. Because clinical beta blockers have cardiovascular action, these agents are discussed in Chapter 26. Another use for beta blockers is for migraine headaches and prophylactically for neurologic conditions as discussed earlier in this chapter (see Table 29-15).

LEARNING TIP

Many beta blockers have names that end in "olol," and several of the alpha blockers have names that end in "osin."

Patient Education for Compliance

1. Adrenergic medications may produce anorexia. Diets high in carbohydrates and proteins and low in fats with small meals are better tolerated.
2. Because insomnia and nervousness accompany adrenergic medications, caffeinated products should be avoided, especially after 5:00 PM. Alternative sleep aids such as relaxation techniques may be tried to reduce insomnia.
3. Patients taking beta-adrenergic blockers should be aware of possible postural hypotension and should use care when changing positions.
4. Pulse should be taken to assess bradycardia that occurs with adrenergic blockers.
5. Alcohol, antihistamines, muscle relaxants, tranquilizers, and sedatives may potentiate CNS depression and sedation that occurs with adrenergic blockers.
6. Sexual dysfunction may result with beta blockers, necessitating dosage regulation or medication change.
7. Beta blockers may increase serum lipid levels; these levels should be tested on regular basis with prolonged therapy.
8. Patients with diabetes should watch glucose levels for hypoglycemia when taking beta-adrenergic blockers because these medications reduce blood glucose levels.
9. Beta blockers may cause headaches, mental confusion, and nightmares, which should be reported to health professional.
10. Weakness, fatigue, dizziness, and sedation are common side effects of beta blockers.

TABLE 29-14 ADRENERGIC AGONISTS (SYMPATHOMIMETIC AGENTS)

GENERIC NAME/ TRADE NAME	USUAL ADULT DOSE, ROUTE, AND FREQUENCY	INDICATIONS FOR USE	DRUG INTERACTIONS
ALPHA-ADRENERGIC AGONISTS			
epinephrine (Adrenalin, Primatene,* Bronkaid*)	0.001% as topical hemostatic with local anesthetics Inhalation 0.3-0.5 mL 1% IM	Bronchospasm, asthma, anaphylaxis, cardiac arrest, elevate BP, prolong local anesthesia	MAOIs, tricyclic antidepressants, anesthetics, beta blockers, sympathomimetics
Epi-Pen	Inject as needed for allergies	Anaphylaxis prevention	
ephedrine (Efedron)	25-50 mg PO qd-qid 12.5-50 mg IM, IV, SC	Bronchodilators, nasal decongestion, increase BP, epistaxis, myasthenia gravis, urinary incontinence	Same as epinephrine and norepinephrine
(Pretz-D and others)*	2-4 drops or small amount of gel in nostril		
methoxamine (Vasoxyl)	5-20 mg IM	Same as metaraminol	Same as ephedrine
norepinephrine (Levophed)	8-12 mcg/min IV	Same as metaraminol	Same as ephedrine
phenylephrine (Neo-Synephrine,† Sinex,* Sinarest Nasal, Neo-Synephrine*)	1-10 mg IV 10 mg PO 2 or 3 drops of spray in nostril—0.25-0.5% solution	Increase BP, nasal decongestant, vasoconstriction, mydriasis	Same as ephedrine
(Neo-Synephrine gel*)	Small amount into each nostril		
pseudoephedrine (Sudafed, Novafed, PediaCare, others*)	60 mg PO q4-6h	Nasal decongestant	Other sympathomimetics, MAOIs, beta blockers

Major Side Effects of Alpha-Adrenergic Agonists:

Palpitations, tachycardia, nervousness, tremors, cardiac arrhythmias, anginal pain, hypertension, hyperglycemia, headaches, insomnia; irritation of nasal sinuses and eyes when used as decongestants

GENERIC NAME/ TRADE NAME	USUAL ADULT DOSE, ROUTE, AND FREQUENCY	INDICATIONS FOR USE	DRUG INTERACTIONS
BETA-ADRENERGIC AGONISTS			
epinephrine (see under Alpha-Adrenergic Agonists)		Bronchodilator	
albuterol (Proventil Ventolin)	2-4 mg PO q6-8h 1 or 2 inhalations q4-6h prn	Bronchodilator	epinephrine, MAOIs, tricyclic antidepressants, beta blockers
isoproterenol (Isuprel)	0.02-0.06 mg IV 0.15-0.2 mg SC 10-15 mg SL	Also used as cardiac stimulator	Same as for albuterol
metaproterenol	2 or 3 inhalations 20 mg PO tid-qid	Bronchodilator	Same as for albuterol
terbutaline (Brethine, Brethaire)	2.5-5 mg PO tid 0.25 mg SC	Also used as muscle relaxant in premature labor	Same as for albuterol
salmeterol (Serevent)	2 inhalations bid	Bronchodilator Prevent exercise-induced bronchospasm	beta blockers
dopamine (Intropin)	IV, based on body weight	Vasopressor for shock	Same as for albuterol

BP, Blood pressure; *IM,* intramuscularly; *IV,* intravenously; *MAOI,* monoamine oxidase inhibitor; *PO,* orally; *SC,* subcutaneously; *SL,* sublingually.
*OTC medication.
†Prescription required.
Note: See Chapter 21 for ophthalmic uses of these medications.

TABLE 29-15 ADRENERGIC BLOCKING AGENTS

GENERIC NAME/ TRADE NAME	USUAL ADULT DOSE, ROUTE, AND FREQUENCY	INDICATIONS FOR USE	DRUG INTERACTIONS
ALPHA BLOCKERS			
doxazosin (Cardura)	1-16 mg PO qd	Benign prostatic hypertrophy, hypertension	ACE inhibitors, indomethacin, verapamil, nifedipine
(Cardura XL)	1-8 mg PO qd		
phentolamine (Regitine)	2-5 mg IM, IV	Peripheral vascular disease	Same as for doxazosin
prazosin (Minipress)	1-5 mg PO qd	Hypertension	ACE inhibitors, NSAIDs, verapamil, beta blockers
terazosin (Hytrin)	1-20 mg PO qd	Hypertension	ACE inhibitors, NSAIDs, propranolol

Major Side Effects of Alpha Blockers:
Miosis, nasal congestion, increased GI activity, tachycardia, orthostatic hypotension, fainting

BETA BLOCKERS			
labetalol (Normodyne)	100-400 mg PO bid	Hypertension and angina pectoris	cimetidine, NSAIDs, epinephrine
nadolol (Corgard)	80-240 mg PO qd-bid		adenosine, ampicillin, antacids, calcium channel blockers, clonidine, lidocaine, neostigmine, NSAIDs, prazosin, tacrine, verapamil
pindolol (Visken)	15-40 mg PO/day in 3-4 divided doses	Hypertension	Same as nadolol and multiple others
propranolol (Inderal)	160-480 mg PO IV/day in 2-3 divided doses	Also used with angina pectoris, arrhythmias, migraines	NSAIDs, antidiabetic agents, barbiturates, calcium channel blockers, digoxin, epinephrine
timolol (Timoptic)	10-60 mg PO bid, ophthalmic as directed	Hypertension Glaucoma	diuretics, NSAIDs
acebutolol (Sectral)	200-800 mg PO qd bid	Hypertension, ventricular arrhythmias	ampicillin, antacids, local anesthetics, digoxin, epinephrine, NSAIDs
atenolol (Tenormin)	25-100 mg PO qd	Hypertension, angina pectoris	neuroleptics (see literature for others)
bisoprolol (Zebeta)	2.5-10 mg PO qd	Hypertension	Same as for acebutolol and atenolol
metoprolol tartrate (Lopressor)	100-450 mg PO tid	Hypertension, angina pectoris, myocardial infarction	Same as for acebutolol and atenolol
metoprolol succinate (Tropol XL)	25-100 mg PO qd		

Major Side Effects of Beta Blockers:
Hypotension, bradycardia, fatigue, lethargy, nausea and vomiting, hypoglycemia, confusion

ACE, Angiotensin-converting enzyme; *GI*, gastrointestinal; *IM*, intramuscularly; *IV*, intravenously; *NSAIDs*, nonsteroidal antiinflammatory drugs; *PO*, orally.
Note: Please see appropriate chapters by body system for more information on alpha and beta blockers including: Chapter 21, Ophthalmic Preparations; Chapter 26, Cardiovascular Conditions; and Chapter 27, Urinary Tract Conditions.

Important Facts about Adrenergic Blockers

- Adrenergic agonists or sympathomimetics are classified as catecholamines or noncatecholamines to mimic "fight-or-flight" actions occurring with sympathetic nervous system stimulation. Naturally occurring adrenergic agonists are epinephrine, norepinephrine, and dopamine.
- Sympathomimetics are used to restore cardiac rhythm, elevate blood pressure, and control bleeding by vasoconstriction.
- Epinephrine is added to local anesthetics for vasoconstriction and to prolong anesthesia effects.
- Sympathomimetics are used for mydriasis in ophthalmology.
- Alpha-adrenergic blockers, or sympatholytic agents, are used to reduce hypertension and for benign prostatic hypertrophy.
- Major adverse effects of alpha blockers are orthostatic hypotension, nasal congestion, tachycardia, and sexual dysfunction.
- The first dose of alpha blocker may cause fainting because of orthostatic hypotension, called "first-dose effect."
- Beta blockers have many drug interactions that should be checked before any other medications are added. OTC nonsteroidal antiinflammatory drugs (NSAIDs) have strong interactions with beta blockers.
- Principal indications for beta blockers—hypertension, angina pectoris, and dysrhythmias from tachycardia (see Chapter 26)—cause postural hypotension.
- Beta blockers must be used with caution in patients with chronic obstructive pulmonary disease (COPD) and asthma because of bronchoconstriction.
- Beta blockers reduce conversion of glycogen to glucose in liver or muscles to reduce blood glucose levels—a problem for people with diabetes.
- Beta blockers are administered once or twice a day and cannot be discontinued abruptly.

DRUGS SPECIFIC FOR STROKE PREVENTION

Antiplatelet medications (see Chapter 26) are indicated in the prevention of arterial thrombi and are used in cerebral thrombi or stroke prevention. *Aspirin* is used for prophylaxis of thrombi, as is *dipyridamole* (Persantine), by preventing platelet aggregation. A combination product of *aspirin 25 mg* and *dipyridamole 200 mg* (Aggrenox) is used for prevention of recurrent strokes in people who have experienced transient ischemic attacks or who have had ischemic attacks from thrombosis. Combined agents reduce stroke risk by a greater margin than either agent used alone but may cause headaches as a side effect.

SUMMARY

The nervous system is composed of two divisions: the CNS (the brain and spinal cord) and the PNS (nerves outside the CNS). The ANS, composed of sympathetic and parasympathetic nervous systems, controls body functions without specific conscious effort by the individual. The CNS receives information from peripheral nerves for interpretation and then returns stimuli to the peripheral system for response. The ANS has either "fight-or-flight" responses or "feed-or-breed" functions needed for maintenance of homeostasis. Medications are used to assist with functions of these systems when secretions responding to stimuli are either too sparse or too great.

Analgesics are used for pain, a worldwide health symptom that disables and distresses people on a daily basis. Important is the fact that pain therapy should be available to all people at a level needed for relief. If opioids or potent analgesics are used for prolonged periods, abuse, misuse, and tolerance are possible. Short-term pain relief until the cause is treated does not cause these effects. Terminally ill persons should be given long-term methods of pain relief and should be kept as pain free as possible. Everyone has a right to be pain free.

Anesthetics are used to interfere with conduction of nerve impulses to the CNS. General anesthesia is used in surgical procedures and may be given IV or by inhalation. Local or regional anesthesia is achieved by topical application or through infiltration of a selected site. Local anesthesia is used to render a body part insensitive to pain. Additives such as epinephrine are included with local anesthetic agents to prolong effects and to cause vasoconstriction to reduce bleeding, but these medications may also cause nervousness, palpitations, and other stimulations to body functions. These side effects are expected, but patients should be aware that these are a normal reaction.

Benzodiazepines are commonly used to treat anxiety and insomnia. These agents, because of their greater effectiveness and safety, have replaced many of the sedatives of the barbiturate family that were used in the past. Geriatric patients are often persons needing medications; therefore care should be taken because of their increased sensitivity to medications. Short-acting medications should be used in the elderly because of decreased metabolism and excretion abilities.

Before medications are prescribed for insomnia, the cause should be considered and appropriate actions taken to reduce this factor. Medications prescribed for insomnia are habit forming when used for prolonged times; therefore a limited prescription with close monitoring of use is recommended to reduce a risk. Allied health professionals should take a complete history to attempt to find the underlying cause of insomnia, possibly preventing medication need.

Seizures are symptoms showing disorganized electric impulses in brain. Classification of seizures is by causative factors and symptoms produced. Several drug groups are used to treat seizures—barbiturates, hydantoins, succinimides, benzodiazepines, and some miscellaneous medications. These drugs produce various side effects that necessitate lifestyle changes for the person with epilepsy. Patients must be taught the importance of taking medications as prescribed and the necessity of reporting seizure activity that occurs while taking medications.

Medications are used with diseases such as parkinsonism, RLS, and myasthenia gravis to treat typical progressive symptoms. Muscle spasticity, inability to ambulate safely, and tremors associated with these diseases are treated to allow patients to function as independently as possible for as long as possible.

With parkinsonism, the ideal is to correct the disease-causing imbalance of dopamine and ACh. Medications such as anticholinergics and antihistamines are used for central effect, and medications that increase dopamine levels in the brain may be prescribed.

Myasthenia gravis is a debilitating disease characterized by skeletal muscle weakness and fatigue. Treatment is to control symptoms using medications that inhibit cholinesterase to provide the ACh necessary for muscle contractility.

Medications that affect cholinergic receptor sites, "feed-or-breed" medications, are used to mimic, intensify, or inhibit parasympathetic nervous system effects.

Medications that affect ACh receptors affect smooth muscle, glands, and cardiac muscles that are essential body functions. Cholinergic medications are used to stimulate the intestinal tract and urinary bladder, lower intraocular pressure, dilate peripheral blood vessels, stimulate muscle contractility, and promote salivation and sweating. Anticholinergic medications are used to treat other illnesses that have spasticity as a symptom such as irritable bowel syndrome and urinary disorders.

The sympathetic nervous system, or adrenergic system, is responsible for the body's "fight-or-flight" response. Medications affecting alpha or beta receptors are used to mimic the sympathetic nervous system (sympathomimetic or adrenergic drugs) with direct or indirect action or both.

Other medications—adrenergic blockers or sympatholytic drugs—block receptor sites and inhibit sympathetic response. Blocking agents are discussed in chapters that cover the systems where the specific action occurs, such as hypertensives in Chapter 26. Adrenergic blockers (sympatholytics) may be alpha, beta, or alpha-beta blockers and are used for treatment of hypertension as well as other conditions such as benign prostatic hypertrophy and glaucoma.

Epinephrine, an important sympathomimetic drug that stimulates alpha and beta receptors, is used to keep the body in homeostasis with treatment of asthma, in emergency conditions such as anaphylaxis and cardiac emergencies, to achieve local hemostasis, and in treatment of open-angle glaucoma.

Norepinephrine is used for peripheral vascular constriction to raise both systolic and diastolic blood pressure and for vasodilation to treat circulatory shock.

CRITICAL THINKING EXERCISES

Scenario

Joseph, age 25, has had three tonic-clonic seizures in the past month. Until now, he has been seizure free for 2 years.

1. What questions should you ask Joseph about taking his medications?
2. Joseph tells you that he has not had the money to buy his medications for 2 weeks. Would this be important to tell the physician? Why or why not?
3. Joseph has taken Dilantin for more than 10 years. What does Joseph need to know about mouth and gum prophylactic care? Why?

DRUG CALCULATIONS

1. Order: phenobarbital 97.5 mg IM stat
   Available medication:

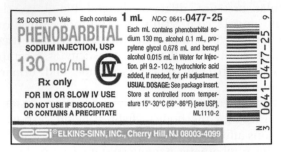

   Dose to be administered: _____
   _____

   Show the amount to be administered on the syringe shown.

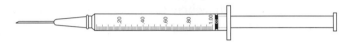

2. Order: Dilantin 60 mg PO
   Available medication:

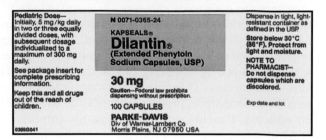

   Dose to be administered: _____
   _____

REVIEW QUESTIONS

1. What is the blood-brain barrier? Why is this important in pharmacology? _____
   _____
   _____

2. What are the two groups of local anesthetics? What are typical examples of each? _____
   _____
   _____

3. Why is epinephrine added to local anesthetics? _____
   _____
   _____

4. What are the actions of barbiturates? _____
   _____
   _____

5. How do hydantoins (Dilantin) work for seizure control? _____
   _____
   _____

6. What are the three pharmacologic categories used to treat Parkinson's disease? _____
   _____
   _____

7. What medication is used prophylactically for cluster headaches? _____
   _____
   _____

8. What diseases with spasticity can be treated with baclofen? What medications are not effective in treating skeletal muscle spasticity? _____

   _____

   _____

   _____

   _____

9. How do cholinergic medications work? Anticholinergics? Adrenergics? Adrenergic blockers? _____

   _____

   _____

   _____

   _____

10. Cholinergics are used for what medical conditions? What are their side effects? _____

    _____

    _____

    _____

    _____

11. What are the side effects of anticholinergic agents? _____

    _____

    _____

12. Can anticholinergic medications be bought OTC? If so, which ones? _____

    _____

    _____

CHAPTER 30

Drugs for Mental Health and Behavioral Disorders

OBJECTIVES

After studying this chapter, you should be capable of doing the following:

- Describing mental health and deviations diagnosed as mental illness.
- Identifying medications used to treat anxiety.
- Recognizing medications used to treat psychotic diseases.
- Identifying principal signs of depression and drugs used as treatment.
- Recognizing agents used as antimanics and medications for bipolar disorder.

- Describing behavioral disorders found in adults and children and drugs indicated in treatment.
- Understanding role of medications in treating Alzheimer's disease.
- Identifying drugs for attention-deficit disorder and attention-deficit/hyperactivity disorder.
- Providing patient education for compliance with medications used to treat conditions and diseases of mental health and behavioral disorders.

Mrs. Jones, age 76, has become more and more disoriented and confused. Dr. Merry has made a tentative diagnosis of Alzheimer's disease. Betty, Mrs. Jones's daughter, wants Dr. Merry to give her mother a medication to cure the disease.

Is this possible? Explain your answer.
If not, why are medications given for Alzheimer's disease?
If Aricept is prescribed, what side effects should Betty be told to look for while caring for her mother?
What are the indications for memantine (Namenda)?

KEY TERMS

Affect	**Bipolar disorder**	**Neuroleptic**	**Psychotherapy**
Affective disorders	**Compulsions**	**Neurosis**	**Schizophrenia**
Akathisia	**Delirium tremens**	**Obsession**	**Tardive dyskinesia**
Alzheimer's disease	**Delusion**	**Psychoanalysis**	**Tourette's syndrome**
Anxiolytic	**Drug holiday**	**Psychologic drug**	**Tranquilization**
Attention-deficit/	**Dystonia**	**dependence or**	
hyperactivity	**Extrapyramidal effects**	**habituation**	
disorder (ADHD)	**Hallucinations**	**Psychosis**	

EASY WORKING KNOWLEDGE OF INDICATIONS AND SIDE EFFECTS

Common Signs and Symptoms of Mental Disorders

Stress, anxiety, depression
Withdrawal from society
Disorganized thinking, hallucinations
Inappropriate or violent behavior
Crying, mood swings
Sleep disturbances, fatigue, agitation
Loss of concentration
Inability to experience pleasure
Forgetfulness
Inability to place self in environment, person, place
Paranoia

Common Side Effects of Medications for Mental Disorders

Hypotension, restlessness
Tachycardia
Dry mouth
Decreased motor and cognitive abilities
Alterations in sleep patterns
Hangover effect
Increased or decreased libido
Impotence
Dizziness, drowsiness, confusion
Extrapyramidal symptoms
Tardive dyskinesia

EASY WORKING KNOWLEDGE OF MEDICATIONS USED FOR MENTAL DISORDERS

DRUG CLASS	PRESCRIPTION	OTC	PREGNANCY CATEGORY	MAJOR INDICATIONS
Anxiolytics, antianxiety, minor tranquilizers	Yes	No	B, C, D	Anxiety
Antipsychotics, neuroleptics, major tranquilizers	Yes	No	B, C, D	Psychotic disorders
Antidepressants				
Unipolar	Yes	No	B, C, D	Depression
Bipolar	Yes	No	D	Mania, depression
Medications for cognitive ability	Yes	No	C, X	Alzheimer's disease
Central nervous system stimulants	Yes	No	B, C	Attention-deficit/hyperactivity disorder

The ability to cope with different types of stressors during a lifetime is part of normal living or mental health. Defining "normal" is difficult because the terms *normal* and *abnormal* are relative to the local environment. What is considered normal can and does vary from culture to culture, country to country, town to town, and even within towns. Daily stressors may even change normal to abnormal within short periods of time.

individuality by integration of the physical, cognitive, and affective domains. In the social dimension the ability to interact with family or community members effectively is dominant. Environmental factors are everything outside of the person. These components interact to form a continuum for mental health throughout life. Mental health is not a concrete achievable goal; rather, a lifelong process forms a sense of personal harmony and balance.

WHAT IS MENTAL HEALTH?

Mental health is a person's interaction among physical, cognitive, affective, behavioral, and social realms as well as interactions with the environment to choose and act with regard to a purpose in life. The physical dimension includes physiologic aspects, whereas the cognitive dimension involves formulation of thoughts, processing of information, and problem solving. The affective domain involves the ability to experience and express feelings and emotions. The behavioral dimension is

WHAT IS A MENTALLY HEALTHY PERSON?

Mentally healthy people are able to perceive reality accurately and control the manner in which emotions are experienced and expressed. Clear and logical thinking allows effective communication while anticipating events and solving problems. Persons can then initiate and maintain meaningful relationships, develop a positive self-concept, and behave in ways to promote personal growth and development.

Mental disorders affect almost everyone at some time during life, either personally or by association with a friend or family member. Factors that produce mental instability include congenital deficiencies, hereditary factors, accidents, traumatic events in one's life, or drug-related toxicity. In many cases, the exact cause of instability is unknown, but most mental disorders are related to stress and pressures imposed by modern society. The pain of mental illness is real and intense, altering a person's ability to adjust to societal stress. When self-esteem is decreased, coping skills are reduced, affecting behavior. Mental disorders may result in mild to severe disruption of the ability to function in interpersonal relationships, self-care, and ability to maintain a job to be self-sufficient. When a person is able to cope and adapt to the stresses of everyday life, he or she is considered to be mentally healthy.

ANXIETY AND DAILY LIVING

Anxiety, a lifelong emotion from infancy to older adulthood, is the major factor in motivating one's emotional life. A person usually takes a course of action to reduce stress, apprehension, tension, and uneasiness that threaten one's well-being or sense of control in a given situation. The way in which a person confronts anxiety-causing situations, from mild anxiousness to states of panic, is an ultimate sign of mental health. Not all anxiety is harmful; mild anxiety increases alertness and increases productivity. Moderate anxiety diminishes cognitive abilities and makes learning and decision making difficult. When a person is unable to adapt to anxiety or stress, homeostasis may be affected, causing changes in mechanisms of protection and defense in an effort to maintain equilibrium. When stress presents a crisis with adaptation and function being affected, medications may be prescribed to decrease stress and anxiety to allow needed adaptation.

Prolonged anxiety, tension, and nervousness result in behavioral and emotional changes or neurosis, while allowing psychosomatic conditions and panic disorders to occur. **Anxiolytics,** formerly called *minor tranquilizers,* are used as treatment to calm the individual and reduce unpleasant symptoms of severe anxiety.

ROLE OF MEDICATION THERAPY IN PSYCHOTHERAPY

Medications in modern psychotherapeutic care are used to reduce or alleviate symptoms of stress and allow tense or psychotic persons an opportunity to participate in other psychotherapeutic treatment. Drugs temporarily modify behavior, whereas **psychotherapy** may permanently change behavior. Psychotherapeutic medications

are chosen by diagnosis (e.g., medications are specific for **schizophrenia,** manic depression, psychosis, or other mental illness) because drugs have additive, potentiating, or antagonistic effects on one another. Selection is based on behavioral actions, pharmacologic effects, and potential adverse reactions, as well as individual and environmental factors present. Elderly patients are often inappropriately prescribed psychotropic agents. In fact, about 10% of all medical visits by elderly patients result in prescriptions for psychotropic agents, leading to increased risk of adverse or serious drug reactions and interfering with cognitive and functional status.

Treatment of mental health has taken giant steps in the United States in the past 60 years with the introduction of tranquilizers. The first antipsychotic agent, **chlorpromazine** (Thorazine), was released in the early 1950s and remains typical of phenothiazines used to calm agitated or anxious patients. Rather than being institutionalized for years, as in the past, many psychotic people are today treated at community mental health centers as outpatients. For those who are hospitalized, the hospitalization course is usually short term—only for the length of time necessary to stabilize the condition and medications.

Newer medications that are more selective in their action on the brain tend to result in **tranquilization** without causing sedation or depressing the entire central nervous system (CNS). Medications are used for treating both basic categories of mental disorders—**neurosis** and **psychosis.**

NEUROSIS VERSUS PSYCHOSIS

Both basic categories—neurosis and psychosis—are treated with tranquilizers in individuals who display agitation, hyperactivity, and inappropriate and sometimes violent behavior. The mentally ill individual is unable to communicate with others and to function in normal activities.

Neurosis is found in the fearful individual who is still in contact with reality but cannot adjust favorably to surroundings or life situations. Many situations in life produce fear or anxiety from either real or unknown danger with stimulation of the "fight-or-flight" response of the sympathetic nervous system, resulting in sleeplessness and either an increase or a decrease in appetite. The accumulation of anxiousness and tension may cause neurosis to occur. Treatment involves **psychoanalysis** to determine the cause of the anxiety and drug therapy using anxiolytics to alleviate symptoms. Types of anxiety-related conditions are generalized anxiety disorder (GAD), social anxiety disorder, and obsessive-compulsive disorder.

GAD, a chronic condition characterized by uncontrollable worrying for 6 months or more, is accompanied by depression with insomnia, trembling, apprehension, and poor concentration. Physical symptoms include tachycardia, sweating, and palpitations. The most commonly used drugs are benzodiazepines such as *lorazepam* (Ativan) and *diazepam* (Valium), *buspirone* (BuSpar), *venlafaxine* (Effexor), and selective serotonin reuptake inhibitors (SSRIs) such as *paroxetine* (Paxil CR).

Social anxiety disorder has characteristics of intense, irrational fear in situations where scrutinizing or humiliation may occur. Symptoms include blushing, stuttering, sweating, palpitations, muscle tension, and dry throat. SSRIs such as paroxetine are drugs of choice for treatment of these disorders.

Obsessive-compulsive disorder is characterized by obsessions and compulsions interfering with daily living. Patients may perform such actions as excessive hand washing, placement of objects, or hoarding. Treatment includes use of SSRIs such as *fluoxetine* (Prozac) and *sertraline* (Zoloft) and tricyclic antidepressants (TCAs) such as *clomipramine* (Anafranil).

In psychosis, the person has lost contact with reality, resulting in the inability to communicate satisfactorily. The personality breaks down, with thought patterns and responses to the environment unrelated to real-life situations. Treatment for this severe mental illness may require hospitalization.

Important Facts about Mental Health

- Mental health is difficult to define and may change from person to person, culture to culture, and time to time. Mental health is ability to live with daily stressors.
- Psychotherapeutic agents are among the most frequently prescribed medications.
- Natural, temporary situations promoting sadness, anxiety, or restlessness do not always need to be treated with psychotherapeutic agents.
- Proper diet, exercise, and a pleasant environment are important in treating emotional disorders.
- Neurosis is found in the individual who is in contact with reality but is unable to adjust favorably to surroundings or situations. Anxiety is major symptom of neurosis.
- Psychosis occurs when a person is out of touch with reality.

ANXIOLYTICS OR DRUGS FOR ANXIETY (MINOR TRANQUILIZERS)

Drugs used for the relief of anxiety may also be used as hypnotics or sedatives to promote sleep (see Chapter 29). The difference between using medications as anxiolytics and as hypnotics is based on dose—a lower dose to relieve anxiety and higher doses for hypnotic effects; a single medication may be prescribed for both uses. These medications may also be used for skeletal muscle relaxants for chronic muscle pain, especially back pain and/or muscle spasms. Occasionally, minor tranquilizers are also used for seizures to reduce the number of convulsions and as adjunctive medication in alcohol withdrawal. These medications, classified as Schedules III and IV drugs, are for short-term use and are contraindicated for long-term use and carry the possibility of tolerance and physical or psychologic drug dependence or habituation, especially in larger doses. Sudden withdrawal of minor tranquilizers may result in seizures, agitation, psychosis, insomnia, and gastric distress. This information is an important warning in patient education. Some of these drugs may be unclassified under the Controlled Substances Act (Table 30-1).

Benzodiazepines

Benzodiazepines, first introduced in the 1960s, are the drugs of choice in treating anxiety and insomnia. Today benzodiazepines are among the most widely prescribed medications in the United States, with *diazepam* (Valium) being the most familiar. Because these medications have few actions outside the CNS, thus having lower potential for abuse and producing less tolerance and physical dependence, they are safer than some CNS depressants. With benzodiazepines, calmness occurs without excessive sedation. Increasing doses cause sedation that may progress to hypnosis and stupor.

Taken via the oral route of administration, benzodiazepines are readily absorbed from the gastrointestinal tract. Diazepam and *lorazepam* (Ativan) may also be given by injection when more rapid action is desired or required. Duration of action is the major difference in benzodiazepines. Long-acting agents have half-lives of more than 29 hours, whereas short-acting drugs have half-lives of 5 to 20 hours. Tremors and extrapyramidal effects may occur with persistent use of these drugs, especially in the elderly. Excessive use of benzodiazepines may lead to interference with memory and to psychotic behavior. Aggressive behavior could become violent with prolonged drug use. Patients who operate machinery including driving a car should be careful of sedating actions.

Patients must realize that anxiolytics only relieve symptoms and do not cure anxiety. The reason for anxiety must be found and eliminated for symptoms to be alleviated. Drug dependency with antianxiety agents comes more from habituation than from physical dependence; thus care should be taken that the medication does not become a crutch for relieving stress and unhappiness. Abuse of benzodiazepines is more likely to occur with patients who take larger than therapeutic doses. Benzodiazepines should be avoided during pregnancy and used with extreme caution in patients who are suicidal, are severely depressed, or have depressed vital signs (Box 30-1).

TABLE 30-1 SELECT MEDICATIONS USED AS ANXIOLYTICS OR ANTIANXIETY MEDICATIONS

GENERIC NAME (SCHEDULE)/ TRADE NAME	USUAL ADULT DOSE, ROUTE, AND FREQUENCY	INDICATIONS FOR USE	DRUG INTERACTIONS
SHORT-ACTING BENZODIAZEPINES		Anxiety, panic disorders	Other CNS depressants, alcohol, cimetidine, anticoagulants, corticosteroids, digitalis, phenytoin, oral contraceptives
alprazolam (III) (Xanax, Xanax XR, Niravam)	0.25-1 mg PO tid		
lorazepam (III) (Ativan)	0.5-1 mg PO, IM, IV bid-tid		
quazepam (IV) (Doral)	7.5-15 mg PO qhs		

Major Side Effects of Short-Acting Benzodiazepines:
Drowsiness, confusion, ataxia, nausea, constipation, dry mouth, GI disturbances, rashes, photosensitivity, menstrual irregularities, loss of libido

GENERIC NAME (SCHEDULE)/ TRADE NAME	USUAL ADULT DOSE, ROUTE, AND FREQUENCY	INDICATIONS FOR USE	DRUG INTERACTIONS
LONG-ACTING BENZODIAZEPINES			Same as short-acting Benzodiazephines
chlordiazepoxide (III)	5-10 mg PO tid-qid	Anxiolytic, alcohol withdrawal	
			Antiseizure
clonazepam (III) (Klonopin)	0.5 mg PO bid		Antiseizure, other anxiolytics, alcohol withdrawal
clorazepate (III) (Tranxene-T)	7.5-15 mg PO in divided doses		
diazepam (III) (Valium)	2-10 mg PO bid-qid, IM, IV		Same as for clorazepate, muscle relaxant and preoperative medication
oxazepam (III)	30-120 mg PO in divided doses		Same as for clorazepate, alcohol, CNS depressants, MAOIs
MISCELLANEOUS ANXIOLYTICS			Same as for short-acting Benzodiazepines
buspirone (BuSpar)	5-10 mg PO qd	Anxiety	
hydroxyzine (Vistaril)	25-100 mg PO, IM qid	Anxiety, emesis, antipruritic, preoperative medications	
paroxetine (Paxil)	10-50 mg PO qd	Anxiety, depression, obsessive-compulsive disorder, panic disorder	MAOIs, cimetidine, phenytoin, risperidone
venlafaxine (Effexor XR)	37.5-225 mg PO qd	Anxiety, depression	MAOIs

Major Side Effects of Miscellaneous Anxiolytics:
buspirone—dizziness, tinnitus, lightheadedness, rashes, fatigue, nausea, chest pain, nasal congestion, sore throat, CNS disturbance; hydroxyzine, paroxetine, trazodone—drowsiness, dry mouth, pain at injection site; in addition: diaphoresis, tremors, vomiting with paroxetine; unpleasant taste, headache with trazodone

CNS, Central nervous system; GI, gastrointestinal; INH, isoniazid; IM, intramuscularly; IV, intravenously; MAOIs, monoamine oxidase inhibitors; PO, orally.

BOX 30-1 OTHER COMMON ANXIOLYTICS

- *Buspirone* (BuSpar) is solely an antianxiety medication, having no anticonvulsant or muscle-relaxing properties or sedative effect. Not substantially impairing psychomotor function, it is more effective for cognitive and interpersonal relationship issues such as anger and hostility, whereas benzodiazepines are more effective for somatic symptoms. BuSpar, not a controlled substance, is well tolerated, and dosage may be increased progressively as needed because its potential for tolerance and drug dependency is low.
- *Hydroxyzine* (Vistaril, Atarax) has many uses as an antihistamine, anxiolytic, antiemetic, or sedative. This medication may be given by mouth or by injection. When given by injection, it must be given deep intramuscularly to prevent irritation to tissue.
- Three medications introduced as miscellaneous anxiolytics and for treatment of hypertension—*paroxetine* (Paxil) and *venlafaxine* (Effexor)—are not Drug Enforcement Administration (DEA)–scheduled drugs and are all used for anxiety and depression. Paroxetine is also used for obsessive-compulsive and panic disorders. Venlafaxine is used for generalized anxiety disorder (see Table 30-1).

Important Facts about Anxiolytics

- Drugs used to treat anxiety are called *antianxiety agents, anxiolytics,* or *minor tranquilizers* and most may also be used as hypnotics.
- Elderly persons generally require lower doses of psychotherapeutic agents and may experience excessive sedation when given the usual adult dose.
- OTC medications such as antihistamines and cough preparations may cause excessive sedation when combined with minor tranquilizers.
- Alcohol should not be combined with any anxiolytic.
- The potential for abuse and addiction is high when tranquilizers are used for a prolonged period of time.
- The principal indications for benzodiazepines are anxiety, insomnia, and possibly seizure disorders. These drugs are safer than barbiturates, have a lower abuse potential, and cause less tolerance and dependence.
- Benzodiazepines may cause severe respiratory depression when mixed with other central nervous system depressants.
- All benzodiazepines have essentially the same pharmacologic action; therefore selection is based on the differences in action time. Benzodiazepines, the drugs of choice for transient insomnia, should be administered intermittently for only 2 to 3 weeks.
- Benzodiazepines should not be used during pregnancy or by persons with sleep apnea. Schedule IV under the Controlled Substances Act, these drugs have a possibility of dependence.
- Care should be taken when using any anxiolytic or psychotherapeutic medication in persons with suicidal tendencies.

✎ **LEARNING TIP**

Note that many of the benzodiazepines have generic names that end in "pam" or "lam."

Patient Education for Compliance

1. Benzodiazepines should be taken with food if gastrointestinal symptoms occur.
2. Patients should take anxiolytic medications as ordered and should not increase dosage or discontinue medications without consulting a physician. Relaxation techniques may also help reduce stress.
3. Transient insomnia usually will be relieved once the precipitating stressor has been eliminated.
4. Drowsiness occurs with benzodiazepines, so hazardous activities should be avoided until effects of the medication can be evaluated by the patient.
5. Physical dependence is rare with most benzodiazepines, but persons using alprazolam (Xanax) have reported substantial dependence factors.
6. Benzodiazepines should not be used with pregnancy.
7. Abrupt discontinuation of anxiolytics may lead to seizures, agitation, psychosis, insomnia, and gastric upset.

NEUROLEPTICS OR DRUGS FOR PSYCHOSIS (MAJOR TRANQUILIZERS)

Psychosis does not have a single diagnosis but is clinically described as being out of touch with reality. The two major forms of psychosis are schizophrenia and severe depression, although other conditions are classified as psychosis.

Persons with schizophrenia have symptoms of withdrawal from the social environment with **hallucinations, delusions,** and inappropriate or unpredictable behavior. Psychotic symptoms may be caused by medications used to treat illnesses, causing the patient to lose contact with reality. The patient with schizophrenia has deterioration in social functioning, with disorganized thoughts, changes in **affect,** and inability to perform tasks needed for daily living. Speech may be incoherent, repetitive, and reflective of wandering thoughts. Tangents, or inability to get to the point in communication, are not uncommon. With persecution delusions, the individual feels threatened and that others are trying to cause personal harm in some way. With delusions of grandeur an exaggerated feeling of importance, knowledge, or identity is present. Treatment for both delusions and hallucinations involves psychotherapy and use of antipsychotic medications, also called **neuroleptics** or major tranquilizers.

The patient with severe depression has strong feelings of hopelessness and is often suicidal and should be evaluated regularly when taking antipsychotics.

Uses for Antipsychotics or Neuroleptics

In general, antipsychotics are effective in three major areas: (1) to relieve the symptoms of psychosis or severe neurosis such as delusions, hallucinations, agitation, and combativeness; (2) to therapeutically relieve nausea and vomiting (see Chapter 24); and (3) to potentiate analgesics, for example, as promethazine does (see Chapter 15).

Dosage of antipsychotics is regulated to modify disturbed behavior and to relieve symptoms of severe anxiety without profound impairment of consciousness. Antipsychotic medications, also called *neuroleptics* (formerly called *major tranquilizers*), do not cure acute or chronic psychosis but are used to control the related symptoms. The most important classes of antipsychotic medications—phenothiazines, butyrophenones, and thioxanthenes—are used to suppress symptoms of schizophrenia and other psychotic conditions. The exact mechanism of action is not well understood, but it is thought that these agents act on dopamine, a neurotransmitter in the brain. Serotonin, another neurotransmitter, is also involved in the control of psychotic behavior. Some drugs block serotonin to act as antipsychotic

agents and are considered *atypical* antipsychotic drugs because their main action is not against dopamine but rather on serotonin (Table 30-2).

Potency and Neuroleptics

Antipsychotics can also be classified by *potency*—not to be confused with drug effectiveness. *Effectiveness* measures therapeutic response to individual medications. *Potency* refers to drug quantity necessary to produce an equivalent effect when compared with a medication of the same drug classification. Antipsychotics are classified by their potency—low potency, intermediate potency, and high potency. An example is ***chlorpromazine*** (Thorazine), a low-potency drug. Thorazine 100 mg is considered to be the equivalent of ***mesoridazine*** (Serentil) 50 mg (an intermediate-potency drug) or ***haloperidol*** (Haldol) 2 mg (a high-potency agent) (See Table 30-2).

Side Effects of Neuroleptics

As patients take antipsychotic medications from months to a prolonged period of time, medications tend to cause extrapyramidal effects by blocking dopamine receptors. **Tardive dyskinesia,** a more serious condition, includes involuntary movements such as tics; movements of the lips, jaws, and tongue; and jerking movements of extremities that cause postural imbalance. Often, tardive dyskinesia appears when the medication is discontinued, and either restarting the drug or increasing the dosage may suppress symptoms, but with further prolonged use the dyskinesia worsens and becomes unresponsive to treatment. These symptoms may then become permanent and irreversible; therefore frequent office visits to assess progression of dyskinesia are important (Figure 30-1).

TABLE 30-2 SELECT DRUGS USED TO TREAT PSYCHOSIS

GENERIC NAME/ TRADE NAME (POTENCY)	USUAL ADULT DOSE, ROUTE, AND FREQUENCY*	INDICATIONS FOR USE	DRUG INTERACTIONS
TRADITIONAL ANTIPSYCHOTICS			
PHENOTHIAZINES		Psychosis	antihistamines, alcohol, analgesics, tranquilizers, narcotics, guanethidine, beta blockers, barbiturates, insulin, oral hypoglycemics, anticholinergics, levodopa, epinephrine
chlorpromazine (LP)	25-50 mg PO bid-qid, IM, IV	Psychosis, emesis, and hiccups	
	May be up to 1000 mg		
fluphenazine HCl	2.5-10 mg PO qd-qid		
fluphenazine decanoate (HP)	12.5-25 mg IM as depot q1-4wk		

TABLE 30-2 SELECT DRUGS USED TO TREAT PSYCHOSIS—cont'd

GENERIC NAME/ TRADE NAME (POTENCY)	USUAL ADULT DOSE, ROUTE, AND FREQUENCY*	INDICATIONS FOR USE	DRUG INTERACTIONS
perphenazine (IP)	8-24 mg PO tid, 5-10 mg IM, IV	Psychosis, emesis	
prochlorpcrazine	5-10 mg PO tid-qid, 10-20 mg IM, IV	Psychosis, emesis	
(Campro) (IP)	25 mg rectal suppository		
thioridazine (LP)	50-800 mg PO qd		
trifluoperazine (HP)	5-40 mg PO in divided doses		

Major Side Effects of Phenothiazines:

Postural hypotension, tachycardia, bradycardia, vertigo, dry mouth, blurred vision, fever, constipation, urinary retention, anorexia, rashes, photosensitivity, insomnia, agitation, restlessness, depression, headaches, confusion, drowsiness, weakness

BUTYROPHENONE

haloperidol (Haldol) (HP)	0.5-2 mg PO bid-hd 2.5 mg IM	Psychosis, mania, schizophrenic	alcohol, lithium, CNS depressants, levodopa, epinephrine

THIOXANTHENE

		Psychosis	Same as for haloperidol
thiothixene (Navane) (HP)	2 mg PO tid		

DIBENZODIAZEPINES DERIVATIVES

			Same as for haloperidol
clozapine (Clozaril Fazaclo) (AT)	75-450 mg PO qd	Psychosis, schizophrenia mania, depression	
loxapine (Loxatine)	60-100 mg PO qd-bid		

ATYPICAL ANTIPSYCHOTIS BENZISOXAZOLE

			Same as for haloperidol
risperidone (Risperdal) (AT)	1-6 mg PO, IM in divided doses	Psychosis, irritability of autism; bipolar disorder	

THIENOBENZODIAZEPINE

			carbamazepine, levodopa, antihypertensives
olanzapine (Zyprexa) (AT)	10 mg PO qd	Schizophrenia	

MISCELLANEOUS

lurasidone (Latuda)	40-80 mg PO qd	Schizophrenia	
iloperidone (Fanapt) (AT)	1-12 mg PO bid	Schizophrenia	paroxetine and ketoconazole
aripiprazole (Abilify) (Abilify Dismelt) (AT)	15-30 mg PO, IM 15-20 mg (oral disintegration tablet)	Schizophrenia, bipolar disease	Antifungals, carbamazepine, paroxetine, fluoxetine, alcohol
ziprasidone (Geodon) (AT)	20-160 mg PO bid, IM	Schizophrenia, bipolar mania	Same as aripiprazole
quetiapine (Seroquel) (AT)	25-50 mg PO qd	Psychosis, depression, mania	alcohol, opioids, lorazepam, dopamine

AT, Atypical agent; *CNS,* central nervous system; *HP,* high potency; *IM,* intramuscularly; *IP,* intermediate potency; *IV,* intravenously; *LP,* low potency; *PO,* orally; *SL,* sublingually.

*Given in divided doses unless otherwise noted.

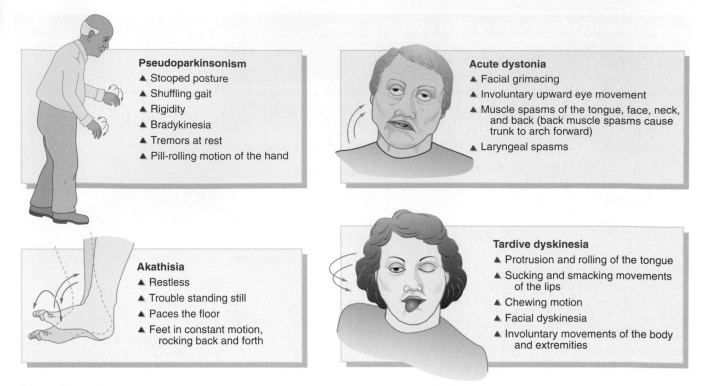

Pseudoparkinsonism
- ▲ Stooped posture
- ▲ Shuffling gait
- ▲ Rigidity
- ▲ Bradykinesia
- ▲ Tremors at rest
- ▲ Pill-rolling motion of the hand

Acute dystonia
- ▲ Facial grimacing
- ▲ Involuntary upward eye movement
- ▲ Muscle spasms of the tongue, face, neck, and back (back muscle spasms cause trunk to arch forward)
- ▲ Laryngeal spasms

Akathisia
- ▲ Restless
- ▲ Trouble standing still
- ▲ Paces the floor
- ▲ Feet in constant motion, rocking back and forth

Tardive dyskinesia
- ▲ Protrusion and rolling of the tongue
- ▲ Sucking and smacking movements of the lips
- ▲ Chewing motion
- ▲ Facial dyskinesia
- ▲ Involuntary movements of the body and extremities

Figure 30-1 Extrapyramidal adverse effects of neuroleptic medications. (From Kee JL, Hayes ER, McCuistion LE: *Pharmacology: a nursing process approach,* ed 6, St Louis, 2009, Saunders.)

Elderly patients taking neuroleptics seem more prone to *parkinsonian symptoms* such as tremors, drooling, tongue protrusion, muscular rigidity, and dysphagia. Antiparkinsonism medications used prophylactically, such as anticholinergic drugs with antipsychotic medications, will not prevent extrapyramidal symptoms, and symptoms only continue to worsen. Although seen in adults, dystonic reactions including muscle spasms of the head with twitching, facial grimacing, torticollis or wryneck, and twisting of the face, neck, and back are more prone to occur in children.

Dystonia usually appears early in treatment and subsides rapidly with medication discontinuation. Anticholinergics are used for treating dystonia. **Akathisia,** or motor restlessness, also more common in children, is manifested by continuous body movement with restlessness, pacing, and insomnia.

Antipsychotics, contraindicated with seizure disorders, severe depression, parkinsonism, and pregnancy, must be used with caution in children and the elderly, patients with hepatic or renal disease, men with prostatic hypertrophy, and patients with glaucoma. Boxes 30-2 and 30-3 list implications in elderly patients and children. Box 30-4 lists the classes of drugs used as antipsychotics.

✏ LEARNING TIP

Generic names for most phenothiazines end in "zine."

BOX 30-2 PEDIATRIC IMPLICATIONS FOR USE OF PSYCHOTHERAPEUTIC AGENTS

- Children are at greater risk of developing extrapyramidal side effects, especially dystonia.
- Pediatric patients with chickenpox, central nervous system infections, measles, dehydration, gastroenteritis, or other acute illnesses are more at risk of developing severe adverse reactions and even Reye's syndrome.
- Tricyclic antidepressants are usually not recommended for depression in children younger than age 12. Some agents such as amitriptyline (Elavil), desipramine (Norpramin), and imipramine (Tofranil) may be used in children older than 6 who have major depression.
- Children are sensitive to acute overdosage, which may be serious and even fatal.
- Increased nervousness, sleeplessness, complaints of being tired, hypertension, and stomach distress are found in children taking tricyclic antidepressants.
- Lithium may decrease bone density and bone formation when used with children.
- SSRI agents have been approved for children and adolescents.
- SSRIs have black box warnings for suicidal ideation in children.

Atypical antipsychotic medications are agents blocking serotonin and dopamine receptors. **Clozapine** (Clozaril), a typical drug, causes sedation, hypotension, and anticholinergic effects, but extrapyramidal effects occur only with large doses. Atypical agents have the advantage

- Older persons tend to have higher serum levels of antipsychotic and antidepressant drugs because of changes in drug distribution from a decrease in lean body mass, less total body water, lower serum albumin, and usually an increase in body fat. These patients need lower doses.
- Geriatric patients are more likely to have orthostatic hypotension, anticholinergic side effects, extrapyramidal effects, and sedation.
- Elderly patients should receive half the recommended adult dose. When clinical improvement is noted, attempts to taper or discontinue medications should be instituted.
- Tricyclic antidepressants may cause increased anxiety in geriatric patients. The tricyclic antidepressant increases the risk of inducing dysrhythmias, tachycardia, stroke, congestive heart failure, and myocardial infarction in persons with cardiovascular disease.
- Lithium is more toxic for geriatric patients. The elderly are more prone to central nervous system toxicity, lithium-induced goiter, and clinical hypothyroidism.

BOX 30-4 CLASSES OF DRUGS USED AS ANTIPSYCHOTICS

- *Chlorpromazine* (Thorazine), the first antipsychotic agent, remains typical of phenothiazines that possess anticholinergic, antiemetic, antihistaminic, and alpha-adrenergic blocking effects and antipsychotic actions. These drugs are also used for treatment of nausea, vomiting, pruritus, and allergic reactions, although they are not the drugs of first choice. Phenothiazine derivatives may also be used as adjuvant therapy with tetanus and intractable hiccups, as well as for **bipolar disorder,** agitation, and **delirium tremens.**
- Butyrophenone derivatives, chemically different from phenothiazines, have the same antipsychotic effects. Haloperidol (Haldol), the main drug in this group, is used as an antipsychotic and antiemetic and for severe behavioral problems in children. **Tourette's syndrome,** a CNS disease with rapid, involuntary, repetitive motor movements of muscles and involuntary vocal tics or noises, can also be controlled by this drug. Low doses of haloperidol have been used to treat severe agitation, combativeness, and psychosis in demented persons. Because butyrophenones cause greater movement disturbances than phenothiazines, elderly patients should receive lowered doses (see Table 30-2).
- Thioxanthenes are chemically similar to phenothiazines. *Thiothixene* (Navane), the typical drug in this group, exerts antipsychotic effects by blocking dopamine in the brain but is more selective in causing extrapyramidal effects.
- *Loxapine* (Loxitane), a dibenzodiazepine and similar to phenothiazines, causes a moderate degree of sedation with a high incidence of extrapyramidal symptoms.

of not causing tardive dyskinesia and so are well suited for patients who previous experienced extrapyramidal symptoms. *Olanzapine* (Zyprexa), a typical thienobenzodiazepine, is used to treat schizophrenia by blocking serotonin and dopamine. Newer miscellaneous atypical antipsychotic agents, such as *aripiprazole* (Abilify) and *ziprasidone* (Geodon), have fewer side effects, such as sedation, extrapyramidal effects, and hypotension, making them more patient friendly (see Table 30-2).

Treatment of Psychosis with Parenteral Medications

For long-term maintenance therapy of schizophrenia, depot injectable antipsychotics with long-acting capabilities are used for patients who may not be compliant on a daily basis or tend to be generally noncompliant. Parenteral medication prevents relapses and maintains the highest possible level of functioning with no greater risk of side effects than found with oral preparations. Risk of tardive dyskinesia is actually reduced. The most commonly used medications for depot administration are *haloperidol* (Haldol) and *fluphenazine* (Prolixin). With long-term therapy, the depot method may be more effective, with fewer withdrawal symptoms, fewer side effects, and better compliance.

Treatment of Schizophrenia

Treatment for schizophrenia is chronic and prolonged and has three major objectives: (1) suppress acute episodes of psychosis, (2) prevent acute disease exacerbations, and (3) maintain the highest possible functional level.

Unless contraindicated, high-potency traditional agents are used. The exact drug depends on patient response, as some patients respond more successfully to a specific medication. Selection may even require a medication trial to determine the drug with fewest side effects, maximum comfort, and greatest promotion of compliance.

Patients should be allowed an attempt at treatment discontinuation after a year of therapy; approximately 25% of patients will not need drug continuation. The time chosen for attempted tapered discontinuation should not be a stressful time.

Important Facts about Antipsychotics

- Antipsychotics are effective in three major areas: to relieve psychosis or severe neurosis, to relieve nausea and vomiting, and to potentiate analgesics.

Continued

Important Facts about Antipsychotics—cont'd

- Antipsychotic medications fall into two groups, traditional and atypical. Traditional drugs are thought to relieve symptoms by blocking neurotransmitter receptors such as dopamine. Atypical medications block other neurotransmitters such as serotonin.
- Major indication for antipsychotics is schizophrenia, a chronic illness marked by hallucinations, delusions, and agitation along with disorganized thoughts and loss of reality. Social withdrawal is often seen.
- Low-potency to high-potency traditional antipsychotics have equal therapeutic effect.
- Low-potency agents produce more sedation, orthostatic hypotension, and anticholinergic effects than high-potency agents.
- Therapeutic effects of antipsychotic medications develop slowly, often taking several weeks to be effective.
- Traditional antipsychotic medications may cause three types of extrapyramidal effects: tardive dyskinesia, acute dystonia, and akathisia.
- Atypical antipsychotics cause few or no extrapyramidal effects.
- Depot parenteral antipsychotic agents are used for long-term schizophrenia maintenance therapy and for those who tend to be noncompliant.
- Chlorpromazine (Thorazine) was the first low-potency agent and is the prototype for antipsychotic medications. Haloperidol (Haldol) is the prototype for high-potency agents.

Patient Education for Compliance

1. Patients should be aware of the psychologic and physical dependence potential with prolonged use of psychotropic medications. Medicines should be taken at prescribed dosage for the time set.
2. No CNS depressants—analgesics, alcohol, muscle relaxants, antihistamines, antiemetics, cardiac medications, and antihypertensives—should be taken with psychotropics unless ordered by a physician.
3. Be careful when taking any medications with antipsychotics because of many drug interactions, especially with OTC antihistamines and sleeping aids.
4. Patients taking psychotropic medications should be educated about orthostatic hypotension and the dangers of changing positions rapidly.
5. Avoid sun exposure with antipsychotics because of sunburn danger with prolonged sun exposure.
6. Report restlessness, muscle spasms, rigidity, tremors, drooling, visual disturbances, weakness, and faintness when taking antipsychotics.
7. Oral antipsychotic liquid medications should be protected from light.

Patient Education for Compliance—cont'd

8. Dilution of oral liquid antipsychotics should be achieved using fruit juice to increase palatability.
9. Oral antipsychotic liquids may cause contact dermatitis, so avoid skin contact.
10. Patients should have written and verbal instructions on dosage and timing of medications. Have family members assist with medication compliance.
11. Educate patients about early signs of extrapyramidal symptoms such as spasticity in the face, neck, and tongue and restlessness.
12. Dry mouth, blurred vision, photophobia, urinary hesitancy, and constipation are possible and should be reported. If symptoms become severe, medication may have to be stopped or a reduced dosage attempted. Mouth dryness may be relieved by chewing gum or sucking on hard candy.
13. Sexual dysfunction is possible with antipsychotics and should be reported for reduction of dosage or change in medication.
14. Patients should attend all psychotherapeutic sessions when taking medications for psychotic conditions.
15. Antipsychotics cause drowsiness. Tasks that require mental alertness should not be attempted until medication effects are known.
16. High-fiber diets are important and a stool softener may be needed when taking antipsychotics because of their constipating effects.

DEPRESSION AND ITS TREATMENT

Depression, one of the most common psychiatric disorders, is characterized by feelings of intense sadness, helplessness, and worthlessness causing impaired functioning. Appetite disturbances such as anorexia or overeating, sleep disturbances, and loss of interest in previously enjoyed activities, including family and work, are physical and psychologic symptoms of depression. Diagnosis of depression generally includes psychologic symptoms of mood changes with despondency, anxiety, self-pity, low self-esteem, hopelessness, and helplessness. Physiologic manifestations include either insomnia or hypersomnia, headaches, loss of energy, and complaints of fatigue, and thought alterations, including decreased concentration, poor memory, confusion, and delusions. Mood swings are often diurnal or related to specific times of day and are often worse in mornings.

Mood disorders, also called **affective disorders,** include depression as well as mania or elation. Many factors including genetics, psychosocial events, physiologic stress, and personality traits precipitate affective disorders such as depression. Major depression is presently referred to as *unipolar affective disorder.* Disorders

BOX 30-5 RECOGNIZING DEPRESSION

Signs of depression include the following:

- Minor fluctuations in mood, becoming an overall "down" feeling
- Feeling overwhelmed by responsibilities
- Future seems dismal
- Negative opinion of self
- Criticizing and blaming self repeatedly
- Smallest incidents of life are bothersome

BOX 30-6 SELECTION OF ANTIDEPRESSANT MEDICATIONS FOR DEPRESSED PATIENTS

A. First- and second-line choices
   1. Secondary amine tricyclic antidepressants
   2. bupropion (Wellbutrin, Zyban)
   3. fluoxetine (Prozac)—SSRI
   4. paroxetine (Paxil)—SSRI
   5. sertraline (Zoloft)—SSRI
   6. trazodone (Desyrel)
B. Alternative agents for patients with special medical considerations
   1. Tertiary amine TCAs for the following:
      a. Absence of serious medical illness including cardiac disease
      b. Need for rapid sedation
   2. MAOIs
      a. Unresponsiveness or intolerance to at least one TCA
      b. Family or personal history of response to MAOI
      c. Atypical depression symptoms
   3. Select anxiolytic medications
      a. Medical contraindications to FDA-approved antidepressant medications
      b. No adverse cardiovascular effects
      c. Low side-effect profile
      d. No history of substance abuse
      e. Need for quick action
      f. Short, limited exposure time needed for medication

FDA, Food and Drug Administration; *MAOI,* monoamine oxidase inhibitor; *SSRI,* selective serotonin reuptake inhibitor; *TCA,* tricyclic antidepressant.

that include mixed-type reactions or mood changes from elation to depression are called *bipolar disorder* (previously known as *manic-depressive disorder*). Dysthymia, a milder form of depression, is typical of those who are sad or "down in the dumps." This person is chronically depressed, finding little joy or excitement in life and having had more days of depression than not for at least 2 years. Dysthymia is a common condition—approximately 6% of the entire population experiences dysthymia in their life, with about 3% affected at any given time. These processes have no single cause, but it is believed that stressful events or mental conflicts precede depression (Box 30-5).

Antidepressant Medications

Major antidepressant drug classes include monoamine oxidase inhibitors (MAOIs), TCAs, SSRIs, and selective norepinephrine uptake inhibitors (SNRIs). Some herbal supplements, called *natural reuptake inhibitors* (NRIs), have also been indicated as antidepressants. The therapeutic response rate with all antidepressants is similar, so agent selection is dependent on drug side effects associated with patient drug experiences in the past. Selection must be based on potential side effects compared with the individual's medical conditions. Some patients will need sedation for agitation, so a sedating antidepressant is ordered. The Depression Guideline Panel in 1993 established medication selection manner (Box 30-6).

Tricyclic Antidepressants

TCAs, so named because of their triple-ring structure, are used with major depression because they are inexpensive, effective, easy to administer, and relatively safe. TCAs block uptake of serotonin and norepinephrine to result in stimulation. The first tricyclic agent, **imipramine** (Tofranil), was introduced in the 1950s, leading to a group of medications to relieve depressive symptoms by blocking reuptake of endogenous neurohormones. TCAs may also assist with pain control, chronic insomnia, and attention-deficit/hyperactivity disorder (ADHD)

and are also used for obsessive-compulsive disorders and enuresis in children.

TCAs are equally effective. Geriatric patients are usually started on one third to one half of the usual adult dose, followed by dosage evaluation and adjustment based on therapeutic response and presence or absence of undesirable side effects (Table 30-3).

Atypical Antidepressants

Atypical antidepressants are second-generation antidepressants; first available in the 1980s, they are used with major depression, reactive depression, and anxiety. These medications affect one or two of the neurotransmitters—serotonin, norepinephrine, and dopamine—and should not be taken with MAOIs (Box 30-7).

Monoamine Oxidase Inhibitors

MAOIs, such as **phenelzine** (Nardil), are antidepressants used only for atypical depression when other medications have not been effective. These medications have numerous interactions with prescription and OTC medications as well as caffeine- and tyramine-containing

TABLE 30-3 DRUGS USED TO TREAT DEPRESSION

GENERIC NAME/ TRADE NAME	USUAL ADULT DOSE, ROUTE, AND FREQUENCY	INDICATIONS FOR USE	DRUG INTERACTIONS
TRICYCLIC ANTIDEPRESSANTS (TSAs)		Depression	alcohol, amphetamines, anticholinergics, antihistamines, antiseizure medications, barbiturates, MAOIs, phenothiazines, antidysrhythmics
amitriptyline	25-300 mg PO qd		
clomipramine (Anafranil)	25-250 mg qd PO	Obsessive-compulsive disorder, depression	
desipramine (Norpramin)	100-300 mg PO qd	Depression	
doxepin	10-300 mg PO qd		
imipramine (Tofranil)	50-150 mg PO qd		
maprotiline	100-150 mg PO tid		
nortriptyline (Pamelor)	25 mg tid to 150 mg PO qd		
protriptyline (Vivactil)	15-40 mg PO tid		
trimipramine (Surmontil)	100-200 mg PO tid		

Major Side Effects of Tricyclic Antidepressants:
Dry mouth, constipation, urinary retention, tachycardia, orthostatic hypotension, blurred vision, drowsiness, restlessness, tremors, mania, sexual dysfunction

ATYPICAL ANTIDEPRESSANTS		Depression	anticholinergics, guanethidine, phenothiazines
amoxapine	50-100 mg PO tid		
bupropion (Wellbutrin, Zyban)	100-450 mg PO qd		
mirtazapine (Remeron)	15-30 mg PO oral dissolving tablet qhs		
trazodone	100-400 mg PO qd in divided doses		and terfenadine, astemizole
(Oleptro)	150-300 mg PO qhs		

Major Side Effects of Atypical Antidepressants:
amoxapine—EPSs, tardive dyskinesia *bupropion*—same as for tricyclic antidepressants plus agitation, insomnia; *mirtazapine*—somnolence with unusual dreams, increased appetite, weight gain, elevated cholesterol, flulike symptoms; *nefazodone*—somnolence, sexual dysfunction; *trazodone*—sedation, nausea, vomiting; *venlafaxine*—diastolic hypertension.

MONOAMINE OXIDASE INHIBITORS (MAOIs)		Neurosis or atypical depression	See Table 30-5
phenelzine (Nardil)	45-90 mg PO tid		
tranylcypromine (Parnate)	10-40 mg PO tid		

Major Side Effects of MAOIs:
Postural hypotension, dry mouth, constipation, urinary retention, blurred vision, impotence, insomnia, tremors, convulsions

SELECTIVE SEROTONIN REUPTAKE INHIBITORS (SSRIs)		Depression, obsessive-compulsive disorder	alcohol, digitalis, anticholinergics, MAOIs, phenytoin, tryptophan
citalopram (Celexa)	20-40 mg PO qd		and cimetidine
duloxetine (Cymbalta)	60 mg PO qd		and thioridazine
escitalopram (Lexapro)	20-60 mg PO qd		
fluoxetine (Prozac, Sarafem)	10-80 mg PO qd		

DR, Delayed release, *EPSs,* extrapyramidal symptoms; *GI,* gastrointestinal; *IM,* intramuscularly; *MAOIs,* monoamine oxidase inhibitors; *NSAIDs,* nonsteroidal antiinflammatory drugs; *PO,* orally.

TABLE 30-3 DRUGS USED TO TREAT DEPRESSION—cont'd

GENERIC NAME/ TRADE NAME	USUAL ADULT DOSE, ROUTE, AND FREQUENCY	INDICATIONS FOR USE	DRUG INTERACTIONS
fluvoxamine (Luvox CR)	100-200 mg PO qd		
paroxetine (Paxil, Paxil CR, Pexeva)	20-40 mg PO qd		
sertraline (Zoloft)	50-100 mg PO qd		

Major Side Effects of Selective Serotonin Reuptake Inhibitors:

All except duloxetine—sexual dysfunction, nausea, headache, nervousness, insomnia, anxiety, dizziness, fatigue, diarrhea, anorexia, diaphoresis; *duloxetine*—nausea, dry mouth constipation, decreased appetite, sleepiness

SELECTIVE NOREPINEPHRINE REUPTAKE INHIBITOR (SNRIs)

nefazodone	50-300 mg PO bid-tid		Benzodiazipanes, propranolol, digoxin, statins, MAOIs

Major Side Effects of Selective Norepinephrine Reuptake Inhibitors:

Dry mouth, tremors, hypotension, constipation, decreased libido, urinary retention, dizziness, headache, insomnia, diaphoresis

MEDICATIONS FOR BIPOLAR DISORDER

aripiprazole (Abilify)	15-30 mg PO qd	Manic depression disorder, agitation, major depression	See in Table 30-2 also multiple others
carbamazepine (Tegretol)	200-400 mg PO bid initially, up to 1200 mg PO qd		
lithium carbonate (Lithobid)	300-600 mg PO dose varies by formulation	Mania	diuretics, fluoxetine, antithyroid, haloperidol, anticholinergics, phenytoin, NSAIDs
lithium citrate (syrup)	Varies with individual		
divalproex sodium (Depakote)	500-1000 mg PO qd	Manic schizophrenia, aggression in children, epilerpsy, migranes	alcohol, aspirin, warfarin, cimetidine, clonazepam
valproic acid (Depakene) (Stavzor) (DR)	500-1000 mg PO qd 750 mg PO qd	Schizophrenia, epilepsy	erythromycin

Major Side Effects of Bipolar Disorder Medications:

lithium carbonate—nausea, tremors, vomiting, diarrhea, drowsiness, loss of equilibrium, tinnitus, frequency of urination; *carbamazepine*—sedation, GI disturbances, tremors, leukopenia; *valproic acid*—sedation, nausea, tremors, hair loss

foods and beverages (Tables 30-4 and 30-5). Food products cause sudden and severe hypertension that may progress to vascular collapse if untreated.

MAOIs inhibit breakdown of norepinephrine and serotonin to permit an increase of these neurotransmitters, allowing stimulation of the CNS for clinical depression improvement. Initially, after 2 weeks of therapy these drugs cause decrease in appetite and insomnia that continues for approximately 2 weeks after discontinuation of therapy. MAOIs are indicated primarily for resistant depression and anxious hostile depression, especially those with panic attacks or when phobic symptoms are involved. In general, MAOIs are most effective in reversing dysphoric states, but bulimia and obsessive-compulsive disorders may also be treated with these medications (see Table 30-3).

Selective Serotonin Reuptake Inhibitors

SSRIs are newer antidepressants that block reuptake of serotonin to inactivate its brain action, causing stimulation to reverse depression. But unlike TCAs, SSRIs have little action to block cholinergic, adrenergic, or

BOX 30-7 COMMON ATYPICAL ANTIDEPRESSANTS

- **Bupropion** (Wellbutrin, Zyban), one of the drugs of choice for smoking cessation therapy, weakly blocks reuptake of neurotransmitters in people who are unresponsive to other antidepressants.
- **Mirtazapine** (Remeron), a drug in a well-tolerated class of medications, increases release of serotonin and norepinephrine to relieve depression, anxiety, and insomnia.
- **Trazodone** (Desyrel), a second-line agent for depression, can be helpful for patients with antidepressant-induced insomnia. A major side effect is priapism.
- **Venlafaxine** (Effexor), used for anxiety and depression, blocks norepinephrine and serotonin and weakly blocks dopamine, with potential to produce a complete remission.
- An agent that has both antidepressant and antipsychotic properties is **amoxapine** (Asendin). Because of side effects, this medication should be used only for psychotic depression (see Table 30-3).

TABLE 30-4 FOODS THAT ARE UNSAFE AND SAFE TO CONSUME WHEN TAKING MONOAMINE OXIDASE INHIBITORS

CATEGORY	UNSAFE	SAFE
Cheeses, milk products	Practically all cheeses, sour cream, yogurt	Milk, cottage cheese, cream cheese
Meats, fresh sausage	Beef and chicken liver; fermented, smoked, aged meats; bologna, pepperoni, salami; dried or cured fish	Fresh meats, fresh fish
Fruits and vegetables	Avocado, fava beans, figs, raisins, bananas, sauerkraut	Most fruits and vegetables
Foods with yeast	Yeast extract	Baked goods with yeast
Beer, wine	Imported beer, Chianti wine, ale	Domestic beers and wines
Other foods	Protein dietary supplements, soups, shrimp paste, soy sauce	Most other foods
Caffeinated beverages	Colas, tea, coffee, chocolate drinks	Noncaffeinated beverages
Chocolate	Any chocolate product	Nonchocolate products
Ginseng	Herbal products containing ginseng	Nonginseng herbals

TABLE 30-5 MEDICAL REACTIONS OF MAOIS WITH DRUGS AND FOODS

DRUG	POSSIBLE EFFECTS
alcohol, CNS depressants	Enhanced CNS depression
local anesthetics	Severe hypertensive reaction
antidepressants	Elevated temperatures, hypertensive crisis, seizures, death
hypoglycemic agents	Enhancement of hypoglycemics
bupropion	Increased risk of toxicity
buspirone	Hypertension
caffeine	Cardiac dysrhythmias, hypertension
dextromethorphan	Increased excitability, increased fever, hypertension
fluoxetine	Agitation, restlessness, gastrointestinal distress, seizures, hypertensive crisis
guanadrel, guanethidine, *Rauwolfia* alkaloids	Severe hypertension
levodopa	Severe, sudden hypertensive crisis
meperidine and other opioids	Severe hypertension, increased excitability, sweating, and rigidity
methyldopa	Severe headaches, hypertension, hallucinations
methylphenidate	Hypertensive crisis
systemic sympathomimetics	Severe hypertensive crisis, increased temperature, cardiac arrhythmias, headache, vomiting

FOOD (See Box 30-8)	POSSIBLE EFFECTS
tryptophan and tranylcypromine	Hyperventilation, increased temperature, disorientation, mania
tyramine or foods containing large amounts of pressors	Sudden, severe hypertensive crisis

CNS, Central nervous system; *MAOIs,* monoamine oxidase inhibitors.

histamine receptors. Therefore SSRIs have fewer side effects and are the most widely used antidepressant drugs (Box 30-8). SSRIs should be orally administered in the morning because of the chance of nervousness and insomnia. Used primarily to treat major depression, the SSRIs are also approved for obsessive-compulsive disorders. Care should be taken with participation in hazardous activities until symptoms of dizziness as a side effect can be evaluated (see Box 30-8).

BOX 30-8 SELECTIVE SEROTONIN REUPTAKE INHIBITORS

- *Fluoxetine* (Prozac) is often prescribed for this class because it is as effective as tricyclic antidepressants with fewer side effects and is less dangerous when taken in overdose. Although not approved for these uses by the Food and Drug Administration, Prozac is the preferred agent for panic disorders and premenstrual syndrome. Other uses include bulimia, alcoholism, attention-deficit/hyperactivity disorder, bipolar disorder, premenstrual migraine headaches, and obesity. It should be used with care in patients with diabetes mellitus and those with suicidal tendencies.
- *Sertraline* (Zoloft) is also frequently used for posttraumatic stress syndrome, obsessive compulsive disorder, panic disorder, premenstrual syndrome disorder, and seasonal affective disorder.
- *Citalopram* (Celexa) is a medication used only with depression. This agent does not produce a sympathomimetic response or anticholinergic activity and thus have fewer side effects. This medication can be used with monoamine oxidase inhibitors (MAOIs) and should not be given until 2 weeks after MAOIs have been stopped (see Table 30-3).

BOX 30-9 ANTIMANIC MEDICATIONS

- *Lithium,* the most commonly used medication for mania, acts as a mood stabilizer. Used prophylactically to reduce the frequency and severity of mania, lithium appears to reduce hyperactivity and excitement while allowing organization of thought patterns. Indicated for treatment of individuals who experience large shifts in mood, mania, or alternating cycles of depression and mania, lithium can control symptoms in both phases. In the acute manic state, lithium reduces hyperactivity without sedation and may be combined with benzodiazepines or antipsychotic agents that suppress symptoms until lithium can be effective. If depression occurs, an antidepressant, such as a tricyclic antidepressant, must be given because lithium does not prevent episodes of depression, although early symptoms may be controlled.
- *Carbamazepine* (Tegretol), *valproic acid* (Depakene), and *divalproex sodium* (Depakote), originally marketed for seizure disorders, have recently been used to treat bipolar disorder. Carbamazepine reduces symptoms during manic and depressive attacks and is used prophylactically for repeated attacks. Valproic acid, antipsychotics, and divalproex sodium are promising alternatives for lithium for those who have not responded to lithium or cannot tolerate its side effects. Both of these medications control acute manic episodes and may prevent recurrent episodes of mania and depression while being especially useful with rapidly cycling bipolar disorder. For more information about carbamazepine, valproic acid and divalproex sodium, see Chapter 29 under antiseizure medications.

Selective Norepinephrine Reuptake Inhibitors

SNRIs are not related to TCAs, MAOIs, or SSRIs; rather, the two medications in this category, **reboxetine** (Vestra) and **atomoxetine** (Strattera), enhance transmission of norepinephrine. These medications induce remission when used for short-term therapy and prevent relapses in long-term use. The chief indication for these drugs is for patients with severe depression who also have difficulty with social functioning (see Table 30-3).

Natural Reuptake Inhibitors

In recent years, increased interest in herbal supplements acting as NRIs for treatment of depression by stabilizing serotonin and norepinephrine has developed. Studies have shown that St John's wort is helpful for mild to moderate depression but not for severe depression. However, herbals do interact adversely with many drugs. Other natural products, including SAM-e and 5-HTP, increase production of serotonin to regulate mood and emotion. Ginseng and *Ginkgo* have also been tried to treat depression.

Antimanic Medications

Antimanic medications are used for the patient with bipolar disorder, in which alternating episodes of mania and depression typically occur. In the manic state, a heightened mood, with hyperactivity, excessive enthusiasm, overactivity at work or play, and a reduced need for sleep, is apparent. Extreme self-confidence, excessive sociability, and extreme talkativeness are characteristic signs. Thoughts and ideations are unrealistic in the manic phase.

Ideally, bipolar disorder is treated with a combination of medications and psychotherapy because drug therapy alone is not optimal (Box 30-9). Poor patient compliance is often found during manic episodes because the patient sees nothing wrong with his or her thinking or behavior. Furthermore, the manic episode may not be an unpleasant experience. Family is an important factor to ensure patient compliance with medication administration during mania and depression.

Patient Education for Compliance

1. Patients taking monoamine oxidase inhibitors (MAOIs) should keep a list of foods and OTC medications that contain caffeine or tyramine so these can be avoided (see Table 30-4).
2. MAOIs cause dizziness, low blood pressure, dry mouth, constipation, and blurred vision, and impotence in males.
3. Patients should report feelings of faintness, difficulty with urination, agitation, or jaundice when taking MAOIs.

Continued

Patient Education for Compliance—cont'd

4. Patients should monitor blood pressure and pulse when taking tricyclic antidepressants.
5. Anyone taking tricyclic antidepressants should not take any medications, especially OTC medications, without permission from the physician.
6. Insomnia, nausea, loss of appetite, headaches, and nervousness are common side effects of SSRIs.
7. Because of noncompliance, common with any psychotropic or antidepressant medication, patients should be encouraged to take medications as prescribed.
8. Therapeutic effects of psychotropic medications may not occur for several weeks.
9. Patients should inform all health care professionals of current antidepressant therapy.
10. Antidepressants should be taken on a daily basis, not as needed.
11. All selective serotonin reuptake inhibitors (SSRIs) should be administered with food.
12. Patients taking lithium should be monitored for hyperglycemia.
13. Patients must maintain adequate sodium intake when taking lithium; a reduced sodium level causes an increased lithium level.
14. Patients taking lithium should drink at least 10 glasses of fluid a day.

Important Facts about Antidepressants and Antimanics

- Antidepressants are slow to provide therapeutic responses. Initial responses develop in 1 to 3 weeks, but maximum response develops in 1 to 2 months. Therapy should continue for 6 to 12 months after relief of symptoms.
- Tricyclic antidepressants (TCAs) cause sedation, orthostatic hypotension, dry mouth, and constipation.
- TCAs and monoamine oxidase inhibitors (MAOIs) cannot be combined because of the danger of hypertensive crisis.
- Selective serotonin reuptake inhibitors (SSRIs) have fewer side effects and are safer in overdose than TCAs.
- SSRIs may cause insomnia and nervousness. TCAs may cause sedation.
- Sexual dysfunction is more common with SSRIs than with other antidepressants.
- TCAs and MAOIs may cause orthostatic hypotension, whereas SSRIs do not.
- Suicidal tendencies should be evaluated in all depressed patients, especially when medications are being prescribed and taken.
- Lithium, used for bipolar disorder, is teratogenic.

DRUGS FOR ALZHEIMER'S DISEASE

Alzheimer's disease is a devastating illness characterized by progressive memory failure, impaired thinking, confusion, disorientation, personality changes, restlessness, speech disturbances, and inability to perform routine tasks. Tragically, the disease is incurable and affects about 250,000 new individuals per year. Clinically, progressive decline of intellectual functions and reduction or deterioration of nerve pathways have recently been shown to respond to therapy with cholinesterase inhibitors and **memantine** (Namenda) (Table 30-6). Most pharmacotherapy is focused on improving cognitive functioning or limiting disease progression, and control of symptoms. In Alzheimer's disease, acetylcholine (ACh) is decreased (ACh is necessary for neurotransmission and for forming memories) and thus cholinesterase inhibitors are used. With memory loss comes confusion, wandering, agitation, and pacing, which seem to intensify in the early evening—a phenomenon called "sundowning." No specific test for Alzheimer's disease exists; therefore a definitive diagnosis is possible only on autopsy and possibly with brain tissue changes as seen on computed tomography scans. When all other causes of dementia have been ruled out, Alzheimer's disease is a probable diagnosis (Box 30-10).

Investigation is being done into the use of NSAIDs and vitamin E to decrease the risk of the disease and to prevent and treat early symptoms. Evidence indicates that a link exists between the disease and inflammation. Estrogens appear to reduce disease risk in postmenopausal women because estrogens seem to improve memory. If needed, medications for delusions, agitation, depression, or anxiety may be used in patients with Alzheimer's disease; however, TCAs must be used with care because of significant anticholinergic actions.

Did You Know?

Razadyne, a medication for slowing of Alzheimer's disease, is derived from daffodil bulbs.

Important Facts about Medications for Alzheimer's Disease

- Alzheimer's disease is a relentless illness characterized by progressive memory loss, impaired thinking, personality changes, and progressive inability to perform routine tasks.
- Tacrine causes modest improvement in 30% of Alzheimer's disease patients; the other 70% do not respond.
- Several medication categories are being investigated for use to slow the disease in Alzheimer's patients.

TABLE 30-6 DRUGS USED WITH ALZHEIMER'S DISEASE

GENERIC NAME/ TRADE NAME	USUAL ADULT DOSE, ROUTE, AND FREQUENCY	INDICATIONS FOR USE	DRUG INTERACTIONS
donepezil (Aricept)	5-10 mg PO qd	Alzheimer's disease	anticholinergics
ergoloid mesylates	1 mg PO tid	Alzheimer's disease	None
rivastigmine (Exelon)	1.5-3 mg PO bid	Alzheimer's disease	None
	4.6-9.6 mg patch qd		
memantine (Namenda)	5-20 mg PO bid	Alzheimer's disease	carbonic anhydrase inhibitors
galantamine (Razadyne)	4-12 mg PO bid	Alzheimer's disease	cimetidine, ketoconazole, paroxetine, erythromycin
(Razadyne ER)	8-16 mg PO bid		

Major Side Effects*: donepezil*—nausea, diarrhea; *memantine*—dizziness, headache, confusion, constipation, hypertension, cough

NSAIDs, Nonsteroidal antiinflammatory drugs; *PO,* orally.

BOX 30-10 DRUGS FOR ALZHEIMER'S DISEASE

- ***Donepezil*** (Aricept) is similar in mechanism of action to tacrine and has the same effectiveness. Approved by Food and Drug Administration (FDA) for Alzheimer's disease, donepezil does not affect the underlying disease process. Unlike tacrine, donepezil does not cause liver damage.
- ***Galantamine*** (Razadyne), antidementia medication, elevates brain's acetylcholine concentrations to slow degeneration.
- ***Memantine*** (Namenda), recent medication approved as anti-Alzheimer's agent, is used to reduce deterioration of cholinergic nerve pathways with moderate to severe Alzheimer's disease (see Table 30-6).
- ***Rivastigmine*** (Ekelon) is a cholinesterase inhibitor that acts much like Razadyne.

DRUGS USED FOR ATTENTION-DEFICIT/HYPERACTIVITY DISORDER

Attention-deficit/hyperactivity disorder (ADHD) is a common behavioral disorder in children, with an average of one ADHD child in each classroom. Symptoms of inattention, hyperactivity, and impulsivity begin between the ages of 3 to 7 and persist into the teenage years. Boys are four to eight times more likely to have ADHD than girls. Children with ADHD are fidgety and unable to complete tasks, jumping from one activity to another with an inability to concentrate on schoolwork; they tend to be impatient in class, never waiting their turn. Diagnosis is made when symptoms occur before 7 years of age and last for 6 months.

The exact underlying pathology for ADHD is unknown, but symptoms do respond to stimulant medications (see Chapter 29). CNS stimulants should be used for a year or less with an interruption because growth suppression caused by these medications occurs. More important, continued treatment should be assessed yearly. Summer break is a good time for long-term interruption, and weekends and holidays are good times for short-term interruption.

The mainstay drugs for ADHD are **methylphenidate** (Ritalin, Concerta), **dextroamphetamine** (Dexedrine), **amphetamine sulfate** (Adderall), **atomoxetine** (Strattera), and **lisdexamfetamine** (Vyvanse) (Table 30-7). These drugs will have increased warnings for children because of heart disease and psychiatric effects found to happen in later life (Box 30-11).

Patient Education for Compliance

Children taking medications for ADHD who require more than one dose per day should take morning dose after breakfast and last dose by 4:00 PM to prevent insomnia.

TABLE 30-7 DRUGS USED FOR ATTENTION-DEFICIT/HYPERACTIVITY DISORDER

GENERIC NAME/ TRADE NAME (SCHEDULE)	USUAL ADULT DOSE, ROUTE, AND FREQUENCY OF ADMINISTRATION	INDICATIONS FOR USE	DRUG INTERACTIONS
		ADHD, narcolepsy	Other CNS stimulants and MAOIs
amphetamine sulfate (Adderall) (II)	5-30 mg PO qd in AM to bid		
atomoxetine (Strattera)	40 mg PO qd		
dextroamphetamine (Dexedrine) (II)	5-15 mg PO bid		
lisdexamfetamine (Vyvanse) (II)	30 mg-70 mg PO qd		
methylphenidate (Ritalin) (II)	20-30 mg PO* qd in 2-3 divided doses		
(Daytrana)	10 mg transdermal patch x9h daily		
(Ritalin-SR)	20-40 mg PO daily in divided doses		
(Concerta)	18-36 PO qd		

Major Side Effects: insomnia, restlessness, tachycardia, anorexia, dry mouth, diarrhea, talkativeness; *methylphenidate*—insomnia, growth suppression, headache, abdominal pain, lethargy, listlessness, weight loss, dry mouth, irritability; *atomoxetine*—headache, dyspepsia, nausea and vomiting, fatigue, decreased appetite, dizziness, altered mood

ADHD, Attention-deficit/hyperactivity disorder; *CNS,* central nervous system; *MAOIs,* monoamine oxidase inhibitors; *PO,* orally.
*May be given twice a day in morning and midafternoon.

BOX 30-11 MEDICATIONS FOR ATTENTION-DEFICIT/HYPERACTIVITY DISORDER (ADHD) AND ATTENTION-DEFICIT DISORDER (ADD)

- ***Methylphenidate*** (Ritalin), Schedule II medication, is the most commonly prescribed drug. Cognitive functions of memory, reading, and arithmetic improve significantly. Use of a stimulant would seem to be the opposite of the expected. Children respond dramatically to this drug with an increased attention span and well-focused behavior, with decreased distractibility, hyperactivity, restlessness, and impulsiveness. Because the child can concentrate on the task at hand, impulsiveness and hyperactivity decline. Methylphenidate does not suppress rowdy behavior but improves attention and focus. The drug comes in sustained-release tablets that are administered once a day in the morning. Also available are standard tablets, taken two or three times per day in the morning and at noon but may be given at 4:00 PM if behavior is impulsive at home after school. Dosage is individualized according to improvement in symptoms and appearance of side effects. If possible, the medication is not given on weekends and during the summer, known as a **drug holiday.**
- ***Dextroamphetamine*** (Dexedrine and others), also a Schedule II drug, is as effective as methylphenidate; in fact, some children who do not respond to Ritalin will respond to dextroamphetamine. Dexedrine has a rapid time of action, with administration occurring at 8:00 AM and 4:00 PM.
- Another amphetamine-based central nervous system (CNS) stimulant is ***lisdexamfetamine*** (Vyvanse), which provides consistent 12-hour ADHD control. Only one dose per day is needed for therapeutic effects.
- Tricyclic antidepressants may be used to decrease hyperactivity but have little effect on impulsivity and inattention. Tolerance frequently develops within a few months, and patients taking these medications should have a drug holiday. Less effective and more dangerous than CNS stimulants, these medications are the second choice for treatment.
- ***Clonidine*** (Catapres), a medication for hypertension, reduces hyperactivity and impulsiveness. Sedation and hypotension that occur with this medication make it an alternate medication to be used only if absolutely needed (see Chapter 26).
- A new medication used for ADHD, ***atomoxetine*** (Strattera), not a Drug Enforcement Administration (DEA) scheduled medication, selectively inhibits uptake of norepinephrine, causing a calming effect (see Table 30-7).

Important Facts about Medications for Attention-Deficit/Hyperactivity Disorder (ADHD)

- Most medications for ADHD, Drug Enforcement Administration (DEA) Schedule II medications, should be treated with proper precautions.
- Goals of ADHD medications are to reduce symptoms of hyperactivity and reduce sleep attacks in patients with narcolepsy.
- Common side effects of amphetamines are insomnia and weight loss.

SUMMARY

The ability to cope with life's stressors at different life stages is the basis for mental health. "Normal" can be difficult to define; it varies from time to time, culture to culture, and person to person. Mental illness affects almost everyone during life stages, either themselves or their family members. Causes of mental illness may be congenital deficiencies, hereditary factors, or traumatic events. Treatment of mental illness has made giant steps in the past 60 years with introduction of new psychiatric medications. Today, most mentally ill persons are treated as outpatients rather than institutionalized.

Two main mental illness categories are neurosis and psychosis, both of which produce such symptoms as agitation, hyperactivity, and inappropriate behavior. Neurosis produces fear or anxiety from either real or unknown dangers, with responses producing many symptoms; drug therapy involves anxiolytics, or minor tranquilizers. Anxiolytics, used to treat prolonged anxiety, may also be used as hypnotics and sedatives, muscle relaxants, adjuvant medications for convulsions, and treatment for alcohol abuse withdrawal. Antianxiety medications cannot be used for prolonged periods of time because tolerance, habituation, and physical and psychologic dependence may occur. Benzodiazepines were introduced in the 1960s and continue to be some of the most widely prescribed anxiolytic medications.

Psychosis occurs when a person is out of control, out of touch with reality, and unable to communicate. Treatment for psychosis includes psychotherapy and antipsychotic medications, also called *neuroleptics* or *major tranquilizers*. The first antipsychotic agents, introduced in the 1950s, changed mental health treatment because of their ability to suppress schizophrenic symptoms and other psychotic conditions by acting on the neurotransmitter dopamine in the brain. Major side effects with these drugs are extrapyramidal symptoms, tardive dyskinesia, parkinsonism-like symptoms, akathisia, and dystonic reactions that are more likely to occur in children. In general, antipsychotics are used to relieve psychotic symptoms or severe neurosis, to relieve nausea and vomiting, and for potentiation of analgesics. Children and geriatric patients require special care when using these drugs.

Depot antipsychotics are used for long-term maintenance therapy. With these injectable medications, patient compliance is enhanced and the patient is maintained at the highest possible level of functioning.

Antidepressants are used for both endogenous and exogenous depression. In many depressed people, neurotransmitters—serotonin and norepinephrine—are in short supply, keeping nerve cells from functioning. Drugs are used to increase levels of these monoamines to elevate moods. Groups of medications used for depression include TCAs, MAOIs, SSRIs, and SNRIs. The TCAs are the usual first line of medication, followed by SSRIs or SNRIs. MAOIs have many side effects, have many drug interactions, and require severe dietary restrictions; therefore they are used only when other antidepressants do not provide relief. In recent years, herbal supplements have been studied and used to relieve mild to moderate depression.

Lithium, a slow-acting drug, is the medication of choice for bipolar or manic-depressive disorder especially in acute manic attacks and may be used prophylactically to prevent these attacks. Benzodiazepines or other antipsychotic agents may be used until lithium becomes effective.

Alzheimer's disease, a progressive illness, causes a decline in intellectual and physical functions. Medications for use to slow advance of the disease have been specifically approved but are not cures for the progressive devastation caused by brain changes. Investigation is being done to study use of NSAIDs, vitamin E, and estrogens with Alzheimer's disease.

Methylphenidate is the drug of choice for ADHD, but amphetamine sulfate, dextroamphetamine, or lisdexamfetamine may be used. These drugs increase children's attention span and enable goal-oriented behavior but require drug holidays, on weekends and during summer to overcome growth suppression, a major side effect. One of the newest drugs for this condition, atomoxetine (Strattera), does not have an amphetamine base and causes calming by inhibiting uptake of norepinephrine.

Within the past half-century, with the introduction of anxiolytics and antipsychotics, use of mental health medications has increased rapidly and has changed health care in many ways; perhaps the greatest of these is that now most mentally imbalanced persons are able to live, work, and contribute in their home communities.

CRITICAL THINKING EXERCISES

Scenario

Lakeesha is a 10-year-old who has been diagnosed with ADHD and is treated with methylphenidate three times a day. Her mother calls to tell you that she is giving the medicine in the morning, at school, and at supper. Lakeesha has been unable to sleep.

1. At what times do you think Dr. Merry intended Lakeesha to take the medication?
2. Her mother also wants to know why Lakeesha cannot take the medications on weekends and during the summer to help with her hyperactivity. What reasons do you think Dr. Merry would give Lakeesha's mother?
3. What side effects from the drug can Lakeesha and her mother expect?
4. In what class of controlled substances is methylphenidate?
5. What does that mean to her family when prescriptions for Lakeesha are necessary?
6. How is the drug effective against ADHD?

DRUG CALCULATIONS

1. Order: Ativan 1 mg stat then bid
   Available medication:

   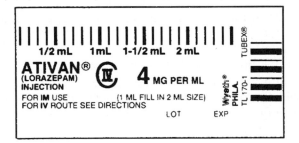

   Dose to be given: _____
   _____

2. Mellaril 15 mL
   Available medication:

   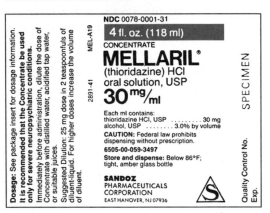

   Dose to be given: _____
   _____

   How should this medication be diluted before administration? _____
   _____
   _____

   Show the amount of medication for dilution and the amount of diluent on the utensil provided.

   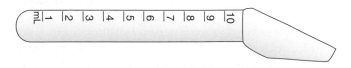

REVIEW QUESTIONS

1. What classes of drugs are used to treat neurosis? Psychosis? _____

_____

_____

_____

2. What are other names used for anxiolytics? _____

_____

3. What are three uses for anxiolytics other than reduction of anxiety? _____

_____

4. What three drug classes are used to treat psychosis? _____

_____

5. What are the uses of neuroleptics? How are they effective in the treatment of schizophrenia? _____

_____

_____

_____

6. What is meant by a low-potency antipsychotic? Intermediate-potency? High-potency? _____

_____

_____

_____

7. What is an atypical antipsychotic medication? How are these effective? _____

_____

8. What is a depot antipsychotic agent? What is the main indication for use of a depot antipsychotic? ____

_____

9. What are the three classes of major antidepressants? _____

_____

10. What is the use of lithium, and what condition does it treat? _____

_____

11. Why are medications effective only in slowing signs and symptoms of Alzheimer's disease? _____

_____

CHAPTER 31

Misused, Abused, and Addictive Drugs

OBJECTIVES

After studying this chapter, you should be capable of doing the following:

- Discussing dangers of drug abuse.
- Recognizing medications used for treatment of alcohol abuse.
- Discussing illegal abused drugs and their effects.
- Identifying misused or abused prescription medications.
- Describing actions leading to misuse or abuse of prescription and nonprescription medications and identifying factors of possible misuse and abuse.
- Providing patient education for compliance with medications used to treat diseases and conditions in the misuse, abuse, and addiction to drugs.

Mr. Goddio, age 45, has lower back pain and early emphysema. You find Mr. Goddio's blood pressure to be elevated, and laboratory tests show an elevated lipid profile. He is known to smoke one to two packs of cigarettes per day.

How does this habit increase Mr. Goddio's chance of cardiovascular disease?
What would you tell Mr. Goddio if he asks why it is important for him to stop smoking?
What types of products are available for prescribing to help Mr. Goddio stop smoking? What are their side effects?
How would you answer Mr. Goddio if he wants to know why the dosage of medication is gradually decreased throughout the program?
Will the medication be effective if he does not want to stop smoking? Why or why not?

KEY TERMS

Cirrhosis	**Dysphoria**	**Inebriation**
Delirium tremens	**Euphoria**	**Leukoplakia**

EASY WORKING KNOWLEDGE OF MEDICATIONS USED TO TREAT SUBSTANCE ABUSE				
DRUG CLASS	**PRESCRIPTION**	**OTC**	**PREGNANCY CATEGORY**	**MAJOR INDICATIONS**
Substance abuse deterrents	Yes	Yes	C, D, X	Cessation of alcohol and nicotine use
Narcotic antagonists	Yes	No	B, C	Detoxification in narcotic abstinence

EASY WORKING KNOWLEDGE OF INDICATIONS AND SIDE EFFECTS

Common Signs and Symptoms of Drug Abuse and Misuse	Common Side Effects of Abused and Misused Drugs
Changes in weight and sleep habits	Drowsiness, constipation
Impaired memory	Hallucinations
Illogical thinking	Lightheadedness, dizziness, headache
Mood swings, irritability, depression, anger	Impotence
Defensiveness	Cardiac arrhythmias
Anxiety and overreaction to difficult situations	Nausea, sore mouth and throat, diarrhea
Changes in vital signs	Respiratory distress
Runny nose, nasal stuffiness, bloodshot eyes, sweating	Erythema, pruritus, local edema, rash
Changes in friends and appearance	Mental confusion

All drugs, prescription or over the counter (OTC), including those used for self-medication, have the potential for abuse and misuse. Each patient's actual needs should be evaluated, and only appropriate medications should be prescribed. Physicians who indiscriminately prescribe medications without looking into physical complaints and the patient's medical conditions are misusing medication. Prolonged and unsupervised taking of medications is also drug misuse. Drug abuse, however, is self-medication on a chronic basis in quantities causing physical or psychologic dependence and inability to function within socially acceptable norms. Taking antihistamines or analgesics either too frequently or in doses not recognized as acceptable is an example of every day drug abuse. Some patients just enjoy feeling high and will take medications to achieve this feeling.

Drug abuse and misuse are not new phenomena; they have occurred throughout history as a way to relieve personal, physical, psychologic, social, and/or economic problems. Since the dawn of civilization, mind-altering drugs have held fascination as a means to elevate mood, induce hallucinations, and modify thinking. Abuse is not related to any certain socioeconomic, cultural, or ethnic group but is found at all societal levels.

Did You Know?

Mind-altering medications, still used in some cultures today during religious ceremonies, may come from sources considered socially or religiously acceptable, such as herbals.

WHAT IS DRUG MISUSE? ABUSE?

Drug abuse may be described as using a drug inconsistently with medical, social, and/or cultural norms while, drug misuse relates to using a medication in an

BOX 31-1 DEFINITIONS OF TERMS USED IN DRUG ABUSE AND MISUSE

- Drug misuse—Nonspecific or indiscriminate use of drugs
- Drug abuse—Drug use not prescribed by a physician, or improper or excessive use of any drug
- Drug habit—Frequent indiscriminate drug use, causing a problem when attempting to stop use
- Drug dependency—Physical or psychologic need to use a drug to achieve a sense of well-being or to avoid withdrawal symptoms; not the same as addiction
- Drug habituation—Drug use so frequent that it is part of daily activities
- Drug addiction—Compulsive, excessive, or constant use of drugs to achieve a desired state, with results being harmful to the person, society, or both
- Drug tolerance—Condition in which an increased amount of a drug is necessary to produce the original effect because the drug produces less effect than when previously taken
- Withdrawal—Effect experienced when drugs of physical or psychologic dependence have been discontinued

inappropriate manner. Each instance of drug use must be evaluated for potential drug misuse and abuse. Large dosages of psychotherapeutic medications may be necessary in certain populations, whereas these dosages could very well be abused in another population. An instance of acceptable medicinal use versus abuse would be use of opioids for relief of acute or chronic pain found with cancer and other painful conditions, which is an acceptable use, versus use of the same drugs by healthy persons to get high, which would be considered abuse. Drug abuse also has degrees of severity from occasional use to habitual, compulsive, and routine use. Box 31-1 shows the terminology of substance abuse.

Drug and alcohol misuse, abuse, and addiction are major social problems in the United States today. One can pick up any newspaper and find articles concerning abused drugs, from stimulants to depressants, from agents causing a high to those bringing abusers down. One major social concern today is theft of medications such as analgesics and antidepressants by children, usually from family members, for personal use or illicit sale. Drug abuse is defined as use of a drug for purposes other than therapeutic. Drug misuse or abuse is indiscriminate use of a drug.

The most frequently misused and abused chemical substances are xanthines and caffeine, found in coffee, tea, caffeine-containing soft drinks, and chocolate, which produce mild stimulation, euphoric effects, and physical dependence—that is, the substance is necessary for performance of daily tasks without experiencing symptoms such as headaches, sleepiness, and lethargy. This abuse is shown in the person who must have a caffeine-laden beverage in midafternoon to be able to complete the day's work.

Did You Know?

Drug or substance abuse is a multibillion-dollar-a-year problem with a significant impact on all aspects of society and affecting people of all cultural and economic backgrounds. Substance misuse or abuse affects every person in the United States, either directly or indirectly, in social, economic, medical, or interpersonal ways. Assaults, rape, and child abuse are often related to substance abuse, whereas traffic accidents and fatalities often involve alcohol and drug impairment.

Factors that Contribute to Drug Misuse and Abuse

Several factors contribute to drug abuse or progressive use of drugs. Curiosity concerning medicinal effects often leads to psychoactive drug use. Drug abuse may begin with occasional misuse for feeling good and then lead to a compulsive need for drugs—or progression from experimentation with drugs to compulsive need for and use of substances (Box 31-2).

Did You Know?

Different abused drugs can be detected in the urine over different lengths of time. For certain drugs, prolonged use can extend these times (Table 31-1).

BEHAVIORS FOUND WITH DRUG ABUSE

Drug misuse or abuse is often unplanned, beginning with experimentation and steadily increasing from there. The person who starts with weekend use may start to rely

BOX 31-2 FACTORS IN DRUG ABUSE AND MISUSE

- People might first try a drug out of *curiosity* or *peer pressure*, but "feeling good" leads to continued use. If the drug had caused negative feelings, drug use would stop.
- *Physical dependence* is based on the size of the dose and the length of time used. The more physically dependent the individual is, the more likely withdrawal symptoms will occur. Physical dependence plays an important role when a person's need is to alleviate symptoms, although other reasons may lead to dependencies. When withdrawal symptoms begin, another dose of drug is taken for relief of symptoms, resulting in ongoing drug abuse.
- *Psychologic dependence*, a craving for the drug with a strong need for a feeling of well-being, leads to addiction, the next step past abuse.
- *Social status* and *social approval*, related to peer pressure, may cause continued use of medications even when the drug causes an unpleasant result. This is often the reason for continued experimentation with substances of abuse.
- *Drug availability* allows drug abuse development and continued use of agents.
- *Vulnerability* to drugs allows some people to be more likely to become drug abusers or misusers. Individual differences lead some people to experiment with a drug once and never try it again; others will try a drug one time and immediately develop a compulsive desire. Once an abuser of one drug, the more likely a person will abuse other drugs.
- *Psychosocial disorders* such as depression and anxiety tend to cause persons who are impulsive with little tolerance for frustration to become rebellious toward social expectations, leading to abuse.
- *Genetics*, especially with alcohol use, have been proven to play a role in drug abuse and misuse. Alcoholism and drug abuse are seen as diseases with familial tendencies.
- *Tolerance to otherwise intolerable situations* occurs when drug use allows a person to alter his or her state of consciousness, with a rapid onset of desired effects but with withdrawal symptoms if the drug is discontinued abruptly. Feelings of shame and inadequacy, personal conflicts, and predisposition to depression are avoided with drug abuse, with the abuser believing he or she can function acceptably in society.

on drugs to assist with difficult situations during the week. Weekend use becomes insufficient and increases to several times a week or daily, until drugs become a crutch in any uncomfortable or tension-producing situation. Often, family members become aware of the problem only when daily drug use becomes the user's mode of surviving, or the norm (Box 31-3).

TABLE 31-1 LENGTH OF TIME FOR WHICH A DRUG CAN BE DETECTED IN THE URINE

DRUG	DURATION
alcohol	<1 day
amphetamines	Up to 1 day
barbiturates	Up to 1 day
benzodiazepines	Up to 2 days
cocaine	Up to 2 days
marijuana—single use	Up to 6 days
marijuana—multiple uses	Up to 1 mo
opioids (short-acting)	Up to 1 day
phencyclidine (PCP)	Up to 6 days
phenobarbital	Up to 6 days

BOX 31-3 SIGNS OF DRUG ABUSE

Physical Signs
- Changes in sleeping habits and in weight and vital signs
- Lack of muscle coordination, with slurring of words
- Lethargy and illnesses on a more frequent basis

Psychologic Signs
- Depression and apathy
- Anxiety and overreaction
- Concentration impairment and shortened memory
- Inability to organize and inflexibility to changes in planned schedules
- Illogical thinking and confusion

Social Signs
- Mood swings, irritability, anger
- Defensiveness and overreaction to social situations
- Decreased school or work performance and absenteeism
- Feelings of inadequacy
- Disrespect for authority and discipline
- Often, the casting aside of old friends

Drug withdrawal symptoms include nervousness, runny nose and stuffiness, sweating, bloodshot or puffy eyes, inability to stay still, and changes in vital signs including variations in blood pressure and pulse with rapid respirations. Death from rapid withdrawal is possible. Withdrawal symptoms cause the abuser to become desperate for the next dose and willing to engage in any activity to obtain the needed drug.

Important Facts About Drug Abuse

- Drug abuse is using a drug in a way that is inconsistent with medical, cultural, and social norms within a given population.
- Drug abuse is not a new phenomenon but has occurred throughout history, involving herbals and prescribed or OTC medications as well as street drugs.
- Drugs used for self-medication are often those most abused or misused because chronic use and excessive dosages are not detected.
- Curiosity is a leading reason for beginning drug use. A desirable feeling after drug use is usually a reason for continued drug abuse or misuse.
- Physical dependence has built-in conditions such as tolerance levels and withdrawal symptoms when the drug is stopped.
- Psychologic dependence leads to addiction because of craving for the medication or agent.
- Drug availability, social status, and social acceptance are reasons for continued use of drugs.
- Parents should watch for loss of prescription medications, as this may be a sign of theft by children for use or illicit sale.

DRUGS OF ABUSE NOT REQUIRING A PRESCRIPTION

Some drugs are easily obtained legally in society. Often not considered drugs, nicotine and alcohol are readily available for persons of legal age. Because of the ease of procuring these legal substances, dangers are often ignored until abuse occurs and treatment is indicated.

Nicotine

The chief source of nicotine, a liquid alkaloid, is tobacco. Nicotine has only one therapeutic use: to provide products for smoking cessation assistance (which seems ironic). However, nicotine is of great pharmacologic and toxicologic interest. Readily absorbed through the skin and the gastrointestinal and respiratory tracts, components of tobacco smoke include potentially dangerous materials, such as carbon monoxide, hydrogen cyanide, ammonia, and coal tar, which are known carcinogens.

Smoking cigarettes, pipe tobacco, or cigars is the greatest single cause of preventable illnesses and premature death, producing complex and unpredictable pharmacologic effects. Secondhand smoking—inhalation of cigarette smoke by nonsmokers—has been shown by the Food and Drug Administration (FDA) to lead to as many health risks and harmful effects (or more than) as

TABLE 31-2 EFFECTS OF NICOTINE ON THE BODY

BODY SYSTEM	EFFECTS
Cardiovascular system	Initially slows heart rate but later causes acceleration Peripheral blood vessels constrict but later dilate, causing drop in blood pressure Causes coronary heart disease, myocardial infarctions, arteriosclerosis
Nervous system	Affects vital organ function regulated by CNS Causes tolerance and physical dependence Increases levels of cortisol and catecholamines
Urinary system	Acts as antidiuretic
Gastrointestinal system	Increases gastric acids Increases gastric muscle tone and motility Causes gastric ulcers and chronic dyspepsia Causes loss of appetite
Immune system	Decreases immunity Causes mutation of cells leading to precancerous cells
Respiratory system	Decreases lung volume Decreases air flow Causes pulmonary emphysema, acute and chronic bronchitis Increases risk of sudden infant death syndrome (SIDS)
Reproductive system	Results in low birth weights of infants born to smokers Increases chance of congenital abnormalities Increases risk of prematurity

BOX 31-4 DRUGS SPECIFIC FOR SMOKING CESSATION

- **Bupropion** (Zyban), which has the same active ingredient as the antidepressant Wellbutrin, reduces craving for nicotine and reduces nicotine withdrawal symptoms. To be effective, treatment takes about a week while the person is still smoking, so an attempt to stop smoking should not be made until the second week of treatment. This medication should be taken for 7 to 12 weeks. If the smoking has not stopped by the seventh week, it is unlikely this medication will be effective.
- **Varenicline** (Chantix) partially activates brain's nicotine receptors to reduce craving for and withdrawal symptoms of nicotine. The medication reduces the urge to smoke and blocks the effects of nicotine if smoking resumes. Treatment takes 12 weeks and may be repeated for a second 12-week period. This medication should also be taken for 7 days prior to an attempt to stop smoking is made.

increased insulin effect, so insulin dosage may need to be decreased to prevent hypoglycemia.

Early signs of nicotine overdose are nausea and vomiting, severe abdominal pain, diarrhea, cold sweat, and severe headaches. Disturbed hearing and vision; confusion; hypotension; and fast, weak, or irregular pulse are found with advanced overdose.

Smoking Cessation Products

Nicotine smoking cessation products come as tablets, gums, lozenges, nasal sprays, and transdermal systems to prevent the experience of acute nicotine withdrawal. Products are available as prescription and OTC items. Tablets, to assist with abstinence, are taken over several months (for at least 3 months but no longer than 6 months), with reduced dosage as the person adjusts to nonsmoking. Buccal absorption of nicotine is slower than inhalation, so instead of smoking, nicotine gum is chewed, with the number of pieces per day decreased over a period of 2 to 3 months. Transdermal patches are worn for 16 to 24 hours daily to mimic daily use of cigarettes with lowering of serum nicotine at night. Nicotine nasal spray, which more closely simulates smoking, is faster than gum or patches and has the same efficacy. Patients should not smoke while using spray, nor should it be used with other nicotine products. The latest smoking deterrent is a vaccine (NicVAX) used to reduce pleasurable effects of smoking (Box 31-4).

Smoking cessation agents should not be used by patients who have angina pectoris, cardiac dysrhythmias, insulin-dependent diabetes mellitus, hypertension, peripheral vascular disease, peptic ulcer, or a history of myocardial infarction (Table 31-3).

smoking itself. Nicotine may cause acute toxicity in children who ingest or inhale tobacco products, or chronic toxicity may occur from long-term use or association with products. Use of chewing tobacco and snuff leads to **leukoplakia** and cancer of oral cavity mucous membranes, a traumatic disease. See Table 31-2 for effects of nicotine on body systems.

Nicotine interacts with other drugs. Smoking increases metabolism of **acetaminophen** (Tylenol), **caffeine**, **oxazepam** (Serax), **pentazocine** (Talwin), **propranolol** (Inderal), and **theophylline,** requiring higher or more frequent doses. Cessation of smoking may result in

TABLE 31-3 DETERRENTS TO DRUG ABUSE AND MISUSE

GENERIC NAME/ TRADE NAME	USUAL ADULT DOSE, ROUTE, AND FREQUENCY	INDICATIONS FOR USE	DRUG INTERACTIONS
NICOTINE DETERRENTS		Use of nicotine products	
nicotine			None indicated except other nicotine products
(Nicotrol)	1 mg = 2 sprays per nostril (1 or 2 doses per hour up to 40 doses per day)		
	1 transdermal patch per day (16 hr)		
	oral inhaler 4 mg		
(Nicorette NicoRelief, Thrive) (OTC)	9-12 pieces of gum at 1- to 2-hr intervals (up to 30 pieces per day)		
(Commit)	Dissolve lozenges in mouth		
(NicoDerm CQ)	1 transdermal patch per day (24 hr)		
(NicVAX)	Injectable		
varenicline (Chantix)	0.5 mg-1 mg tab PO bid		
bupropion (Zyban, as well as others)	150 mg PO qd-bid		alcohol, TCA, ritonavir, tramadol

Major Side Effects of Nicotine Deterrents:

All—Nausea, tachycardia, headaches, dizziness, increased appetite, indigestion, insomnia; *gums and lozenges*—damage to mouth, teeth, and dental work; *transdermal patches*—local rash or pruritus

ALCOHOL AND OPIOID DETERRENTS			
acamprosate (Campral)	666 mg PO tid	Alcoholism	
disulfiram (Antabuse)	125-500 mg PO qd	Alcoholism	alcohol, isoniazid, warfarin
methadone (Dolophine)	20-120 mg PO qd, SC, IM	Opioid abuse	alcohol, warfarin, cimetidine, selegiline, furazolidone
naloxone	0.4-2 mg SC, IM, IV	Opioid abuse	Decrease effect of opioids
naltrexone (Revia, Depade)	50 mg PO qd	Alcoholism, opioid misuse	analgesics, cough preparations, any preparation with alcohol base
(Vivitrol)	380 mg IM q4wk		

Major Side Effects of Alcohol and Opioid Deterrents:

disulfiram—drowsiness; side effects such as nausea and vomiting are desired; *acamprosate*—diarrhea, gas, loss of appetite, dizziness, weakness, itching; *naloxone*—tachycardia, drowsiness, nervousness

IM, Intramuscularly; *IV,* intravenously; *PO,* orally; *SC,* subcutaneously; *TCA,* tricyclic antidepressants.

Physical dependence causing use of larger and larger amounts of alcohol with denial and tolerance is common with chronic use. Those with physical dependence to alcohol tend to have cross-dependence on other CNS depressants such as barbiturates and benzodiazepines. When alcohol is discontinued after physical dependence, **delirium tremens** may occur. With chronic use of alcohol, detrimental effects to body systems will shorten life expectancy (Table 31-4).

Drug Interactions with Alcohol

Drug interactions of alcohol with other medications may be additive, or alcohol may just change the effectiveness of medications, causing many detrimental symptoms, even life-threatening ones (Table 31-5). For patient safety, a general rule to be followed with medications is that alcohol should be avoided when taking prescription or OTC medications unless the physician is aware of the patient's alcohol consumption.

ETHYL ALCOHOL OR ETHANOL

Alcohol, one of the oldest and most abused drugs in the United States, is a central nervous system (CNS) depressant. Alcohol does have some medicinal uses—for example, as a vehicle for cough suppressants and as a germicidal in mouthwashes. Alcohol is often misused or abused through use of OTC medications such as nighttime cough and cold preparations containing antihistamines; some have as much as 25% alcohol (or 50 proof). Elderly individuals may use ethyl alcohol–based medications as appetite stimulants during periods of disability or convalescence or may use alcohol preparations for rest when other hypnotics cannot be tolerated. Effects are dose dependent, with high doses causing depression of the medulla and thus basic life functions. The most common concern is nonmedical chronic use by heavy drinkers, causing atrophy of the cerebrum and loss of intellectual functions. In extreme doses, alcohol may produce anesthesia that could be lethal.

TABLE 31-4 EFFECTS OF ALCOHOL ON THE BODY	
BODY SYSTEM	**EFFECTS**
Gastrointestinal system	Liver damage by accumulation of fats and proteins, leading to cirrhosis and hepatitis
	Erosion of gastric mucosa with gastric bleeding
	Esophageal varices
	Pancreatitis
Nervous system	Hepatic encephalopathy
Urinary system	Acts as diuretic by suppressing antidiuretic hormone
Respiratory system	Depresses respirations
Nervous system	Produces tolerance
	Central nervous system depressant

TABLE 31-5 INTERACTIONS BETWEEN MEDICATIONS AND ALCOHOL

ALCOHOL COMBINED WITH	MAY CAUSE
Medication for sleep, tranquilizers	Increased physical and psychologic dependence
Antidepressants	Rapid intoxication
Motion sickness medications	Excessive drowsiness
Pain relievers, muscle relaxants, antiallergics, antihistamines	Mental confusion
Medications for angina pectoris	Dizziness, fainting
Antihypertensives	Lack of skeletal muscle coordination
Agents such as aspirin, NSAIDs, anticoagulants, potassium supplements	Increased gastric irritation and bleeding
Some antibiotics, metronidazole	Nausea, vomiting, and flushing
Oral hypoglycemics	Tachycardia, dyspnea
Anticoagulants, seizure medications, hypoglycemics	Changes in effectiveness of medications in controlling specific illness

NSAIDs, Nonsteroidal antiinflammatory drugs.

Drugs Used to Treat Alcoholism

For those who have chronic alcohol intake with dependence or alcoholism, certain medications may assist with withdrawal symptoms. Benzodiazepines (tranquilizers; see Chapter 30), **atenolol** (Tenormin; see Chapter 26), and **naltrexone** (Revia) are used to suppress these symptoms. Research has shown decreased craving for alcohol, fewer drinks consumed, and fewer instances of relapse with use of naltrexone. Once abstinence has been accomplished, continued abstinence may be maintained if needed by the use of **disulfiram** (Antabuse) or **acamprosate** (Campral).

- Disulfiram's only use is its known interactions with alcohol, discouraging persons from drinking and causing severe side effects when mixed with alcohol. Desired side effects include nausea, copious vomiting, flushing, palpitations, headache, thirst, sweating, chest pain, blurred vision, weakness, and hypotension that may be severe and may last from 30 minutes to several hours with even the smallest absorption of alcohol (as little as 7 mL). The person who does not have the desire to stop alcohol use should not be treated with disulfiram because of its severe adverse effects (see Table 31-3). Patient education with disulfiram is extremely important, as any alcohol consumption (e.g., cough syrups; cooking sauces; mouthwashes, products applied to the skin such as liniments, aftershave lotions, perfumes; and any product containing alcohol) may produce severe and potentially fatal reactions.
- Acamprosate is used along with counseling and social support to help persons avoid craving for and drinking of large amounts of alcohol. A delayed-release tablet must be administered three times a day but does not cause alcohol aversion as found with disulfiram and does not cause a reaction when alcohol is ingested. However, this medication does increase suicidal tendencies.

Other Alcohol Preparations

Toxic alcohols include isopropyl alcohol and methyl or wood alcohol. When unable to purchase ethyl alcohol or ethanol, some alcoholics will substitute isopropyl (rubbing) alcohol or methyl alcohol (antifreeze) for consumption. Either of these will prevent alcohol withdrawal symptoms but potentially cause poisoning or death.

Patient Education for Compliance

1. Disulfiram should not be administered until at least 12 hours have passed since the last ingestion of alcohol. Patients should avoid all alcohol products, no matter what form, while taking Antabuse.
2. Many OTC and home remedies containing alcohol cause sedation and hypnosis without the person taking the medication being aware of this content.
3. People may become less self-conscious when drinking alcohol and may not realize the dangers of excessive drinking.
4. Some states require a witness for administration of disulfiram in patients with a history of driving under the influence.

Important Facts about Medications for Alcoholism

- Alcohol is a depressant drug.
- Alcohol increases blood pressure in direct correlation to the amount of alcohol consumed. Alcohol depresses respirations and leads to hepatitis, cirrhosis of the liver, and erosive gastritis.
- Chronic use of alcohol produces tolerance to many of alcohol's effects and to central nervous system (CNS) depressants except opioids.

Continued

PRESCRIPTION DRUG ABUSE

Use of prescription medications for pain, such as opioids and opiates, and stimulants such as amphetamines and use of anabolic steroids, for example, by body builders, may lead to misuse or abuse when directions for prescription are not followed. Persons with tendencies toward drug dependence often fall victim to misuse and abuse and finally addiction. Therefore careful screening including a familial history is important before pain or stimulant medications are prescribed. The allied health professional should also be aware of the dangers of personal use of easily available prescription medications, as well as the abusers' needs for these drugs. Indications of the abuser's drug seeking should also be evaluated in the medical office.

Opiates and Opioids

Drugs that are frequently misused and abused are synthetic opioids (such as hydrocodone, methadone, oxycodone), opiates from natural sources (such as opium alkaloids of heroin and morphine), and semisynthetic drugs (hydromorphone, oxymorphone) (see Chapter 15 for more information as analgesics). These medications may be taken by mouth, by percutaneous means for absorption through mucous membranes or skin, by injection, by direct administration into veins (or mainlining), or by sniffing and snorting. The most frequently abused prescription pain relievers are **meperidine** (Demerol), **oxycodone** (OxyContin, Percodan, and Percocet), and **morphine.** The most frequently abused street drugs are marijuana, heroin, cocaine, and oxycodone. Oxycodone and meperidine are prescription drugs most frequently abused by health care professionals because of ease of availability.

The beginning of opioid use that may lead to misuse occurs either socially or for pain management in a medical setting, whereas most abuse starts with illegal use of a street drug or inappropriate use of prescription pain medications. Opioids relieve pain; elevate mood; relieve tension, fear, and anxiety; and produce tranquility and peace with **euphoria.** Other effects include suppression of cough and appetite. All these effects can lead to psychologic and physical dependence. Long-term continued use is based on feelings of "all is well" rather than a rush that occurs with earlier administration. The user or abuser has the perception that the world is rosy and bright with no problems. Researchers believe that psychologic dependence continues throughout life, although desire may be controlled with strong willpower and personal desire to remain drug free.

Toxicity levels, often found with abuse of these medications, cause signs such as slow, shallow breathing leading to cyanosis and hypoxia; cold, clammy, skin; pinpoint pupils; depressed blood pressure; and depressed sensory perception. Because these agents also tend to decrease gastric motility and reduce peristalsis, increased amounts of medication may be absorbed.

Signs and Symptoms of Opioid and Opiate Withdrawal

Withdrawal from dependency on opioids or alcohol will produce symptoms that start approximately 2 to 48 hours after the last dose, depending on the abused drug. Feelings of restlessness, chills, hot flashes, restless sleep, piloerection (goose bumps), rhinorrhea (runny nose), tearing, and dilation of eye pupils occur during first

24 hours. Sneezing, yawning, leg cramping, vomiting, diarrhea, loss of appetite, sweating, muscle twitches, insomnia, elevated vital signs, and drug craving follow when these early symptoms subside. In some cases, withdrawal symptoms may progress to cardiovascular collapse.

Withdrawal programs provide therapeutic means for handling symptoms of abrupt, or "cold turkey," withdrawal by tapering the drug dosage over a period of days, using a substitution of methadone for the opioid or opiate. Methadone, a synthetic opioid analgesic, permits substitution by cross-tolerance, stalls the euphoric effects of heroin and other opioids, and reduces craving without physical and mental effects. Methadone treatment programs change dependence to methadone, but withdrawal symptoms for methadone are less severe (see Table 31-3).

Important Facts about Opioid and Opiate Abuse

- One of the most misused and abused groups of drugs is the opioids and opiates, used as pain relievers. Morphine, OxyContin, meperidine, and hydromorphone are prescription items abused most frequently.
- Opioids and opiates, depressant drugs, produce mental depression and analgesia, as well as cough and appetite depression. The abuser likes the feelings of well-being and euphoria rather than the rush occurring immediately after administration.
- Withdrawal symptoms such as restlessness, cramping of the legs, vomiting, diarrhea, insomnia, and craving occur with prolonged use of opioids.
- Methadone is used in withdrawal programs for opioid abuse.

ABUSED CENTRAL NERVOUS SYSTEM STIMULANTS

Some CNS stimulants have specific medical uses but are also used illegally and illicitly, including manufacture of these drugs in the person's home environment. Those most commonly seen are discussed so that the allied health professional has knowledge of the dangers and signs and symptoms of the user or abuser.

Amphetamines

Amphetamines, called "uppers" or "speed," have both medical and illegal uses. Medically prescribed, amphetamines are classified as Drug Enforcement Administration (DEA) Schedule II drugs, used to treat chronic fatigue syndrome, obesity, narcolepsy, attention deficit disorder, and mental depression, and to combat side effects of narcotics in terminally ill patients (see Chapters 29 and 30). When used illegally, they increase physical performance and provide psychologic stimulus. The most frequently abused amphetamines are methamphetamine ("ice" or "crystal meth"), which may be smoked or taken orally or intravenously. A rapid rise in methamphetamine use and manufacture using OTC medications such as cold and allergy products containing pseudoephedrine has caused the FDA to place limits on OTC sales of products containing pseudoephedrine. Stores have moved these drugs into the pharmacy or behind the checkout area for safekeeping, with a limit on purchases per person to once in 48 hours.

Amphetamines provide more confidence, alertness, and talkativeness, with hyperactivity and a feeling of euphoria and a sense of arousal. Amphetamines are also anorexics, so the person feels no need for food and therefore weight loss occurs. Other symptoms of possible illicit use include irritability, confusion, social withdrawal, chewing or teeth grinding, photophobia, and paranoia. Compulsive behaviors drive users to repeat drug use again and again to maintain euphoria. Physical dependence is moderate, but psychologic dependence may be intense.

Signs of toxicity with amphetamines are flushing or pallor, palpitations, tremors, extreme fluctuations of pulse and blood pressure, chest pain, sweating, dilated pupils, and mental disturbances. Treatment is symptomatic, as no antidote is available for amphetamines. Abrupt withdrawal will produce a disagreeable and depressed mood—an experience known as a "crash." These manifestations, especially the depression, may persist for months, causing resumption use of amphetamines.

Cocaine

Cocaine has been used for years by native Indians of South America to ward off fatigue and hunger. In the nineteenth century cocaine was considered a "wonder drug" for numerous medical conditions, but in 1914 legislation restricted its use. However, its use as a recreational drug dramatically increased beginning in the 1970s, causing numerous social and medical problems. The only approved medicinal use of cocaine is as a local anesthetic applied topically, usually for nasal procedures, because of anesthetic and vasoconstrictive properties.

Did You Know?

Coca-Cola originally contained cocaine from the coca plant—hence the name and nickname *Coke.*

Effects of cocaine are similar to those of amphetamines, with the intensity and duration of the effects being dependent on purity of preparation and method of administration. Cocaine, because of its derivation from coca leaves, can be converted to a water-soluble hydrochloride salt in a powder form for oral, intranasal, and intravenous administration. When it is used as a drug of abuse, the usual route is intranasal—"snorted"—for rapid nasal mucosal absorption.

Cocaine base, which is a crystalline rock form, gets the name "crack" from the cracking sound it makes as it burns. Powdered, pure cocaine is cut by adding such substances as cornstarch or baking soda to raise drug volume, thus increasing its street value. Unfortunately, drug purity or the amount of cocaine is not predictable, and potency will vary greatly from one dose to the next. When cocaine base ("crack") is smoked (or freebased), rapid absorption occurs through the lungs. Euphoria ("high") received from smoking crack cocaine is rapidly replaced by **dysphoria,** ("down"), and the cocaine user repeats doses to maintain euphoria.

The half-life of cocaine is short, with symptoms subsiding in 1 to 2 hours, leading to acute intoxication. As a person uses cocaine, tolerance develops, causing an increase in need for the drug or in amount used to obtain the same euphoria. For this reason cocaine addiction is difficult to treat, and no antidote is available for toxicity (Table 31-6).

Important Facts about Medications Used as Stimulants

- Amphetamines, nicotine, and cocaine are CNS stimulants that are often abused.
- Amphetamines are called "uppers" or "speed" and have both medicinal and illicit implications.
- Amphetamines produce compulsive behaviors, causing users to repeat drug use again and again.
- Treatment for amphetamine or cocaine toxicity must be symptomatic, as no antidote is known.

ABUSED CENTRAL NERVOUS SYSTEM DEPRESSANTS

Barbiturates and benzodiazepines (as well as alcohol, discussed earlier) are often abused CNS depressants. These agents have many safe therapeutic applications when used as designed by the manufacturer and prescribed by a physician. However, because of the potential for abuse, tolerance, and physical dependence, these medications are regulated under the Controlled Substances Act.

TABLE 31-6 EFFECTS OF COCAINE ON THE BODY

BODY SYSTEM	EFFECTS
Cardiovascular system	Tachycardia Hypertension Myocardial infarction and thrombi
Respiratory system	Lung infections and abscesses Pulmonary edema Pneumonitis Atrophy of nasal mucosa with snorted cocaine with a loss of smell Necrosis and perforation of nasal passages with intranasal use Severe respiratory system damage occurs when other substances of abuse are used in conjunction with cocaine
Urinary system	Acute renal failure
Nervous system	Seizures Strokes and increased intracranial pressure
Reproductive system	Leads to stillbirths and preterm labor Congenital deformities Acute withdrawal symptoms in the infant, with behavioral delays throughout life
Psychologic health	Paranoia and depression Psychosis Suicide Dependence with severe anxiety and auditory, visual, and tactile hallucinations

Barbiturates

Barbiturates (see Chapter 29) typify the CNS depressants used for illicit purposes. Depressant effects are dose dependent and range from mild sedation to sleep or coma.

Used indiscriminately, barbiturates are called "downers." They produce symptoms including drowsiness, confusion, impaired judgment, slurred speech, and lack of facial expression. Route of administration is oral, or intravenous injection in a liquid form. Acute toxicity produces three expected signs: respiratory depression, coma, and constriction of pupils to pinpoints. Symptoms include nausea and loss of appetite. Rebound rapid-eye-movement sleep and nightmares occur on withdrawal of medications. No specific antidote is available for barbiturate intoxication.

Benzodiazepines

Benzodiazepines, commonly prescribed for anxiety and insomnia (see Chapter 30), are safer than barbiturates and are rarely lethal when taken alone. Danger comes when drugs are combined with other CNS depressants such as alcohol. Benzodiazepines are generally not considered street drugs, but misuse, abuse, and dependencies have been reported, especially with *diazepam* (Valium), *alprazolam* (Xanax), and *lorazepam* (Ativan). As a rule, tolerance and physical dependence are only minimal when these drugs are taken for medicinal indications, but a substantial problem can occur with misuse or abuse.

For the patient who has built a tolerance and abuse level, gradual withdrawal by changing to a long-acting benzodiazepine is recommended. Symptoms of withdrawal include increased anxiety and irritability, twitching, aching, muscle weakness, tremors, headaches, nausea, anorexia, depression, lethargy, hypersensitivity to stimuli, blurred vision, and sleep disturbances. Health care professionals should be aware that prolonged use of benzodiazepines is dangerous even for therapeutic reasons, especially in elderly patients who use these medications for insomnia and daily anxieties. *Flumazenil* (Romazicon) is specific as an antagonist for benzodiazepine toxicity and sedation reversal.

Important Facts about Abused Central Nervous System Depressants

- Barbiturates and benzodiazepines are commonly abused prescription medications because of their use for anxiety relief as "downers."
- Tolerance, a common effect of barbiturate and benzodiazepine use, leads to physical dependence.
- Withdrawal from barbiturates and benzodiazepines should be gradual when the drugs have been used for prolonged lengths of time.

Marijuana and Hashish

Marijuana and hashish, classified as CNS depressants, cause euphoria, sedation, and hallucinations. Drug potency of tetrahydrocannabinol (THC) varies with conditions under which the hemp plants, *Cannabis sativa*, were grown. Resin from female plants is known as *hashish*, whereas the dried plant (seed, flower, twigs, and leaves) is the basis for marijuana. These drugs, known as *cannabinoids*, have street names such as *grass*, *weed*, *hemp*, *Mary Jane*, *pot*, and *dope*; marijuana cigarettes are known as *stogies*, *joints*, or *reefers*.

When smoked, marijuana has its effect in 5 to 15 minutes, peaking at 30 to 90 minutes, with a duration of 3 to 4 hours. Because of fat solubility, THC is taken up in fatty body tissues and thus metabolizes slowly, with 30% to 50% of the drug remaining a week later. When smoked, hashish is rapidly absorbed through the lungs. A major side effect of marijuana is lung damage, with a greater risk of cancers. Marijuana produces a greater amount of tar than its equivalent weight in tobacco and contains more carcinogens than tobacco smoke.

Marijuana produces three subjective effects: sedation, euphoria, and sometimes hallucinations. No other drug produces all three responses, placing marijuana in a class by itself. When the drug is taken orally, practically all the THC is absorbed but is inactivated by first pass through the liver, so three to 10 times as much marijuana or hashish is required to obtain the same effect as found with smoking. When ingested, marijuana may have some effectiveness for up to 12 hours (Table 31-7).

Tolerance occurs with marijuana use, with rapid reversal after product cessation. Abrupt cessation after prolonged use is associated with psychologic symptoms from the physical dependence. Symptoms include dysphoria, anxiety, tremors, eating and sleeping disturbances, and increased sweating. Psychotic reactions and acute panic-anxiety reactions occur with inexperienced users who are not familiar with the effects or with those who have taken high doses or have experienced prolonged marijuana use.

Important Facts About Marijuana Use

- Marijuana is considered to be a central nervous system depressant, although it causes euphoria before sedation and hallucinations.
- Marijuana is fat soluble, leading to absorption in fatty body tissues, providing prolonged effects.
- Marijuana produces three effects—euphoria with gaiety and heightened sense of humor, sedation with lethargy and memory loss, and sometimes hallucinations caused by perceptual inadequacies and increased sensory stimuli.
- Tolerance occurs with marijuana and is rapidly reversed with cessation of use.

HALLUCINOGENS, PSYCHEDELICS, AND PSYCHOTOMIMETICS

Hallucinogens and psychedelics (mind-altering drugs) are agents that produce auditory and visual hallucinations, or a "psychedelic" state. Psychoactive effects occur 1 to 2 hours after administration and may range from euphoria to panic and severe depression. Persons often

TABLE 31-7 EFFECTS OF MARIJUANA ON THE BODY

BODY SYSTEM	EFFECTS
Cardiovascular system	Tachycardia
Gastrointestinal system	Increased appetite
Respiratory system	Bronchodilation
	Lung irritations and cough
Sensory system	Conjunctival redness
	Increased sense of taste, touch, and smell
	Distortion of time perception
	Perceptual inaccuracies
Nervous system	Short-term memory loss
	Impaired learning with decreased intellectual performances
	Impaired reflex reaction with inability to multitask
Reproductive system	Decreased sperm counts and reduced testosterone levels
	Irregular menses and sporadic ovulation
	Reduced estrogen levels
	Teratogenic to fetus; lower birth weights
Psychologic health	Euphoria and relaxation with gaiety and heightened sense of humor
	Apathy, dullness, lethargy, poor grooming
	Reduced interest in achievement (amotivational syndrome)
	Paranoia and depression
	Psychosis
	Suicide
	Dependence with severe anxiety and auditory, visual, and tactile hallucinations

do not realize the difference in self and nonself, have an increased awareness of sensory stimuli, and often believe the world is harmonious and beautiful. Psychedelics have the ability to bring about the types of alterations in thought, perception, and feeling that otherwise occur in dreams, or psychedelics can cause dreaming without loss of consciousness, effects not seen with other drugs. Lysergic acid diethylamide (LSD), dimethyltryptamine (DMT), phencyclidine (PCP), mescaline, psilocybin, and MDMA (ecstasy) are examples of these agents, with LSD considered the prototype.

LSD is a potent hallucinogenic street drug, to which tolerance develops rapidly. As with most street drugs, strengths vary, causing many user problems. Unpredictable effects take place in 20 minutes including hypertension, dilated pupils, hyperthermia, tachycardia, and enhanced awareness of activities. Unpleasant experiences are frequent, such as altered states of consciousness that cause psychosis to develop, or the drug may trigger latent psychosis to become observable. Homicidal thoughts may be a result of acute panic or paranoia. After alternating and altering levels of consciousness, a complete state of exhaustion results as drug's effects wear off—a time when suicide is a risk. Significant unfavorable reactions induced by LSD may be prolonged and/ or delayed with recurrent flashbacks ("bad trip"), including paranoia, depression, and schizophrenic psychotic reactions.

Mescaline, from flower heads of the peyote cactus, produces effects similar to those of LSD. The flower may be dried and smoked, or a soluble crystalline powder may be ingested either as a tea or capsule. Effects of mescaline include vivid, colorful hallucinations with physical effects of abdominal pain, nausea, vomiting, and diarrhea. Anxiety, stimulation of reflexes, tremors, and psychic disturbances occur with drug use.

Psilocybin, from Mexican mushrooms, produces hallucinogenic dysphoria similar to that from mescaline but of shorter duration. Mood may be pleasant for some people, but apprehension may be produced in others. The capacity to make critical judgments is poor, performance abilities are impaired, and compulsive hyperkinetic movements, laughter, dilation of pupils, vertigo, ataxia, paresthesia, muscle weakness, drowsiness, and sleep occur.

MDMA (3,4-methylenedioxymethamphetamine), or "ecstasy," became prominent in the mid-1980s. At first it was not a regulated drug, but it soon became classified as a Schedule I controlled substance, indicating no medicinal use. Ecstasy acts as both a psychedelic and a psychostimulant agent. Taken orally, this amphetamine derivative produces CNS stimulation, euphoria, and visual disturbances. Those who use MDMA report a sense of closeness with people, lowering of defenses, reduced anxiety, enhanced communication skills, and increased sociability. With large doses, panic, anxiety, paranoia, and signs of sympathetic nervous system stimulation such as increased heart rate, irregular pulse and respirations, dilated pupils, and, caused by decreased body temperature, vasoconstriction of the blood vessels in the skin are seen.

PCP, or "angel dust," "acid," or "purple haze," was first studied for use as a general anesthetic. Human use was subsequently dropped because of a high incidence of delirium, but the drug is still used in veterinary practices. Use and cheapness of the agent's production at the street level have led to abuse. Effects of PCP make it one of the most dangerous and most unpredictable of abused street substances. PCP may be administered orally, intranasally, intravenously, and by smoking. Because of its high solubility, PCP is rapidly absorbed from all sites. Absorption begins in the stomach, followed by recirculation of the blood back to the acid environment of the stomach, where the drug reenters the intestines for reabsorption again into the blood. This constant recycling through the body leads to prolonged drug action.

Low PCP doses cause CNS stimulation, euphoria, and sympathetic nervous system stimulation, similar to the effects of amphetamines or alcohol. With increased doses, disorientation, motor incoordination, and slurred speech occur. Euphoria leads to rapid release of inhibitions and emotional swings. Bizarre behavior may occur with high doses, progressing to dysphoria, catatonia, muscle rigidity, hypertensive crisis, coma, and death. Treatment for PCP use includes protection by removing the person from external stimuli because antipsychotics and psychotherapy are rarely effective. Symptoms of withdrawal must be treated to provide life support.

> ## Important Facts about Hallucinogens, Psychedelics, and Psychotomimetics
>
> - Hallucinogens and psychedelics produce auditory and visual hallucinations owing to increased awareness of sensory stimuli.
> - Lysergic acid diethylamide (LSD) is a potent hallucinogen that causes unpredictable responses, some pleasant and some unpleasant.
> - LSD may produce prolonged, delayed, and recurrent reactions of depression and schizophrenic and psychotic reactions, with rapid tolerance developing.
> - Mescaline is similar to LSD, causing vivid, colorful hallucinations.
> - Psilocybin produces hallucinogenic effects that are less prolonged than those of LSD or mescaline.
> - MDMA, or ecstasy, a derivative of amphetamine, acts as a psychedelic and psychostimulant.
> - Phencyclidine (PCP) produces stimulation and euphoria, similar to alcohol or amphetamines. Euphoria leads to release of inhibitions and produces emotional changes on a rapid basis.

INHALANTS

Benzine (used in dyes and drug production), acetone (nail polish and paint removers), carbon tetrachloride (dry cleaning fluid), gasoline, trichloroethylene (anesthetic), and toluene are volatile hydrocarbons used for sniffing. Many of these chemicals are found in common household products using hydrocarbons as propellants. These products are relatively inexpensive and easily

bought legally—for example, gasoline, kerosene, ink correction fluids, gas found in aerosol containers, and even helium found in balloons. Therefore these agents have become more popular with young people and those who cannot afford illicit substances. Although children and teens are most likely to use hydrocarbons for sniffing, adults are also abusers.

Bagging, huffing, and sniffing processes are used for inhalation. Bagging is performed by pouring solvents in a plastic bag and inhaling vapors. Huffing is pouring the solvent on a rag to inhale vapors. Sniffing is inhaling the solvent from its original container. All three means of inhalation produce rapid general CNS depression with marked inebriation, dizziness, lightheadedness, and intense feelings of well-being similar to alcohol intoxication. Euphoria and hallucinations usually lasting for 15 to 45 minutes are the desired and expected results. Some users experience feelings of reckless abandonment and increased power, with resultant aggressiveness, headaches, vertigo, and ataxia. High doses lead to confusion, brain damage, and coma, causing permanent disability or death. Sudden death is possible, caused by anoxia, respiratory depression, increased heart rates, and dysrhythmias. For persons in poverty or economic deprivation, glue sniffing may be the drug of choice. Tolerance to inhalants commonly occurs; those starting with a single tube of glue per day may progress to three, four, or more tubes to maintain the same effect.

> ## Important Facts about Inhalants
>
> - Commonly found inhalants such as cleansing products, glue, hairsprays, lacquers, and paints are abused, especially by young people and economically depressed individuals.
> - Inhalants provide euphoria and hallucinations.

ANABOLIC STEROIDS

Many anabolic-adrenergic steroidal preparations are available for oral or parenteral use. They are therapeutically prescribed, especially for males with low testosterone levels and specifically for underweight individuals, but are also used nontherapeutically by individuals who want an athletic edge. Misuse and abuse of these drugs, a growing problem, includes the use of anabolic (adrenergic) steroids by athletes to enhance athletic performance and increase their chances of winning in sports events, to gain strength, and simply to "look good."

> ### Did You Know?
>
> *Steroids* refers to a class of drugs; *adrenergic* refers to increased masculine characteristics; and *anabolic* refers to muscle building.

Many organizations, such as the National Collegiate Athletic Associations, the International Olympic Committee, and major league sports, have banned the use of these drugs. The U.S. Congress has even had hearings because of the increased use of these products. Misuse led to the addition of anabolic steroids to the DEA's controlled substance list in 1982.

Readily available on the Internet, anabolic steroids are known by names such as D-bol, Sten, Deca, and Anadrol. Some persons use these drugs by "cycling," involving taking multiple doses of drug over a period of time, stopping for a time, and then starting again to increase effectiveness. "Stacking" of steroids, or taking multiple metabolic steroids at one time, is still a practice used illegally and unethically by some athletes. Coinciding with the steroid use, a program of strenuous exercise and a high-protein diet are used to increase muscle mass and stamina. Short-term effects include increased aggressive behavior and masculinization in females. Long-term use leads to aggression, extreme mood swings, and other psychiatric effects, such as paranoia, depression, delusions, and impaired judgment. Because of misuse and abuse, steroids are Schedule III drugs in all states, with some states making these drugs Schedule II agents with a high potential for misuse or abuse (see Table 28-2).

Important Facts about Anabolic Steroids

- Anabolic steroids are misused by athletes to increase body weight and strength.
- Anabolic steroids are prepared from the male hormone testosterone, thus tending to masculinize users.

CARING FOR PATIENTS WITH DRUG MISUSE AND ABUSE PROBLEMS

Health care professionals need knowledge of psychotropic drugs, their actions, and their side effects. When giving care to persons with drug misuse or abuse problems, professionals should be nonjudgmental but willing to work with the patient, family, and members of the community to provide support needed for treatment. Through education and recognition of signs and symptoms of drug abuse, proper referrals for care may be made. Some of the more common signs of drug misuse or abuse include the following:

- Abrupt changes in work or school attendance, quality of work, work output, grades, and discipline
- Unusual flare-ups or outbreaks of rage or temper
- Withdrawal from responsibility
- General changes in overall attitude
- Deterioration in physical appearance
- Wearing sunglasses at inappropriate times

- Continual wearing of long-sleeved garments, particularly in hot weather, or reluctance to wear a short-sleeved garment
- Association with known drug abusers
- Secretive behavior about actions and behaviors; poorly concealed attempts to evade attention and suspicion, such as frequent trips to restrooms, basements, and like areas
- Stealing items including prescription medications from home, work, or school
- Glazed appearance in eyes
- Odor on breath
- Changes in health habits
- Asking for particular medications for pain and accepting only those medications

Knowledge of symptoms of drug use will enable the health care professional to assess drug usage (Table 31-8). Through asking questions, assistance with interventions may break the drug abuse cycle, uncomfortable withdrawal symptoms may be eased, and severe or life-threatening effects may be avoided. Remember that substance abuse is not limited to street drugs but may be found with use of prescription medications also.

Low self-esteem, a feeling of not belonging in society, a strong need for social approval, and inadequate

TABLE 31-8 SYMPTOMS SPECIFIC TO ABUSED DRUGS

SUBSTANCE	SYMPTOMS
inhalants	Nausea, dizziness, headaches, lack of coordination, odor of substance on breath
heroin and narcotics	Euphoria, drowsiness, nausea, vomiting, pinpoint pupils, needle tracks on arms
cocaine and amphetamines	Talkativeness, hyperalert state, increased blood pressure, history of weight loss, hyperactivity, ulcers in nose and throat, hallucinations and paranoia
barbiturates and benzodiazepines	Slow pulse and respiratory rates, doctor-hopping with vague complaints, slurred speech
hallucinogens (PCP, LSD)	Mood/mind alteration, panic, extreme focus on details, symptoms of fear and paranoia, unpredictable violent behavior
marijuana	Red eyes, dilated pupils, dry mouth, altered perceptions of surroundings, euphoria, inappropriate laughing and manner, smell of burnt rope, panic reactions, impaired memory

LSD, Lysergic acid diethylamide; *PCP*, phencyclidine.

communication skills are risk factors that increase drug misuse and abuse. Inability to feel gratification and non-bonding with families and friends predispose an individual to substance abuse. A person with a family history of alcoholism or drug abuse is also more likely to become an abuser as a way of avoiding personal confrontation.

Patient Education for Compliance

The best patient education is teaching prevention of misuse and abuse of substances, including therapeutic medicines such as analgesics and steroids.

SUMMARY

Drug abuse is self-medication on a chronic basis, using excessive quantities that may cause physical and/or psychological dependence. Drugs, from therapeutically prescribed medications to street drugs, may be misused or abused. Before a medication is prescribed, a definite need for the drug should be established.

Not a new phenomenon, drug abuse is using a medication in a way inconsistent with medical, social, and cultural norms of a certain population. It is important to note that the definition of drug abuse is related to social and cultural norms and to specific situations in which medications are prescribed. No socioeconomic, ethnic, and cultural classes are exempt from drug and substance abuse.

Physical and psychologic dependence occurs with misuse or abuse of drugs, with tolerance leading to greater doses. Drug availability is another factor leading to dependency and continued use; abuse can occur only if drugs can be obtained. Vulnerability to abuse can be a familial tendency; dependence can be a crutch to cope with everyday tensions.

Physical signs of drug abuse include weight loss, changes in sleep habits that cause lethargy, and frequent illnesses. Psychologic signs include inability to concentrate, lack of memory, apathy, and inability to function caused by illogical thought processes. Socially, mood swings, irritability, anger, and isolation from the environment including changes of surroundings and friends are apparent. Drug abusers may become anxious in social situations and may overreact, for instance, with defensiveness and unexplained anger.

The two most abused drugs are readily available and legally purchased by adults—nicotine and alcohol. Dangers from addiction to these drugs far outweigh any positive effects. Tolerance occurs with both drugs. Alcohol has interactions with many other drugs, causing severe physiologic effects. Disulfiram and acamprosate are specific therapeutic treatment for alcohol abuse. Patient education is absolutely necessary when these medications are prescribed.

Use of illicit drugs is a societal and personal major problem in the United States today. Some abused substances are easily obtained, such as glue, household chemicals, or acetaminophen, whereas others are more difficult to obtain, such as narcotics and amphetamines, making these agents expensive at street level. Some problems of misuse arise from patient administration of medications or even from unintentional misuse of prescribed medicines.

The theft of prescription drugs for illegal street use is one of today's social concerns.

One of the main dangers of illicit drugs consists of variability in drug strength caused by manufacture at street level—cutting drugs for increased profits. Because each dose is different and there is no control of these illegal substances, users are at risk for overdose. The health care professional must be aware of and recognize the many schemes used to obtain prescription medications such as opiates and opioids for illicit use. A physical disease may be replaced by psychologic dependence with medication tolerance, in which more and more drug use is needed to achieve the same results.

Of great importance for the health care professional to remember is that all medicinal agents have potential for misuse and abuse. Innocently using medications when there are insufficient symptoms is abusing drugs—that is, using drugs too frequently or using excessive dosages. These misuse and abuse problems are frequently seen in health care facilities today.

CRITICAL THINKING SCENARIO

Mrs. Svensdottir comes to the physician's office because of a migraine headache. Dr. Merry prescribes a narcotic medication for pain. Mrs. Svensdottir mentions that she has been drinking wine nightly with her dinner and has another glass of wine before bedtime when she feels she will not sleep well.

1. Does Dr. Merry need this information? Why or why not?
2. Could the use of wine at night be a kind of drug misuse? Why or why not?
3. Mrs. Svensdottir denies that she has an alcohol abuse problem and states that she has "everything under control." How is this a typical response from someone who is alcohol dependent?

REVIEW QUESTIONS

1. What is drug abuse? Drug misuse? Why are these so prevalent? _____

_____

_____

_____

2. How can a drug be used therapeutically and abused by the same person? _____

_____

_____

3. How does drug availability affect drug abuse? _____

_____

_____

4. What are the psychologic symptoms of drug abuse? Physical signs? Social effects? _____

_____

_____

_____

_____

5. What is the effect of alcohol on the body? What groups should avoid the use of alcohol? _____

_____

_____

6. What distinct patient education must occur with disulfiram? _____

_____

_____

_____

_____

7. Explain what tolerance to medications means and how this increases the dangers of drug abuse. _____

_____

_____

_____

_____

8. What is a hallucinogen/psychedelic? Why are these agents dangerous? _____

_____

_____

9. Have anabolic steroids been placed on the DEA's list of scheduled drugs? If so, which schedule, and why?

_____

_____

10. What are the implications for the medical assistant when confronted by a drug abuser or misuser? _____

_____

_____

_____

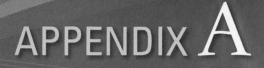

Check Your Understanding Answers

Chapter 6

6-1

1. E
3. I
5. E
7. P
9. E
11. $\frac{1}{3}$, $\frac{2}{6}$, $\frac{3}{9}$, $\frac{5}{15}$, $\frac{6}{18}$, $\frac{10}{30}$, $\frac{15}{45}$
13. $\frac{1}{4}$, $\frac{3}{12}$, $\frac{5}{20}$
15. $\frac{1}{4}$, $\frac{2}{8}$, $\frac{5}{20}$

6-2

1. $4\frac{2}{3}$
3. $6\frac{1}{5}$
5. $7\frac{6}{7}$
7. $4\frac{1}{6}$
9. $6\frac{1}{3}$
11. $\frac{7}{5}$
13. $\frac{13}{2}$
15. $\frac{29}{6}$
17. $\frac{69}{4}$
19. $\frac{57}{10}$
21. $8\frac{3}{4}$
23. $4\frac{1}{3}$
25. $3\frac{1}{2}$
27. $1\frac{1}{2}$
29. $4\frac{3}{8}$

6-3

1. 40
3. 12
5. 42
7. 6
9. 35
11. $1\frac{1}{4}$
13. $\frac{3}{8}$
15. $\frac{12}{35}$
17. $\frac{15}{28}$
19. $\frac{19}{21}$

6-4

1. $\frac{9}{28}$
3. $\frac{5}{8}$
5. $\frac{17}{63}$
7. $\frac{7}{16}$
9. $\frac{1}{2}$
11. $12\frac{1}{6}$
13. $5\frac{15}{28}$
15. $1\frac{11}{24}$
17. $1\frac{3}{4}$
19. $\frac{11}{30}$

6-5

1. $\frac{1}{2}$
3. $\frac{1}{8}$
5. $\frac{1}{14}$
7. $\frac{6}{1}$
9. $\frac{12}{1}$
11. $\frac{5}{12}$
13. $\frac{7}{9}$
15. 12
17. $\frac{1}{12}$
19. $13\frac{1}{5}$

6-6

1. $\frac{19}{5}$
3. $\frac{5}{4}$
5. $\frac{51}{5}$
7. 11
9. $2\frac{1}{3}$
11. $4\frac{4}{5}$
13. $1\frac{20}{57}$
15. $8\frac{4}{25}$

6-7

1. $\frac{7}{5}$
3. $\frac{2}{4}$, $\frac{1}{2}$
5. $\frac{1}{3}$
7. $3\frac{1}{2}$
9. $6\frac{3}{4}$

6-4 (cont.)

11. $1\frac{5}{6}$
13. $4\frac{2}{3}$
15. $1\frac{7}{8}$
17. $\frac{1}{8}$
19. $1\frac{19}{45}$

6-8

1. 1
3. 1
5. 68
7. 56.8
9. 121.3
11. 233.33
13. 88.89
15. 100.06
17. 234.557
19. 357.975

6-9

1. 0.625
3. 0.167
5. 0.375
7. 1.9
9. 2.7
11. 3.5
13. 4.75
15. 2.64

6-10

1. 125.72
3. 1345.151
5. 655.541
7. 912.29
9. 782.454
11. 6.242
13. 39.94
15. 3.37
17. 90.038
19. 0.14

6-11
1. 269.07
3. 770.76
5. 521.11
7. 0.01
9. 6874.47

6-12
1. 2.3
3. 6.1
5. 3
7. 2.2
9. 6.2

6-13
1. $32\frac{84}{100}$
3. 33
5. 1
7. 3.7
9. 0.38
11. 68.247
13. 1047.322
15. 17.4
17. 100.39
19. 204.1
21. 1491
23. 1.183
25. 2.882

6-14
1. 0.01
3. 0.05
5. 0.31
7. 0.08
9. 0.18

6-15
1. 359%
3. 6%
5. 4.7%
7. 117%
9. 5.5%

6-16
1. 3.92
3. 5.34
5. 14.25
7. 48
9. 15.58

6-17
1. 83.3%
3. 18.2%
5. 42.9%
7. 15.4%
9. 9.1%

6-18
1. 10
3. 25
5. 50
7. 125
9. 30

6-19
1. 0.005
3. 0.0144
5. 0.3333
7. 7234%
9. 5%
11. 0.5
13. 32.7
15. 16.8
17. 34%
19. 67%
21. 60
23. 50
25. 3
27. 32
29. 48

6-20
1. $x = 25$
3. $x = 22$
5. $x = 150$
7. $x = 7$
9. $x = 16$
11. $x = 6$
13. $x = 9$
15. $x = 2$
17. $x = 125$
19. $x = 400$

6-21
1. 60
3. 9
5. 20
7. 188
9. 27
11. 64
13. 125
15. 19
17. 47
19. 80

6-22
1. $x = 4$
3. $x = 20$
5. $x = 0.04$
7. 56 tablets
9. $1\frac{1}{2}$ tablets
11. 0.2 mL
13. 95 kg

15. 2 tablets
17. ¾
19. 900 mg

Chapter 7

7-1
1. less than
3. greater than
5. greater than
7. less than
9. gram
11. 1.001
13. 0.0011
15. 0.10101
17. length; 120 cm
19. length; 3000.75 m
21. solid (weight); 1000 mcg
23. solid (weight); 5 kg
25. length; 750 km

7-2
1. 6.9 m
3. 0.043 m
5. 9 cm
7. 88 mm
9. 120 cm
11. 425 mm
13. 50 cm
15. 100 cm

7-3
1. 0.001 L
3. 6400 mL
5. 0.5 L
7. 1.45 L
9. 0.1 L
11. 2000 mL
13. 1 L
15. 3 L

7-4
1. 1.5 mg
3. 6500 mg
5. 340 g
7. 90 mg
9. 30 g
11. 2200 g
13. 0.5 mg
15. 1 tab = 0.088 mg

7-5
1. tablespoon
3. cup
5. tablespoon
7. greater than

9. less than
11. Dissolve 2 level teaspoons of magnesium sulfate into 1 cup of water and take by mouth.
13. Take 1 teaspoon of Benylin elixir every 4 hours. Do not exceed 6 doses daily.
15. Instill 2 drops of Liquifilm tears in each eye as needed.

Chapter 8

8-1
1. 0440
3. 1102
5. 2245
7. 0033
9. 1533
11. 9:21 PM
13. 12:45 AM
15. midnight
17. 2:10 AM
19. 3:15 PM

8-2
1. 37.6° C = 99.6° F
3. 39.4° C = 103° F
5. 26.7° C = 80° F
7. 100° C = 212° F
9. −17.8° C = 0° F
11. 57.2° F = 14° C
13. 41° F = 5° C
15. 204.8° F = 96° C
17. 108.1° F = 42.3° C
19. 51.8° F = 11° C

8-3
1. $1:5 = \frac{1}{5}$
3. $2:5 = \frac{2}{5}$
5. $9:10 = \frac{9}{10}$
7. $\frac{1}{2} = 1:2$
9. $\frac{1}{100} = 1:100$

8-4
1. 3 tbsp
3. 15 (16)* gtt
5. 90 mL
7. 1 c
9. 500 mL
11. 2 T
13. 2 qt or 64 oz
15. 1 oz

8-5
1. 45 mg
3. 900 mg

5. 0.3 g
7. 6 gr
9. 360 mg
11. 3 lb
13. 4250 mg
15. 75 g

8-6
1. 20 cm
3. 10 ft
5. 2 ft
7. 2 m
9. 1 m
11. 25 mm (2.5 cm); yes
13. 45 cm
15. 0.6 in

Chapter 9

9-1
1. 3 tsp
3. 6 mL
5. 5 mL

9-2
1. $\frac{2}{3}$
3. $\frac{1}{150}$
5. $\frac{2}{7}$
7. 1:250
9. 1:1000
11. $1\frac{1}{2}$ tabs
13. 2 tabs
15. 4 tabs

9-3
1. a. 500 mg
   b. 1000 mg
   c. mL
   d. 2.5 mL
3. a. 160 mg
   b. 320 mg
   c. tablets
   d. $\frac{1}{2}$ tablet
5. a. 400 mg
   b. 200 mg
   c. mL
   d. 10 mL
7. $1\frac{1}{2}$ tabs
9. 20 mL; 4 tsp

9-4
1. 1000 mg/1 g
3. 10 mL/200 mg
5. 1 g/1000 mg
7. $1\frac{1}{2}$ tabs
9. 20 mL; 4 tsp

9-5
1. two 500 mg tablets by mouth twice a day
3. two 50 mg tablets by mouth 4 times a day
5. four 250 mg tablets by mouth daily
7. one half of one 0.05 mg tablet by mouth daily
9. one 300 mg tablet by mouth twice a day

9-6
1. 1200 mg
3. 30 mL
5. Yes, 1 teaspoon = 5 mL; use dose syringe for accuracy
7. 200 mg
9. 6 days
11. 87 mL

9-7
1. 0.35 BSA
3. 1.0 BSA
5. 1.2 BSA

9-8
1. 0.92 m²; 135 mg; 2.7 mL or $\frac{1}{2}$ tsp
3. 1.36 m²; 4 mg or 4 mL
5. 1.08 m²; 318 mg; 6.4 mL or $1\frac{1}{3}$ tsp

9-9
1. 250 mg; 5 mL
3. 380 mg/day; 127 mg/dose or 125 mg/dose; 1 mL; $\frac{1}{5}$ tsp
5. 500 mg/dose; 10 mL/dose; 2 tsp

Chapter 10

10-1
1. 2.3 mL
3. 0.7 mL
5. 2.8 mL
7. draw a line at 0.9 mL
9. draw a line at 1.1 mL
11. draw a line at 0.3 mL
13. draw a line at 1.9 mL
15. draw a line at 2.9 mL

10-2
1. 2.5 mL
3. 0.5 mL
5. 3 mL

10-3
1. 52 units
3. 14 units
5. 26 units
7. show 46 units insulin
9. show 0.5 mL

10-4
1. 35 units
3. 84 units
5. 15 units
7. 1 mL IM four times a day (every 6 hours)
9. 1.8 mL

10-5
1. 0.5 mL
3. 1.5 mL
5. 2 mL
7. 0.9 mL
9. 0.2 mL

Drug-Nutrient and Drug-Drug Interactions

DRUG-NUTRIENT INTERACTIONS

calcium carbonate (Tums): dairy products, bran and other whole grains

erythromycin, penicillins: acidic juices, citrus fruits, soft drinks

all statins (Mevacor, Zocor): grapefruit juice

tetracyclines: calcium-containing foods such as ice cream, cheese, and milk

warfarin sodium: beef liver, spinach, cabbage, Brussels sprouts, broccoli

Monoamine oxidase inhibitors (MAOIs): foods high in tyramine such as cheese, sour cream, yogurt, meat tenderizers, beer and wine, aged meats

CLINICALLY SIGNIFICANT DRUG-DRUG INTERACTIONS

carbamazepine (Tegretol): charcoal, erythromycin, clozapine

chlorpropamide (Diabinese): ethyl alcohol

clonidine (Catapres): propranolol (Inderal)

clozapine (Clozaril): carbamazepine (Tegretol)

digitoxin: rifampin (Rifadin)

digoxin (Lanoxin): amiodarone (Cordarone), erythromycin base, quinidine, tetracycline, verapamil (Calan)

diltiazem (Cardizem): cyclosporine (Neoral)

erythromycin: cyclosporine (Neoral)

ethyl alcohol: disulfiram (Antabuse)

gentamicin (Garamycin): carbenicillin (Geocillin), cephalothin (Keflin)

heparin: aspirin

insulin: propranolol (Inderal)

ketoconazole (Nizoral): cyclosporine (Neoral)

lidocaine (Xylocaine): cimetidine (Tagamet)

lincomycin (Lincocin): kaolin

lithium carbonate (Lithobid): acetazolamide (Diamox), chlorothiazide (Diuril)

meperidine (Demerol): phenelzine (Nardil)

methotrexate (Folex): aspirin, probenecid (Benemid), sulfamethoxazole-trimethoprim (Septra, Bactrim)

phenelzine (Nardil): levodopa (l-dopa)

phenytoin (Dilantin): cimetidine (Tagamet), disulfiram (Antabuse), dopamine (Dopastat, Entropion), fluconazole (Diflucan)

propranolol (Inderal): cimetidine (Tagamet), epinephrine

pyridoxine (vitamin B_6): levodopa (l-dopa)

quinidine: amiodarone (Cordarone), verapamil (Calan)

rifampin (Rifadin): cyclosporine (Neoral), oral contraceptive agents

spironolactone (Aldactone): potassium chloride (K-Tabs)

tetracycline: aluminum hydroxide (Amphojel), ferrous sulfate

theophylline (Elixophyllin, Theo-Dur): charcoal, cimetidine (Tagamet), erythromycin, tobacco

triazolam (Halcion): ketoconazole (Nizoral)

warfarin (Coumadin): amiodarone (Cordarone), aspirin, cimetidine (Tagamet), clofibrate (Atromid-S), disulfiram (Antabuse), erythromycin, glucagon, methyltestosterone, nalidixic acid (NegGram), phenobarbital, phenylbutazone (Alka Butazolidin), phytonadione (vitamin K), rifampin (Rifadin), sulfamethoxazole (Gantanol), sulfinpyrazone (Anturane), thyroid (Synthroid)

Source for drug-drug interactions: Pocket guide to evaluations of drug interactions, ed 4, Washington, DC, 2002, American Pharmaceutical Association.

Glossary

Absence or petit mal seizures Loss of consciousness for a short period of time caused by seizure activity

Absorption Uptake of medications for distribution in the body through or across tissues

Accommodation Change in shape of the lens of the eye to adjust to viewing objects at different distances

Acetylcholine (Ach) Chemical neurotransmitter in the parasympathetic nervous system

Acid Any substance with a hydrogen ion that is released in a solution and reacts with metals to form salts; pH below 7

Acid rebound Increase in gastric acid secretions to neutralize antacids that have been taken for a prolonged period of time

Acne Inflammation of the hair follicles and sebaceous glands characterized by comedones, pustules, and papules (raised areas)

Acquired immunity Immunity that is the result of exposure to a disease antigen, the injection of immune globulins, or immunizations

Actinic keratosis Horny, premalignant lesions of the skin caused by excessive exposure to sunlight

Action onset Time at which the desired function begins to produce an effect, such as with medications

Action peak Time at which the desired function reaches the highest potential, such as the highest level of medication in the blood stream during drug administration cycle

Active immunity Immunity resulting from the development of antibodies within a person's body that renders the person immune; may occur from exposure through a disease process or from immunizations

Active ingredient Medicinal ingredient in a pure, undiluted form of the chemical that has effects on body functions

Addiction Compulsive, uncontrollable dependence on a chemical substance, habit, or practice to such a degree that either the means of obtaining or ceasing may cause emotional, mental, or psychologic reactions

Adenocarcinoma A malignant tumor arising from glandular tissue

Adjuvant medication Medication used to increase or hasten the action of the principal medications

Administer To give to or apply medication on a person

Adrenergic agonist Also called sympathomimetic agent or agonist; agent that stimulates the action of the sympathetic nervous system or mimics the action of the sympathetic nervous system

Adsorbent Liquid or gas substance that readily adheres the surface of a solid material to the surface of another substance

Adverse reaction Unintended, undesirable, and often unpredictable effect of a medication that cause pain, discomfort, or unwanted symptoms; more severe than a side effect

Aerobic bacteria Bacteria that live in an environment containing oxygen

Aerochamber A hollow, closed tube added to inhalation medications to increase the availability of the medication

Aerosol Liquid in a pressurized container that dispenses medication to sites of absorption

Aerosol foam Water-in-oil emulsion that dispenses into a foam when mixed with air

Affect Emotion or emotional response

Affective disorders Group of disorders characterized by disturbances in mood, from partial to full mania or depression

Aggregation Clustering or clumping of substances, such as blood cells

Agitate To shake a container vigorously

Agonist Medication that binds to the receptor site and stimulates the function of that site; drug that mimics a function of the body

Akathisia Restlessness, inability to sit still, urgent need to move

Alkaline A substance having a pH below 7; a substance that combines with acids to form salts

Alkaloid Organic compound that is alkaline in nature and is combined with acids to make salts; a group of alkaline organic substances obtained from plants

Alkylating agent Substance that interferes with cell metabolism and growth by introducing an alkyl agent or compound; agent used to treat malignancies

Allergic reaction Hypersensitivity to a drug that may occur after only one dose has been taken (see *Hypersensitivity reaction*)

Alopecia Loss of hair

Alternative medicine Practice of using products for which scientific evidence of safety and efficacy is lacking (e.g., most herbal preparations, copper bracelets for arthritis)

Alzheimer disease Disease characterized by progressive impairment in memory and cognitive function that may lead to a vegetative state and death

Ampule Small glass container that is sealed and holds a single dose of medication, usually for injection

Amyloid Abnormal neuronal lipoprotein; starchlike complex that is deposited in tissues, such as the brain; possible cause of Alzheimer disease

Amyloid blockers Drugs that prevent the formation of amyloids

Anabolic steroids Synthetically produced androgens

Anabolism Constructive metabolic process by which substances are converted by an organism into other components of the organism's chemical structure; in the example of anabolic steroids such as testosterone, the result is greater muscle mass

Anaerobic bacteria Bacteria that live in an environment free of oxygen

Analeptics Drugs that stimulate the central nervous system

Analgesic Medication with pain-relieving property

Anaphylaxis Severe allergic reaction, possibly fatal, to a drug that occurs a short time after the drug has been administered to a person who is hypersensitive to it

Anaplastic Characterized by loss of cell differentiation

Anatomy Branch of science that deals with structure of organisms

Androgen Any male sex hormone

Anesthesia Loss of sensation, either of the entire body or of certain body areas

Angina pectoris Insufficient blood flow to the heart, with resultant spasm of the cardiac muscle, causing chest pain

Ankylosing spondylitis Change in spine, similar to rheumatoid arthritis, that causes stiffening of the back

Ankylosis Immobility of joints, caused by congenital conditions, surgery, trauma, or diseases

Anomaly Any deviation from normal

Anorectal Pertaining to the anus and rectum

Anorexia Loss of appetite

Anorexiant Medication used to suppress appetite

Anosmia Lack of sense of smell

Antagonism Cancellation or reduction of one drug's effect by another drug

Antagonist Medication that binds at receptor sites to prevent other medications from binding to those same sites

Anthelmintics Agents used for treatment of intestinal worms

Antibacterial drugs Drugs with the ability for destruction or inhibition of growth of bacteria

Antibiotic Natural or synthetic substance, originally derived from plant or animal sources, that kills or inhibits the growth of microorganisms

Antibody Protein that develops in response to the presence of an antigen in the body and reacts with the antigen on the next exposure; may be formed from infections, immunizations, transfer from the mother to a child, or from no known antigen stimulation

Antibody titer Quantity of viable antibodies required to respond to a given quantity of antigen as determined by a laboratory (serologic) test

Anticholinergic agents Also called *anticholinergics*; agents that block the parasympathetic nerve impulse (e.g., causing dilation of the pupil)

Anticholinergics See *Anticholinergic agents*

Antidiarrheal Agent or substance that prevents or treats diarrhea

Antidote Drug or substance given to stop a toxic effect

Antiemetic Agent that prevents or relieves nausea or vomiting

Antiflatulent Agent that decreases excessive gas in the stomach or intestines

Antigen Substance that is either introduced into the body or formed by the body to induce the formation of antibodies specific to that antigen

Antigen-antibody response Neutralization or destruction of antigen by antibodies

Antihistamine Agent that decreases histamine release

Antiinflammatory Medication with inflammation-reducing property

Antimetabolite Agent that disrupts essential cell metabolic processes and is used to treat malignancies by opposing the actions of or replacing a metabolite necessary for cell growth by interfering with DNA metabolism

Antimicrobial Pertaining to destruction or inhibition of growth of microorganisms; when said of drugs, includes both those of organic origin (*antibiotics*) and those of nonorganic origin (e.g., silver, sulfur, and mercury)

Antineoplastic agent Drug used to prevent development, growth, or proliferation of malignant cells

Antipyretic Medication with fever-reducing property

Antisecretory agent Agent that inhibits secretions of a gland or organ

Antiseptic Agent that reduces, prevents, or inhibits the growth of microbial flora of the skin and mucous membranes without necessarily killing them

Antiserum Serum containing antibodies to a specific antigen; usually of human or animal origin

Antispasmodics Agents that prevent or decrease intestinal spasms

Antitoxin Agent that provides antibodies produced in response to a specific toxin that has the ability to neutralize that same toxin in another person (e.g., tetanus antitoxin)

Antitumor antibiotics Drugs that hold to DNA to inhibit synthesis of DNA and RNA

Antitussive Agent that relieves or suppresses coughing

Antiviral Agent that opposes the action of a virus; medication specifically for treating viral conditions

Anxiolytic Medication to relieve anxiety; minor tranquilizer

Aperture An opening or hole in an object

Apothecary Pharmacist or druggist

Apothecary system One of the oldest measurement systems used to calculate drug orders; based on grains and drams

Aqueous Like water, watery

Aqueous solution Water-soluble solution; when referring to injections, the aqueous solution is considered to be thin or watery

Arrhythmia Irregular rhythm (i.e., irregular heartbeat)

Arteriosclerosis Thickening of walls of arterioles causing loss of elasticity and loss of ability to contract

Arthritis Inflammation of joint, accompanied by pain, swelling, and bony changes in the joint

Articulate To join bones in joints

Artificial active immunity Long-term immunity provided by immunization with a specific agent to develop antibodies to a specific disease process

Artificial passive immunity Short-term immunity provided from other persons or animals that have the antibodies for a specific disease (e.g., immune globulins, antitoxins)

Ascites Accumulation of serous fluid in peritoneal cavity

Aspirate Drawn in or out by suction; to pull on plunger of syringe to withdraw air

Asthma Disease of tracheobronchial tree with paroxysmal constriction of bronchial airways

Astringent Agent that causes shrinking or constricting action, usually applied topically or locally

Ataxia Difficulty with balance

Atelectasis An airless condition in the nonexpanded lung

Atherosclerosis Form of arteriosclerosis characterized by buildup of fatty plaques on the walls of arteries and arterioles

Attention-deficit/hyperactivity disorder (ADHD) Disease found most frequently in children that is characterized by inattention, hyperactivity, and impulsiveness

Attenuated Lessened, abbreviated; in reference to immunity, lessened virulence of a pathogen

Aura Neurologic visual phenomena (e.g., light flashes, blank areas in the field of vision) that may precede epileptic seizures and migraine headaches

Auralgia Ear pain; also called *otalgia* or *otodynia*

Automaticity Automatic spontaneous initiation of a heart impulse

Autonomic nervous system Self-governing, involuntary nervous system

Auxiliary label Label added to prescription bottle to provide additional information

Avirulent Inability to produce disease or pathogenicity

Avitaminosis Any disease caused by lack of vitamin production or intake

Bacteria (singular, *bacterium*) One-celled organisms that can synthesize DNA, RNA, or other essential products and can reproduce, but live on food supplied by a host or by a supportive environment

Bactericidal Pertaining to destruction of bacteria; drugs or chemicals with this ability

Bacteriocidal agent Substance with the ability to destroy bacteria

Bacteriostatic Inhibiting or retarding the growth of bacteria; drugs or chemicals with this ability

Bacteriostatic agent Substance with the ability to inhibit or retard growth of bacteria

Base Any substance that combines with hydrogen to form a salt; pH above 7 or alkaline in nature

Bath Method of cleansing the body or its parts or treating the body therapeutically with a cleansing agent

Benign Nonmalignant

Bevel Slanted surface on the end of a hypodermic needle, including the point and the lumen

Bioequivalence State or property of having the same strength and availability for absorption in the body as the same dosage of another available source of that drug

Biotherapy System of cancer therapy that uses interferons and mitogen stimulated lymphocytes

Biotransformation Chemical changes a substance undergoes in the body

Bipolar disorder Psychiatric condition characterized by alternating periods of mania and depressive states; previously called *manic-depressive disorder*

Bleb Irregularly raised elevation of the epidermis

Blepharitis Inflammation of the eyelids from bacterial infections or allergies

Blood-brain barrier Capillary walls of the brain, which can act to prevent potentially harmful substances from moving out of the bloodstream and entering the meninges in the brain or cerebral spinal fluid

Body surface area (BSA) Total body surface area based on the relationship of height to weight

Body surface area (BSA) calculation Process of calculating dosages based on weight and height using a nomogram

Bolus Concentrated amount of medication given rapidly intravenously

Brand-name drug Proprietary drug with a trademark (such drugs are marked with ®)

Broad-spectrum antibiotic Antibiotic effective against a variety of gram-positive and gram-negative microorganisms

Bronchiectasis Abnormal condition of bronchial tree characterized by irreversible dilation and destruction of bronchial walls

Buccal Inside of cheek, surface of tooth, or gum

Buccal tablet Tablet placed in the mouth between cheek and gum (buccal area) for absorption

Buffered tablet Medication combined with an antacid to reduce irritation to the stomach when ingested

Bureau of Narcotics and Dangerous Drugs (BNDD) Government agency that existed from 1968 to 1973 and had responsibilities for regulation of controlled substances

Bursitis Inflammation of the bursa of joints

Cancer Malignant neoplasm; uncontrolled growth and spread of abnormal cells

Caplet Long, oblong tablet with a smooth film-coated covering for ease of swallowing

Capsule Small gelatin container filled with medication in powder or granule form

Carbuncle Lesion of the skin with inflammation of the skin and deeper tissues that produces suppuration and sloughing of the tissue; similar to a boil or furuncle

Carcinogenic Potential to produce cancer or increase the risk of cancer; agent with carcinogenic potential

Caries Cavities in teeth

Carminative Agent that helps prevent formation of gas in the gastrointestinal tract

Cataplexy A condition characterized by sudden muscular weakness and hypotonia caused by anger, fear, or surprise

Cataract Opacity (loss of transparency) on or in the lens or capsule of the eye

Catecholamines Epinephrine, norepinephrine, and dopamine, derived from tyrosamine

Cathartics Active agents that cause a bowel movement

Ceiling effect Dose beyond which no further response occurs (e.g., an analgesic ceiling effect)

Cell cycle phase Steps that occur in the growth and development of a cell

Celsius Temperature scale in which 0° is freezing and 100° is boiling point of water at sea level

Central nervous system Brain and spinal cord

Cerumen Ear wax

Chalazion Hard eyelid cyst resulting from chronic inflammation of a meibomian gland

Chelator Agent used to treat metal poisonings

Chemotherapy Treatment of disease using chemical agents

Chewable tablet Tablet with a sugar or flavored base, designed to be chewed

Chloasma Darkening of the skin around the eyes

Cholelithiasis Formation or presence of calculi or bile stones in the gallbladder

Cholinergic agent (or parasympathomimetic agent) Drug that mimics the parasympathetic nervous system; agent that acts to transmit nerve stimulations in the parasympathetic nervous system (e.g., causing constriction of the pupil in the eye)

Cholinesterase Enzyme to inhibit the action of acetylcholine

Chronotropic effect Increase or decrease in the heart rate

Cirrhosis Chronic liver disease frequently found in persons with long-term alcohol abuse

Clinical pharmacology Study of drug effects in humans

Clonic Pertaining to alternating contracting and relaxing of muscles

Closed-angle glaucoma Elevated pressure in eye caused by obstruction of outflow of aqueous humor that occurs with a narrowing of angle between the iris and cornea to block exit of aqueous humor

Coanalgesia Administration of two or more medications (analgesics) together for synergistic effect

Coitus Sexual union of two people of the opposite sex in which the penis is introduced to the vagina

Colloid suspension/solution Suspension with alcohol, water, or ether as a solvent; a thin layer of medication is left on the skin when the solvent evaporates

Comedones (singular, *comedo*) Skin lesions found with acne vulgaris; commonly called *whitehead* or *blackhead*

Compatible Suitable for mixing without unfavorable actions; in pharmacology, refers to mixing two or more medications

Complementary medicine Alternative medical techniques that have been proved effective by scientific research as a basis for use and that are accepted as part of good medical practice (e.g., acupuncture, massage therapy)

Compounding Mixing a prescription according to the physician's order

Compulsion An irresistible, repetitive, irrational, impulse to perform an act that results in overt anxiety if act is not done

Concentration Ratio of mass or volume of a solute to the mass or volume of the solution or solvent

Conjunctivitis Acute inflammation of the conjunctiva from bacterial or viral infection, usually self-limiting; also called *pinkeye*

Contraception Prevention of fertilization of the ovum and the subsequent onset of pregnancy

Contraindication Condition in which use of given medication should be avoided

Controlled substance Medication that is controlled by the Drug Enforcement Administration because of its potential for abuse and misuse

Conversion factor Known equivalency of two values in different measurement systems; may be written as a fraction or a ratio

Convert Change from one form to another

Convulsion Abnormal motor movements, such as the jerking movement of a grand mal seizure

Corticosteroids Any one of the hormones (except the sex hormones) from the adrenal cortex that control body processes

Coryza Inflammation of the mucous membranes of the nose with a profuse nasal discharge; commonly called a "head cold"

Cream Semisolid preparation in a base that is absorbed into the tissue for slow, sustained release

Crepitus Crackling sounds in joints resulting from arthritis

Cryptorchidism Developmental defect in which one or both testicles fail to descend into the scrotum

Cumulation (accumulation) Increasing storage of a medication in the body caused by the body's inability to metabolize or excrete the medication before another dose is taken

Curative (healing) medication Medication prescribed to kill or remove the causative agent of a disease

Cycloplegia Paralysis of the ciliary muscle

Cytotoxic agent Compound that causes cell destruction

Dangerous drug Drug that can cause addiction or that is detrimental to the body

DEA number Identification number supplied to medical professionals, pharmacies, and the like by the Drug Enforcement Agency to allow the agency to enforce regulations controlling scheduled substances

Decimal A fractional part of a number

Decongestant Agent that reduces swelling and congestion in the respiratory tract

Defecation Passage of feces from the body; bowel movement

Delayed-action capsule Capsule prepared to release drug at a particular site or to provide a steady release of medication over a period of time

Delirium tremens Restlessness, confusion, insomnia, and irritability, with visual, tactile, and auditory hallucinations, caused by abstinence of alcohol consumption in an alcohol abuser

Delusion False belief that cannot be changed with reason

Demulcent Drug used to soothe a body part or to relieve symptoms of irritation

Denominator Term for number below or to the right of the line in a fraction indicating the number of equal parts into which the while is divided

Dentifrice Substance for cleaning teeth

Dentition Development and eruption of teeth; arrangement, number, and kind of teeth as they appear in the mouth

Dependence Total psychophysical state of addiction to drugs or alcohol; state in which an increasing amount of a substance is needed to prevent the onset of withdrawal symptoms

Depot form of medication Drug injected or implanted to be slowly absorbed into circulation, usually into a fatty tissue area where the drug is stored and distributed

Depot injectable Medication given parenterally that is stored in the fatty tissue for slow release in the body

Depressant Drug that acts to lower or lessen the activity of a body part

Desired therapeutic effect or desired effect Intended response to a medication

Destructive agent Substance that destroys cells and tissues, from bactericidals to chemotherapy

Diagnostic agent Medication used to assist in diagnosing diseases

Diaphoresis Excessive perspiration

Diffusion Process in which particles in a fluid moves from an area of higher concentration to an area of lower concentration, resulting in an even distribution of the particles in the fluid

Digitalization Rapid administration of digitalis to reach a therapeutic level

Diluent Agent that dilutes a substance; in pharmacology, the liquid added to a powder to change the powder to a liquid form for parenteral administration or for unstable oral preparations

Dimensional analysis Extended rates used to calculate doses for medications when two medication measurement systems are used

Disease-modifying antirheumatic drug (DMARD) Drug that modifies rheumatic diseases

Disinfectant or germicidal agent Agent that decreases the number of microorganisms on inanimate objects and prevents infection by killing bacteria on inanimate surfaces

Dispense To give medications to a patient to be taken at a later time

Dispersion Scattering of medication particles throughout the body or throughout a liquid

Distribution Dispersion of medication to sites in the body

Diuresis Loss of water in the body

Dividend Number or quantity to be divided

Divisor Number or quantity by which the dividend is divided to produce the quotient

Documentation Written notation in a medical record of information obtained from a patient and procedures that have been performed in the medical setting

Dosage Regimen of administering individual doses of medication, expressed in quantity per unit of time

Dosage strength (weight) Strength or weight of medication in the dose(s) of administered medication(s)

Dose Exact amount of a medication to be given or taken at one time

Dose spoon A spoon-like device used to administer doses of liquid medications orally

Dose syringe A syringe-like device used to administer liquid doses of oral medications

Douche A procedure in which a liquid medication or solution is introduced into the vagina

Dram Unit of measure for liquid volume in the apothecary system

Dromotropic effect Increase or decrease in the conduction of cardiac electrical impulses

Drug Any chemical that has an effect on living processes

Drug abuse Misuse or overuse of drugs in a manner that deviates from the prescribed manner, which might lead to physical or psychologic dependence, usually by self-medication

Drug addiction Compulsive use of drugs or substances that results in physical, psychologic, or social harm

Drug blood level Amount of a drug circulating in the bloodstream; also known as the *reference value* in laboratory reports

Drug dependence Compulsion to take a drug, either continuously or periodically, to relieve a real or imagined physical or psychologic need

Drug efficacy Ability of a drug to produce the desired chemical change in the body

Drug Enforcement Administration (DEA) Agency in the Department of Justice with the legal responsibility to enforce the statutes of the Comprehensive Drug Abuse and Prevention Act of 1970

Drug Facts and Comparisons Publication updated monthly by Facts and Comparisons giving in-depth information concerning medications; usually used by pharmacists

Drug habituation Taking of medication as a matter of course, not out of need

Drug half-life Time in which half of the available drug is metabolized by the body for excretion

Drug holiday Period during which drug doses are withheld to allow reversal of side effects or adverse reactions

Drug interaction Effects of medications taken together

Drug misuse Nonspecific or indiscriminate use of drugs; the use of drugs for purposes other than therapeutic intentions

Drug nomenclature System of naming drugs (i.e., chemical, generic, and brand names)

Drug purity Quality or state of having the type and concentration of substances set forth by FDA standards for production of a drug

Drug quality State or condition of ensuring that each time a medication is taken as ordered or in compliance with the manufacturer's directions, it meets the same drug standards

Drug sample Medication left by a manufacturer's representative in a physician's office to be given, not sold, to a patient with the main purpose of ensuring the patient can effectively take the medication

Drug standardization Process in which a pharmaceutical preparation or chemical substance of know quantity, ingredients, and strength is the same quantity, ingredients, and strength in a comparable pharmaceutical preparation

Drug standards Rules and regulations to assure consumers that they are receiving medications with therapeutic consistency

Drug strength or potency Concentration of active ingredient(s) in a medicinal preparation

Drug tolerance Accustomization to a medication resulting in a decreased response to the usual dose

Dry powder inhaler (DPI) Drug delivery system that dispenses a given amount of medication as a dry powder directly to the mucous membranes of the respiratory tract

Dyskinesia Excessive involuntary body movements

Dyspareunia Painful sexual intercourse

Dysphonia Difficulty speaking or hoarseness

Dysphoria Exaggerated feeling of depression or unrest

Dyspnea Difficulty breathing; a subjective sensation of stressful breathing due to respiratory and cardiac exercise or anxiety

Dysrhythmia A disturbance or abnormality in normal rhythmic pattern as with heart rhythm

Dystonia Weak, slow body movements caused by lack of muscle coordination or impaired muscle tone

Dysuria Painful urination

Ectopic beats An event of heart beats occurring at the wrong time, such as premature beats

Eczema Acute or chronic skin irritation that has erythema, papules, vesicles, pustules, scales, crusts, or scabs, either alone or in combination

Edema Excessive amount of tissue fluid; swelling

Effervescence Formation of gas bubbles on the surface of a liquid

Effervescent powder Coarsely ground medicinal agent that has been mixed with an effervescent salt to release carbon dioxide when a liquid is added

Electrolyte Substance that uncouples into ions in solution and can then conduct an electrical charge; in human physiology, an ionized salt such as sodium and chloride found in blood, tissue fluids, and cells

Elixir Clear, sweetened, flavored medication containing alcohol and water

Embolus Obstruction of a blood vessel by a foreign substance or a blood clot

Emesis Act of vomiting

Emollient Agent that softens and soothes the surface to which it is applied, usually the skin

Emphysema Abnormal condition of respiratory system characterized by overinflation and destructive changes in alveolar walls resulting in loss of lung elasticity and decreased gas exchange

Empiric Method of treating disease based on observations and experience without an understanding of the cause or mechanism of the disorder or the way therapeutic agent affects improvement or cure

Emulsion Water-and-oil mixture containing medication in pharmacology

Endemic Pertaining to continuous or cyclic presence of disease in a given geographic area

Endogenous Arising from within a cell, an organ, or an organism itself

Endorphin Naturally occurring opioid-like substance, produced by the body, that blocks pain stimuli

Enema Instillation of a liquid into the rectum

Enteral Pertaining to gastrointestinal tract route of medication administration (i.e., oral or rectal); the medication is absorbed from the gastrointestinal tract

Enteric-coated tablet Tablet coated with a film, formulated to pass through the stomach into the small intestines for absorption; prevents irritation of the gastric mucosa

Enuresis Involuntary discharge of urine after an age when bladder control should be achieved; usually called *bedwetting* because the person does not wake up at night

Epistaxis Nosebleed

Equivalent fractions Fractions of the same value

Eschar Sloughing of skin after a burn

Estrogen Female sex hormone

Euphoria Exaggerated feeling of well-being

Exacerbate To aggravate symptoms or cause increased symptomatology of a disease

Excoriation Abrasion of the skin

Excretion Elimination of medication from the body through respiration, perspiration, urination, or defecation

Exogenous Originating outside an organ or organism itself

Expectorant Agent that assists with the removal of mucous secretions from the lower respiratory tract

Expectoration The act of spitting out saliva or cough materials from the air passages

Extract and fluid extract Highly concentrated preparation of liquid medication achieved through evaporation of a solution

Extrapyramidal symptoms (effects) Tremors, dystonia, or slow irregular, involuntary movements of the upper extremities, especially hands and fingers; symptoms of motor imbalance and lack of muscle tone

Extravasation Escape of fluid from vessels into surrounding tissues; in pharmacology, refers to drugs that escape from blood vessels into tissues

Factors Numbers being multiplied; any of two or more quantities which form a product when multiplied together

Facultative bacteria Pertaining to bacteria with the ability to thrive in dissimilar environments; bacteria that are able to live in either aerobic or anaerobic conditions

Fahrenheit Scale of measurement of temperature in which the boiling point is 212° and the freezing point is 32° at sea level

Fibromyalgia Debilitating disease with chronic pain of muscles and soft tissues surrounding the joints

Filter needle Hypodermic needle that contains a small filter system to prevent aspiration of small glass particles from ampules into the syringe; should be removed from the syringe and replaced with a hypodermic needle before injection

First-pass effect Rapid inactivation of some oral medications as they pass through the liver for the first time before entering the systemic circulation

Focal (partial) seizure Seizure with limited spread in the brain, usually affecting a single muscle group

Folk medicine Remedies for illnesses passed down from generation to generation in families or in a culture for the treatment of specific symptoms (e.g., cobwebs to stop bleeding, meat tenderizer to relieve the itching of insect bites)

Food and Drug Administration (FDA) Agency responsible for the safety, efficacy, and purity of drugs marketed in the United States

Formula method Substitution of information into a formula

Free drug Drug that has reached the bloodstream and is ready for use in the body; synonym for *unbound drug*

Fungicidal Drug with ability to kill fungi

Fungistatic Drug with ability to inhibit growth of fungi

Fungus (plural, *fungi*) Spore-forming, plantlike, single-celled microorganism that thrives on dead organic matter; usually part of normal body flora

Furuncle Acute, deep-seated inflammation of the skin that begins in a hair follicle or sweat gland and produces suppuration and necrosis; boil

Fusion Joining together of two lines, such as bone fusion, in which two sections of bone are permanently joined together

Galactorrhea Excessive secretion of milk

Gastroesophageal reflux disease (GERD) Condition in which acidic contents of the stomach flow backward into the esophagus

Gauge Standard of measurement indicating the diameter of the lumen of a hypodermic needle

Gel Semisolid in a water base with a thickening agent for absorption through the skin

Gelcap Soft gelatin shell filled with liquid medication

Generalized seizure Seizure with loss of consciousness

Generic drug Drug not protected by a trademark but regulated by the FDA

Genetic immunity (inborn or natural immunity) More or less permanent immunity present from birth as a result of genetic factors

Germicide Agent with the ability to destroy germs or microorganisms

Germistatic agent Agent that prevents growth of microorganisms

Gingivitis Inflammation of the gums

Glaucoma Disease of the eye characterized by increased intraocular pressure

Glucocorticoid Hormone secreted by the adrenal cortex that protects against stress and is used in protein and carbohydrate metabolism

Glycoside Active plant substance that yields a sugar (*glyco-*) plus an active ingredient

Goiter Enlargement of the thyroid gland

Grain Basic unit of measure for solid weight in the apothecary system; compared with one grain of wheat or rice

Gram Basic unit of measure for solid weight in the metric system

Grand mal seizure Generalized tonic-clonic seizure

Granule a small particle of dry mass capable of free-flowing movement

Growth hormone Hormone secreted by the anterior pituitary that regulates cell division and protein synthesis needed for growth

Gum Sticky substance that dries to a solid mass that is soluble in water

Habituation psychologic and emotional dependence on a drug, tobacco, or alcohol that results from repeated use of the substance but without the addictive need to increase dosage

Halitosis Bad breath

Hallucination Perception that has no basis in reality; may be visual, auditory, tactile, or olfactory

Helminths Worms

Hematuria Blood in urine

Hemoptysis Cough that contains blood expectorated from either the oral cavity or another part of the respiratory tract

Hemostasis Arrest of bleeding

High-density lipoprotein (HDL) Simple protein that is combined with lipids—cholesterol, phospholipids, and triglycerides; a high level of HDL lipoproteins is desirable

Hirsutism Excessive body hair in masculine distribution pattern as a result of heredity, drugs, hormonal dysfunction, or the like

Hives Vascular skin condition characterized by papules and wheals, producing intense itching

Home remedy Treatment devised and applied at home without professional medical advice; may or may not have therapeutic value (e.g., preparations from plants grown in herb gardens to treat toothache, itching from poison ivy, nausea, and the like)

Homeostasis Equilibrium of the body that is maintained by ever-changing feedback and regulation processes in response to external or internal changes; state of equilibrium in the internal environment of the body

Hordeolum Localized, purulent, inflammatory bacterial infection of sebaceous glands of the eyelids, usually with small abscesses; also called a *stye*

Hormone Substance originating in an organ, gland, or body part that is secreted directly into the bloodstream and carried to another part of the body to begin a chemical action, to increase the activity of that part, or to increase another secretion

Host Organism that provides nourishment for a parasite

Household system System of measurement that uses common kitchen measuring devices

Hyperglycemia Elevated blood glucose level

Hypersensitivity reaction Heightened immune reaction or allergic reaction to a medication

Hypertension Elevation of blood pressure above normal limits

Hyperuricemia Excessive amounts of uric acid in blood

Hypervitaminosis Condition resulting from the excess intake of vitamins, usually vitamin compounds; usually found with lipid-soluble vitamins

Hypnotic Medication used to induce or maintain sleep

Hypoglycemia Decreased blood glucose level

Hypogonadism Deficiency in secretions from ovary or testes

Hypothalamus Portion of the brain that lies directly under the thalamus; it has many functions including secretion of, releasing, and inhibiting hormones

Hypovitaminosis Condition resulting from a deficiency or lack of absorption or use of one or more dietary vitamins

Ideal drug Drug that is both effective and safe, producing no side effects or adverse reactions; only a theoretical construct

Idiosyncratic drug reaction Unexpected, unusual response to a drug

Immune serum Serum from an animal immune against a specific pathogen for injection into a patient with the disease from the same organism; a blood component

Immunity Antibody protection against a disease, especially infectious diseases

Immunodeficiency Decreased or compromised ability of the body to respond to an antigen with an appropriate immune response

Immunoglobulins or immune globulins Blood products that contain disease-specific antibodies for passive immunity

Immunomodulator A substance that alters the immune response by augmenting or reducing the ability of the immune system to produce antibodies that recognize and react with the antigen that caused the reaction

Immunostimulant Agent that stimulates the activity of the immune system

Immunosuppressant Agent that interferes with the normal reactions of the immune system to an antigen; used in arthritis treatment and organ transplantation to prevent the production of antibodies to foreign antigens

Impetigo Inflammatory skin disease with isolated pustules that become crusted and break down; usually caused by streptococci or staphylococci

Implant Form of medication placed under the skin for long-term, controlled release; also called a *pellet*

Improper fraction Fraction with the numerator equal to or greater than the denominator

In situ Localized, in place

Inactivated vaccines Suspension in which the virus or microorganisms have been treated so they are no longer capable of reproduction

Incontinence Inability to hold or retain urine

Indication Reason to use a particular drug for a particular disorder

Inebriation State of intoxication or drunkenness

Inert ingredient Ingredient that has little or no effect on body functions; used to provide substance to active ingredient

Inotropic effect Increase or decrease in the force of myocardial contraction

Inscription Part of the prescription that indicates the name of a drug and the dosage prescribed

Instillation Procedure by which fluid is introduced into a body cavity to expose tissue of the area to the fluid or medication

Insulin pen Device for administering insulin using a cartridge containing insulin that inserts into a penlike container for ease of administration

Intermittent claudication Severe pain in the calf muscles that occurs during exercise because of inadequate blood supply to the lower extremities

International Standard ISO 8601 Internationally accepted standard date and time notation; yyyy-mm-dd and hh-mm-ss

Intraarticular within a joint

Intradermal Into or within the dermis of the skin

Intramuscular Into or within a muscle

Intravenous Into or within a vein

Ion Atom or molecule bearing a positive (cation) or negative (anion) electric charge; in aqueous solutions and in body fluids, ions are charged electrolytes

Irritant Drug applied to produce inflammation at the site of administration

Ischemia Decreased supply of oxygenated blood to a body part causing pain and organ dysfunction

Islets of Langerhans Clusters of cells in the pancreas that produce insulin

Isotonic Referring to solutions with the same tonicity; in physiology, solutions that are compatible with normal body tissue on the basis of having the same concentration of solutes as is found in that body tissue (e.g., physiologic salt solution and normal saline)

Keratin Tough protein substance in the hair, nails, and stratum corneum

Keratitis Inflammation of the cornea

Keratolytic agent Agent that causes or promotes the shedding of skin

Killed vaccines Vaccines made from whole killed microbes and their components

Kyphosis Abnormal condition of spine characterized by increased convexity (outward curve) in the curvature of the thoracic spine as viewed from the side

Laxative Substance that acts to promote and facilitate the evacuation of bowel contents, thus alleviating constipation

Legend drug Drug that requires an order from a licensed health care provider for dispensing (synonym: prescription drug)

Lethargy Feeling of sluggishness

Leukoplakia Formation of white spots or patches on mucous membrane of the tongue or cheek

Leukotrienes Group of metabolites that function as chemical mediators of allergic reactions and inflammation that are implicated in the inflammatory responses in asthma

Liniment Medication that combines oil, soap, water, or alcohol and is placed on the skin to produce heat

Lipodystrophy Abnormality in the distribution and metabolism of fats

Liter Basic measurement unit of volume (liquid or gas) in the metric system

Live vaccines or live attenuated Vaccines composed of live microbes that have been rendered avirulent

Local action Drug action of a medication at the site of administration or in the surrounding tissues

Lotion Free-flowing liquid or formulation with ingredients suspended in water for application to the skin

Low-density lipoprotein (LDL) Simple protein that is combined with lipids-cholesterol, phospholipids, and triglycerides; a high level of LDL lipoproteins is undesirable

Lowest common denominator (LCD) The lowest number or integer that is exactly divisible by each fractional denominator in a set of fractions

Lowest common multiple (LCM) The lowest number that is a multiple of two or more numbers

Lozenge Hard, dry medication held in the mouth to dissolve

Lumen A tabular space within a hypodermic needle

Macrophage Phagocytic cell of reticuloendothelial system

Magaldrate Mixture of aluminum and magnesium compound

Magma Suspension of fine particles in small amount of water

Maintenance medication Medication prescribed to maintain a condition of health; usually used with a chronic disease process

Malaise Discomfort or a nonspecific feeling of uneasiness, often a sign of illness

Malignant Cancerous

Masticate To chew, tear, or grind food with teeth

Medicated enema Enema that provides medication for absorption in the rectum

Medication administration Introduction of a medication into the body or its application to the body; the giving of a dose of medicine

Medication error Mistake made in prescribing, administering, or dispensing a medication; may include administering the wrong medicine or the incorrect dose, using the incorrect route, failing to administer a medicine that has been ordered, giving the medicine at the incorrect time, or giving the medicine to the wrong patient

Medication order Written or verbal (oral) order for administration of a medication in a health care setting

Medication(s) A drug or other substance that is used as a medicine

Meniscus Concave curvature made by a solution when poured into a container; in pharmacology, the liquid is poured into a calibrated measuring cup

Metabolism Physical or chemical processes in the body that inactivate a drug for excretion from the body; biotransformation

Metastasis Change in the location of a disease or its manifestations from one body organ or area to another; a secondary growth of malignant cells in a new location

Meter Basic measurement unit of length in the metric system

Metered dose inhaler (MDI) Breath-activated device that delivers a given amount of a fine mist of medication directly to the mucous membranes of the respiratory tract

Metric system Measurement system based on powers of 10, considered to be the international standard for scientific and industrial measurements; uses grams, liters, and meters

Microbe Unicellular or small multicellular organism

Microbiology Study of microscopic organisms

Micronutrient Dietary element essential in minute amounts for normal physiologic function, such as vitamins and minerals or chemicals

Milliequivalent Weight of a drug (usually in milligrams) in a volume (usually liters) of solution

Mineral Inorganic (neither plant nor animal) solid substance, usually a component of the earth's crust

Mineralocorticoid Hormone secreted by the adrenal cortex that is primarily involved in the regulation of fluid and electrolytes through actions on ion transport and the renal tubules

Minim Smallest unit of volume (liquid) in the apothecary system; approximately a drop in household measure

Miosis Constriction of the pupil

Miotic Agent that causes the pupil to constrict (contract)

Mitotic alkaloids Group of alkaline materials obtained from plants that interfere with cell division

Mitotic inhibitors Drugs that decrease all division by preventing division and migration of cell chromosomes or cell mitosis

Mixed number Number containing a whole number and a fraction

Morbidity Illness or disease state

Morphology Study of the structure and form of organisms without regard to the function

Mortality Death

Mucokinetic agent Medication that removes excessive or abnormal secretions from the respiratory tract

Mucolytic Agent that decreases the viscosity or thickness of sputum or other secretions of the respiratory tract

Mucosal Pertaining to mucous membrane

Mucus Viscid fluid secreted by mucous membranes and glands containing mucin, white cells, epithelial cells, and water and salts, such as the fluids from the mucous glands of the mouth

Muscle spasm Sudden involuntary muscular contraction

Muscle spasticity Increased tone or contractions of muscle, causing stiff and awkward movements

Mutagenic Causing a change in genetic structure

Myasthenia gravis Disease with symptoms of great muscular weakness (without muscle atrophy) and progressive fatigue on exertion

Mydriasis Dilation of the pupil

Myocardial infarction (MI) Deprivation of the myocardium of blood supply to the heart caused by blockage of the coronary arteries with resultant necrosis of the myocardium; heart attack

Myopia Visual refractive error; nearsightedness

Narcolepsy Syndrome characterized by sudden sleep attacks, cataplexy, and visual/auditory hallucinations at the onset of sleep

Narcotic Older term for a controlled drug that depresses the central nervous system to relieve pain and has the potential to cause habituation or addiction

Narrow-spectrum antibiotic Antibiotic effective against only a few or specific microorganisms

National Drug Code (NDC) Number on drug label that identifies the manufacturer, product substances, and size of container

National Formulary **(NF)** List of officially recognized names of drugs that have an established usefulness

Natural active immunity Immunity that is more or less permanent by species or results from the formation of antibodies after disease processes

Natural immunity Immunity that is genetically determined by species, families, or populations

Natural passive immunity Immunity passed from mother to child, either in utero or in breast milk; immunity from natural inherent factors

Nebulizer Breath-activated device that delivers a fine spray of micronized powder into the mucous membranes of the respiratory tract

Necrosis Death of tissue or bone in areas that are surrounded by healthy tissue

Negative feedback Control mechanism in which a stimulus produces a response that reverses or reduces a previous stimulation, thereby stopping the initial response

Neoplasm New and abnormal formation of tissue

Neurohormones Hormones found in portions of the nervous system, such as the catecholamines

Neuroleptic Another name for medication used to treat psychosis

Neuron Nerve cell

Neurosis Abnormal behavior from increased anxiety, tension, or emotional imbalance

Nits Eggs of lice

Nocturia Excessive urination at night

Nomenclature A system of naming used in scientific disciplines, the means providing systematic and consistent scientific or technical names

Nomogram Measuring device used to show relationships among numerical values; set up as a graph, it is the most accurate means of calculating the dose of medication based on weight and height; usually used with pediatric and geriatric patients

Nonopioid medications Analgesics that contains no opium, opium derivatives, or synthetic opioid medications

Nonparenteral medications Medications taken by mouth or through mucous membranes or skin, such as ears, eyes, nose, or rectum

Nonproductive cough Cough in which no exudate is expelled

Nonsalicylate Antiinflammatory agent that does not contain salicylic acid (e.g., Tylenol, naproxen)

Nonsteroidal antiinflammatory drug (NSAID) Antiinflammatory medication that does not contain a steroid preparation

Normal flora Bacteria and microorganisms normally found on or within the body; may be potentially pathogenic when the body is not in homeostasis

Novolin pen Prefilled, multiuse cartridge of insulin that allows a dosage to be dialed for administration of correct dose

Numerator Term of fraction that shows how many specific parts of a unit are taken, number written above or to left of line in a fraction

Nutrient Food or substance that supplies the body with the necessary elements for metabolism and body nourishment

Nystagmus Constant involuntary movement of the eye in any direction

Obsession Persistent and recurrent thought or idea with which the mind is continuously preoccupied and cannot be expunged voluntarily

Occlusive dressing Dressing that does not allow air to enter under the dressing (e.g., plastic wrap)

Off-label use Use of drug to treat a condition for which the FDA has not approved treatment

Oil Thick, greasy liquid that is either volatile (having an aroma) or fixed

Ointment Semisolid in greasy base that is not absorbed into the skin, but the medication is absorbed from the greasy base

Oliguria Diminished ability to form and pass urine

Oogenesis Formation of female gametes or ova

Open-angle glaucoma Increased pressure in eye in which the angle permits the drainage of aqueous humor but the function of drainage is inadequate due to overproduction of aqueous humor or outflow obstruction

Ophthalmic preparations Medications used in the eye

Opiate Drug containing or derived from opium; a narcotic

Opioid analgesic Drug that is a synthetic pain medication with the strength of a morphine-like substance but is not derived from opium

Opportunistic infection Infection that is present because the immune system cannot fight the normal flora found on the body or in the environment; resident flora proliferate and infect the body

Orthostatic hypotension Drop in blood pressure that a person experiences when changing from a supine to an upright position

Osteoarthritis Chronic noninflammatory autoimmune disease of the joints, especially weight-bearing joints, that causes destruction of the joints

Osteomalacia Disease in which softening of the bones causes flexibility and brittleness, leading to deformities; the adult form of rickets in children

Osteoporosis Disease involving reduction of bone mass that tends to occur in older adults; bones become porous

Otic preparations Medications used in the ear

Otitis media Infection of the middle ear; also called tympanitis

Ototoxicity Detrimental effect from medications on the eighth cranial nerve or the organ of hearing

Over-the-counter (OTC) drug Drug that does not require a prescription; nonlegend drug

Ovulation Release of ovum from ovary

Ovum Egg; female reproductive cell

Package insert Comprehensive, concise description of a medication developed by the manufacturer that accompanies any legend drug; required by the Food and Drug Administration for all pharmaceutics

Pain perception Point at which a person becomes aware of a painful stimulus

Pain threshold Point at which a person acknowledges that the stimulus is painful

Pain tolerance Person's ability to tolerate pain

Palliative Alleviating a symptom without curing the condition causing the symptom

Pannus Inflamed synovial granulation tissue of joints found in rheumatoid arthritis

Papule Small, red, elevated area on skin that precedes pustules; pimple

Parasite Organism that lives within, on, or at the expense of another without contributing to survival

Parasympathetic nervous system Portion of the autonomic nervous system that conserves energy and restores body resources in rest and digestion ("feed-or-breed" action)

Parasympathomimetic (cholinergic) agent Agent that blocks the action of the parasympathetic nervous system

Parenteral route Route by which medications are given through the skin by injection, such as intramuscular, intradermal, subcutaneous, and intravenous

Paresthesia Sensation of numbness, prickling, or tingling

Parkinson disease Chronic nervous system disease characterized by fine, slowly spreading tremors and muscular weakness and rigidity, accompanied by a characteristic shuffling gait

Passive immunity Immunity acquired from the injection or passage of antibodies from an immune person or animal to another or short-term immunity or immunity passed from mother to child

Paste Stiff, thick, semisolid medicated preparation that adheres to the skin

Patent State in which an object is open, as in an open airway

Pathogen Organism capable of causing disease; usually a microorganism

Pathology Study of the causes of diseases, involving structure or function; condition produced by disease

Pediculicide Agent that kills lice

Pellagra Disease resulting from deficiency of niacin

Pellet See Implant

Percent In, to, or for every hundred

Percutaneous Route through the skin; in pharmacology, refers to medications absorbed through the skin or mucous membranes such as topical, buccal, or transdermal medications

Peripheral nervous system Portions of the nervous system outside the brain and spinal cord

Peripheral vascular resistance Resistance of blood flow through the arterial vascular system, especially arterioles and capillaries

Peristalsis Progressive wavelike involuntary movement that occurs in a hollow tubular body organ; for moving food and waste materials through the gastrointestinal tract

Pharmacodynamic agent Substance that alters normal body function in some way

Pharmacodynamics Interactions of drugs and living tissues

Pharmacognosy Branch of pharmacology dealing with the origins of drugs (natural or manufactured sources)

Pharmacokinetics Processing of drugs by the body

Pharmacology Study of drugs, their uses, and their interactions with living systems

Pharmacotherapeutics Effects of drugs in the treatment of disease

Photophobia Abnormal intolerance of light

Photosensitivity Abnormal response to exposure to light, specifically on exposure to sunlight or its equivalent

Physical dependence Craving for drugs because of extended use, so the drugs have taken over the individual's life and have affected normal body functioning; discontinuation of use of the drug typically results in withdrawal symptoms

***Physicians' Desk Reference* (PDR)** Book, published yearly, that is a compilation of drug package inserts

Physiology Study of normal physical body functions

Placebo Medication with no pharmacologic or therapeutic effect that is used to satisfy a patient's psychologic need for medication

Plant alkaloids Group of organic alkaline substances obtained from plants for medicinal purposes

Plaster Solid or semisolid, medicated or unmedicated preparation that adheres to the skin

Point of maximum impulse (PMI) Landmark in the fifth intercostal space, 2 inches to the left of midline, where the pulse of the heart can be felt most strongly

Polydipsia Excessive thirst

Polyphagia Excessive uncontrolled eating or hunger

Polypharmacy Indiscriminate use, whether intentional or unintentional, of multiple drugs at the same time (commonly found with older adults)

Polyuria Excessive urination

Potency Strength of a medication

Potentiation Prolongation of or increase in the effect of a drug by another drug

Powder Medication in fine particle form; may be reconstituted into other forms of medication or used as a powder

Precaution Specific warning to consider when prescribing or administering medications

Precipitate Insoluble granules or solid particles that separate from a solution

Premeasured cartridge Premeasured, one-dose amount of medication in a disposable cartridge

Presbyopia Inability of the lens to accommodate to near objects because of the rigidity of the lens caused by aging

Prescribe To indicate, either in writing or orally, a medication to be given

Prescription Written order for dispensing or administering medications, usually by a physician, dentist, or other licensed health care provider as allowed by law

Preventive (prophylactic) medication Medication prescribed to prevent a disease or illness or to lessen its severity

Priapism Frequent or continuous erections in the male

Product Result of multiplying

Productive cough Cough in which mucus or an exudate is expelled

Progestin Female sex hormone secreted by the corpus luteum

Progesterone Natural female hormone

Prokinetic agent Agent used to stimulate gastrointestinal motility by reducing esophageal sphincter pressure and accelerating gastric and intestinal emptying

Proliferation Rapid and repeated reproduction by cell division

Proper fraction Fraction in which the numerator is less than denominator

Prophylactic agent Drug used to prevent pregnancy or illness

Proportion Equality between ratios; relationship between four quantities on two ratios

Proportional method Process of setting up dosage problems by comparing the relationships between two ratios that are considered equivalent

Proteolytic enzyme Enzyme that helps break down proteins into usable peptides

Proton pump inhibitors (PPIs) Located in stomach, parietal cells that excretes hydrogen in exchange for potassium to form gastric acids

Protozoa (singular, *protozoan*) Single-celled parasitic organisms

PSD Packaging, storage, and distribution

Pseudoaddiction A syndrome of abnormal behavior developed as a direct consequence of inadequate pain management

Psoriasis Chronic disease of the skin with silvery, yellow-white lesions that form plaques with distinct borders

Psychoanalysis Method of obtaining mental and emotional history of past experiences that are currently affecting mental disorders

Psychologic drug dependence or habituation Accustomization to a drug through frequent use or exposure or repeated administration of medications for the patient's mental sense of well-being; the craving for a drug because of frequent use

Psychosis Mental illness accompanied by bizarre behavior and altered personality with failure to perceive reality

Psychotherapy Treatment of mental illness through mental means rather than physical or chemical therapy

Purine Group of nitrogenous components that are end product of certain proteins while some are synthesized within the body

Pustule Small elevation of the skin filled with lymph or pus

Pyuria Pus in the urine

Quality assurance (QA) Established standards of excellence in patient care and tailoring care to those standards

Quotient Number obtained when one quantity or number is divided by another quantity or number

Radioisotope Radioactive form of an element; used to diagnose or treat neoplasms

Rale Common abnormal respiratory sound consisting of discontinuous babbling noises heard on inspiration

Ratio Expression that compares two quantities; a colon usually separates the two quantities

Rebound congestion Reflex response of nasal congestion that occurs after the prolonged daily use of decongestants; nasal congestion caused by the body's response to prolonged depression of the mucous membranes' secretions by medication

Receptor site Cell component that combines with a drug to alter cell function; in pharmacology, the part of a cell that interacts with drugs

Reciprocal Fraction obtained when inverting a fraction

Recombinant DNA technology Genetic engineering technology used to create new drugs

Reconstitution Process of adding a fluid such as water or saline to a powdered form of a drug, making a specific dosage strength

Refill Additional medication or treatment to be dispensed if prescribed

Regurgitation Backward flow; the return of stomach contents to the mouth, as in vomitus

Replacement therapy Medication therapy used to replace missing chemicals in the body, including hormones, electrolytes, and fluids

Repository action Medication inserted and stored for slow release at body temperature

Respondeat superior Legal premise by which the employer is held responsible or liable for the wrongful actions of an employee that may cause injury or damage as long as the employee works within the scope of practice; literally, "Let the master answer"

Restless legs syndrome Condition of unknown cause marked by intolerable creeping sensation in lower legs causing irresistible urge to move legs

Rhinitis Inflammation of the nasal mucous membranes

Rhinorrhea Runny nose

Rubs Substance applied topically to relieve a symptom, such as muscle ache or rash

Safe drug Drug that causes no harmful effects when taken in high doses over a long period of time

Salicylate Antiinflammatory drug compound containing salicylic acid (e.g., aspirin)

Salt Chemical compound resulting from the interaction of an acid and a base

Sanitization Process of cleaning and removing dirt from objects

Scabicide Agent that kills scabies

Schizophrenia Group of mental disorders of unknown cause that affect thinking, affect, and behavior

Seborrheic dermatitis Inflammatory skin disease of unknown cause that causes yellow or brown-gray greasy scales

Sebum Fatty secretion from the sebaceous glands of the skin

Sedative Medication used to reduce the desire for physical activity and produce a calming effect

Seizure Epileptic event

Semisynthetic A natural substance that has been partially altered by chemical manipulation

Serum Serous fluid that moistens the surfaces of serous membranes; clear watery fluid that has been separated from more solid elements

Shelf life Storage time for medication to maintain drug potency and to ensure drug safety

Side effect Mild or annoying but expected and fairly common undesirable response to a medication

Signature (Sig or Signa) Part of prescription that indicates the proper dosage of medication to be taken

Skin cleanser Agent used as soap to remove debris, bacteria, and waste products from the skin

Solubility Ability of particles to be dissolved

Solute Substance dissolved in a solution or body fluids

Solution Medication dissolved in a liquid vehicle

Solvent Liquid in which substances are dissolved (e.g., water in the body)

Spacer Aerochamber used with metered dose inhalers

Spasticity Phenomenon in which uncoordinated movements are caused by CNS overstimulation

Spermatogenesis Process of development of spermatozoa

Spirits Alcoholic or hydroalcoholic solutions containing volatile aromatic ingredients

Spore Reproduction unit of some fungi and protozoa

Spray Set of fine medicated vapor applied to a diseased part or discharged into the air

Sputum Substance obtained and expelled from coughing or clearing of the throat containing a variety of materials from the respiratory tract

Standardization See Drug standards

Standard protocol Written description of one or more steps to be taken in treating specific medical problems; this should be signed by the appropriate health care provider

Standing order Request for a procedure that is routine for certain medical treatments under certain conditions

Sterilization Process of destroying all microorganisms and spores

Steroid Hormone produced by the adrenal cortex

Stimulant Drug that acts to increase the function or activity of a body part

Stomatitis Inflammation of the mouth

Subcutaneous Beneath the skin; injected into the subcutaneous tissue

Sublingual Under the tongue

Sublingual tablet Tablet designed to dissolve under the tongue

Subscription Part of the prescription containing the directions for the pharmacist with the information for compounding ingredients if necessary

Summation Combining of drugs to achieve the expected effect of each drug

Superinfection New infection that appears during the course of treatment for a primary infection

Superscription Portion of a prescription designated with the symbol R_x

Supplemental medication Medication used to avoid deficiencies or to achieve necessary levels of existing body chemicals

Supportive medication Medication prescribed to assist with maintenance of homeostasis until a disease process can be resolved

Suppository Medication carried in cocoa butter, hydrogenated vegetable oil, or glycerinated gelatin to form a solid dose for insertion into a body orifice such as the vagina, urethra, or rectum

Suspension Medication in the form of undissolved particles dispersed in a liquid vehicle

Sustained-release (controlled-release) tablet Tablet form of medication in which the medication is released over a period of time; also called *controlled-release tablet*

Sustained-release capsule Capsule form of medication in which the medication is released over a desired period of known duration

Sympathetic nervous system Portion of autonomic nervous system that mobilizes a person in an emergency situation ("fight-or-flight" reaction)

Sympatholytic (or adrenergic blocking) agent Agent that blocks the action of the sympathetic nervous system

Sympathomimetic (adrenergic or adrenergic-acting) agent Agent that acts to simulate or mimic the sympathetic nervous system

Synergism Working together of two or more drugs to produce a stronger effect than could be achieved with each drug taken alone

Synthetic Substance produced by artificial rather than natural process or material

Synthetic or manufactured drug Drug that has been created chemically in the laboratory without the use of plant or animal products

Syrup Aqueous solution sweetened with sugar or a sugar substitute to disguise taste

Systemic action Drug action found at more than the site of administration, usually tissues throughout the body

Tablet Dried powder form of medication that has been compressed into a small disk

Tampon Packed cotton sponge or other material for checking bleeding to an organ or part of the body by pressure

Tardive dyskinesia Slow, rhythmic, involuntary movement as a result of the use of psychotropic drugs

Target organ Site to which the effects of a drug, hormone, or therapeutic agent are primarily directed

Tenacious Thick, viscous

Tenacious cough Stubborn, retentive, or persistent cough with thick, viscous exudates

Teratogen Agent that adversely affects the development of an embryo or fetus

Teratogenic Capable of causing abnormal cellular development of an embryo or fetus

Testosterone A naturally occurring androgenic hormone

Tetany Hyperexcitability of nerves and muscles characterized by spasms, cramps, and twitching

Therapeutic(s) Pertaining to beneficial treatment

Therapeutic medication/agent Medication used in the treatment of a condition or disease to relieve symptoms or effect a cure

Thromboembolism Embolism; the blocking of a blood vessel by a detached embolus

Thrombus Blood clot that obstructs the lumen of a blood vessel

Tincture Alcohol-based liquid used as a skin disinfectant

Tinnitus Ringing in the ears

Tolerance Decreased response to a medication after prolonged use

Tonic Pertaining to muscular tension or contraction

Tonometry Measurement of intraocular pressure; used to diagnose glaucoma

Topical Adjective denoting surface; in pharmacology, refers to medications applied to a surface area or locally to the skin or mucous membrane

Tourette syndrome Rare disease of unknown cause characterized by lack of muscle control, tics, purposeless movements, and incoherent grunts and barks

Toxic Poisonous

Toxicology Study of poisonous effects of drugs

Toxoid Bacterial toxins that have been changed to a nontoxic state for immunization

Trade name Brand name given to a drug by its manufacturer

Tranquilization State of reduced mental tension characterized by calmness but without significant sedation or mental confusion

Transdermal Through the skin; in pharmacology, refers to medications that are applied to the skin for local or systemic effect

Transdermal patch or disk Drug-containing patch or disk that is applied to the skin, through which the drug is absorbed

Triglycerides Simple fat compound consisting of three molecules of fatty acid and glycerol

Troche Hard disk of medication designed to dissolve in the mouth for local effect; similar to lozenge

Tropic hormone Hormone secreted by the pituitary gland that stimulates the production of another hormone; also known as a *stimulating hormone* (e.g., thyroid-stimulating hormone)

Tumor Swelling or enlargement; new growth formation

Tumor necrosis factor (TFN) A protein produced by white blood cells to provide signals for regulation of cell growth and function during an immune response and inflammation

Tympanic membrane Eardrum

Ulcer Open sore including sores of mucous membranes, as in the stomach and duodenum

Ulceration Lesion of the skin or mucous membrane accompanied by sloughing of the inflamed necrotic tissue

Unit Basic quantity used when calculating desired dosages to indicate the strength of a particular medication; the unit is unique for each drug, based on the drug's strength in a basic measurement system (e.g., grain, gram, milligram)

United States Pharmacopoeia (USP) Official guide prepared by a national group of pharmaceutical professionals and issued every 5 years (with periodic supplements) by the U.S. government giving the approved formulas and information on the preparation and dispensing of medications found in the United States

United States Pharmacopoeia/Dispensing Information (USP/DI) Compendium of practical information about medications approved by USP

United States Pharmacopoeia/National Formulary (USP/NF) Official drug reference book for medications approved in the United States; combination of USP and NF

Urgency Sudden, uncontrollable need to urinate

Urinary frequency Frequent urination or urgency while not increasing daily urinary output

Usage Application or administration of a medication for a given purpose

Uveitis Inflammation of the uveal tract (iris, choroid, and ciliary body)

Vaccination Process of immunization for prevention of diseases

Vaccine Preparation containing a suspension of whole or fractionated microorganisms that on administration causes the recipient to form antibodies to a disease

Vasocongestion Congestion of the blood vessels

Vasoconstrictor Agent that narrows or constricts blood vessels

Vasodilator Agent that increases size or dilates blood vessels by relaxation of vascular smooth muscles

Vector Carrier, usually an insect, that transmits pathogens (disease-causing organisms) from infected to uninfected individuals without the carrier itself acquiring the disease

Vehicle Inactive agent that carries an active medicinal ingredient

Verbal order Request for medications or procedures that is given orally rather than in writing

Vertigo Sense that the environment or oneself is revolving

Very-low-density lipoprotein (VLDL) Simple protein that is combined with lipid-cholesterol, phospholipids, and triglycerides; a high level of these proteins is undesirable

Vial Glass or plastic container with a metal-enclosed rubber seal for injectable medications; may hold single or multiple doses

Virulence Disease-producing strength of a microorganism

Virus Bundle of genetic material in a protein coat that requires a host for nutrition and reproduction; sometimes considered to be a one-celled microorganism

Viscosity Ability or inability of a fluid to flow easily; fluid that is thick and flows slowly

Viscous Thickness of a substance

Viscous solution Thick, often oil-based solution; when referring to injections, a solution with a viscous base is much thicker than an aqueous solution and is therefore given intramuscularly

Viscous suspension Thick, gummy or gelatinous compound made up of solid particles mixed, but not dissolved, in a fluid

Vitamin General term for a number of organic substances necessary in trace amounts for normal growth, development, metabolism, and release of energy from food; exclusive of proteins, carbohydrates, fats, and organic salts

Volume Space occupied by a gas or liquid

Wheal Round or elongated elevation of the skin, which can be produced by intradermal injections

Xerostomia Dry mouth

Index

Page numbers followed by f, figures; t, tables.